COMPLICATIONS OF INTERVENTIONAL CARDIOVASCULAR PROCEDURES

A Case-Based Atlas

COMPLICATIONS OF INTERVENTIONAL CARDIOVASCULAR PROCEDURES

A Case-Based Atlas

Editors

Issam D. Moussa, MD
Division of Cardiovascular Diseases
Mayo Clinic College of Medicine
Jacksonville, Florida

Steven R. Bailey, MD
Janey Briscoe Divison of Cardiology
University of Texas Health Sciences Center
San Antonio, Texas

Antonio Colombo, MD
EMO-GVM Centro Cuore Columbus
Milan, Italy

demosMEDICAL
New York

Visit our website at www.demosmedpub.com

ISBN: 9781936287185
e-book ISBN: 9781617050473

Acquisitions Editor: Rich Winters
Compositor: Newgen Imaging

Medicine is an ever-changing science. Research and clinical experience are continually expanding our knowledge, in particular our understanding of proper treatment and drug therapy. The authors, editors, and publisher have made every effort to ensure that all information in this book is in accordance with the state of knowledge at the time of production of the book. Nevertheless, the authors, editors, and publisher are not responsible for errors or omissions or for any consequences from application of the information in this book and make no warranty, express or implied, with respect to the contents of the publication. Every reader should examine carefully the package inserts accompanying each drug and should carefully check whether the dosage schedules mentioned therein or the contraindications stated by the manufacturer differ from the statements made in this book. Such examination is particularly important with drugs that are either rarely used or have been newly released on the market.

Library of Congress Cataloging-in-Publication Data
Library of Congress Control Number: 2012932170

Printed in the United States of America at Bradford & Bigelow.
12 13 14 15 / 5 4 3 2 1

Contents

Preface

Sergeant Lewis: They don't make any sense.
Morse: Things never do until you find out.
Colin Dexter

With increased experience and improved technology, complications of catheter-based cardiovascular interventions have steadily declined over the past 3 decades, but complications still occur in a significant minority of patients, with occasionally tragic consequences. Although training in interventional cardiovascular medicine is structured to provide trainees with adequate conceptual and technical skills to enter practice with confidence, the same cannot be said about preparedness to anticipate and manage complications. Furthermore, because they are uncommon, complications and their management are seldom given proper attention in traditional cardiovascular texts. The agenda in texts and the literature is weighted heavily toward technical and scientific advances in the field. Technical advances have reduced complications, but it does not eliminate them. On the contrary, some "advances" have created a new type of complication and may have increased the severity as well.

The very nature of cardiovascular interventions leaves room for many sources of error, including technique and judgment. Such errors may occur in any phase of the planned intervention. Errors during the preintervention assessment phase may occur due to overlooking or underinterpreting important data, such as abnormal glomerular filtration rate in a low-weight elderly woman with "normal" creatinine and missing an abnormal femoral pulse in a patient scheduled for transfemoral intervention. Errors during the technical execution phase may occur due to inappropriate choice of interventional devices (type, size, length, etc.), misuse of devices due to lack of training or lack of attention to associated therapy or downstream effects, and so on. Errors can also occur when assessing procedural completion and success. Errors in this phase are cognitive rather than technical in nature. On one hand, the operator may not take corrective action because he overlooked subtle findings, such as a distal wire perforation in a hemodynamically stable patient or a nonflow limiting stent edge dissection. On the other hand, the operator may not take corrective action for identifiable problems, such as a suboptimally expanded stent in the proximal LAD, by invoking the concept that "perfect is the enemy of good." Alternatively, the operator may take corrective action in pursuit of perfection when perfection is not feasible, such as insisting on a 0% residual stenosis in a difficult-to-dilate lesion.

So, how do we avoid complications? Some adopt the attitude of "avoidance," where the physician avoids treating patients in whom the risk of complications is high. Complication avoidance should not mean "treatment avoidance"! Occurrence of a complication, as regrettable as it is, should be viewed as a learning opportunity. The first question the interventionalist should ask is, "Did I do the best procedure I could?" This question should lead to an introspective critical assessment of the event(s) precipitating the complication. The physician learns from this exercise, thereby improving in technique and becoming better prepared for subsequent procedures. Complications signify the physician's vulnerability, and as such demands a reckoning of personal limitations.

The goal of this book, *Complications of Interventional Cardiovascular Procedures,* is to present the reader with a patient-centered approach to clinical and technical decision making on how to avoid and manage complications. To bring this product to fruition, we relied on experts who shared with us real-life complications, their reflections on the event(s) that led to the complication, and how they managed it. This book is replete with images and video loops corresponding to the case presentations to enhance the learning experience. The first chapter discusses the parallels between complications of cardiovascular interventions and accidents in the aviation industry. The first section of the book addresses complications of PCI, including access-site complications; the second section addresses complications of structural and valve heart disease interventions; and the final section addresses complications of peripheral and carotid interventions. A concentrated emphasis was placed on a common presentation format, as well as an emphasis on providing actionable tips and tricks to avoid complications and to manage them.

Ultimately, we hope that this book will highlight the importance of strategic thinking to avoid complications, and if they occur, the importance of creativity to manage complications. It is important to remember that although "experience is the best teacher," one should always strive to "learn from others' mistakes." Physicians should pattern their practice on that of their mentors, but we should never stop questioning everything we are told and much of what we see. That is how learning never stops.

Issam D. Moussa, MD
Steve R. Bailey, MD
Antonio Colombo, MD

Contributors

Zahid Amin, MD, FAAP, FSCAI, FAHA
Professor of Pediatrics, Director of Hybrid Catheterization Suite, Rush Center for Congenital and Structural Heart Disease, Rush University Medical Center, Chicago, Illinois
Complications of Transcatheter Closure of Atrial Septal Defects and Patent Foramen Ovale
Complications of Ventricular Septal Defect Closure
Complications of Patent Arterial Duct Closure
Complications of Transcatheter Treatment of Aortic Coarctation

Gary M. Ansel, MD, FACC
Director, Center for Critical Limb Care, McConnell Heart Hospital/Riverside Methodist Hospital, MidOhio Cardiology and Vascular Consultants, Columbus, Ohio
Complications of Infrapopliteal Complications

Dabit Arzamendi, MD
Interventional Cardiology Division, Montreal Heart Institute, University of Montreal, Montreal, Canada
Complications of Mitral Valvuloplasty

Steven R. Bailey, MD, FSCAI, FACC
The University of Texas Health Science Center, Janey and Dolph Briscoe Division of Cardiology, San Antonio, Texas
Abrupt Coronary Occlusion, Slow Flow, and No Reflow

Mandy Jo Binning, MD
Staff Cerebrovascular/Endovascular Neurosurgeon, Department of Neurosurgery, Capital Health Institute for Neurosciences, Trenton, New Jersey
Avoiding Complications During Percutaneous Cardiovascular Interventions: What Should We Learn From the Aviation Industry?

Jeffrey D. Booker, MD
Fellow, Mayo Graduate School, Division of Cardiovascular Diseases, Mayo Clinic, Rochester, Minnesota
Complications of Paravalvular Leak Closure Interventions

Charles F. Botti, Jr., MD
MidOhio Cardiology and Vascular Consultants, Athens, Ohio
Complications of Infrapopliteal Complications

Carlo Cernetti, MD
Chief, Cardiology Division, Ospedale San Giacomo, Castelfranco Veneto, Italy
Complications of Carotid Artery Stenting

Antonio Colombo, MD
Interventional Cardiology Unit, San Raffaele Scientific Institute, and EMO-GVM Centro Cuore Columbus, Milan, Italy
Coronary Perforations
Trapped Devices in the Coronary Arteries
Stent Thrombosis

Konstantinos P. Donas, MD, PhD
Department of Vascular Surgery, St. Franziskus Hospital Münster and Münster University Hospital, Münster, Germany
Complications of Endovascular Thoracic Aortic Aneurysm Repair

Luca Favero, MD
Catheterization Laboratory, Cardiology Department, Mirano Public Hospital, Mirano, Italy
Complications of Transcatheter Aortic Valve Implantation
Complications of Carotid Artery Stenting

Thomas J. Forbes, MD, FSCAI, FAHA, FAAP, FACC
Director, Cardiac Catheterization Suites, Department of Cardiology, The Children Hospital of Michigan, Detroit, Michigan
Complications of Ventricular Septal Defect Closure

Lawrence A. Garcia, MD, FACC, FAHA
Chief, Section Interventional Cardiology; Associate Director, Vascular Medicine Program; Director, Interventional Cardiology Fellowship Program, St. Elizabeth's Medical Center, Tuft's University School of Medicine, Boston, Massachusetts
Complications of Iliac and Superficial Femoral Artery Interventions

Kevin "Chaim" Herman, MD
Teaneck, New Jersey
Complications of Renal Artery Interventions

Leo Nelson Hopkins, MD
Chairman and Professor, Department of Neurosurgery, Millard Fillmore Gates Hospital, Buffalo, New York
Avoiding Complications During Percutaneous Cardiovascular Interventions: What Should We Learn From the Aviation Industry?

Akhilesh Jain, MBBS, MD
Clinical Fellow, Section of Vascular Surgery, Yale University, Yale New Haven Hospital, New Haven, Connecticut
Transfemoral Access Complications
Closure Device Complications

Alfonso Ielasi, MD
Interventional Cardiology Unit, San Raffaele Scientific Institute, Milan, Italy
Stent Thrombosis

Damien Kenny, MB, ChB, MRCPCH
Rush Center for Congenital and Structural Heart Disease, Rush University Medical Center, Chicago, Illinois
Complications of Ventricular Septal Defect Closure
Complications of Transcatheter Treatment of Aortic Coarctation
Complications of Patent Arterial Duct Closure

Azeem Latib, MB, BCh
Interventional Cardiology Unit, San Raffaele Scientific Institute, and EMO-GVM Centro Cuore Columbus, Milan, Italy
Coronary Perforations
Trapped Devices in the Coronary Arteries
Stent Thrombosis

Elad I. Levy, MD
Professor, Department of Neurosurgery & Radiology and Toshiba Stroke Research Center, School of Medicine and Biomedical Sciences, University at Buffalo, State University of New York and Department of Neurosurgery, Millard Fillmore Gates Hospital, Kaleida Health, Buffalo, New York
Avoiding Complications During Percutaneous Cardiovascular Interventions: What Should We Learn From the Aviation Industry?

Robin Martin, MB, FRCP
Lead Interventionalist, Department of Cardiology, Bristol Royal Hospital for Children and Bristol Royal Infirmary, Bristol, United Kingdom
Complications of Transcatheter Treatment of Aortic Coarctation

Jeffrey W. Moses, MD
Professor of Medicine, Columbia University, Center for Interventional Vascular Therapy, NewYork Presbyterian Hospital, Columbia University Medical Center, New York, New York
Complications of Coronary PCI: An Overview

Shilesh Nandish, MD
Interventional Cardiology Fellow, Department of Internal Medicine, University of Texas Health Sciences Center, San Antonio, Texas
Abrupt Coronary Occlusion, Slow Flow, and No Reflow

Aravinda Nanjundappa, MD, FACC, FSCAI, RVT
Associate Professor of Medicine and Surgery, West Virginia University, Charleston, West Virginia
Transfemoral Access Complications
Closure Device Complications

Dimitrios Nikas, MD, PhD
Cardiology Division, Ospedale Civile, Mirano - Venice, Italy
Complications of Transcatheter Aortic Valve Implantation
Complications of Carotid Artery Stenting

Andrea Pacchioni, MD
Cardiology Division, Ospedale Civile, Mirano - Venice, Italy
Complications of Transcatheter Aortic Valve Implantation
Complications of Carotid Artery Stenting

Igor Palacios, MD
Director, Interventional Cardiology; Associate Professor, Cardiology Division, Harvard Medical School, Boston, Massachusetts
Complications of Mitral Valvuloplasty

Samir Pancholy, MD
Associate Professor of Medicine, The Commonwealth Medical College, Scranton, Pennsylvania
Transradial Vascular Access–Related Complications During Coronary Interventions

Gianpaolo Pasquetto, MD
Cardiology Division, Ospedale Civile, Mirano - Venice, Italy
Complications of Transcatheter Aortic Valve Implantation
Complications of Carotid Artery Stenting

Tejas Patel, MD, DM, FACC, FESC, FSCAI
Chairman, Apex Heart Institute; Professor and Head, Department of Cardiology, Smt. NHL Municipal Medical College & Sheth VS General Hospital, Gujarat, India
Transradial Vascular Access–Related Complications During Coronary Interventions

Carlo Penzo, MD
Cardiology Division, Ospedale Civile, Mirano - Venice, Italy
Complications of Transcatheter Aortic Valve Implantation
Complications of Carotid Artery Stenting

Paul Poommipanit, MD
Interventional Cardiologist, Department of Cardiology, Trinity Medical Center, Rock Island, Illinois
Complications of Transcatheter Closure of Atrial Septal Defects and Patent Foramen Ovale

Bernhard Reimers, MD
Chief, Cardiology Division, Ospedale Civile, Mirano - Venice, Italy
Complications of Transcatheter Aortic Valve Implantation
Complications of Carotid Artery Stenting

Charanjit S. Rihal, MD, MBA
Chair, Division of Cardiovascular Diseases; Professor of Medicine, Division of Cardiovascular Diseases, Mayo Clinic, Rochester, Minnesota
Complications of Paravalvular Leak Closure Interventions

John H. Rundback, MD
Clinical Director, Manhattan Interventional Radiology, New York, New York, and Director, Interventional Institute at Holy Name Hospital, Teaneck, New Jersey
Complications of Renal Artery Interventions

Salvatore Saccà, MD
Cardiology Division, Ospedale Civile, Mirano - Venice, Italy
Complications of Transcatheter Aortic Valve Implantation
Complications of Carotid Artery Stenting

Sanjay Shah, MD, DM
Director, Department of Cardiology, Apex Heart Institute; Assistant Professor, Department of Cardiology, Smt. NHL Municipal Medical College & Sheth VS General Hospital, Gujarat, India
Transradial Vascular Access–Related Complications During Coronary Interventions

Adnan H. Siddiqui, MD, PhD
Department of Neurosurgery & Radiology and Toshiba Stroke Research Center, School of Medicine and Biomedical Sciences, University at Buffalo, State University of New York and Department of Neurosurgery, Millard Fillmore Gates Hospital, Kaleida Health, Buffalo, New York
Avoiding Complications During Percutaneous Cardiovascular Interventions: What Should We Learn From the Aviation Industry?

Mitchell J. Silver, DO
MidOhio Cardiology and Vascular Consultants, Inc., Columbus, Ohio
Complications of Infrapopliteal Complications

Jonathan Tobis, MD
Director, Interventional Cardiology Research, Division of Cardiology, Department of Medicine, Professor of Medicine, David Geffen School of Medicine at UCLA, Los Angeles, California
Complications of Transcatheter Closure of Atrial Septal Defects and Patent Foramen Ovale

Giovanni B. Torsello, MD, PhD
Department of Vascular Surgery, St. Franziskus Hospital and Centrum for Vascular and Endovascular Surgery, Münster, Germany
Complications of Endovascular Repair of Abdominal Aortic Aneurysms
Complications of Endovascular Thoracic Aortic Aneurysm Repair

Giovanni F. Torsello, CM
Department of Vascular Surgery, St. Franziskus Hospital, Münster, Germany
Complications of Endovascular Repair of Abdominal Aortic Aneurysms

Francesco Versaci, MD
Università Tor Vergata, Rome, and Cardiology Division, Ospedale Civile, Mirano - Venice, Italy
Complications of Transcatheter Aortic Valve Implantation

Giora Weisz, MD
Associate Professor of Clinical Medicine, Center for Interventional Vascular Therapy, NewYork Presbyterian Hospital, Columbia University Medical Center, New York, New York
Complications of Coronary PCI: An Overview

1

Mandy Jo Binning, Adnan H. Siddiqui, Elad I. Levy, and Leo Nelson Hopkins

Avoiding Complications During Percutaneous Cardiovascular Interventions: What Should We Learn From the Aviation Industry?

BACKGROUND

Catheter-based cardiovascular and neurovascular interventions have many similarities with aviation. Both disciplines have made the extraordinary ordinary—through the teamwork of specialists using sophisticated equipment to perform previously inconceivable tasks in life-threatening situations. Perhaps what is most astounding about these two human endeavors is not what they entail, but rather how frequently they occur. On any one day, an estimated 85,000 flights and 550,000 operations are completed worldwide. What are the implications of scaling up life-or-death events to such enormous levels? One consequence of such large throughputs is that even minute risks are magnified. If even a small percentage of patients and passengers die, this amounts to a significant number of families affected by preventable deaths. Every year around 500 people die in aviation accidents, and the World Health Organization (WHO) estimates that 1 million people die in the perioperative period, many due to avoidable mistakes. So, what is being done to minimize these risks in the area of catheter-based cardiovascular and neurovascular interventions? The parallels between catheter-based cardiovascular interventions and aviation make the airline industry an ideal source of ideas for practitioners and researchers alike.

Aviation safety began in 1918, when the federal government began operating the U.S. Air Mail Service. By 1924, the Air Mail Service evolved into a 24-hour service on the transcontinental route between New York City and San Francisco (1). The U.S. Air Mail Service was the first aviation service to place a strong emphasis on safety. As regulations for aviation safety were developing, flight simulation was also in its infancy. One of the best known early flight simulators was the Link trainer, designed in the late 1920s (2). At that time, Army Air Corps pilots were trained to fly by watching the ground to prevent disorientation, rather than using instruments, making flight in adverse weather conditions quite dangerous. During the first week of mail service, nearly a dozen pilots were killed while flying in stormy weather. Suddenly, the Army Air Corps gained interest in a simulator that would train pilots to fly by trusting and reading their instruments. The story goes that on a day with poor visibility in 1934, Link was slated to meet with a group of Army officers in Newark, New Jersey. He was flying from Binghamton, New York. Impressed that Link could fly safely, solely on instruments, the Army Air Corps ordered six of his trainers for $3,500 each (Figure 1.1). During World War II, the ANT-18 Trainer, known to new pilots as the "Blue Box," was standard equipment at every training school in the United States and the allied nations (Figure 1.2). Currently, military, aviation, and aerospace trainees

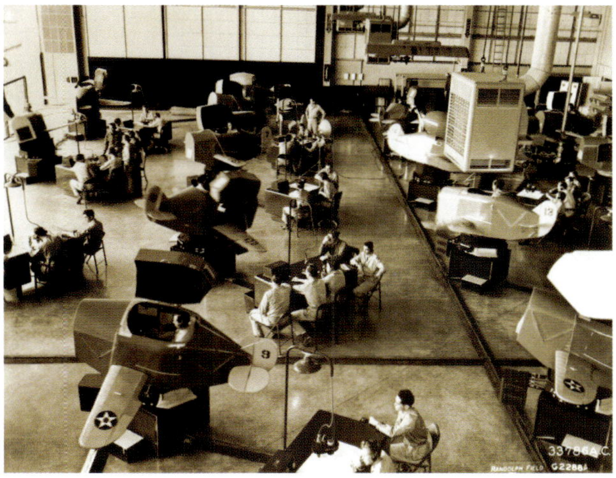

FIGURE 1.1

To train their pilots to fly by using instruments, the Army Air Corps ordered six Link trainers for $3,500 a piece in 1934.

Photo courtesy of L-3 Link Simulation and Training.

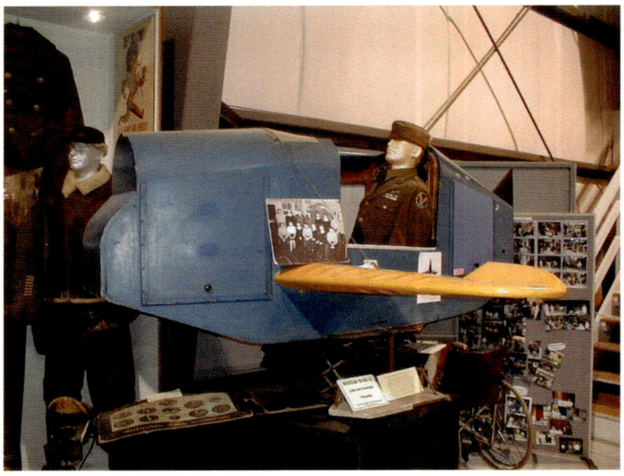

FIGURE 1.2

The Link trainer, also known as the "Blue Box," is a flight simulator produced between the early 1930s and early 1950s by Edwin Link. These simulators were used as a key pilot training aid by almost every combatant nation during World War II.

Source: Wikimedia Commons http://en.wikipedia.org/wiki/Link_Trainer. The copyright holder of this work allows anyone to use it for any purpose, including unrestricted redistribution, commercial use, and modification.

use simulation extensively for training and maintaining skills and for assessing competency. In fact, flight simulation fidelity has reached a point at which commercial pilots may be certified to fly a new type of aircraft with simulator experience alone (3). In addition, simulation allows one to experience infrequent events that have high value but are rarely encountered in real life (e.g., engine failure in flight).

Among other initiatives, the pilots were required to submit a completed 180-item checklist at the end of every trip. Although the safety initiatives required a tremendous amount of manpower [the ratio of mechanics to aircraft was nearly 4:1 (1)], the fatality rate for the Air Mail Service was 1 per 789,000 miles flown between 1922 and 1925, compared with 1 per 13,500 miles flown for other commercial carriers at the time (1). Pilots learn to routinely go through sets of standardized checklists before takeoff, at takeoff, while cruising, and before landing. Each checklist is specific for each type of aircraft. Checklists were developed for systematic review of procedures to reduce errors, and their use is accepted and part of the culture of flying.

In the aviation industry, flight simulation and the use of checklists are the standard for training pilots in routine and hazardous flight conditions to improve safety (4–7). Simulation and extensive use of checklists are two main aspects of aviation safety that lend themselves well to percutaneous cardiovascular intervention. Additional techniques used in aviation that can be applied to intervention include teamwork training to focus on improving communication among physicians, nurses, and other staff members; preoperative briefings/huddle, postoperative debriefings, sterile "cockpit" during critical periods in the procedure, crew resource management, line operations safety audit (LOSA), and time outs (which can also be integrated into a checklist); and nonpunitive incident reporting to allow physicians and nurses to anonymously report adverse events, near mistakes, and unsafe conditions to hospital officials as part of quality assurance and peer review.

MEDICAL SIMULATION

Traditionally, training in catheter-based cardiovascular and neurovascular interventions has been accomplished through mentoring of fellows by an experienced physician during actual procedures. As the emphasis on patient safety and its association with human error and performance has increased, the impetus to utilize simulators in medicine has gained momentum. In 1993, Satava (8) adapted the concept of simulation to surgical application, and since then, many medical and surgical simulators have been developed. Medical and surgical simulation is increasingly being used to improve patient safety and the quality of healthcare in many specialties (4, 9–13). In randomized studies, Seymour et al (14) and Grantcharov et al (15) separately reported improvement in trainee performance after the use of surgical simulators for laparoscopic cholecystectomy. Simulators have also been extensively investigated for training for carotid artery stenting, and simulation training has been shown in randomized studies to lead to improvements in procedural time, fluoroscopy time, and catheter-handling skills, as well as a reduction in contrast volume (16–18). In 2004, the Food and Drug Administration detailed the importance of training of specialists in carotid artery stenting and suggested that simulation may be beneficial prior to allowing training physicians to perform carotid artery stenting (19). Although several studies have shown enhanced proficiency in the performance of surgical procedures and endovascular techniques with simulator training (14–18, 20), whether simulation training for catheter-based cardiovascular procedures provides measurable, real-world benefit remains to be seen.

Simulator training does have some limitations. The tactile feedback of most systems makes them most appropriate for novice operators because the haptics are not sophisticated enough to perfectly model live procedures. In addition, simulator training is not widely available. The best or most realistic simulators may cost up to $500,000, which makes them cost prohibitive to most private centers (7). Regional training centers or shared simulators are, therefore, a likely solution to making simulators available to trainees. However, simulators for practicing cases on a routine basis would be more difficult to make available to all centers.

Virtual reality-based simulation in medicine is still in its infancy but consists of a simulated workspace with multiple sensory feedback mechanisms to simulate the task—this is the next step for simulation for catheter-based cardiovascular interventions. Although simulators that simulate diagnostic angiography, carotid stenting, and aneurysm coiling have been developed, the simulators depend on generic cases with poor haptics, without realistic feedback to the interventionist, and most do not allow patient-specific data to be entered and rehearsed. Patient-specific simulation for carotid artery stenting was described successfully in a single case by Roguin and Beyar (21) using the patient's preoperative computed tomographic angiography (CTA) images on an endovascular simulator and in five separate cases by Hislop et al (22). Both teams utilized the ANGIO Mentor™ (Simbionix, Lod, Israel) simulator (Figure 1.3). The operators were able to determine radiographic projections, measurements, and devices needed prior to the actual procedure, limiting radiation exposure and contrast administration (21, 22). Hislop et al (22) reported that simulated embolic protection devices, stents, and angioplasty balloons chosen based on preoperative imaging of the arteries were typically appropriate for the dimensions measured in the actual procedures. In addition, the devices chosen based on the arch anatomies predicted by preoperative imaging and practiced on the simulator were correct. The simulation correctly identified and predicted difficulties with anatomy and devices in all patients, and all poststent vessel configurations were accurate, except one. Hislop et al (22) concluded that these patient-specific simulations were realistic and had a positive influence on patient outcomes. The disadvantage of the ANGIO Mentor system is that anonymous CTA datasets must be sent to the Simbionix Corporation where they are processed by the PROcedure Rehearsal Studio™ to create simulation files. The turnover time may be as long as 2 weeks. Patients undergoing urgent intervention could, therefore, not benefit from this technology. In addition, not all interventional devices can be represented by this simulator, not all aspects of intervention can be simulated, and the haptics are imperfect.

The Procedicus Vascular Interventional System Trainer (VIST) (Mentice AB, Gothenburg, Sweden) has been used widely in carotid stent training (Figure 1.4). The VIST offers the appearance of real-time digital subtraction angiography with computer-generated images that are responsive to actual hands-on catheter manipulation. It contains a realistic control panel and produces realistic angiographic images with a series of three advanced haptic devices that allow translational and rotational movements of real endovascular instruments.

However, none of the currently available catheter-based interventional simulators have the sophisticated haptics necessary to allow a truly realistic experience. Eventually, interventional simulators will need to have airline simulator quality haptics and imaging datasets. The gold standard would be high-fidelity simulators with exceptional haptics to allow each device to be modeled with software algorithms that simulate accurate shape, stiffness, force, and flexibility in order to predict the behavior of wires, guide catheters, microcatheters, coils, embolizate, and stents in specific anatomy. In addition, the behavior of the devices in relation to each other (e.g., wire to catheter, wire to stent) and in relation to specific anatomy could be modeled. Preprogrammed cases would be available for training purposes, and the software would allow integration and planning of patient-specific datasets.

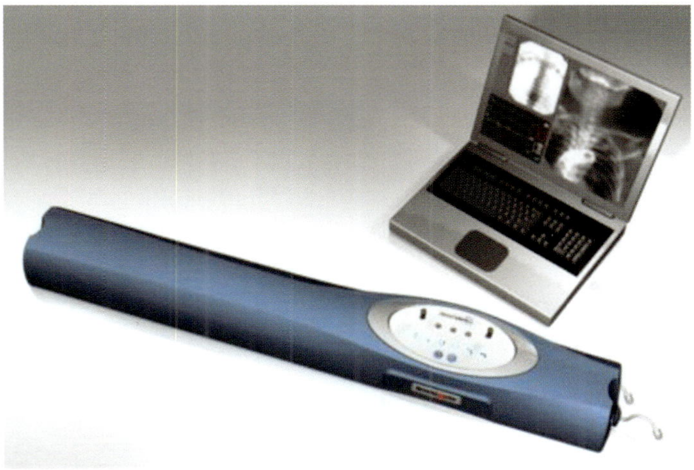

FIGURE 1.3

The ANGIO Mentor™ simulator was designed to provide hands-on practice in a simulated environment of endovascular procedures.

Courtesy of Simbionix: http://simbionix.com/simulators/angio-mentor/

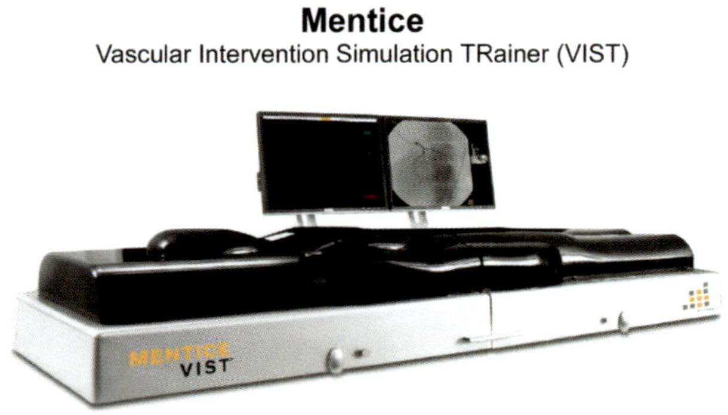

FIGURE 1.4

The Procedicus Vascular Interventional System Trainer (VIST) (Mentice AB, Gothenburg, Sweden).

Courtesy of Mentice AB: http://www.mentice.com/archive/pdf_products/Mentice_A4_broschyr_LR2.pdf.

CHECKLISTS

Another aspect of aviation safety that has not truly been incorporated in intervention is the use of checklists. Data suggest that many surgical complications may be avoidable (23, 24), and teamwork in surgery has been linked to improved outcomes and fewer adverse events (25, 26). In 2009, WHO identified and published their guidelines for recommended practices to ensure the safety of surgical patients (27). On the basis of these guidelines, Haynes et al (28) designed a checklist with elements for "sign in," "time out," and "sign out" intended to be applicable to all surgical procedures to reduce the rate of the major avoidable surgical complications (Table 1.1). Mortality following noncardiac surgery at a diverse group of eight hospitals was 1.5% before implementation of this checklist and 0.8% afterward. Inpatient complications decreased from 11% to 7% after implementation.

Checklists are a way to improve communication within the team of physicians, nurses, and other staff members and ensure that all safety measures have been addressed. Even though many interventionists may perform a mental "checklist" prior to performing each procedure, true checklists should involve the entire team, incorporate basic items to ensure safety for that procedure, and be used every time with every intervention regardless of how routine.

Global safety initiatives including specific checklists for intervention, sterile catheterization laboratory (cath lab), anonymous error reporting, and LOSA have been implemented in pilot trials (R. Minor, personal communication, August 2010); examples of these are as follows.

1. Preoperative briefing/huddle, checklist, and postoperative debriefing

   The interventional team meets to review the "time out" (as in Table 1.1) and also the case details or a preprocedure checklist, which may include the following points:

   A. *Preprocedure checklist* (developed at University at Buffalo Neurosurgery)

   - Review previous films/have them up in the angiography suite if available
   - Review previous operative notes
   - Review indication for the current procedure
   - Confirm which vessels to inject during angiography
   - Perform a baseline neurological examination on ALL patients
   - Review serum creatinine values—if level is *high*
     - Administer a bicarbonate drip
     - Administer oral Mucomyst (no contraindication)
   - Check that patients with known or suspected allergy to contrast media have received a steroid-diphenhydramine hydrochloride preparation
   - Administer a bolus dose of aspirin and clopidogrel if necessary
   - Ensure that metformin hydrochloride has been discontinued in diabetic patients 24 hours preprocedure and will be withheld for 48 hours postprocedure
   - Confirm that warfarin or heparin has been stopped prior to groin stick, when appropriate
   - Ensure the patient has adequate intravenous access

   The team would include a captain (responsible interventionist), residents, fellows, nurses, and technicians.

   B. *Postoperative debriefing* would include a review of what the team did correctly and incorrectly during the procedure.

2. "Sterile cath lab" during critical periods in the intervention: for example, femoral artery access, during key interventional period (defined by team captain; e.g., from catheter entry into heart, kidney, or head until device deployment) and closure. Akin to "sterile cockpit," where all hands are focused on critical parts of the flight with no irrelevant interruptions, "sterile cath lab" would demand that all team personnel completely focus on the patient and procedural steps during critical periods. For example, a sterile cath lab would be maintained during the time in which the team is reviewing a checklist.

TABLE 1.1

Elements of the Surgical Safety Checklist—Modified for Endovascular Intervention.

SIGN IN

Before induction of anesthesia or conscious sedation, members of the surgical team orally confirm:

- The patient's identity, surgical site, procedure, and consent
- The surgical site is marked or site marking is not applicable
- The pulse oximeter is on the patient and functioning
- Known allergies are reported to all members of the team
- If there is a risk of blood loss of at least 500 mL, appropriate access and fluids are available

TIME OUT

Before skin incision or groin puncture, the entire team orally:

- Confirms that all team members have been introduced by name and role
- Confirms the patient's identity, surgical site, and procedure
- Reviews the anticipated critical events
- Confirms that prophylactic antibiotics have been administered if indicated
- Confirms that all essential images are displayed if applicable

SIGN OUT

Before the patient leaves the operating room:

- The following items are read aloud with the team
  - Name of the procedure as recorded
  - That the needle, sponge, and instrument counts are correct, incorrect, or not applicable
  - That the specimen (if any) is correctly labeled, including with the patient's name
  - Address any equipment issues if applicable
- The team discusses the key concerns for the recovery and care of the patient

Adapted from Haynes et al (28), and World alliance for patient safety (29).

Access Checklist (developed at University at Buffalo Neurosurgery)

- Check that distal pulses are present
- Previous punctures (which closure device was used?)
- Previous femoral artery/groin region complications
- Previous groin hematomas
- Verification of needle stick location: femoral head or crease
- Consider a long sheath in the obese patient
- Consider using ultrasound to localize femoral artery in the pediatric patient
- Perform femoral artery run after access is obtained
- Distal pulses postclosure

In fact, specific checklists can be developed to cover all aspects of an interventional procedure, including management of complications.

3. Incident reporting (nonpunitive) to allow physicians and nurses to anonymously report adverse events, near mistakes, and unsafe conditions to hospital officials. A generic reporting form without identifying information could be developed and completed after the procedure.

4. LOSA: An experienced interventionist is invited to the center as a visiting professor who spends 1 or 2 days in the laboratory observing procedures with a particular emphasis on safety procedures, then reports back on findings next year in a peer review format or setting (such as a meeting of his/her peers). This initiative can be part of the center's normal visiting professor program. The interventional

team is not informed of the LOSA mission and assumes that the sole purpose is the visiting professor educational program.

These global safety initiatives, including checklists, help ensure that the equipment, physician, and other members of the team are ready for each intervention and all devices are available. Checklists should exist for each type of intervention to troubleshoot the equipment and devices and for treatment of complications. This systematic process is meant to maximize safety and preparedness while providing a safe environment to report errors so that the team can learn from them, rather than be blamed for them.

CONCLUSIONS

Cardiovascular and neurovascular intervention is an area of medicine that lends itself well to simulation and use of checklists. As in the aviation industry, successful intervention requires assurance that the equipment is in perfect working condition, the proper equipment and devices are available, the patient is ready for the intervention, and the staff is well prepared for routine and nonroutine cases. In the case of an emergency, appropriate measures can be taken to troubleshoot the problem and maximize the chance of a good outcome. The physician and team members—much like the pilot and his/her team—should be able to practice the exact case they will perform based on preoperative imaging data or/and practice drills and checklists to maximize safety. Although this scenario not only seems possible but also is almost expected by today's consumers (i.e., patients), current simulators lack the sophistication of modern-day flight simulators. The technology exists to create realistic, true haptic, virtual reality medical simulators that can simulate any intervention; however, unlike the aviation industry, the medical industry has not mandated their development and therefore their use. Endovascular simulators exist for training, and although they fail to realistically create the angiography suite and the experience of a true intervention, they have been shown to improve proficiency in trainees.

References

1. Air Traffic Organization Operations Planning, Office of Aviation Research and Development. History of aviation safety oversight in the United States, 2008 (DOT/FAA/AR-08/39) http://www.tc.faa.gov/its/worldpac/techrpt/ar0839.pdf. Accessed September 20, 2010.
2. L-3 Communications. Link simulation and training, 2010. http://www.link.com/history.html. Accessed September 20, 2010.
3. Smith BE, Gaba DM. Simulators. In: Lake C, Blitt C, Hines R, eds. *Clinical Monitoring: Practical Applications for Anesthesia and Critical Care*. Philadelphia: W.B. Saunders; 2001:26–44.
4. Dawson DL. Virtual reality training for carotid intervention. *Nat Clin Pract Neurol*. 2007;3:470–471.
5. Helmreich RL, Merritt AC, Wilhelm JA. The evolution of crew resource management training in commercial aviation. *Int J Aviat Psychol*. 1999;9:19–32.
6. Helmreich RL, Wilhelm JA, Gregorich SE, Chidester TR. Preliminary results from the evaluation of cockpit resource management training: performance ratings of flightcrews. *Aviat Space Environ Med*. 1990;61:576–579.
7. Ogilvy CS, Samuelson RM, Bendok BR, et al. Simulation for neurointervention. *Endovasc Today*. 2008; November:71–76.
8. Satava RM. Virtual reality surgical simulator: The first steps. *Surg Endosc*. 1993;7:203–205.
9. Dawson DL, Meyer J, Lee ES, Pevec WC. Training with simulation improves residents' endovascular procedure skills. *J Vasc Surg*. 2007;45:149–154.
10. Gurusamy K, Aggarwal R, Palanivelu L, Davidson Br. Systematic review of randomized controlled trials on the effectiveness of virtual reality training for laparoscopic surgery. *Br J Surg*. 2008;95:1088–1097.
11. Sarker SK, Patel B. Simulation and surgical training. *Int J Clin. Pract*. 2007;61:2120–2125.
12. Schendel S, Montgomery K, Sorokin A, Lionetti G. A surgical simulator for planning and performing repair of cleft lips. *J Craniomaxillofac Surg*. 2005;33:223–228.
13. Tsang JS, Naughton PA, Leong S, Hill AD, Kelly CJ, Leahy AL. Virtual reality simulation in endovascular surgical training. *Surgeon*. 2008;6:214–220.
14. Seymour NE, Gallagher AG, Roman SA, et al. Virtual reality training improves operating room performance: results of a randomized, double-blinded study. *Ann Surg*. 2002;236:458–464.
15. Grantcharov TP, Kristiansen VB, Bendix J, Bardram L, Rosenberg J, Funch-Jensen P. Randomized clinical trial of virtual reality simulation for laparoscopic skills training. *Br J Surg*. 2004;91:146–150.
16. Dayal R, Faries PL, Lin SC, et al. Computer simulation as a component of catheter-based training. *J Vasc Surg*. 2004;40:1112–1117.
17. Hsu JH, Younan D, Pandalai S, et al. Use of computer simulation for determining endovascular skill levels in a carotid stenting model. *J Vasc Surg*. 2004;40:1118–1125.
18. Patel AD, Gallagher AG, Nicholson WJ, Cates CU. Learning curves and reliability measures for virtual reality simulation in the performance assessment of carotid angiography. *J Am Coll Cardiol*. 2006;47:1796–1802.
19. US Food and Drug Administration, Center for Devices and Radiological Health, Medical Devices Advisory Committee, Circulatory System Devices Panel Meeting. http://www.fda.gov/ohrms/dockets/ac/04/transcripts/Pages%20from%204033t1-01.pdf. Accessed September 21, 2010.
20. Gallagher AG, Ritter EM, Champion H, et al. Virtual reality simulation for the operating room: proficiency-based training as a paradigm shift in surgical skills training. *Ann Surg*. 2005;241:364–372.
21. Roguin A, Beyar R. Real case virtual reality training prior to carotid artery stenting. *Catheter Cardiovasc Interv*. 2010;75:279–282.
22. Hislop SJ, Hedrick JH, Singh MJ, et al. Simulation case rehearsals for carotid artery stenting. *Eur J Vasc Endovasc Surg*. 2009;38:750–754.
23. Gawande AA, Thomas EJ, Zinner MJ, Brennan TA. The incidence and nature of surgical adverse events in Colorado and Utah in 1992. *Surgery*. 1999;126:66–75.
24. Kable AK, Gibberd RW, Spigelman AD. Adverse events in surgical patients in Australia. *Int J Qual Health Care*. 2002;14:269–276.
25. Lingard L, Regehr G, Orser B, et al. Evaluation of a preoperative checklist and team briefing among surgeons, nurses, and anesthesiologists to reduce failures in communication. *Arch Surg*. 2008;143:12–18.
26. Mazzocco K, Petitti DB, Fong KT, et al. Surgical team behaviors and patient outcomes. *Am J Surg*. 2009;197:678–685.
27. World Health Organization. *WHO Guidelines for Safe Surgery 2009*. http://whqlibdoc.who.int/publications/2009/9789241598552_eng.pdf. Accessed September 20, 2010.
28. Haynes AB, Weiser TG, Berry WR, et al. A surgical safety checklist to reduce morbidity and mortality in a global population. *N Engl J Med*. 2009;360:491–499.
29. World Alliance for Patient Safety. *WHO Guidelines for Safe Surgery* (1st edition). Geneva: World Health Organization, 2008. http://www.who.int/patientsafety/safesurgery/knowledge_base/WHO_Guidelines%20_Safe_Surgery_finalJun08.pdf. Accessed September 21, 2010.

I

COMPLICATIONS OF PERCUTANEOUS CORONARY INTERVENTIONS

2

Aravinda Nanjundappa and Akhilesh Jain

Transfemoral Access Complications

INTRODUCTION

The femoral artery, due to its relatively large size and easy accessibility, remains the preferred access site for percutaneous coronary and peripheral vascular interventions. In fact, more than 95% of percutaneous peripheral vascular interventions are performed via this route. Percutaneous interventions, when compared to open surgical procedures, are associated with a decreased morbidity and mortality; however, they are associated with some complications that are unique to this mode of intervention. Of these, complications associated with the transfemoral vascular access are a major source of morbidity and potential mortality in some patients.

The reported overall vascular complication rate associated with percutaneous access ranges from 1.5% to 9%, from which 20% to 40% of complications require surgical repair (1). An increased understanding of the variables affecting the incidence of access site complications and subsequent implementation of multiple preventive strategies has led to a decrease in the complications associated with transfemoral access (2).

Vascular access–related complications range from a simple hematoma leading to some discomfort to a life-threatening massive retroperitoneal hemorrhage. These complications can be broadly categorized as secondary to inaccurate vascular access or oversized sheath, or due to inadequate hemostasis at the conclusion of procedure. About 20% to 40% of these complications require surgical intervention. The various complications commonly associated with vascular access include bleeding/pseudoaneurysm formation, arteriovenous fistula (3), vessel perforation, retroperitoneal hemorrhage, and dissection/occlusion.

STEPS TO REDUCE VASCULAR ACCESS COMPLICATIONS

1. Identify of the lower one-third of the femoral head under fluoroscopy.
2. Use a single anterior wall puncture so that the needle enters the common femoral artery (CFA) at the lower one-third of the femoral head.
3. Use Doppler ultrasound to identify CFA in patients with obese body habitués, poor palpable pulse, complex interventional access, such as potential thrombolytic cases, and carotid artery stenting.
4. Use meticulous wire maneuver and sheath placement with the introducer in situ and careful wire handling during sheath exchanges under fluoroscopy.
5. Use anticoagulation after the interventional sheaths are placed.
6. Use weight-based heparin to keep activated clotting time (ACT) between 250 and 300 seconds.
7. A femoral angiogram at completion with 30° ipsilateral angulation will show the puncture site.
8. A puncture too low is more predisposed to pseudoaneurysm, and a puncture above the inferior epigastric artery is associated with an increased risk for retroperitoneal hemorrhage.
9. Vascular access management should be planned either by manual compression or appropriate vascular closure device, depending on the physician's familiarity and choice before the patient leaves the lab.
10. Any active extravasation seen at the completion of angiogram should be dealt with immediately, which usually involves reversal of anticoagulation, coil embolization, covered stent, or surgical repair.
11. Manual pressure should be held based on size of the sheath and anticoagulation used.
12. Post procedure, patients with hypotension, abdominal pain, or groin discomfort need immediate assessment with imaging. Patients with suspected retroperitoneal bleeding will need angiogram and percutaneous intervention, such as coil embolization and covered stent.
13. Multidisciplinary approach involving surgeons early in the case is beneficial.

Figures 2.1 and 2.2 demonstrate the ideal CFA access over the femoral head.

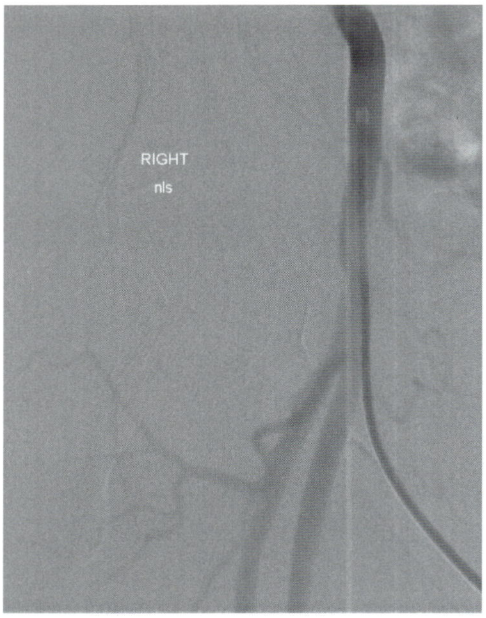

FIGURE 2.1
Sheath angiogram in anterio posterior view unable to demonstrate the correct access site.

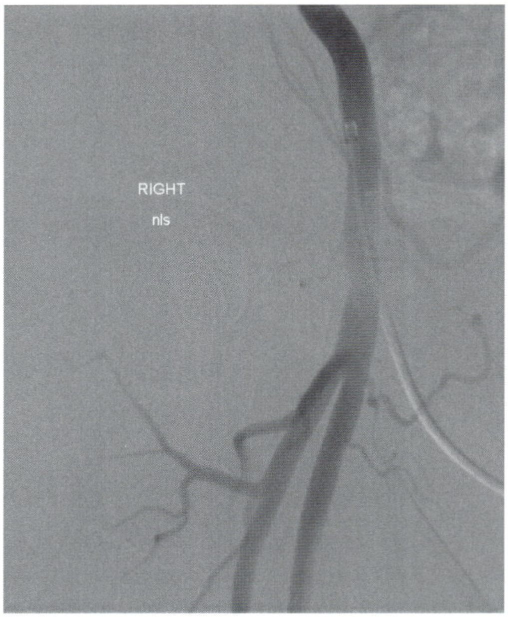

FIGURE 2.2
Sheath angiogram in 30° right anterior oblique view demonstrating the ideal CFA puncture over the femoral head.

TABLE 2.1
Various Complications Following Percutaneous Femoral Artery Access.

COMPLICATION	INCIDENCE	ETIOLOGY	PREVENTION	MANAGEMENT
Pseudoaneurysm	1.2%	Inadequate compression, failure of closure device, obesity	Fluoroscopic guidance to puncture the CFA at the lower one-third of the femur head	Ultrasound-guided thrombin injection or surgical repair (based on size)
Arteriovenous fistula (AVF)	0.6% to 1%	Low arterial puncture	Fluoroscopic guidance to puncture the CFA at the lower one-third of the femur head	Low-flow AVF: observation High-flow AVF: covered stent or surgical repair
Retroperitoneal bleeding	0.5%	High arterial puncture	Fluoroscopic guidance to puncture the CFA at the lower one-third of the femur head	Supportive care, blood transfusion, reversal of anticoagulation: covered stent or open surgical repair for persistent bleeding
Vessel perforation	<1%	Back wall puncture, puncture of inferior epigastric, or circumflex iliac artery	Ensure single front wall puncture; use of micro-puncture needle	Reversal of anticoagulation Covered stent Coil embolization of branch vessel Surgical repair
Vessel occlusion	<1%	Dissection by wire or sheath tip leading to occlusion	Careful wire advancement guided by fluoroscopy (if needed) Ensure sheath and dilator are advanced as one unit	Stenting Surgical repair if stenting is unsuccessful

CASE 2.1

Perforation

CLINICAL HISTORY AND DIAGNOSTIC TESTING RESULTS

An 83-year-old obese woman with a history of hypercholesterolemia and coronary artery disease presented with nonhealing ulcer on the left great toe. Her left lower extremity ankle-brachial index (ABI) was 0.3.

PLANNED PROCEDURE

Diagnostic peripheral angiogram.

PROCEDURE

Right femoral arterial puncture using the modified Seldinger technique was performed after fluoroscopic localization of the femoral head, and a 0.035-inch guidewire was advanced to guide sheath insertion. Diagnostic peripheral angiography was performed per standard technique.

COMPLICATION AND MANAGEMENT

After completion of peripheral diagnostic angiography, a sheath angiogram was carried out to visualize the access site. The angiogram revealed extravasation from the right inferior epigastric artery (Figure 2.3).

At this point, the patient had small hematoma at the access site; however, the patient was hemodynamically stable. It was decided to embolize the inferior epigastric artery via the contralateral approach. Contralateral femoral artery puncture was carried under ultrasound localization, and 6-Fr sheath was inserted in the left CFA. Aortic bifurcation was traversed using a 0.035-inch hydrophilic-angled guidewire in a crossover catheter. Right inferior epigastric artery was cannulated and then embolized using microcoils.

Completion angiography confirmed cessation of bleeding (Figure 2.4) The patient remained hemodynamically stable throughout the procedure and had an uneventful postoperative course.

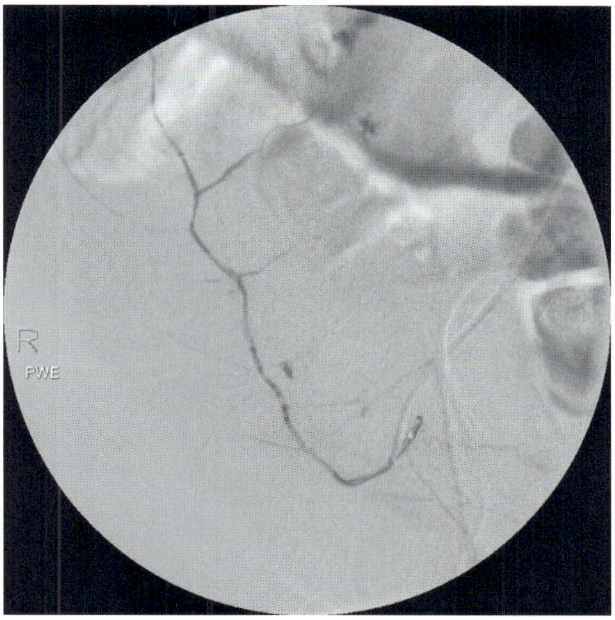

FIGURE 2.3
Extravasation from the right inferior epigastric artery.

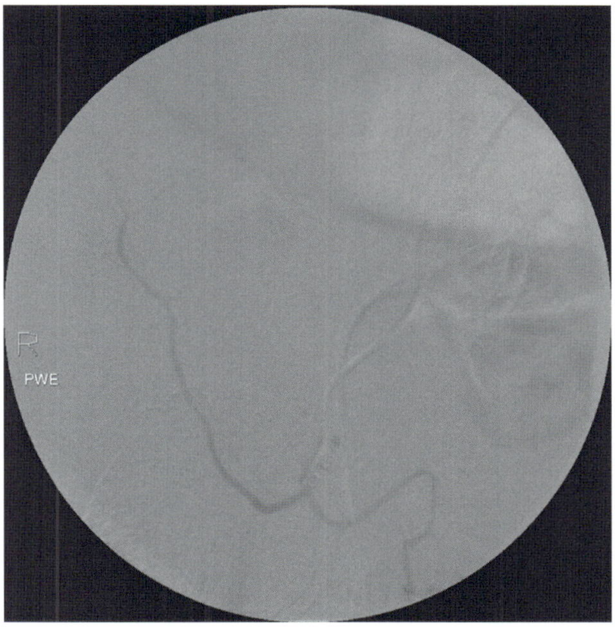

FIGURE 2.4
Deployment of coils in the right inferior epigastric artery with successful control of bleeding.

CASE ANALYSIS

Fluoroscopic guidance should be used in all patients prior to femoral access, and ultrasound guidance should be used selectively to assist in complex cases, such as those associated with administration of thrombolysis. In this case, use of ultrasound guidance to access the CFA might have prevented the inadvertent puncture of the inferior epigastric artery.

LESSONS

- Use fluoroscopic guidance to attain femoral artery access.
- Perform sheath angiography prior to full heparinization.

SUGGESTED READING

Bates MC, Campbell JE. Technique for ipsilateral rescue embolization of common femoral side branch vessel injury. *Catheter Cardivasc Interv.* 2007;70:791–794.

Cherukuri M, Pershad A. Late spontaneous epigastric arterial bleeding associated with abciximab: Successful percutaneous treatment with coil gel-foam embolization. *J Invasive Cardiol.* 2002;14(11):692–693.

CASE 2.2

Retroperitoneal Bleed and Salvage of High Femoral Access

CLINICAL HISTORY AND DIAGNOSTIC TESTING RESULT

A 56-year-old man with a history of right internal carotid endarterectomy 5 years before presented with high-grade restenosis, which was diagnosed using routine follow-up carotid duplex ultrasound.

PLANNED PROCEDURE

Carotid angiography and carotid artery stenting.

PROCEDURE

Right femoral artery access was performed under fluoroscopic guidance, and a long shuttle sheath was inserted over a 0.035-inch guidewire. Patient received 600 mg of Plavix and full-dose anticoagulation to achieve an ACT of > 250 seconds prior to deployment of the carotid stent. Carotid artery stenting was performed per standard technique with a satisfactory completion angiogram of the internal carotid artery.

COMPLICATION AND MANAGEMENT

Immediately after carotid angiography, the patient became hypotensive (systolic blood pressure ~ 70 mmHg). At this point, our differential diagnosis included hypotension secondary to carotid stenting versus access site bleeding. The patient did not respond to intravenous fluid boluses, so intravenous phenylephrine drip was started.

The long shuttle sheath was then exchanged for a 10-cm 6-Fr sheath. Sheath angiography revealed arterial bleeding from a high femoral stick (Figure 2.5). An attempt was made to deploy a suture-based percutaneous closure device to seal the access site, but that was unsuccessful. At this point, it was decided to obtain access from the contralateral side to better define the problem. Contralateral femoral artery access was performed using fluoroscopic and ultrasound guidance, and a 6-Fr sheath was inserted. The aortic bifurcation was traversed using a 0.035 hydrophilic, angled guidewire in a crossover diagnostic catheter. Right external iliac angiography revealed active bleeding at the site of the ipsilateral sheath insertion, with displacement of the bladder indicating retroperitoneal hematoma (Figure 2.6).

The crossover diagnostic catheter was exchanged for a 7-Fr destination sheath over the 0.035 guidewire, and the tip was positioned in the proximal external iliac artery (Figure 2.7). The 0.035 guidewire

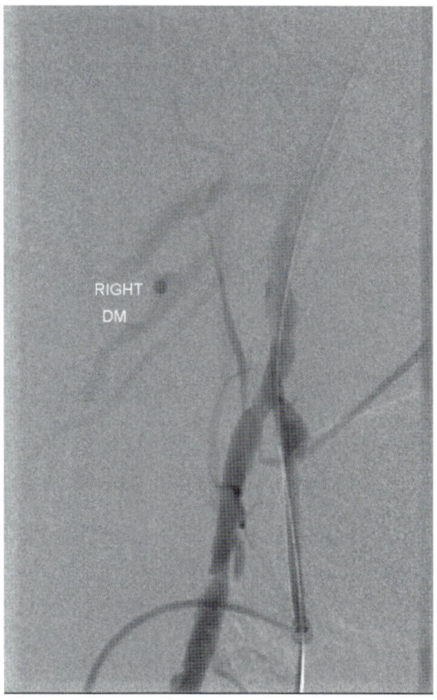

FIGURE 2.5

Femoral angiography demonstrating distal external iliac artery extravasation.

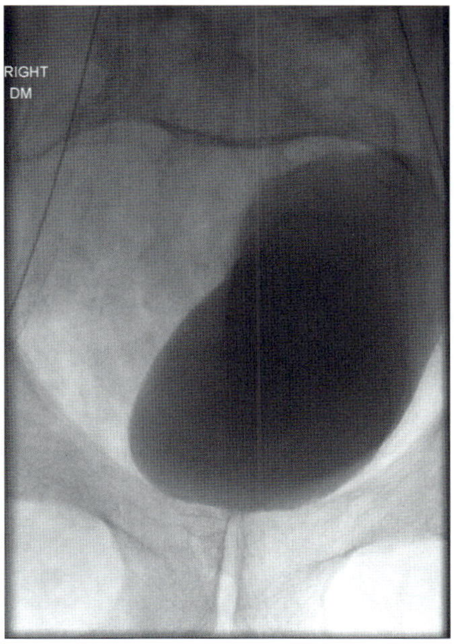

FIGURE 2.6

Displacement of bladder to the left side indicating a retroperitoneal hematoma.

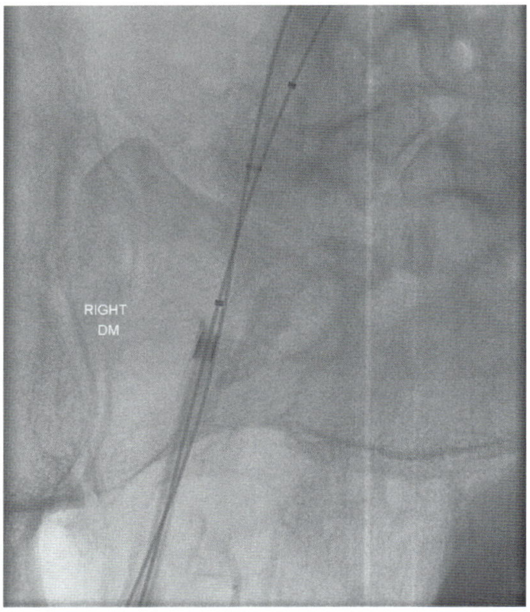

FIGURE 2.7
Guidewire from contralateral femoral artery stationed in the right superficial femoral artery with a covered stent ready to be deployed across the ipsilateral access site.

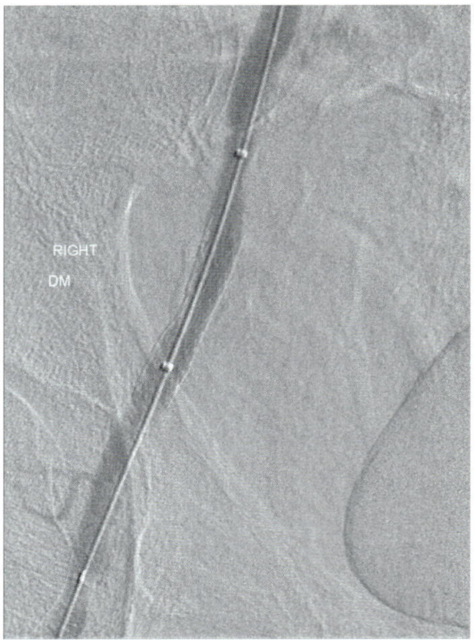

FIGURE 2.8
Completion angiography demonstrating bleeding cessation.

was stationed in the distal superficial femoral artery, and then a self-expanding polytetrafluoroethylene (PTFE)-covered stent was deployed across the access site while the sheath was withdrawn. This led to successful control of bleeding, as demonstrated by completion angiography (Figure 2.8). The contralateral destination sheath was then removed and the access site closed using a suture-mediated percutaneous closure device. The patient had an uneventful postoperative course.

CASE ANALYSIS

Fluoroscopic or ultrasound-guided vascular access would have prevented this complication. Sheath angiography should be performed prior to anticoagulation to detect access-related complications early.

LESSONS

- Always use fluoroscopic guidance to avoid high or low sticks in the femoral artery.
- Always suspect retroperitoneal bleeding in patients with unexplained hypotension.
- Covered stents are valuable tools to control arterial bleeding from high femoral stick.

SUGGESTED READING

Freilich MI, Gossman DE, Applegate RJ, Werns SW, Gips SJ, Turi ZG. The "bladder sign"—An important early marker of retroperitoneal hemorrhage. *Catheter Cardiovasc Interv* [published online ahead of print May 3, 2011]. doi: 10.1002/ccd.23141.

Witz M, Cohen Y, Lehmann JM. Retroperitoneal haematoma—A serious vascular complication of cardiac catheterisation. *Eur J Vasc Endovasc Surg.* 1999;18(4):364–365.

CASE 2.3

Pseudoaneurysm

CLINICAL HISTORY AND DIAGNOSTIC TESTING RESULTS

A 73-year-old patient with history of hypertension, diabetes mellitus, and hypercholesterolemia presented with symptomatic aortic stenosis. Echocardiogram showed severe aortic stenosis with aortic valve area of 0.8 cm^2 with preserved left ventricular ejection fraction. Coronary angiogram did not show any evidence of coronary artery disease. Patient was considered high risk for surgical valve replacement.

PLANNED PROCEDURE

Balloon aortic valvuloplasty (BAV).

PROCEDURE

Left CFA access was obtained under fluoroscopic guidance using standard Seldinger technique, and a 12-Fr short sheath was inserted. Sheath angiography confirmed the puncture to be in the CFA. Heparin was administered to obtain an ACT of >250 seconds. BAV was performed successfully per standard technique. The arterial sheath was then removed and manual pressure applied for 20 minutes.

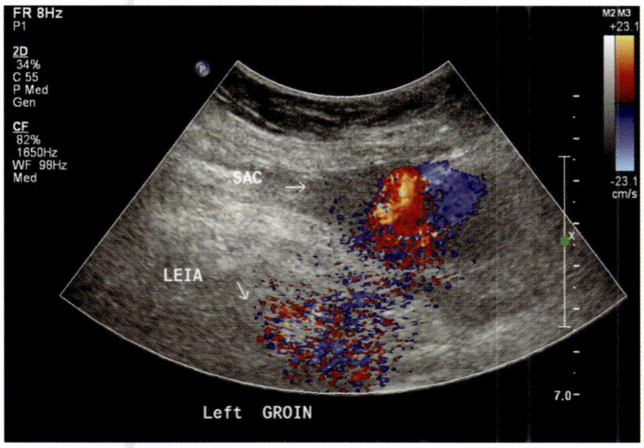

FIGURE 2.9
Duplex ultrasound demonstrating a left CFA pseudoaneurysm as evidenced by to-and-fro motion of blood.

COMPLICATION AND MANAGEMENT

Several hours after procedure completion, the patient complained of left groin pain and swelling. Duplex ultrasound confirmed a left CFA 4-cm pseudoaneurysm (Figure 2.9). Under ultrasound guidance, 1,000 units of thrombin was injected in the pseudoaneurysm sac with successful pseudoaneurysm obliteration (Figures 2.10 and 2.11).

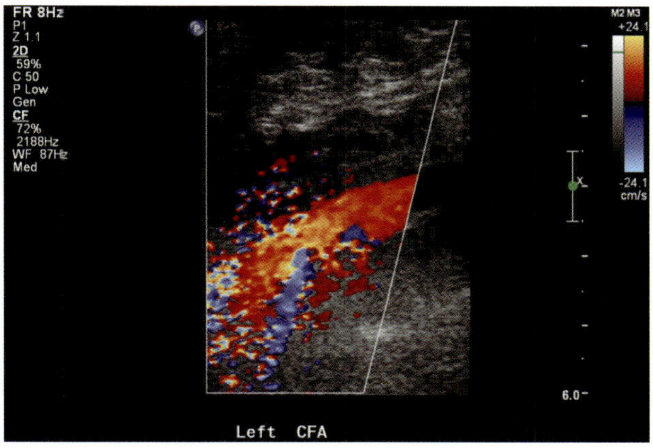

FIGURE 2.10
Successful thrombin injection and obliteration of the pseudoaneurysm.

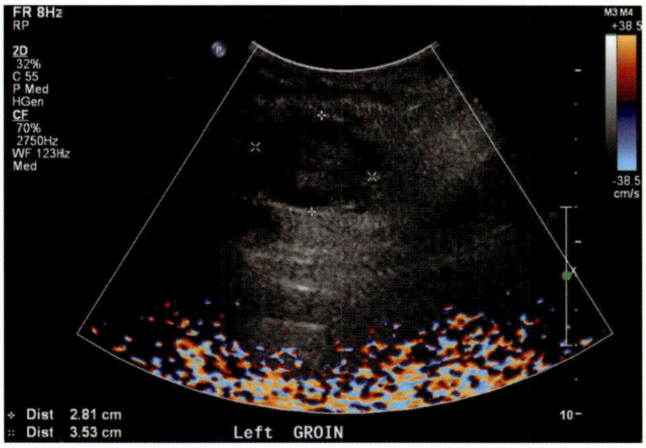

FIGURE 2.11
Thrombosed aneurysm sac.

CASE ANALYSIS

The femoral pseudoaneurysm in this case occurred because of improper (short duration) manual compression. Attaining adequate manual hemostasis after removal of large caliber arterial sheaths requires prolonged compression (30 minutes or more), with close monitoring thereafter. Alternatively, preclosure with suture-based closure devices is also a good technique.

LESSONS

- The duration of manual compression after removal or femoral artery sheaths should be tailored to sheath size.
- For sheaths 10 Fr or larger, manual compression should be applied for 30 minutes or more, with close monitoring thereafter.
- Ultrasound-guided thrombin injection is a valuable technique to treat iatrogenic femoral artery pseudoaneurysms.

SUGGESTED READING

Dean SM, Olin JW, Piedmonte M, Grubb M, Young JR. Ultrasound-guided compression closure of postcatheterization pseudoaneurysms during concurrent anticoagulation: A review of seventy-seven patients. *Journal Vasc Surg.* 1996;23:28–35.

Ahmad F, Turner SA, Torrie P, Gibson M. Iatrogenic femoral artery pseudoaneurysms—A review of current methods of diagnosis and treatment. *Clin Radiol.* 2008;12:1310–1316.

CASE 2.4

External Iliac Occlusion and Profunda Femoralis Perforation

CLINICAL HISTORY AND DIAGNOSTIC TESTING RESULTS

A 65-year-old woman with multiple cardiovascular risk factors presented with an acute inferior wall ST segment elevation myocardial infarction.

PLANNED PROCEDURE

Coronary angiography and primary percutaneous coronary intervention.

PROCEDURE

Right CFA access was obtained per standard technique, and a 6-Fr sheath was inserted. Coronary angiography revealed occluded right coronary artery (RCA). The patients received dual antiplatelet therapy and full-dose anticoagulation. The RCA was successfully recanalized and stented. The arterial sheath was removed and manual compression applied for 30 minutes.

COMPLICATION AND MANAGEMENT

Four hours later, the patient complained of severe right leg pain, and on examination, she was found to have cold right lower extremity with absent pulses (stage IIa acute limb ischemia). The left leg had palpable pulses and an ABI of 0.62.

A left CFA access was obtained, and a 6-Fr sheath inserted. A 5-Fr multipurpose catheter was advanced and positioned at the origin of the right external iliac artery (EIA), where angiography showed dissection of the EIA with flow in the right CFA (Figure 2.12). A 45-cm-long, 6-Fr crossover sheath was placed at the origin of the right EIA over a stiff 0.035-inch wire. The dissection was traversed with an angled stiff 0.035-inch glide wire. A balloon expandable stent was placed in the right EIA (Figure 2.13). Distal vessel angiography showed active extravasation from the right profunda femoris artery (Figure 2.14). Patient became hypotensive, intravenous fluid bolus was given, and a 5- × 20-mm balloon was placed across the profunda femoris artery to attain temporary hemostasis. Then, a 5- × 22-mm PTFE-covered stent was placed in the proximal profunda femoris artery with successful bleeding cessation (Figures 2.15 and 2.16).

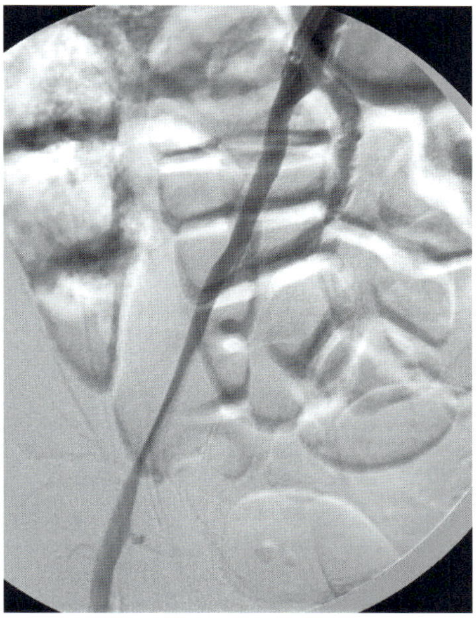

FIGURE 2.12
Left iliac angiography (from contralateral access) demonstrating EIA dissection.

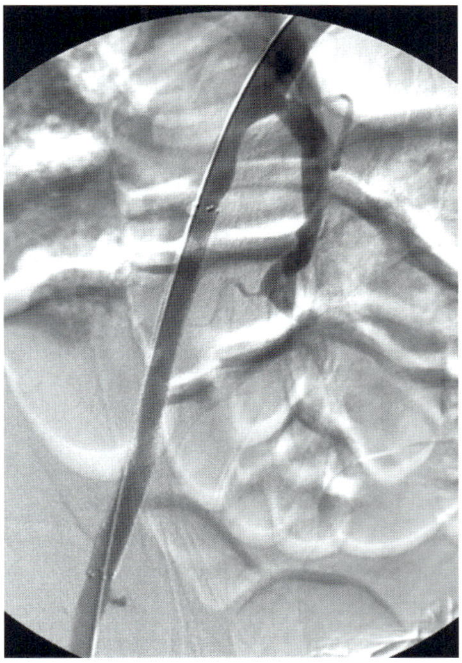

FIGURE 2.13
Iliac angiography after successful deployment of the iliac stent, demonstrating vessel patency.

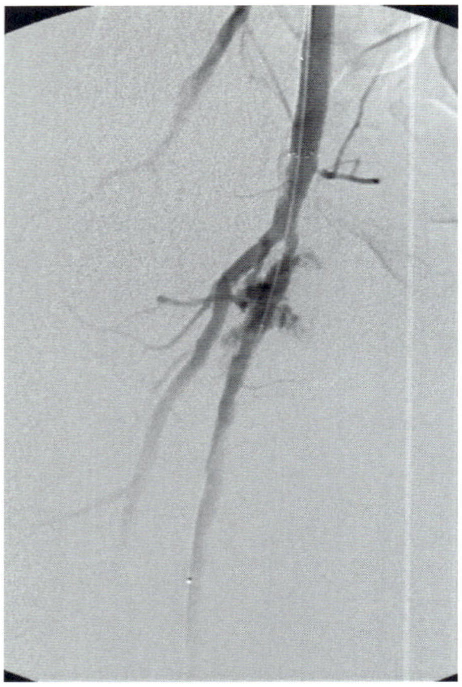

FIGURE 2.14
Femoral angiography showing proximal profunda femoris artery perforation.

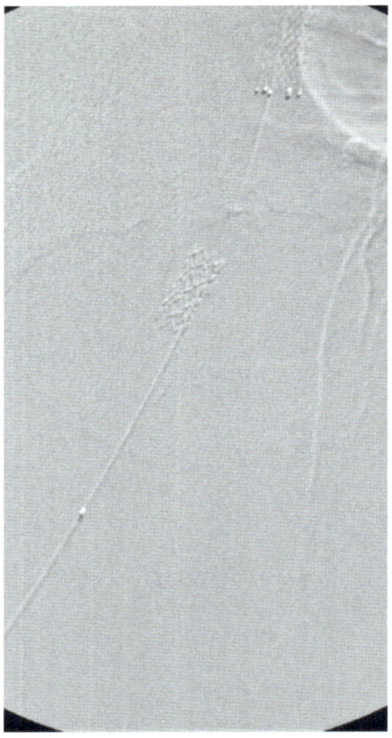

FIGURE 2.15
Deployment of covered stent at the bleeding site in the profunda femoris artery.

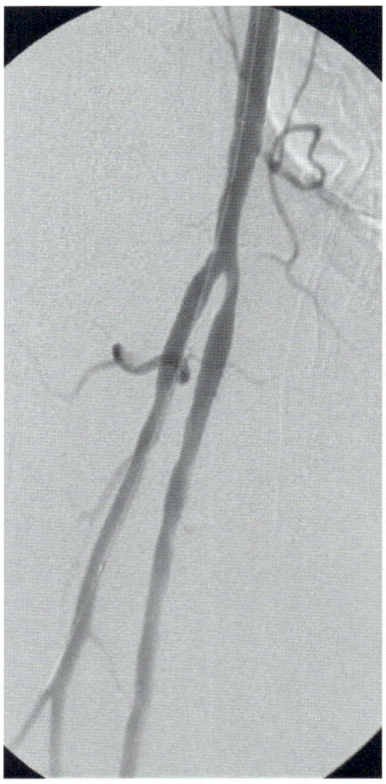

FIGURE 2.16
Completion angiogram showing patent superficial femoral and profunda femoris arteries.

CASE ANALYSIS

In this case, the original puncture for the coronary intervention was made in the right proximal profunda femoris artery, and wire/sheath-induced dissection resulted in occlusion of the right EIA. Again, fluoroscopic guidance would have prevented the low puncture that led to this series of complications.

SUGGESTED READING

Tsetis D. Endovascular treatment of complications of femoral arterial access. *Cardiovasc Intervent Radiol.* 2010 June;33(3):457–468. [published online ahead of print Feb 17, 2010].

Khoo SW, Han DC. The use of ultrasound in vascular procedures. *Surg Clin North Am.* 2011;91(1):173–184.

References

1. Koreny M, Riedmuller E, Nikfardjam M, Siostrzonek P, Mullner M. Arterial puncture closing devices compared with standard manual compression after cardiac catheterization: Systematic review and metaanalysis. *JAMA*. 2004;291:350–357.
2. Applegate RJ, Sacrinty MT, Kutcher MA, et al. Trends in vascular complications after diagnostic cardiac catheterization and percutaneous coronary intervention via the femoral artery, 1998 to 2007. *J Am Coll Cardiol Intv*. 2008;1:317–326.
3. Ohlow MA, Secknus MA, von Korn H, et al. Incidence and outcome of femoral vascular complications among 18,165 patients undergoing cardiac catheterisation. *Int J Cardiol*. 2009;135:66–71.

3

Aravinda Nanjundappa and Akhilesh Jain

Closure Device Complications

INTRODUCTION

Vascular closure devices (VCDs) are used to manage arterial puncture sites following coronary or peripheral vascular interventions. Vascular access management of the arterial puncture sites remains the most important impediment to patient ambulation and/or discharge after diagnostic or interventional procedures. The mainstay of vascular access management for patients undergoing percutaneous femoral arterial access is manual compression. VCDs have been used since 1995 to provide patient comfort and early ambulation and discharge after a diagnostic or interventional cardiovascular procedure. Despite the numerous devices available and ease of use of VCDs, the complications continue to be the Achilles, heel. Several VCDs have been tested over the past decade to replace manual compression. These devices have shown safety comparable to manual compression but have demonstrated improved patient satisfaction and faster ambulation times. The annual projected sales for VCDs is between $500 million and $700 million. There are numerous VCDs, but the most commonly used are Angio-Seal (St. Jude Medical, Inc., St. Paul, MN) and Perclose and StarClose closure systems (Abbott Vascular, Santa Clara, CA).

The most common complications of VCDs are device failure, bleeding, and hematoma. Other serious complications, such as infection, need for vascular surgery, limb loss, and death, are infrequent.

VASCULAR CLOSURE DEVICES

Commercially available VCDs can be categorized as follows:

1. Compression devices (e.g., FemoStop [St. Jude Medical, Inc.] and Safeguard [Maquet Cardiovascular, Wayne, NJ])
2. Topical hemostasis agents (e.g., D-Stat [Vascular Solutions, Inc., Minneapolis, MN], Syvek [Marine Polymer Technologies, Inc., Danvers, MA], and Closure PAD [Scion Cardio-Vascular, Inc., Miami, FL])
3. Invasive suture-based devices (e.g., Perclose and Prostar [Abbott Vascular]); invasive, medicated collagen plugs (e.g., Angio-Seal, Duett [Vascular Solutions, Inc.], and VasoSeal [St. Jude Medical, Inc.]); and clip-based (e.g., StarClose and EVS [expanded vascular stapling] [Angiolink Corp., Taunton, MA])
4. Invasive without a foreign body (e.g., Cardiva Catalyst [Cardiva Medical, Inc., Sunnyvale, CA])

The following table depicts the attributes and potential complications of the various access site hemostasis methods.

	MANUAL COMPRESSION	ANGIO-SEAL	PERCLOSE	MINX
Time to hemostasis	3+	1+	1+	1+
Time to ambulation	3+	1+	1+	1+
Foreign body in the vascular compartment	No	Yes	Yes	No
Foreign body in extravascular compartment	No	Yes	Yes	Yes
Potential for embolism and infection	1+	2+	1+	2+

Advantages of Closure Devices

1. Patients on anticoagulation can achieve faster hemostasis.
2. Patients can be restarted on anticoagulation immediately after the procedure.
3. Faster ambulation times.
4. Increased patient satisfaction.
5. Early discharge.
6. Facilitation of vascular access management of large sheaths (>10 Fr).

The clear contraindications for the use of VCDs are small-sized femoral arteries (<5 mm), severe atherosclerosis or heavy calcification of the common femoral artery (CFA), and high or low common femoral stick.

Disadvantages of Closure Devices

1. There is a learning curve for every device based on experience and the device ease of use.
2. Access site infections can be difficult to treat due to presence of a foreign body.
3. VCDs can result in local discomfort during deployment, some more than others.
4. VCDs are more costly than manual compression.
5. Although serious complications are infrequent, they can result in limb ischemia or loss.

VCD Complications

1. *Hematoma:* Hematomas, both large and small, can result in discomfort, ecchymosis, and possible nidus for infection, but rarely need surgical evacuation. It can occur with both suture-mediated and nonsuture-mediated devices. When hematoma occurs, additional manual compression for 3 to 5 minutes can ameliorate its impact.
2. *Hemorrhage:* Mild oozing from the arterial puncture site is common but can be stopped with manual pressure. Persistent bleeding may require prolonged manual compression or the use of an adjuvant compression device, such as C clamp or femostop. Device failure can lead to both retroperitoneal and surface hemorrhage.
3. *Retroperitoneal bleed (RP):* It is rare to have RP after successful VCD deployment. Nevertheless, RP bleed can occur when VCDs are deployed in cases of unintended use, such as high femoral artery puncture or external iliac artery puncture, concomitant puncture of inferior epigastric artery or lateral circumflex iliac artery, and multiple punctures for access, especially double-wall puncture.
4. *Infection:* Development of localized infection at the site where VCDs are used can be due to the collagen plug in the tissue track or to suture material infection.
5. *Device failure:* This occurs in 1% to 2% of cases, especially during the operator learning curve. Strict adherence to indications and instructions for use for each device can reduce the incidence of device failure.
6. *Embolization:* Device embolization can be seen with anchor devices, such as Angio-Seal, Vasoseal, and Minx. This can lead to acute limb ischemia and limb loss.
7. *Vessel thrombosis:* This is seen primarily as arterial narrowing with suture or staple-mediated devices or as a reaction to collagen material that is exposed to the arterial blood stream.

CASE 3.1

Acute Limb Ischemia Due to Collagen Plug Embolization

CLINICAL HISTORY AND DIAGNOSTIC TESTING RESULTS

An 82-year-old man with hypertension, refractory to medical therapy, was diagnosed with high-grade right renal artery stenosis by magnetic resonance angiography.

PLANNED PROCEDURE

Renal artery stenting.

PROCEDURE

Right CFA access was obtained, and a 7-Fr sheath was inserted. Renal artery stenting was performed per standard technique. The arterial sheath was removed, and an Angio-Seal device (St. Jude Medical, Inc, St. Paul, MN) was deployed.

COMPLICATION AND MANAGEMENT

One hour after closure device deployment, the patient complained of severe right leg pain, and right ankle-brachial index (ABI) was noted to be 0.0 (acute limb ischemia). Emergent right femoral artery angiography through a left femoral artery access showed the collagen plug lodged at the bifurcation of the right CFA (Figure 3.1). The superficial femoral artery (SFA) was noted to have chronic proximal occlusion with distal reconstitution and a two-vessel runoff. A failed attempt was made to snare the collagen plug, and the right CFA appeared to be hazy (Figure 3.2). Patient received 2000 units of heparin, and balloon angioplasty of the CFA into the right profunda was performed with 5- × 20-mm balloon. Repeat angiography showed extravasation at the site of the original puncture (Figure 3.3). This puncture site bleeding was treated with a 5- × 20-mm balloon prolonged sequential inflation for 4 minutes each for a total of 12 minutes Subsequently, the collagen plug was pulled with an internal mammary catheter and pushed into the occluded proximal SFA. Final angiography showed patent right CFA into the right profunda femoris artery (PFA), occluded right SFA, and no further bleeding from the puncture site (Figure 3.4).

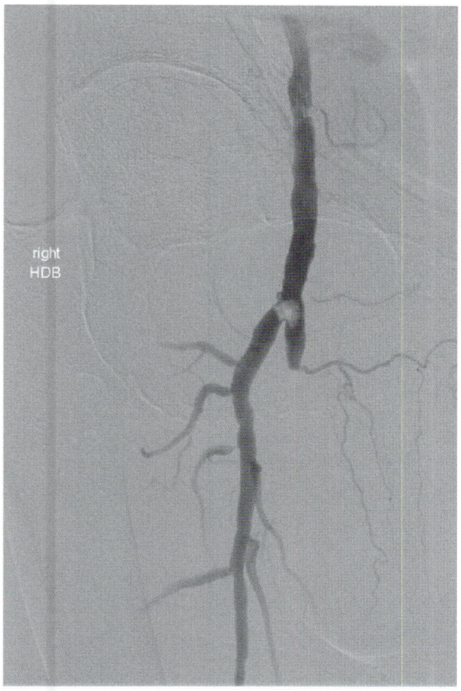

FIGURE 3.1
Angiography showing collagen plug embolization into the right CFA bifurcation.

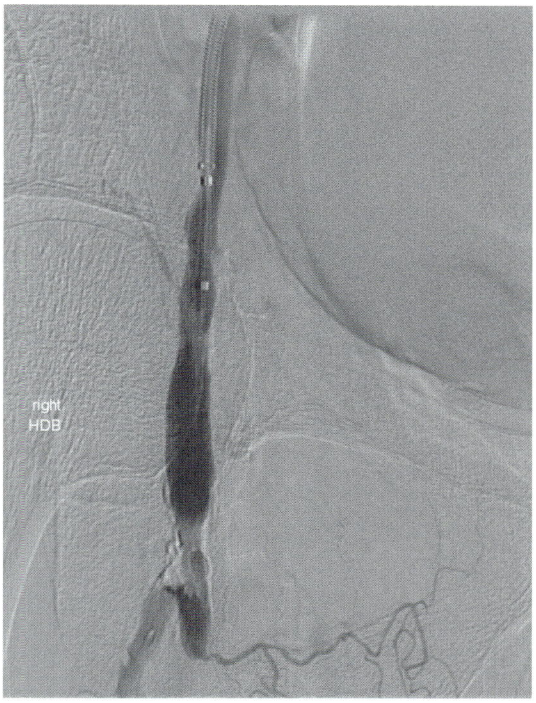

FIGURE 3.2
Angiography demonstrating right CFA bifurcation haziness after failed attempt to snare the plug.

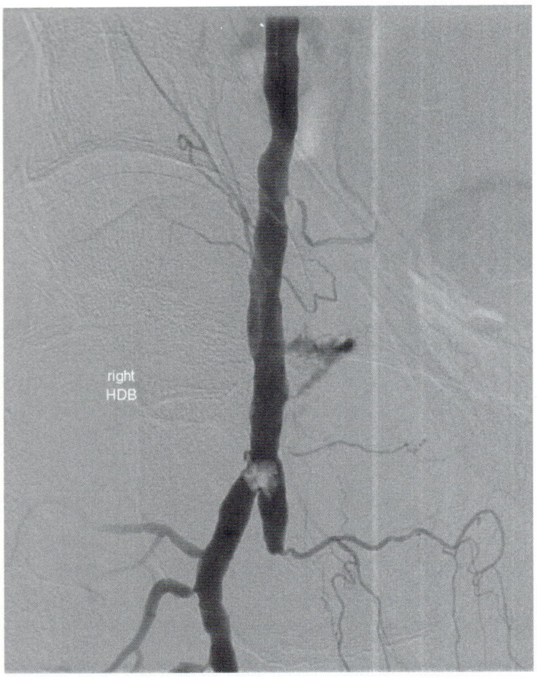

FIGURE 3.3
Angiography demonstrating extravasation from the original puncture site after balloon angioplasty of the femoral artery bifurcation.

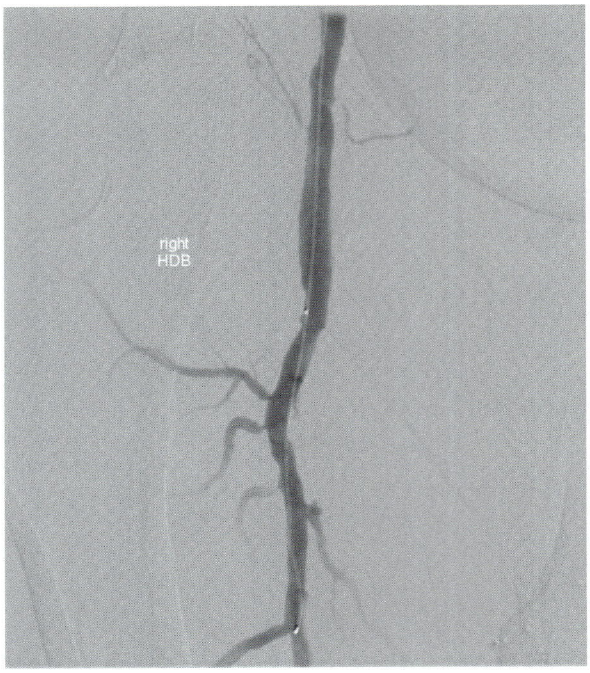

FIGURE 3.4
Angiography after prolonged balloon occlusion of the CFA and redirection of the collagen plug toward the SFA. Note the complete occlusion of the SFA and sealing of the extravasation.

CASE ANALYSIS

When collagen plug embolization occurs, it can result, as demonstrated in this case, in acute limb ischemia. Although the exact cause of embolization is unclear, it is possible that the side puncture will have contributed to this complication; however, device-related malfunction cannot be ruled out. Although catheter-assisted plug removal from the bifurcation has alleviated the acute limb ischemia, subsequent surgical removal would have been preferable.

LESSONS

- Collagen-based closure devices can be associated with collagen plug embolization and subsequent acute limb ischemia.
- Although catheter-assisted redirection of the embolized plug is helpful for immediate relief of ischemia, surgical exploration is necessary for plug removal and definitive arterial repair.

SUGGESTED READING

Dauerman HL, Applegate RJ, Cohen DJ. Vascular closure devices: The second decade. *J Am Coll Cardiol*. 2007;50:1617–1626.
Turi Z. Overview of vascular closure: Endovascular Today annual review current update. *Endovasc Today*. 2008;7:1–7.

CASE 3.2

Acute Limb Ischemia Due to Suture-Based Closure Device

CLINICAL HISTORY AND DIAGNOSTIC TESTING RESULTS

A 72-year-old woman with multiple cardiovascular risk factors presented with acute coronary syndrome.

PLANNED PROCEDURE

Coronary angiography and possible percutaneous coronary interventions (PCI).

PROCEDURE

Left CFA access was obtained per standard technique, and a 6-Fr sheath was inserted. Coronary angiography showed severe stenosis of the left circumflex artery. Stent implantation was performed successfully. A left common femoral sheath angiogram was performed demonstrating moderate to severe calcifications (Figure 3.5). The arterial sheath was removed, and a Perclose closure device (Abbott Vascular, Santa Clara, CA) was deployed.

COMPLICATION AND MANAGEMENT

After closure device deployment, the left femoral pulse was noted to be absent and left leg ABI was 0.3 (stage IIa acute limb ischemia). Arterial access was obtained from the right femoral approach, and left femoral artery angiogram demonstrated left CFA occlusion with faint filling of the superficial femoral artery (SFA) and profunda femoral artery (PFA) (Figure 3.6). The

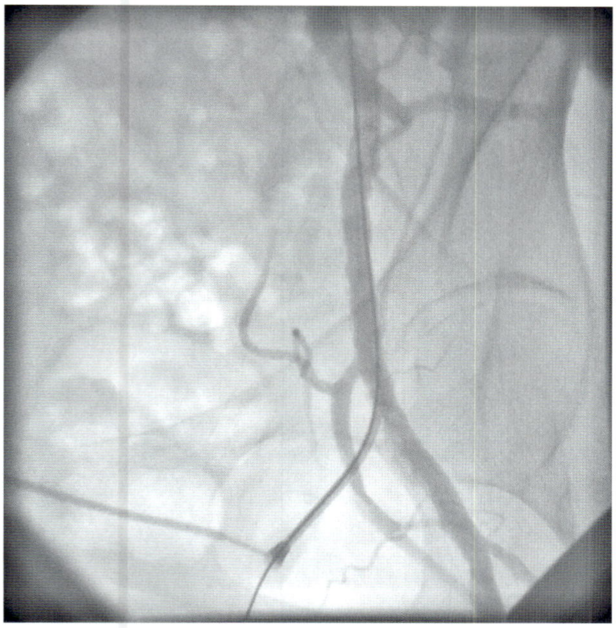

FIGURE 3.5
Postprocedure angiogram showing good femoral access site.

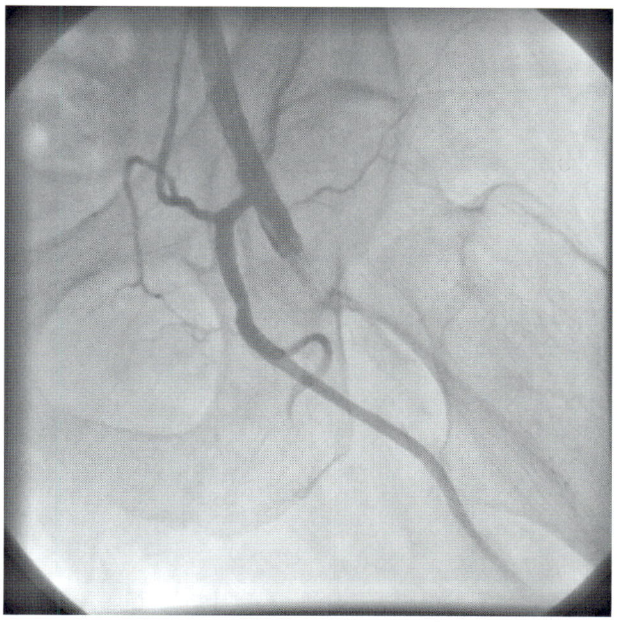

FIGURE 3.6
Post-Perclose deployment occlusion of the CFA.

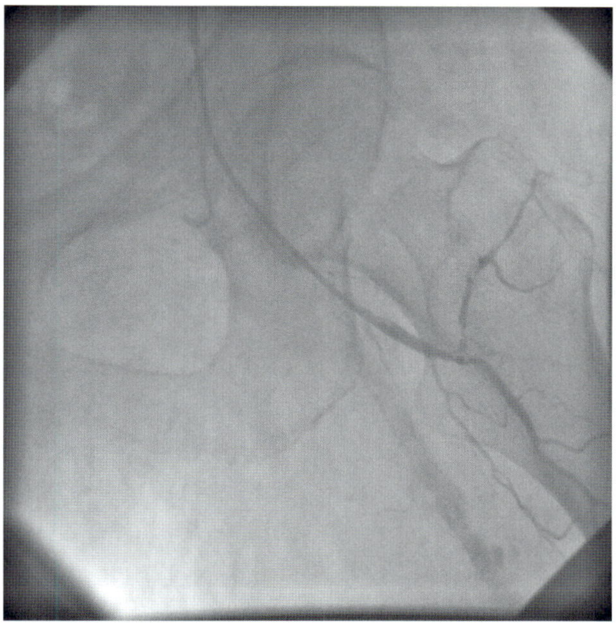

FIGURE 3.7
Crossing into the PFA.

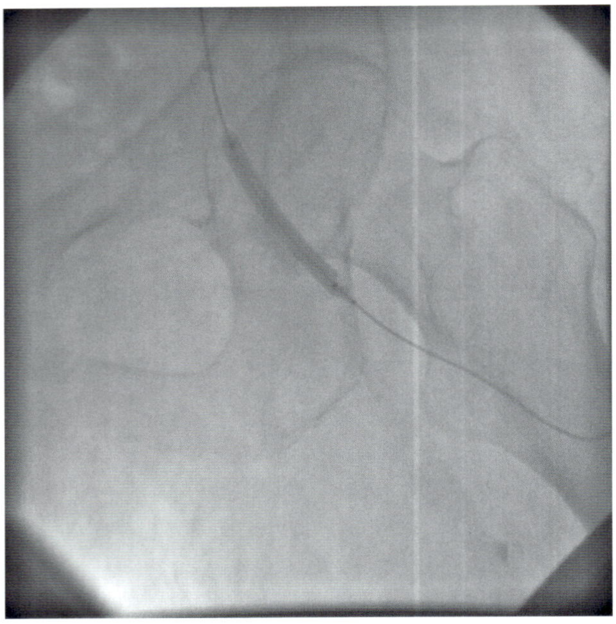

FIGURE 3.8
Balloon angioplasty of the CFA.

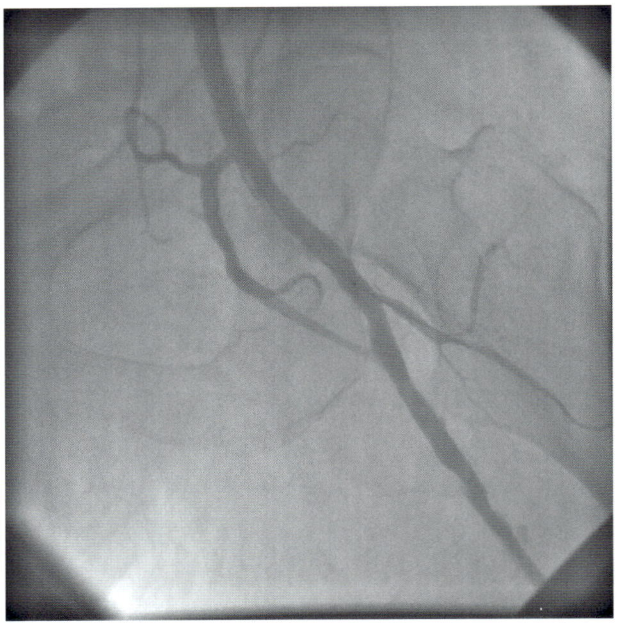

FIGURE 3.9
Completion angiogram showing patent CFA.

occluded left CFA was crossed with a 0.035-inch stiff straight glidewire into the left PFA (Figure 3.7) The left CFA was treated with a 3-minute balloon inflation (5- × 40-mm balloon) (Figure 3.8). Final angiography showed a patent CFA, SFA, and PFA (Figure 3.9).

CASE ANALYSIS

Although the exact cause of the left CFA occlusion after Perclose device deployment is unclear, severe calcification of the CFA may have been the culprit. The success in recanalization of the occlusion and reestablishing vessel patency with catheter-based intervention suggests that the failure mode of suture-based closure devices is more benign than that of collagen-based closure devices.

LESSONS

- VCDs should not be used in severely calcified vessels.
- Catheter-based intervention should be attempted to recanalize occlusions caused by suture-based closure devices.

SUGGESTED READING

Koreny M, Riedmüller E, Nikfardjam M, et al. Arterial puncture closing devices compared with standard manual compression after cardiac catheterization: systemic review and meta-analysis. *JAMA*. 2004;291:350–357.

CASE 3.3

Acute Limb Ischemia From Bioabsorbable Sealant-Based Closure Device

CLINICAL HISTORY AND DIAGNOSTIC TESTING RESULTS

A 34-year-old woman with history of extensive coronary artery disease and status postcoronary artery bypass graft surgery presented with acute ischemic syndrome.

PLANNED PROCEDURE

Coronary angiography and possible PCI.

PROCEDURE

A 6-Fr sheath was inserted via the right CFA. Coronary angiography showed severe stenosis of the saphenous vein graft (SVG) to the right posterior descending artery (PDA). Successful coronary stenting was performed per standard technique. Vascular hemostasis was obtained with a Minx closure device (AccessClosure, Inc., Mountain View, CA).

COMPLICATION AND MANAGEMENT

Five hours after closure device deployment, the patient complained of numbness and discomfort in the right leg. An angiogram of the right CFA from the contralateral left femoral approach showed acute occlusion of the right CFA (Figure 3.10). A contralateral sheath was introduced from the left femoral artery and positioned in the right external iliac artery. The totally occluded right CFA was crossed with straight stiff 0.035-inch glide wire (Figure 3.11), and a thrombolytic catheter was placed across the occlusion (Figure 3.12). Repeat angiography 12 hours after thrombolytic infusion revealed patent right CFA (Figure 3.13). Intravascular ultrasound demonstrated a dissection in the mid–right CFA (Loop 3.14). Prolonged balloon inflation in the right CFA resulted in widely patent right CFA, PFA, and SFA (Figure 3.15).

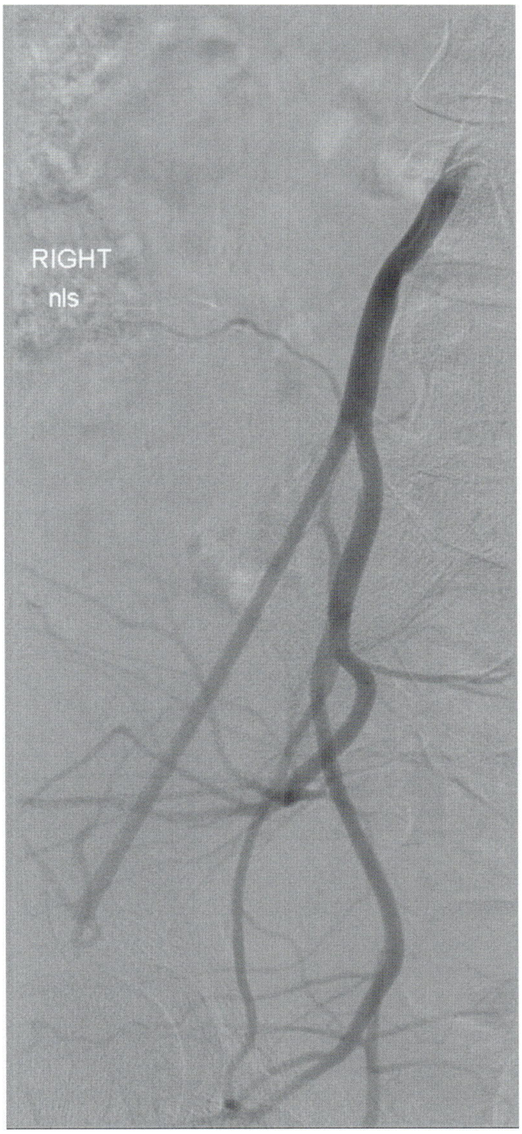

FIGURE 3.10
Angiogram of right external iliac artery showing occlusion of the right CFA.

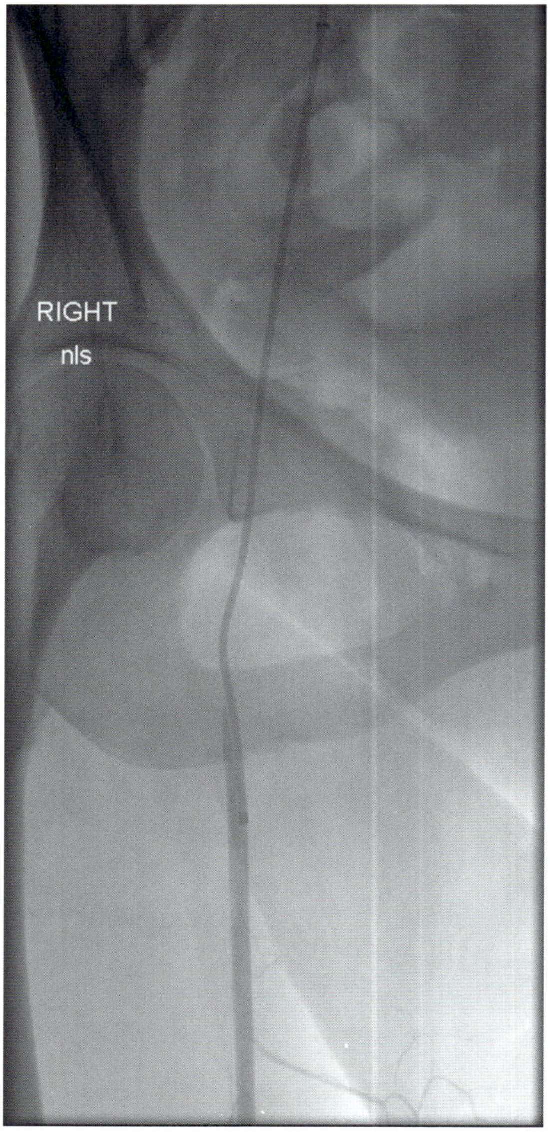

FIGURE 3.11
Successful occlusion recanalization.

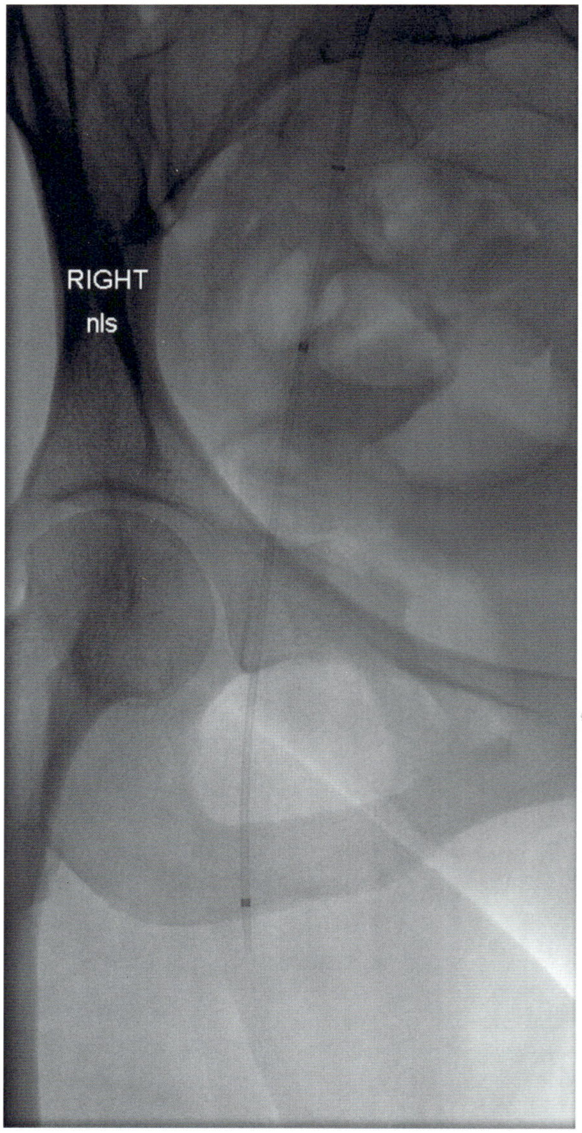

FIGURE 3.12
Catheter-based thrombolytic infusion.

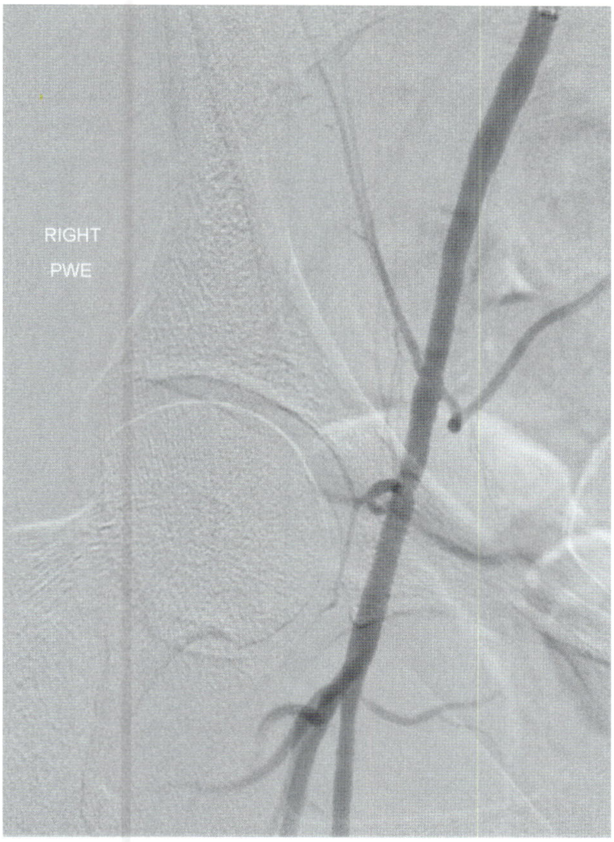

FIGURE 3.13
Angiography 12 hours postthrombolysis showing patent right CFA.

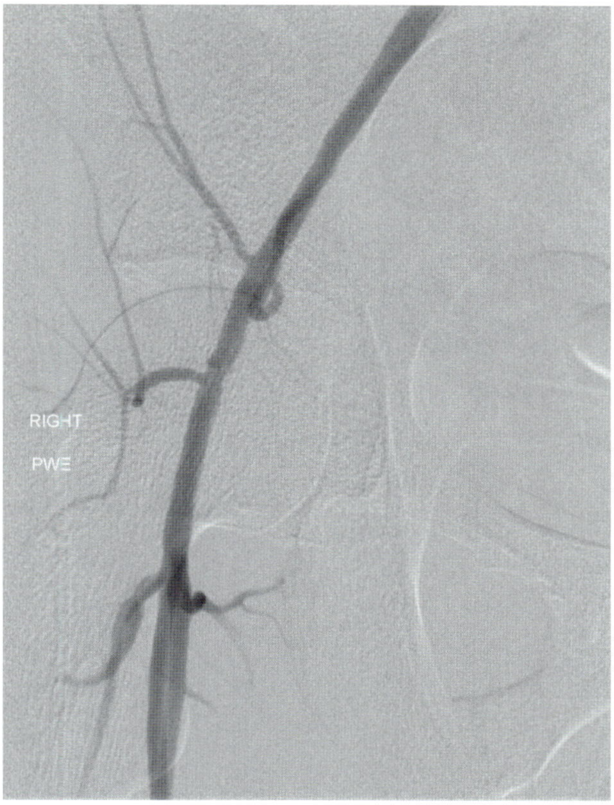

FIGURE 3.15
Completion angiography after prolonged balloon inflation.

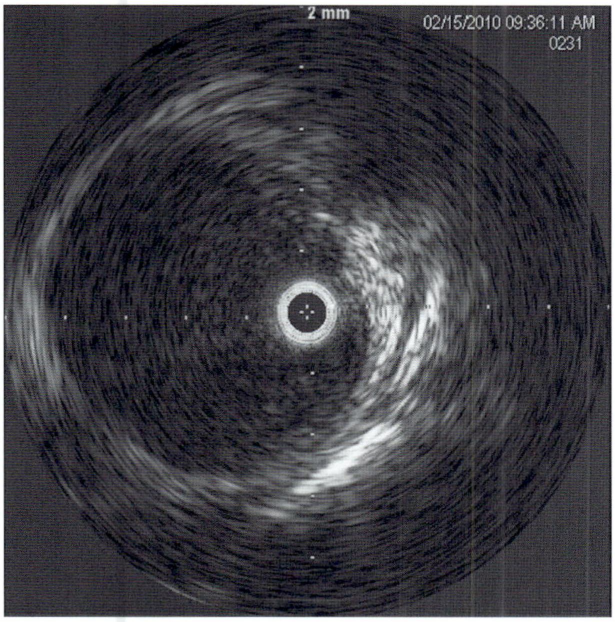

FIGURE 3.14
LOOP 3.14 Intravascular ultrasound interrogation of the right CFA demonstrating intraluminal dissection.

CASE ANALYSIS

In retrospect, it appears that the size of the right CFA is rather small. This is not surprising, given the fact that the patient is a 34-year-old woman. Whether the arterial dissection/occlusion resulted from the small arterial size or technical issues related to closure device deployment is unclear. However a preprocedure sheath angiogram would have shown the small size of the CFA and may have altered the access site closure strategy in this patient.

LESSONS

- Baseline arterial sheath angiography is valuable in determining best access site closure strategy.
- The Minx closure device, similar to other closure devices, can be associated with vessel closure.
- Catheter-based interventions should always be attempted to relieve acute occlusions from closure devices. The need for surgical intervention should be evaluated concomitantly.

SUGGESTED READING

Nikolsky E, Mehran R, Halkin A, et al. Vascular complications associated with arteriotomy closure devices in patients undergoing percutaneous coronary procedures: a meta-analysis. *J Am Coll Cardiol.* 2004;44:1200–1209.

4

Tejas Patel, Sanjay Shah, and Samir Pancholy

Transradial Vascular Access–Related Complications During Coronary Interventions

INTRODUCTION

Campeau in 1989 demonstrated feasibility of transradial approach (TRA) for coronary angiography. In 1993, Keimneij published his data on coronary stent implantation through TRA. In the past 2 decades, TRA has seen a slow but steady global growth. Several studies have shown that TRA reduces bleeding and access site–related complications as compared with the transfemoral approach (TFA). Despite many distinct advantages, there has been relatively slow adoption of TRA for coronary interventions because of the required learning curve. Although the TRA is relatively safe, complications can occur. In this chapter, we will discuss the following potential complications through case studies and tips and tricks to manage them:

1. Radial or brachial artery perforation leading to a hematoma formation
2. Radial artery spasm
3. Guidewire or catheter-induced dissection in the radial, axillary, or subclavian artery
4. Radial artery pseudoaneurysm (PA) and depigmented scar at the puncture site
5. Radial artery occlusion.

CASE 4.1

Radial Artery Perforation and Forearm Hematoma

CLINICAL HISTORY AND DIAGNOSTIC TESTING RESULTS

A 75-year-old woman with known coronary artery disease (CAD) and diabetes mellitus (DM) presented with acute coronary syndrome.

PLANNED PROCEDURE

Diagnostic coronary angiography and possible ad hoc coronary intervention through right TRA.

PROCEDURE

After radial artery puncture, a 5-Fr introducer sheath was inserted using standard technique. Spasmolytic cocktail was given as per standard protocol. A 5-Fr Tiger catheter (Terumo, Japan) was introduced over a 0.032-inch standard guidewire. We encountered resistance to the advancement of the guidewire and diagnostic catheter at the brachio radial junction. Several attempts were made to negotiate the assembly through that junction without success. The patient began to complain of forearm pain, and a progressive local swelling suggestive of hematoma was observed. The guidewire was immediately removed and the catheter pulled back. Diluted contrast injection through the catheter revealed a complex loop and significant extravasation of contrast suggestive of perforation (Figure 4.1a).

COMPLICATION AND MANAGEMENT

Angiography (Figure 4.1a) demonstrated a large perforation in the complex radial loop resulting in an enlarging hematoma in the right forearm. The patient remained hemodynamically stable. A 0.014-inch balanced middle weight (BMW) percutaneous transluminal coronary angioplasty (PTCA) guidewire was used to cross the loop, and subsequently a 5-Fr diagnostic catheter was carefully negotiated over it (Figure 4.1b). Once the diagnostic catheter crossed the arterial loop, where the perforation was located, the extravasation ceased. Coronary angiography revealed a critical proximal left anterior descending artery (LAD) stenosis, and an ad hoc percutaneous coronary intervention (PCI) was planned. The 5-Fr Tiger catheter was exchanged over a 0.035-inch standard guidewire for a 5-Fr EBU guide catheter (Launcher, Medtronic, Minneapolis, MN). Successful stenting of the LAD lesion was performed as per standard technique (Figure 4.1c). After the end of the procedure, the guide catheter was removed, and contrast injection revealed that the perforation was sealed (Figure 4.1d). A compressive dressing was applied to patient's arm (at the hematoma site), and the patient was advised to keep her arm elevated for few hours. The patient was discharged from the hospital at day 3 postprocedure in a hemodynamically stable condition with significant improvement in the forearm hematoma (Figure 4.1e).

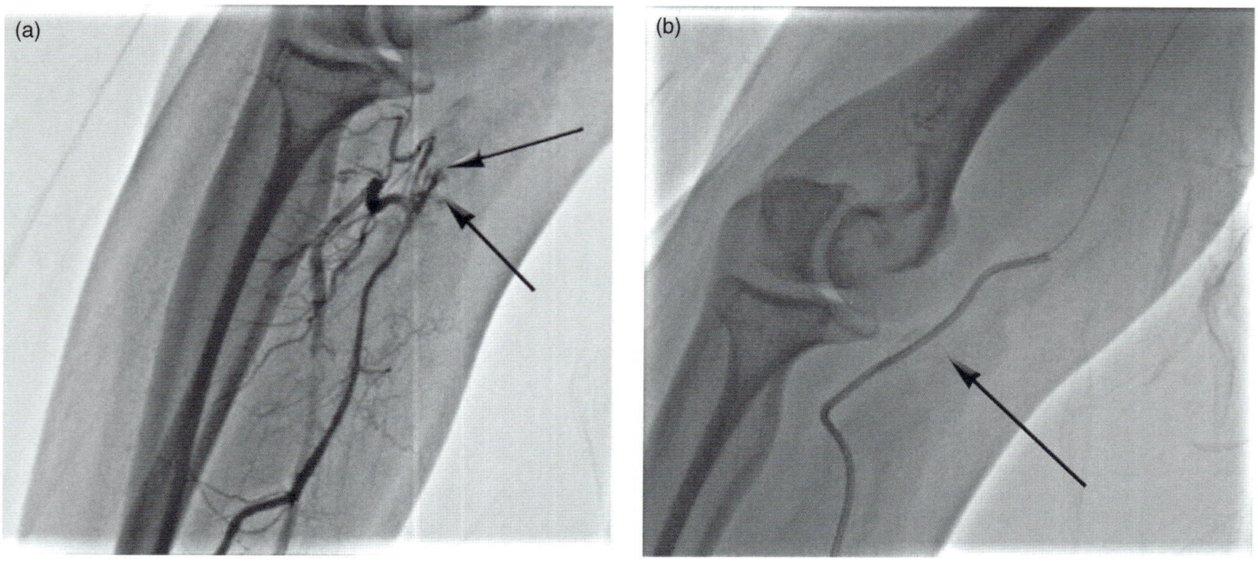

FIGURE 4.1

Continues on next page.

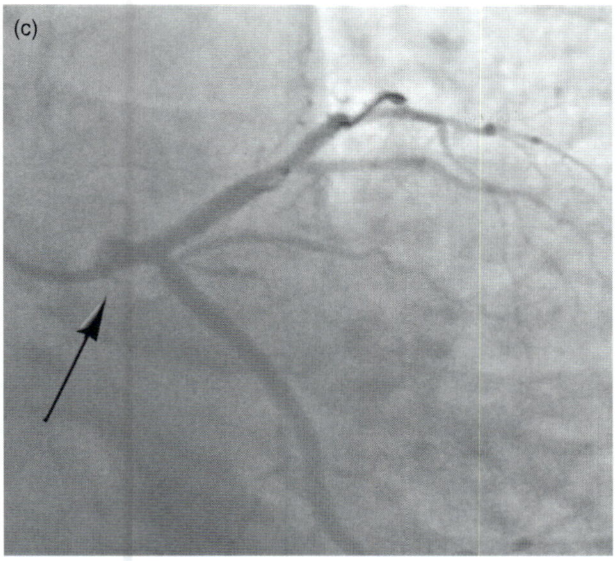

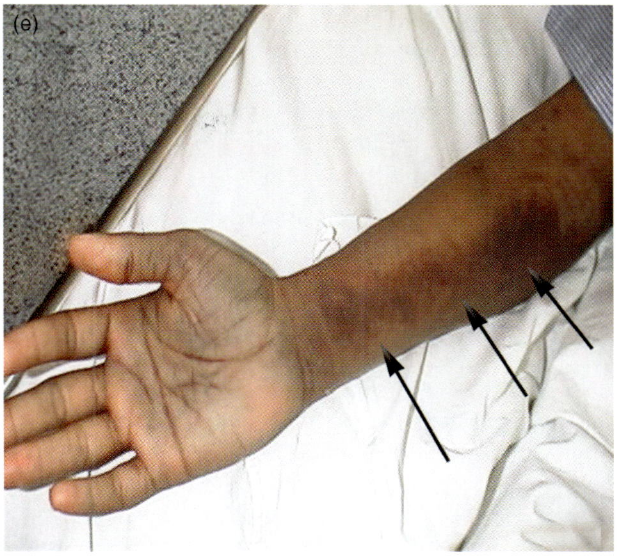

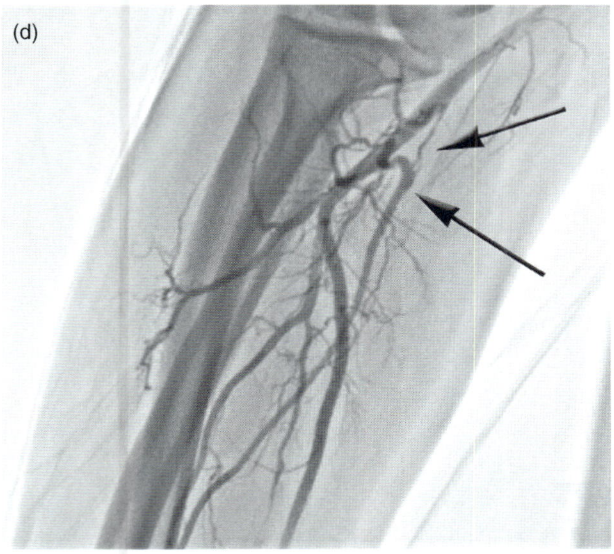

FIGURE 4.1

(Cont.) Radial artery perforation leading to a forearm hematoma. (a) Complex loop with perforation, (b) loop crossed with a 0.014-inch BMW PTCA wire and 5F diagnostic catheter, (c) stenting of LAD lesion, (d) sealed perforation and no extravasation of contrast, and (e) resolving forearm hematoma. **(LOOPS 4.1a, b, c, d)**

CASE ANALYSIS

Guidewire- and/or catheter-induced arterial perforation in the brachio radial region leading to a forearm hematoma is a known complication of TRA.

This Complication Occurred Because

1. The patient had a complex radial arterial loop, which is an anatomical variant, but we were not aware of its presence.
2. Persistence to negotiate the standard 0.032-inch guidewire and the 5-Fr Tiger diagnostic catheter through the arterial loop, despite encountering significant resistance.

This Complication Could Have Been Avoided If

1. The operator already knew about the presence of the radial arterial loop before advancement of the guidewire and diagnostic catheter by performing radial artery angiography through the sheath.

2. The operator stopped making repeated attempts to navigate the loop with the 0.032-inch guidewire after encountering initial resistance. Instead, the operator should have removed the guidewire, pulled the diagnostic catheter proximally while injecting diluted contrast to define the arterial anatomy, and used a 0.014-inch guidewire to navigate the loop.

Courses of Action Once the Complication Was Identified

It is important to remove the guidewire that encounters resistance, with simultaneous pullback of the diagnostic catheter while injecting diluted contrast to help define the anatomy and identify the complication. Once the complication is identified, the operator has one of two choices:

1. If the operator is a beginner radialist, he/she should abort the procedure, reverse the effect of heparin, and apply firm pressure bandage at the hematoma site. This will allow the perforation to seal and prevent the development of a large hematoma. The deferred PCI can be reattempted later using the contralateral radial or a femoral approach.
2. If the operator is an experienced radialist, he/she can proceed with the planned intervention as described above. A diagnostic catheter or guide catheter that is placed across the perforated segment acts as an internal hemostatic device and contributes to sealing of the perforation. In our experience, this technique is predictable and reproducible.

LESSONS

- Baseline arterial angiography through the radial sheath can uncover unexpected anatomic variants and potentially help avoid vessel dissection/perforation.
- If the operator encounters resistance to guidewire advancement through the radial brachial arteries, he/she should avoid repeated attempts at navigating through the segment. Arterial angiography should be performed to uncover the cause of resistance.
- A 0.014-inch soft tip coronary guidewire should be used to navigate through complex arterial anatomy or perforated arterial segments. It is possible to deliver a diagnostic catheter or even a guide catheter over a 0.014-inch wire.
- If the operator encounters difficulty in advancing a catheter through a complex arterial loop or a perforated segment, it is important to downsize the catheter (i.e., use 4-Fr instead of 5-Fr diagnostic catheter).
- In case of radial artery perforation, the catheter itself can serve as an internal hemostatic device and help seal the perforation.

SUGGESTED READING

Patel T, Shah S, Ranjan A. *Patel's Atlas of Transradial Intervention: The Basics*. Seattle, WA: Sea Script Company; 2007.

Louvard Y, Lefevre T. Loops and transradial approach in coronary diagnosis and intervention. *Cathet Cardiovasc Interven*. 2000;51:250–252.

Barbeau GR. Radial loop and extreme vessel tortuosity in the transradial approach: Advantage of hydrophilic-coated guidewires and catheters. *Cathet Cardiovasc Interven*. 2003;59(4):442–450.

Patel T, Shah S, Sanghvi K, Pancholy S. Management of radial and brachial artery perforations during transradial procedures—A practical approach. *J Intven Cardiol*. 2009;21:544–547.

CASE 4.2

Radial Artery Spasm

CLINICAL HISTORY AND DIAGNOSTIC TESTING RESULTS

A 38-year-old man without known cardiovascular risk factors presented with angina pectoris and underwent a stress test that revealed moderate, reversible inferior ischemia.

PLANNED PROCEDURE

Elective coronary angiography through the right TRA.

PROCEDURE

After radial artery (RA) puncture, a 5-Fr introducer sheath was inserted using standard technique. Spasmolytic cocktail was given as per standard protocol. While negotiating a 5-Fr Tiger diagnostic catheter over a standard 0.032-inch guidewire, we encountered significant resistance, and the patient simultaneously complained of significant pain in his forearm. As per our standard protocol, the catheter was pulled back, and diluted contrast was injected to define the arterial anatomy. Angiography revealed occlusive focal spasm in the radial artery (Figure 4.2a).

COMPLICATION AND MANAGEMENT

A guidewire- or catheter-induced focal or diffuse spasm in a radial artery is a well-known complication of TRA procedures. In this patient, after identifying the occlusive spasm in the radial artery, we administered intraarterial diltiazem (5 mg) and nitroglycerin (200 µg) through the catheter. Repeat diagnostic angiography revealed spasm resolution (Figure 4.2b). However, repeat arterial angiography in the right anterior oblique (RAO) and left anterior oblique (LAO) views revealed a complex loop in the brachial artery just distal to the spastic segment (Figure 4.2c, d). Subsequently, the arterial loop was crossed using standard technique as described in Case 1 (Figure 4.2e), and coronary angiography was completed.

CASE ANALYSIS

Radial artery spasm is not uncommon during TRA. Predictors of RA spasm include vessel tortuosity (especially loops), small vessel caliber, high origin of the RA (from the proximal brachial or axillary artery) because RA caliber is almost invariably small with this anomaly, preexisting atherosclerosis, and use of large profile catheters (>6-Fr). The complication in this case occurred because

1. The patient had a complex brachial arterial loop that the operator was not aware of.
2. Persistence in negotiating the standard 0.032-inch guidewire and the 5-Fr Tiger diagnostic catheter through the arterial loop despite encountering significant resistance.

This Complication Could Have Been Avoided If

1. The operator already knew about the presence of the brachial arterial loop before advancement of the guidewire and diagnostic catheter by performing angiography through the sheath.
2. The operator avoided making repeated attempts to navigate the loop with the 0.032-inch guidewire after encountering initial resistance. Instead, the operator should have removed the guidewire and pulled the diagnostic catheter proximally while injecting diluted contrast to define the arterial anatomy and use a 0.014-inch guidewire to navigate the loop.

Course of Action Once the Complication Was Identified

Once the diagnosis of radial spasm was made, the operator administered a dose of spasmolytic cocktail, which relieved the spasm. Occasionally, spasm persists despite two or more doses of spasmolytic cocktail. After spasm relief, the arterial loop should be carefully navigated under fluoroscopic guidance with a 0.014-inch soft-tipped PTCA wire or a 0.025-inch hydrophilic wire (Glidewire, Terumo, Japan) and a 5-Fr diagnostic catheter. The catheter should not be pushed but advanced in a corkscrew fashion until the affected arterial segment is crossed.

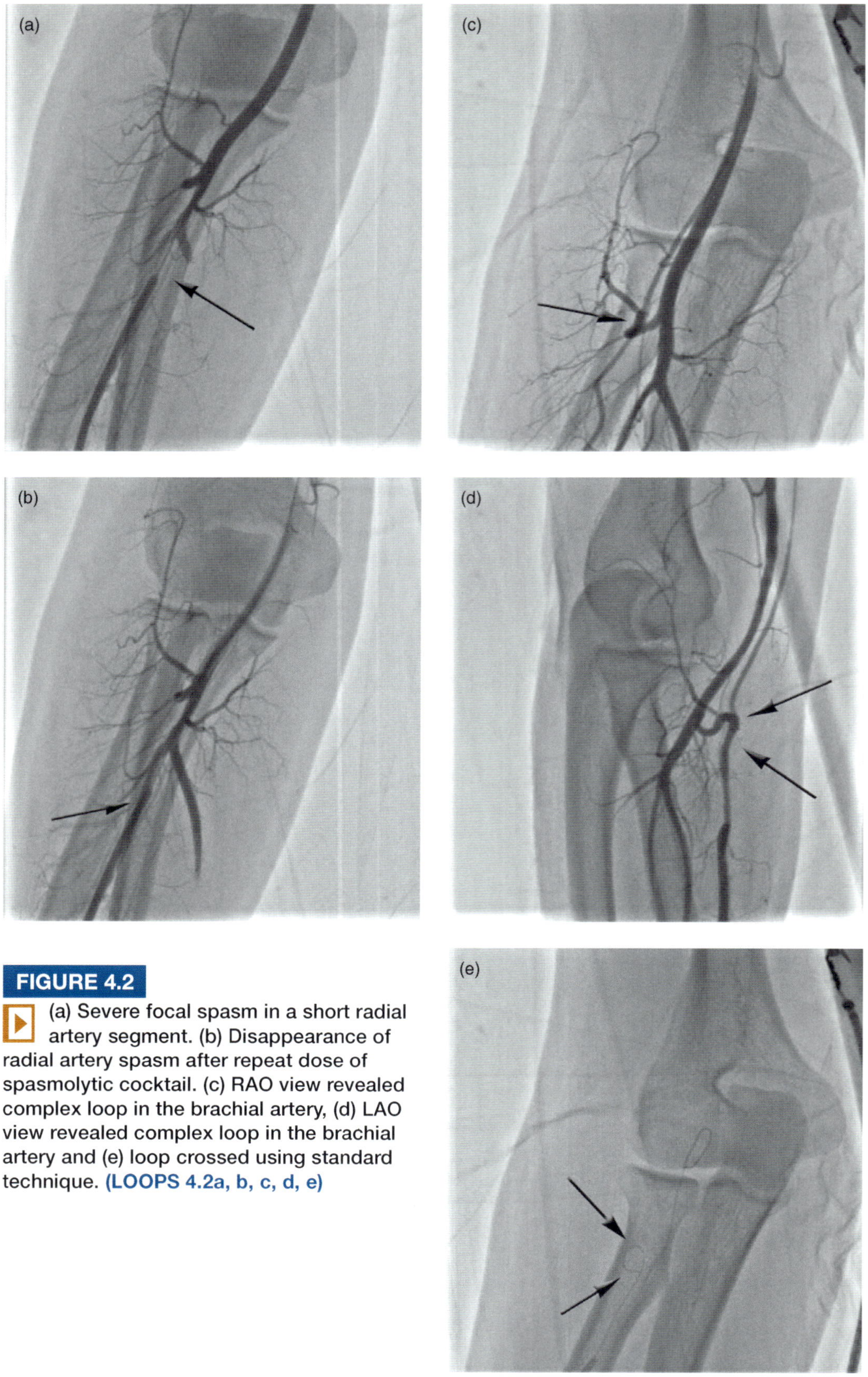

FIGURE 4.2

(a) Severe focal spasm in a short radial artery segment. (b) Disappearance of radial artery spasm after repeat dose of spasmolytic cocktail. (c) RAO view revealed complex loop in the brachial artery, (d) LAO view revealed complex loop in the brachial artery and (e) loop crossed using standard technique. **(LOOPS 4.2a, b, c, d, e)**

LESSONS

- It is important to identify arterial spasm at an early stage of the procedure.
- Keep a low threshold for RA angiography to define the anatomy.
- Spasmolytic cocktail relieves arterial spasm in most cases.
- Mild sedation should be administered to relieve anxiety and/or pain.
- Use either a 0.025-inch hydrophilic guidewire or a 0.014-inch soft-tipped PTCA wire instead of standard 0.032-inch or 0.035-inch guidewires to navigate through tortuosity and spasm.
- Downsize the diagnostic catheter.
- RA spasm is common after multiple failed attempts at RA puncture. It is important to perform the initial puncture carefully to avoid spasm. Sometimes, after repeated RA punctures, the RA pulse disappears. In this situation, the following steps should be taken: Administer local subcutaneous nitroglycerine and wait few minutes. The RA pulse often reappears. If the spasm persists, an experienced operator should attempt a puncture at a higher RA site.

SUGGESTED READING

Patel T, Shah S, Ranjan A. *Patel's Atlas of Transradial Intervention: The Basics*. Seattle, WA: Sea Script Company; 2007.

Pancholy S, Coppola J, Patel T. Subcutaneous administration of nitroglycerin to facilitate radial artery cannulation. *Catheter Cardiovasc Interv.* 2006;68(3):389–391.

Coppola J, Patel T, Kwan T, et al. Nitroglycerin, nitroprusside, or both, in preventing radial artery spasm during transradial catheterization. *J Inv Cardiology.* 2006;18(4):155–158.

Gilchrist IC. Transradial technical tips. *Cathet Cardiovasc Interven.* 2000;49(3):353–354.

CASE 4.3

A Guide Catheter–Induced Dissection of the Subclavian Artery

CLINICAL HISTORY AND DIAGNOSTIC TESTING RESULTS

A 65-year-old man had a history of DM, hypertension, and known CAD with recurrent angina while on medical therapy. The patient underwent transfemoral coronary angiography at another institution, which demonstrated severe proximal LAD stenosis.

PLANNED PROCEDURE

PCI of a proximal LAD artery stenosis through a right TRA.

PROCEDURE

Right RA puncture was performed, and a 6-Fr introducer sheath was inserted using standard technique. A 6-Fr EBU guide catheter (Launcher, Medtronics, Minneapolis, MN) was introduced over a 0.035-inch standard wire. We encountered resistance to the advancement of the wire or guide assembly in the axillo subclavian region. We removed the guidewire, pulled back the guide catheter to the mid-brachial segment, and performed brachial angiography. Angiography revealed a large dissection in the axillo subclavian arterial segment (Figure 4.3a). Patient complained of pain in the axillary region but remained hemodynamically stable and had palpable radial and ulnar pulse.

COMPLICATION AND MANAGEMENT

The patient has a guide catheter–induced dissection involving the axillo subclavian arterial segment. After identifying the dissection, we navigated a 0.014-inch coronary guidewire (BMW) into the true arterial lumen and positioned it in the ascending aorta. During wire advancement, the free movement of the wire tip and the rapid washout of contrast confirmed its intraluminal location (Figure 4.3b). Subsequently, the guide catheter was carefully advanced and positioned in the ascending aorta (Figure 4.3c). PCI of the LAD artery was then performed using standard technique (Figure 4.3d). At the end of the procedure, diluted contrast was injected in the previously dissected arterial segment during the pull-back of the guide catheter, which revealed a sealed dissection and normal blood flow (Figure 4.3e). The patient was discharged the next day in a stable condition.

CASE ANALYSIS

Guide catheter–induced arterial dissection during TRA is an uncommon but important complication that should be promptly identified and treated to avoid forearm/hand ischemia. This complication occurred because of the following reasons:

- Forceful maneuvering of a standard 0.035-inch guidewire through a possibly diseased and tortuous axillary artery probably led to its entry in the subintimal region and was further aggravated by the guide catheter tip.
- The guide catheter tip could have been primarily responsible for the injury and dissection of a tortuous and diseased axillary segment.

LESSONS

- The operator should stop advancing the guidewire or catheter through the upper extremity arterial system during TRA when resistance is encountered.
- Arterial angiography can help identify the problem.
- A 0.014-inch soft-tipped guidewire is useful to reenter the true lumen in dissected arterial segments.
- Even major dissections in the upper extremity arterial system can seal spontaneously at the end of the procedure.

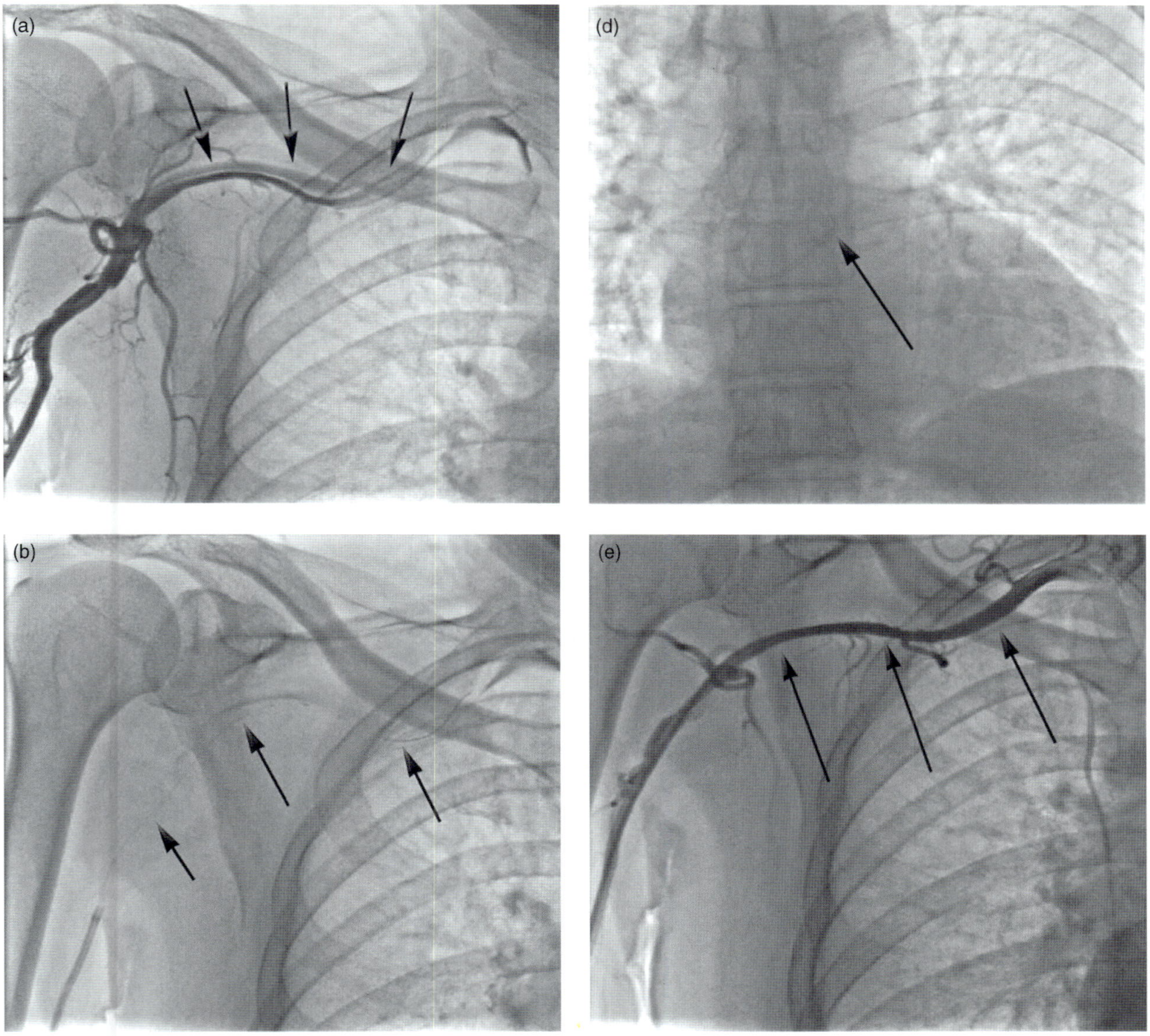

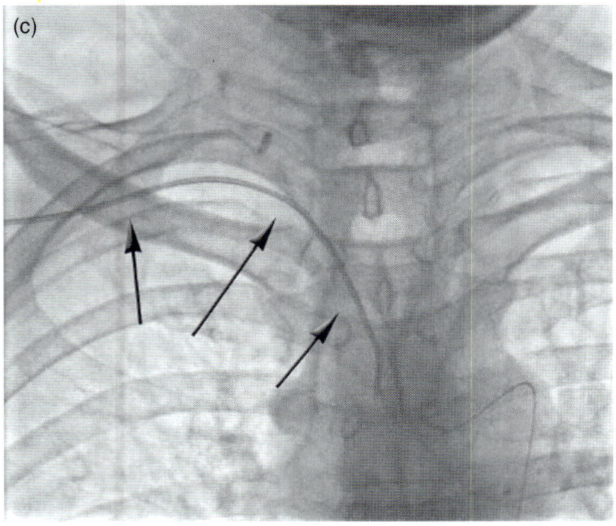

FIGURE 4.3

(a) Major dissection in axillo subclavian region with significant holdup of the contrast. (b) A 0.014-inch BMW PTCA wire found the true lumen. (c) Guide catheter in ascending aorta, (d) LAD stenting done. (e) Sealed dissection and normal blood flow. **(LOOPS 4.3a, b, c, d, e)**

SUGGESTED READING

Patel T, Shah S, Ranjan A. *Patel's Atlas of Transradial Intervention: The Basics*. Seattle, WA: Sea Script Company; 2007.

Gilchrist IC. Transradial technical tips. *Cathet Cardiovasc Interven*. 2000;49(3):353–354.

CASE 4.4

Radial Artery Occlusion

CLINICAL HISTORY AND DIAGNOSTIC TESTING RESULTS

An 82-year-old woman with history of DM, hypertension, and renal insufficiency (GFR was 45 mL/min) was admitted with unstable angina.

PLANNED PROCEDURE

Coronary angiography through a right transradial (TRA).

PROCEDURE

After radial artery puncture, a 5-Fr Radiofocus sheath (Terumo, Japan) was introduced using standard technique. Spasmolytic cocktail was given as per standard protocol. Intravenous unfractionated heparin (5,000 units) was administered. Coronary angiography was performed with a 5-Fr JL3.5 and JR4 catheters, and it demonstrated a 90% eccentric mid-LAD stenosis. PCI was planned as a staged procedure after 72 hours due to renal insufficiency. After sheath removal, a DTR band was applied for 2 hours with successful hemostasis. Upon patient return to the catheterization laboratory 72 hours later, the nurse noted significant reduction in the right radial artery pulse. Barbeau's test revealed RAO. This was confirmed by Doppler evaluation.

COMPLICATION AND MANAGEMENT

When RAO occurs, it can be reaccessed if other access sites are not available. In this case, we reaccessed the occluded radial artery by percutaneous entry into the artery distal to the occlusion (Figure 4.4a) using counterpuncture technique. After arterial access using an 18-gauge needle, a 0.018-inch guidewire was introduced and advanced through the occlusive thrombus (Figure 4.4b). The wire was navigated through the occlusion without resistance, and a 5-Fr introducer sheath was introduced into the radial artery (Figure 4.4c). After removal of the dilator, negative pressure was applied with a 10-cc syringe, and the sheath was gradually pulled back up, leaving the tip 1 to 2 cm into the artery. When blood flow was reestablished through negative pressure suctioning, copious purging of blood was performed until pulsatile flow was reestablished (Figure 4.4d). In cases where blood flow cannot be reestablished by suction and sheath withdrawal, a 0.035-inch guidewire was introduced through the introducer sheath and the sheath was advanced with negative suction and subsequently withdrawn. This maneuver is performed with extreme caution, and it is imperative to not advance the introducer sheath into the proximal radial artery close to the brachial bifurcation. *NO FORWARD INJECTION SHOULD BE PERFORMED UNTIL PULSATILE FLOW IS UNEQUIVOCALLY ESTABLISHED.* We have found the technique described above to be successful in reaccessing the occluded radial artery in 80% of the cases.

CASE ANALYSIS

RAO occurs as a result of thrombosis of the radial artery initiated by intimal injury from sheath insertion and compounded by flow reduction due to presence of the introducer sheath and to the application of hemostatic compression following sheath removal. Technical factors that increase the chances of RAO are large sheath-to-artery ratio, lack of anticoagulation, and prolonged hemostatic compression time. RAO usually presents with asymptomatic absence of radial pulse at the site of previous arterial entry. Occasionally, it causes pain in the forearm, which is believed to be caused by thrombus-related inflammatory reaction. The presence of superficial and deep palmar arches that provide a macrocollateral circuit and a network of microvascular collaterals at the level of the interosseus membrane helps reduce the chances of hand ischemia. However, hand ischemia has been reported after radial artery occlusion in the presence of unknown ulnar artery occlusion.

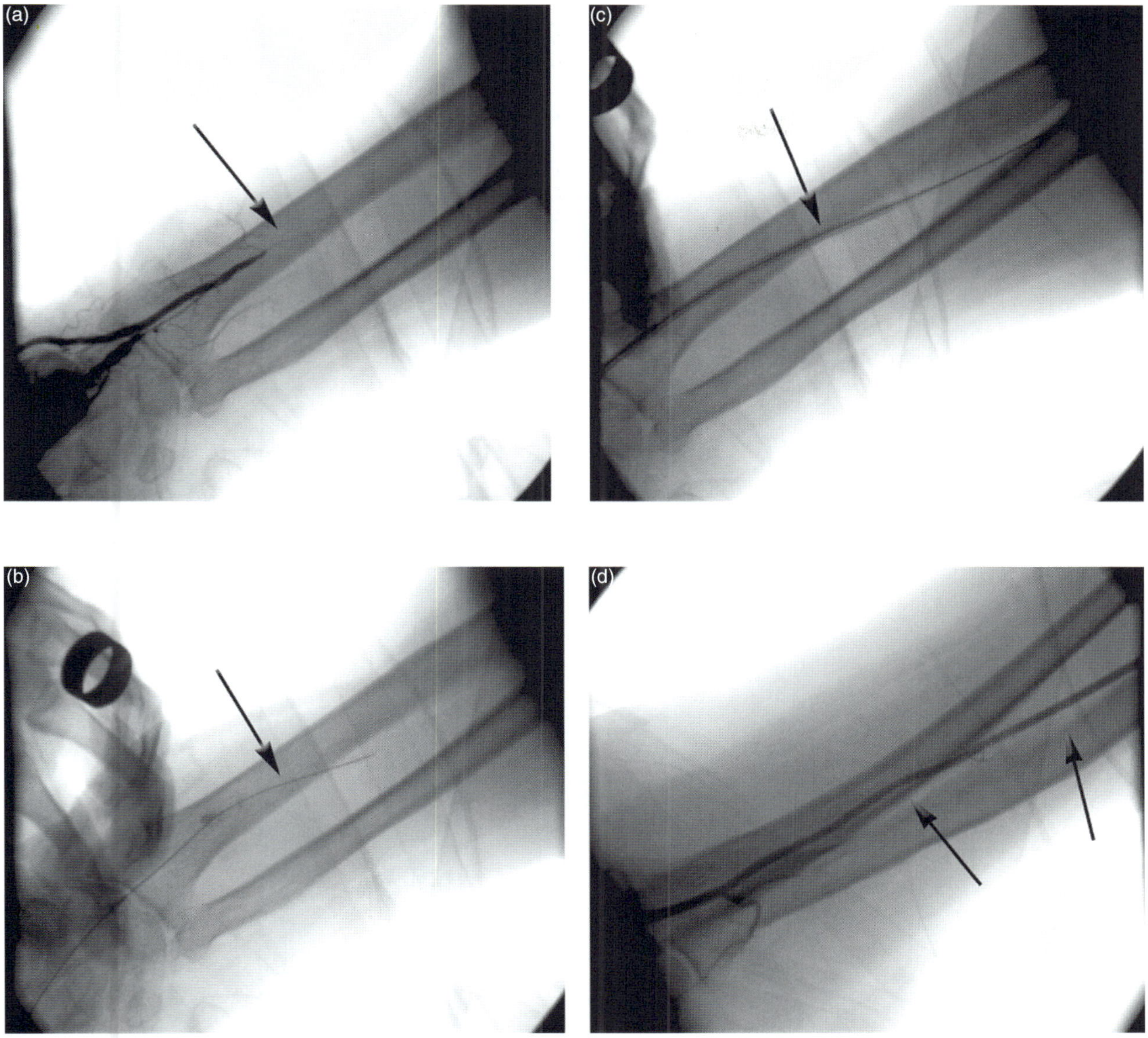

FIGURE 4.4

(a) Occluded radial artery, (b) a 0.018-inch guidewire successfully crossed the occlusion, (c) a 5-Fr introducer sheath negotiated, and (d) occlusion opened up and patency established.

LESSONS

- The incidence of RAO can be significantly reduced by heparinization.
- Maintaining radial artery patency during hemostatic compression is independently effective in reducing RAO. Maintenance of flow is the best prophylaxis against thrombotic occlusion.
- Often, no invasive treatment is required for RAO. As mentioned earlier, this condition is almost always asymptomatic in properly selected patients. In patients with forearm pain, local warm compresses or analgesics may be prescribed. The risk of attempted recanalization grossly outweighs the benefits, and hence instrumentation to relieve occlusion in the absence of limb threatening ischemia is contraindicated.

SUGGESTED READING

Saito S, Ikei H, Hosokawa G, et al. Influence of the ratio between radial artery inner diameter and sheath outer diameter on radial artery flow after transradial coronary intervention. *Catheter Cardiovasc Interv.* 1999;46(2):173–178.

Spaulding C, Lefèvre T, Funck F, et al. Left radial approach for coronary angiography: results of a prospective study. *Cathet Cardiovasc Diagn.* 1996;39(4):365–370.

Pancholy SB. Comparison of the effect of intra-arterial versus intravenous heparin on radial artery occlusion after transradial catheterization. *Am J Cardiol.* 2009;104(8):1083–1085.

Pancholy S, Coppola J, Patel T, et al. Prevention of radial artery occlusion-patent hemostasis evaluation trial (PROPHET study): A randomized comparison of traditional versus patency documented hemostasis after transradial catheterization. *Catheter Cardiovasc Interv.* 2008;72(3):335–340.

Pancholy SB. Transradial access in an occluded radial artery: new technique. *J Invasive Cardiol.* 2007;19(12):541–544.

Stella PR, Kiemeneij F, Laarman GJ, et al. Incidence and outcome of radial artery occlusion following transradial artery coronary angioplasty. *Cathet Cardiovasc Diagn.* 1997;40(2):156–158.

Rhyne D, Mann T. Hand ischemia resulting from a transradial intervention: successful management with radial artery angioplasty. *Catheter Cardiovasc Interv.* 2010;76(3):383–386.

CASE 4.5

Radial Puncture Site–Related Complications

Case 4.5a—*Radial Artery Pseudoaneurysm*

CLINICAL HISTORY AND DIAGNOSTIC TESTING RESULTS

A 79-year-old woman with history of DM and multiple cardiovascular risk factors admitted with unstable angina and angiographically documented multivessel CAD.

PLANNED PROCEDURE

PCI through right TRA.

PROCEDURE

Patient underwent successful multivessel stenting through the right TRA. She was discharged the next day without complications. The patient returned to the hospital 15 days postprocedure with a complaint of painless swelling at the radial puncture site with no tenderness on palpation (Figure 4.5a). Clinical examination was consistent with diagnosis of a PA, which was also confirmed by Doppler ultrasound examination.

COMPLICATION AND MANAGEMENT

Radial artery PA is a rare complication of TRA. In this patient, ultrasound-guided compression was successful in leading to PA regression. Physical examination and vascular Doppler examination at 3- and 6-month follow-up revealed normal radial pulse. In cases where ultrasound-guided compression is not effective, surgery would be required. Typically, a radial artery PA can be repaired using a small incision under local anesthesia in an outpatient setting. In our experience, two of six cases of radial artery PAs required surgical intervention.

Case 4.5b—*Depigmented Scar at Radial Puncture Site*

CLINICAL HISTORY AND DIAGNOSTIC TESTING RESULTS

A 52-year-old woman had a history of multiple cardiovascular risk factors, reversible inferior ischemia on stress testing, and known severe stenosis on the RCA.

PLANNED PROCEDURE

PCI of the RCA lesion via right TRA.

PROCEDURE

PCI of the RCA was performed through the right TRA using standard technique. The radial sheath was removed immediately postprocedure, and a TR Band (Terumo, Japan) was applied to attain hemostasis. The band was removed with complete hemostasis. The patient was discharged the second day without any complications.

COMPLICATION AND MANAGEMENT

At 1-month follow-up, a depigmented scar was noted over the radial puncture site (Figure 4.5b).

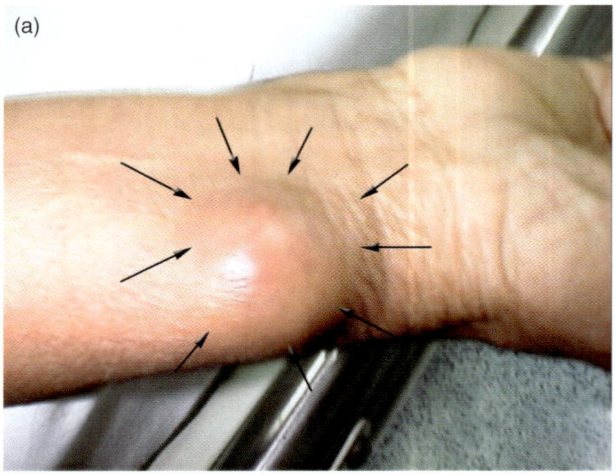

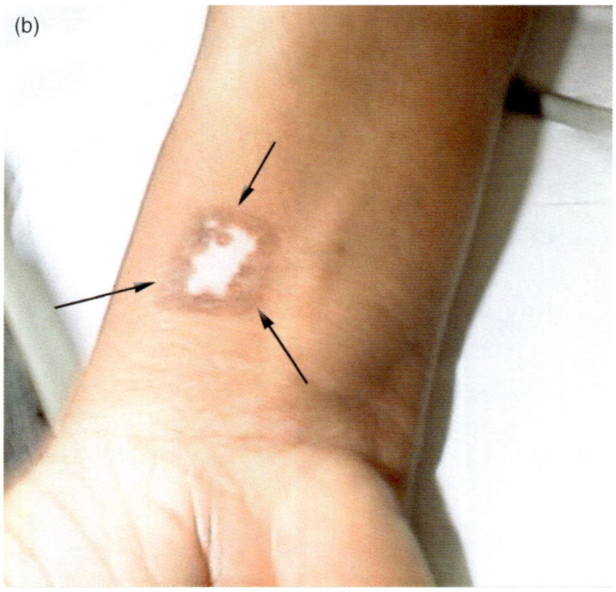

FIGURE 4.5
(a) Pseudoaneurysm at radial puncture site and (b) depigmented scar at radial puncture site.

CASE ANALYSIS

Our standard practice after transradial PCI is to remove the introducer sheath immediately and apply a TR Band. This device has an inflatable cuff, which is filled with 13 to 17 cc of air to create occlusive pressure at the puncture site. Usually, we remove this device after 3 to 4 hours and place a wrist bandage.

If the pressure is significantly higher than required, it may lead to pressure necrosis at the site and subsequent formation of a depigmented scar. Implementing a patency-documented hemostasis technique is the best approach to avoid this complication.

SUGGESTED READING

Patel T, Shah S, Ranjan A. *Patel's Atlas of Transradial Intervention: The Basics*. Seattle, WA: Sea Script Company; 2007.

Pancholy S, Coppola J, Patel T, et al. Prevention of radial artery occlusion-patent hemostasis evaluation trial (PROPHET Study): A randomized comparison of traditional versus patency documented hemostasis after transradial catheterization. *Cathet Cardiovasc Interv*. 2008;72(3):335–340.

5

Giora Weisz and Jeffrey W. Moses

Complications of Coronary PCI: An Overview

INTRODUCTION

Major complications of percutaneous coronary intervention (PCI) have become infrequent because of increased operator experience and tremendous evolution in technology and technique. However, complications still occur, and they contribute significantly to the morbidity and mortality of patients undergoing PCI. Complications after PCI can be categorized into cardiac or noncardiac, early or late, minor or major, and transient or permanent (Table 5.1). Complications that are managed medically (arrhythmias, nonaccess site bleeding, contrast-induced nephropathy, allergies, radiation exposure, etc.) are beyond the scope of this atlas. In this chapter, we will present several case scenarios of complications during PCI of undilatable lesions, bifurcation lesions, unprotected left main coronary artery (LMCA), and diffuse disease. The ensuing chapters will focus on coronary perforations, slow or no reflow, trapped devices in the coronary tree, and stent thrombosis.

TABLE 5.1
Complications Associated With PCI.

Cardiac Complications
Coronary
Perforation
Slow/no reflow
Device entrapment/embolization
Stent thrombosis
Arrhythmias
Tachyarrhythmias
Bradyarrhythmias
Noncardiac Complications
Contrast-induced nephropathy
Access site complications
Hematoma
Retroperitoneal bleeding
Femoral-iliac artery dissection
Pseudoaneurysm
Arteriovenous fistulae
Infection
Nonaccess site–related bleeding
Cerebrovascular events
Thrombocytopenia
Cholesterol embolism
Allergic reactions
Radiation injury

CASE 5.1

Coronary Perforation Caused by Inflating an Oversized Balloon in a Previously Implanted Stent

CLINICAL HISTORY AND DIAGNOSTIC TESTING RESULTS

A 59-year-old woman had a history of type 2 diabetes mellitus, hypertension, hypercholesterolemia, and coronary artery disease (CAD) and with prior drug-eluting stent implantation in the middle and distal left anterior descending artery (LAD). Four months earlier, she was admitted to another hospital and later to us with chest pain and ST segment elevation in leads V3–V5 and was hemodynamically stable. Patient reported compliance with her daily aspirin and clopidogrel. The patient was started on bivalirudin in the emergency room and referred for immediate coronary angiography. Coronary angiography revealed patent right coronary artery (RCA) (Figure 5.1, Loop 5.1) and left circumflex artery (LCX) (Figure 5.2, Loop 5.2) and thrombotic occlusion of the distal-LAD at a previous stent site (Figure 5.3, Loop 5.3). Left ventriculogram showed mild left ventricular (LV) dysfunction with anteroapical hypokinesis.

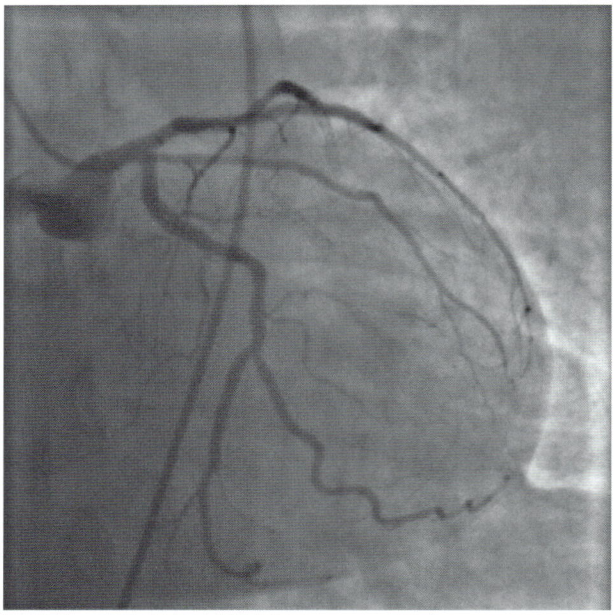

FIGURE 5.2

Patent LCX with luminal irregularities. **(LOOP 5.2)**

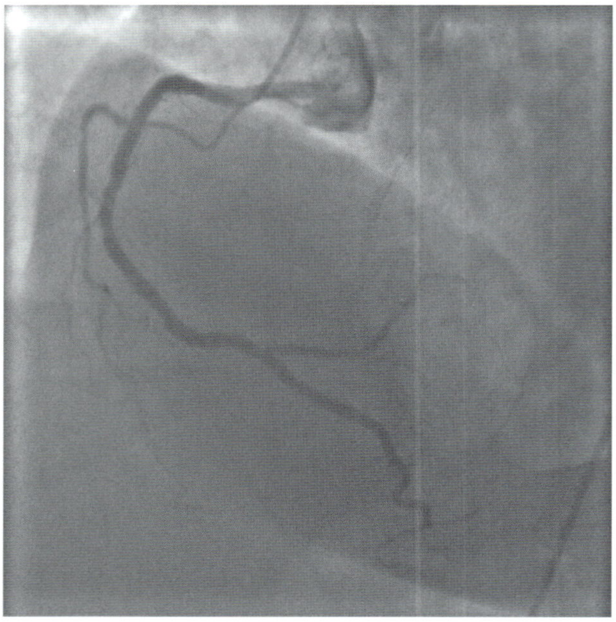

FIGURE 5.1

Patent RCA with luminal irregularities. **(LOOP 5.1)**

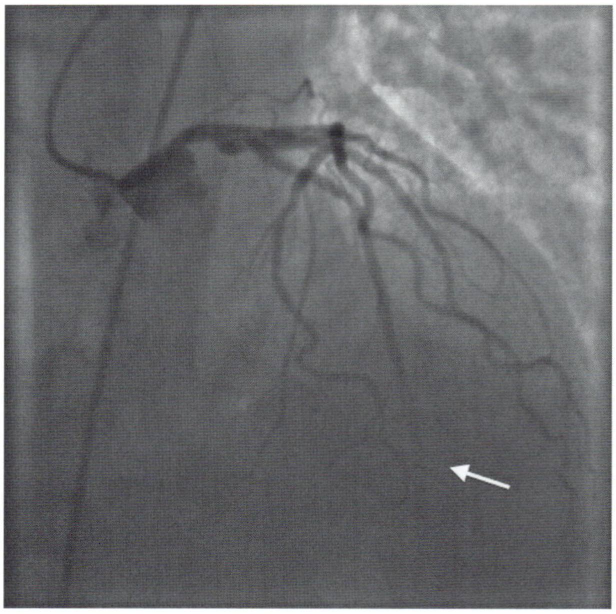

FIGURE 5.3

Thrombotic occlusion in a previously implanted stent in the distal segment of the LAD (white arrow). **(LOOP 5.3)**

PLANNED PROCEDURE

PCI to mid-LAD.

PROCEDURE

An intravenous (IV) bolus and infusion of abciximab was initiated. After the diagnostic catheter was exchanged for a guiding catheter, a 0.014 soft coronary wire was advanced to the LAD across the thrombotic lesion without resistance. Aspiration thrombectomy and dilatation with a 2.0 x 15 mm balloon led to establishment of flow in the LAD (Figure 5.4, Loop 5.4). Intravascular ultrasound (IVUS) interrogation demonstrated stent under expansion (minimal luminal diameter was 1.6 mm, cross-sectional luminal area was 2.5 mm^2), with an adherent thrombus and a vessel diameter of 2.7 mm. The stent was redilated with a 2.5-mm high-pressure balloon, which appeared underexpanded at its center (Figure 5.5). Repeat IVUS interrogation demonstrated only minimal increase in lumen cross-sectional area to 3.0 mm^2. Subsequently, a 2.75-mm high-pressure balloon was inflated within the stent up to 20 atm, resulting in better balloon expansion (Figure 5.6).

COMPLICATION AND MANAGEMENT

Coronary angiography after balloon deflation showed free-flow perforation at the distal part of the stent (Figure 5.7, Loop 5.7). The balloon was immediately reinflated at low pressure at the perforation site, and bivalirudin and abciximab were discontinued. The

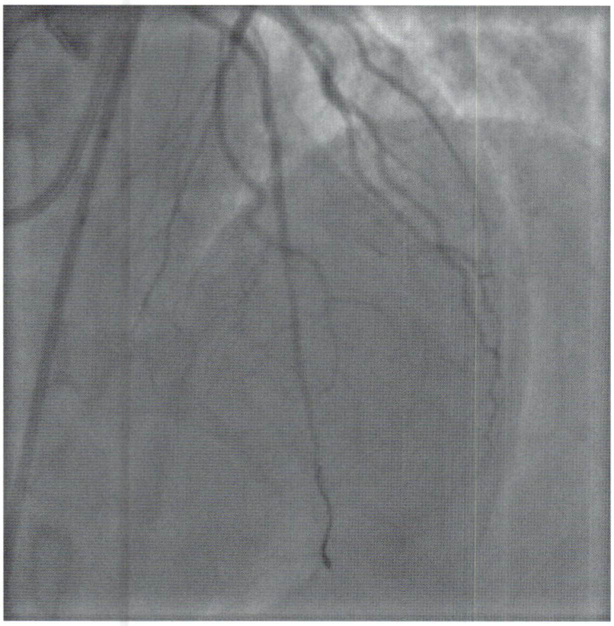

FIGURE 5.4

Coronary angiography after aspiration thrombectomy and balloon dilatation (2 × 15 mm). Note reestablishment of flow in the LAD. **(LOOP 5.4)**

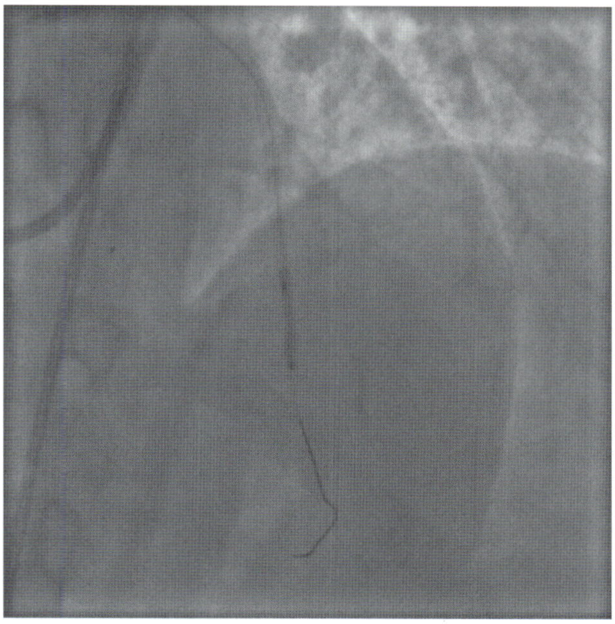

FIGURE 5.5

Stent redilation with a 2.5-mm high-pressure balloon. This step was performed in response to IVUS findings of an underexpanded stent and a vessel diameter of 2.7 mm.

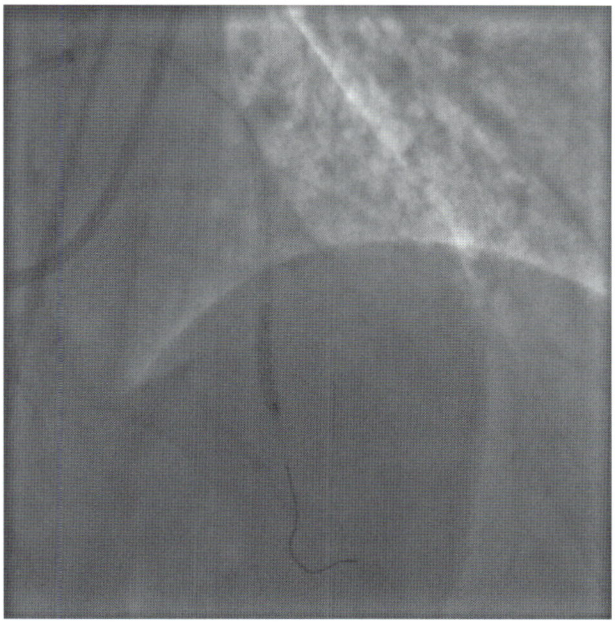

FIGURE 5.6

Stent redilation with a 2.75-mm high-pressure balloon inflated up to 20 atm. This inflation was performed in response to the IVUS findings of continued stent under expansion after the use of the 2.5-mm balloon.

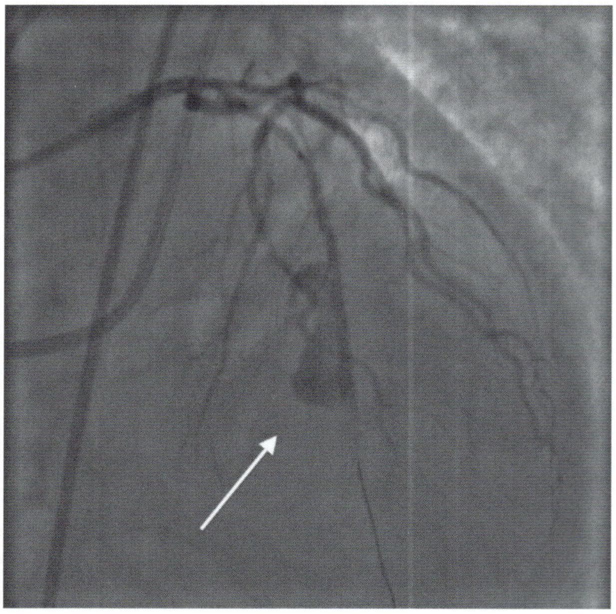

FIGURE 5.7

Coronary angiography after balloon deflation demonstrated free-flow perforation at the distal part of the stent (white arrow). (LOOP 5.7)

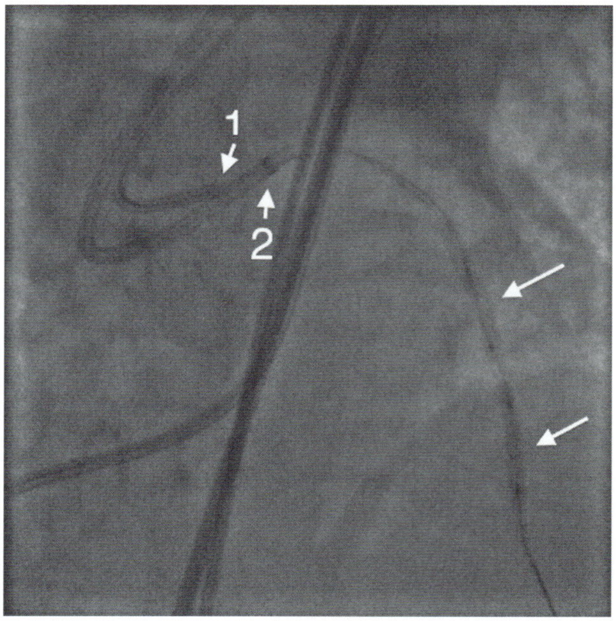

FIGURE 5.8

This figure demonstrates the dual catheter technique. While a balloon is inflated, the guide catheter is slightly withdrawn from the coronary ostium (short arrow 1), and a second 8-Fr guiding catheter is advanced from the contralateral femoral artery to engage the left coronary artery (short arrow 2). A second 0.014-inch coronary wire was used to cannulate the proximal segment of the LAD through the second guide and a coronary PTFE-covered stent was advanced over this wire and positioned proximal to the sealing balloon (long arrows).

balloon was kept inflated for 15 minutes, during which the patient had recurrent chest pain and ST segment elevation in the anterior leads. Prolonged balloon inflation failed to seal the perforation. The operator proceeded to implement the dual-catheter technique. While the balloon was inflated, the guide catheter was slightly withdrawn from the coronary ostium and a second 8-Fr guiding catheter was advanced from the contralateral femoral artery (Figure 5.8). A second 0.014-inch coronary wire was used to cannulate the proximal segment of the LAD through the second guide, and a coronary polytetrafluoroethylene (PTFE)-covered stent (3 × 12 mm—the smallest diameter available in the United States) was advanced over this wire and positioned proximal to the inflated balloon. Then the balloon was deflated and withdrawn proximally with its wire to allow for the passage of the second wire, leading the covered stent to the perforation site where it was deployed. However, the perforation was not sealed despite using high inflation pressure (18 atm) to deploy the covered stent (Figure 5.9, Loop 5.9). A second identical PTFE-covered stent was deployed inside the first stent and expanded up to 22 atm. Poststent deployment, coronary angiography demonstrated successful sealing of the perforation (Figure 5.10, Loop 5.10). However, a proximal LMCA dissection was noted, probably as a result of aggressive guide catheter manipulation, while advancing the covered stent. The LMCA dissection was promptly sealed with a 3.5- × 8-mm sirolimus-eluting stent and postdilated with a short 4.0-mm balloon. Final angiography showed thrombolysis in myocardial infarction grade 3 (TIMI-3) flow with patent LMCA and LAD (Figures 5.11 and 5.12, Loops 5.11 and 5.12). The patient remained stable throughout the procedure. Bedside echocardiography showed only a small amount of pericardial effusion. At 1-year follow-up, the patient was asymptomatic, with good functional capacity and nonischemic stress test.

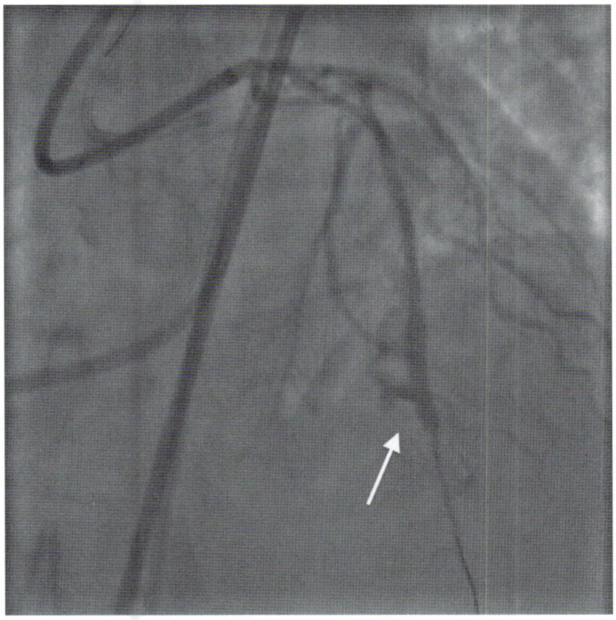

FIGURE 5.9

The sealing balloon was deflated and withdrawn proximally with its wire to allow passage of the second wire leading the PTFE-covered stent to the perforation site where it was deployed. Despite using high inflation pressure (18 atm) to deploy the covered stent, the perforation was not completely sealed (arrow). **(LOOP 5.9)**

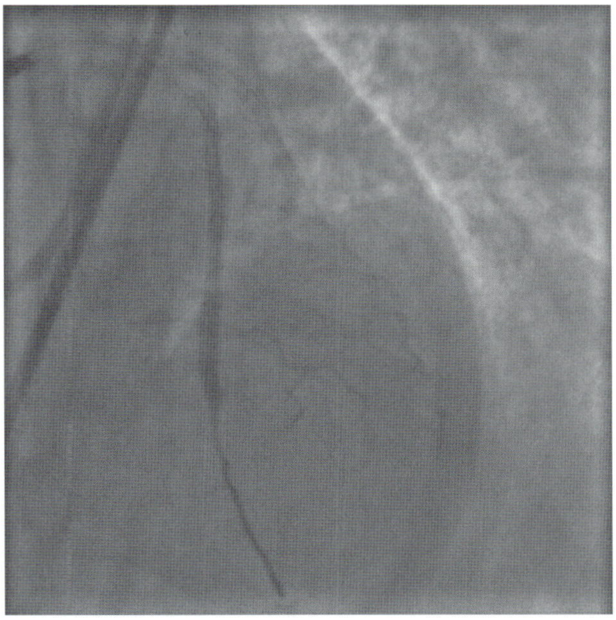

FIGURE 5.10

A second identical PTFE-covered stent was placed inside the first one and expanded up to 22 atm. This led to successful sealing of the perforation, but aggressive guide engagement led to LMCA dissection. **(LOOP 5.10)**

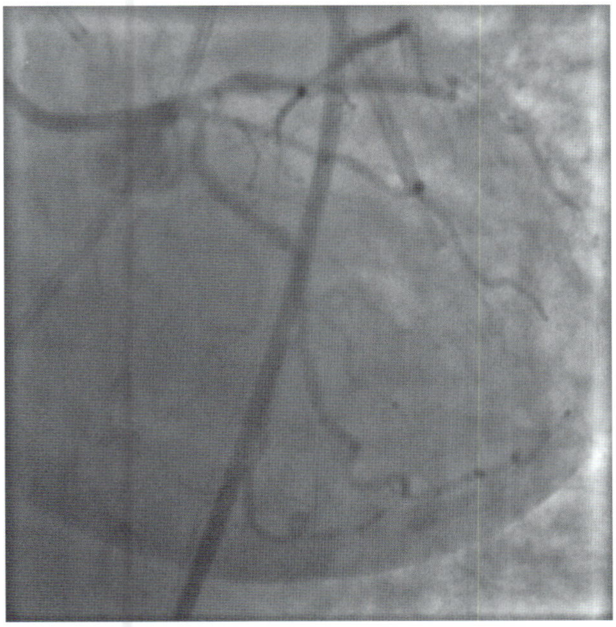

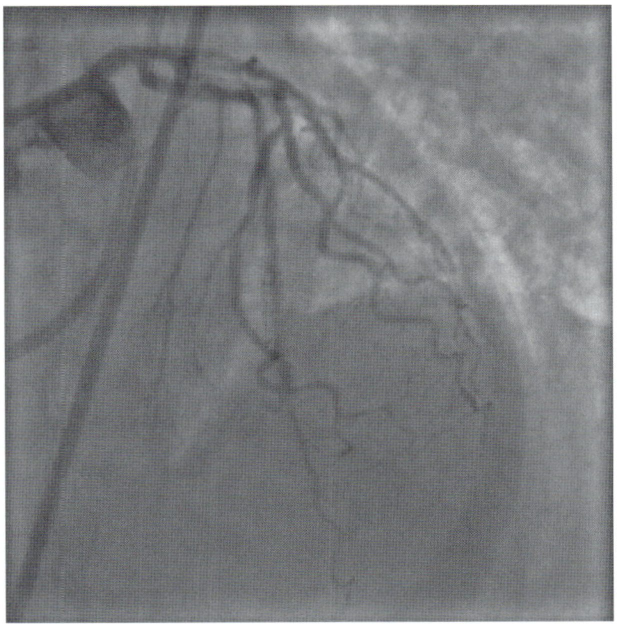

FIGURES 5.11 AND 5.12

Final coronary angiography after LMCA stenting with a 3.5- × 8-mm sirolimus-eluting stent (postdilated with 4-mm balloon) demonstrated TIMI-3 flow with patent LMCA and LAD. **(LOOPS 5.11 AND 5.12)**

CASE ANALYSIS

The perforation in this case occurred as a result of using an oversized balloon (2.75-mm balloon in a 2.7-mm vessel) to dilate an underexpanded stent. Although there is a belief that using an oversized balloon inside a previously deployed stent is safe, this case tells a different story. Expanding a previously implanted underexpanded stent to a more desirable diameter is often challenging because, typically, the underlying plaque is either severely fibrotic or calcified. When faced with a previously implanted underexpanded stent, it is safer to use a balloon that is smaller than the media-to-media diameter (in this case, a 2.5-mm balloon) and inflated to very high pressure. In cases where this technique fails, some operators have reported on the effective use of laser energy at the site of under expansion followed by high-pressure balloon inflation.

Once a coronary perforation has occurred, prompt management is critical. Immediate reinflation of the balloon at the perforation site, reversal of anticoagulation, and utilizing a dual-guide catheter technique to deliver covered stents were very effective in limiting the clinical sequelae of this event.

LESSONS

- When attempting to expand a previously implanted underexpanded stent, never use a balloon larger than the media-to-media diameter. Alternatively, use an undersized noncompliant balloon inflated at very high pressure. After deflating the balloon, always perform angiography before removing the balloon to ensure absence of perforation.
- Once a perforation has occurred, the dual-guide catheter technique is an effective strategy to deliver covered stents because it allows for continuous hemostasis at the perforation site until the stent is delivered proximal to the perforated segment.

SUGGESTED READING

Ben-Gal Y, Weisz G, Collins MB, et al. Dual catheter technique for the treatment of severe coronary artery perforations. *Catheter Cardiovasc Interv.* 2010;75:708–712.

Ellis SG, Ajluni S, Arnold AZ. Increased coronary perforation in the new device era. Incidence, classification, management, and outcome. *Circulation.* 1994;90:2725–2730.

Lansky AJ, Yang YM, Khan Y, et al. Treatment of coronary artery perforations complicating percutaneous coronary intervention with a polytetrafluoroethylene-covered stent graft. *Am J Cardiol.* 2006;98:370–374.

Noble S, Bilodeau L. High energy excimer laser to treat coronary in-stent restenosis in an underexpanded stent. *Catheter Cardiovasc Interv.* 2008;71(6):803–807.

CASE 5.2

Wire-Induced Coronary Perforation During PCI of a Bifurcation Lesion

CLINICAL HISTORY AND DIAGNOSTIC TESTING RESULTS

A 71-year-old man with a history of hypertension, hyperlipidemia, and CAD, and with complaints of severe exertional angina pectoris despite maximal medical therapy was referred for coronary angiography. Coronary angiography showed double-vessel disease involving the mid-LAD-diagonal bifurcation (Medina class 1,1,1) and the obtuse marginal (OM) branch (Figures 5.13 and 5.14, Loops 5.13 and 5.14).

PLANNED PROCEDURE

PCI of the mid-LAD bifurcation lesion.

PROCEDURE

Patient received aspirin and clopidogrel prior to intervention, and IV bivalirudin was initiated at the outset of the procedure. A 7-Fr broad-transition guide catheter was positioned at the ostium of the left coronary artery, and two soft-tip coronary wires were advanced to the LAD and the diagonal branch (Figure 5.15, Loop 5.15). After balloon predilatation of the LAD and the diagonal branch, the bifurcation was treated with two paclitaxel-eluting stents, using the mini-crash technique, resulting in good angiographic result (Figures 5.16 and 5.17, Loops 5.16 and 5.17). Subsequently, the operator had difficulty in rewiring the diagonal branch but was eventually able to do so using a hydrophilic wire. After successful PCI of the LAD-diagonal bifurcation, a stent was implanted in the OM branch (Figure 5.18, Loop 5.18). The patient was asymptomatic and hemodynamically stable at the end of the procedure.

COMPLICATION AND MANAGEMENT

Three hours after the end of the procedure, the patient complained of weakness and diaphoresis. His heart rate was 112 beats per minute and blood pressure was 65/30 mmHg. His jugular veins were distended. Bedside echocardiogram demonstrated a moderate amount of pericardial effusion with right atrial and ventricular collapse. The patient was transferred back to the catheterization laboratory, where pericardiocentesis was performed (350 mL of blood was drained, with immediate stabilization of the patient) and a pigtail catheter placed in the pericardial space. Repeat coronary angiography demonstrated a pericardial stain in the anterior-lateral wall (Figure 5.19, Loop 5.19). The stain did not enlarge with additional contrast injections and appeared to be stable. The pericardial catheter was left in place overnight without any additional bleeding into the pericardium.

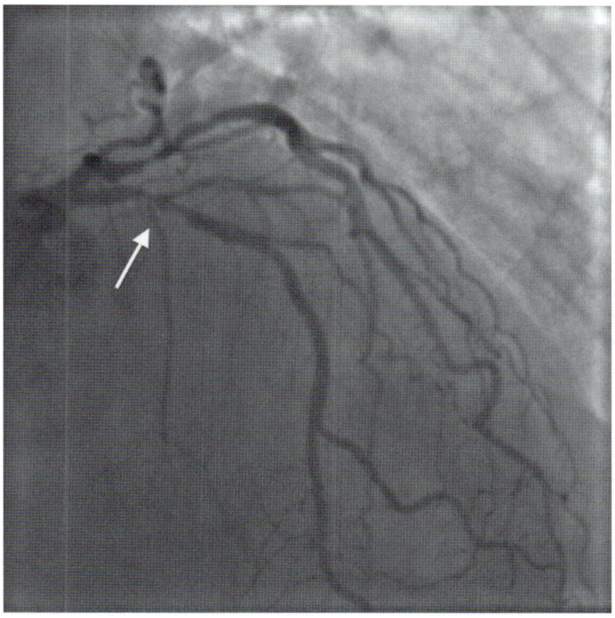

FIGURE 5.13

Anteroposterior (AP) cranial view. LAD-diagonal bifurcation disease (Medina class 1,1,1) (white arrow). (LOOP 5.13)

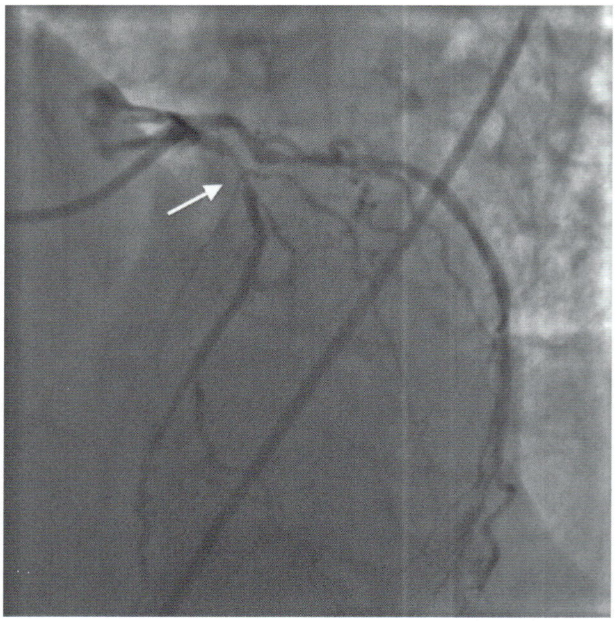

FIGURE 5.14

Left anterior oblique cranial view. LAD-diagonal bifurcation disease (Medina class 1,1,1) (white arrow). (LOOP 5.14)

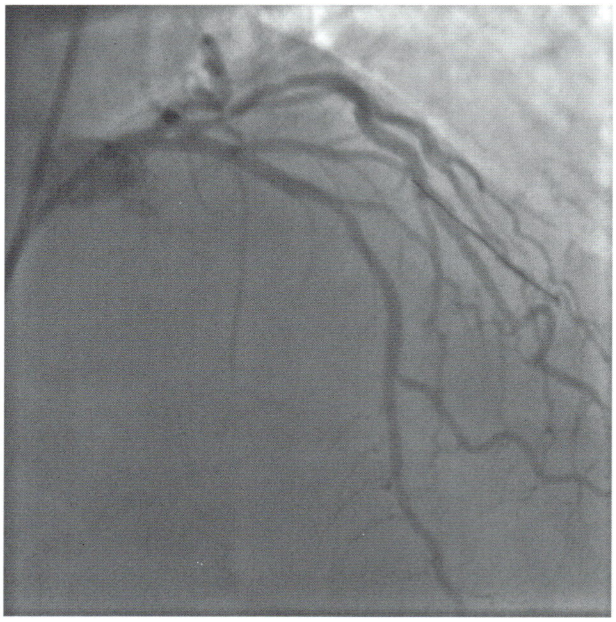

FIGURE 5.16

Anteroposterior (AP) cranial view. Coronary angiography after stents deployment in the LAD-diagonal bifurcation using the mini-crush technique. (LOOP 5.16)

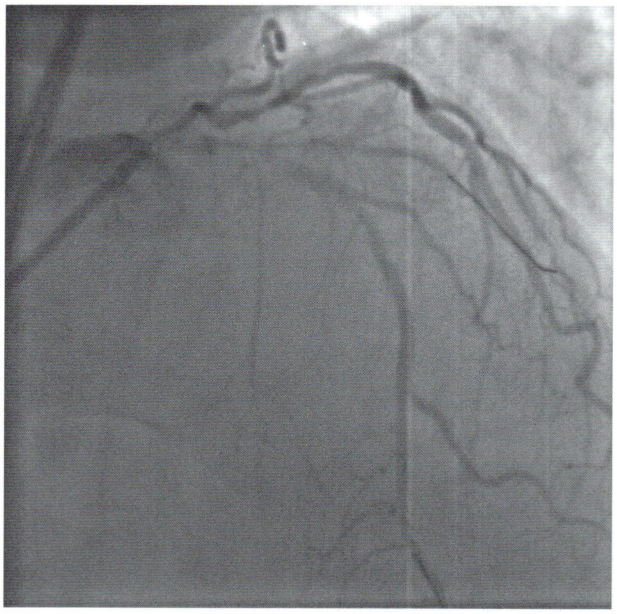

FIGURE 5.15

Soft-tip, 0.014-inch coronary wires in the LAD and diagonal branch. (LOOP 5.15)

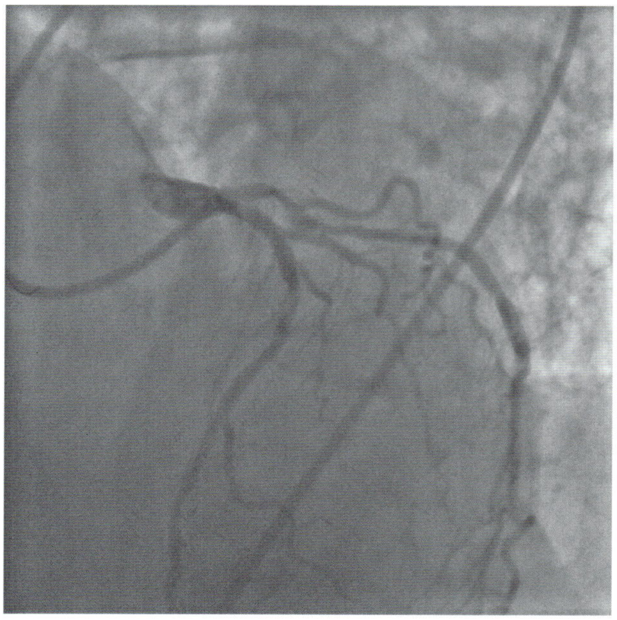

FIGURE 5.17

Left anterior oblique cranial view. Coronary angiography after stents deployment in the LAD-diagonal bifurcation using the mini-crush technique. (LOOP 5.17)

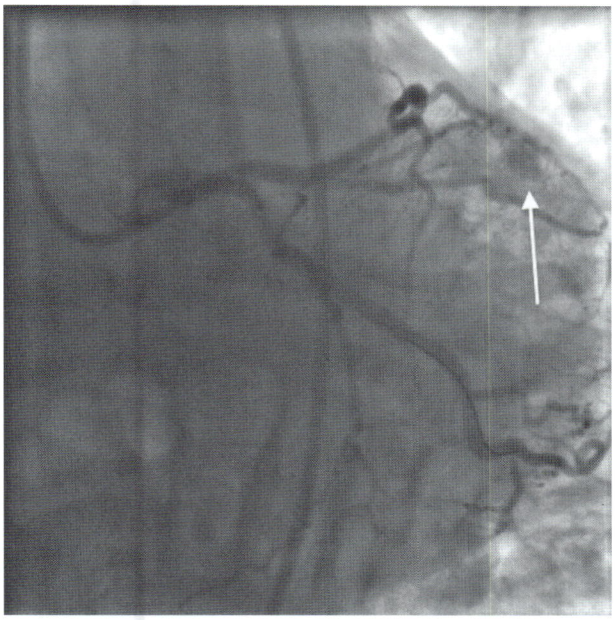

FIGURE 5.18

Anteroposterior (AP) caudal view. Coronary angiography after stent deployment in the mid-LCX and OM branch. Note a small localized contrast staining in the lateral wall (white arrow). **(LOOP 5.18)**

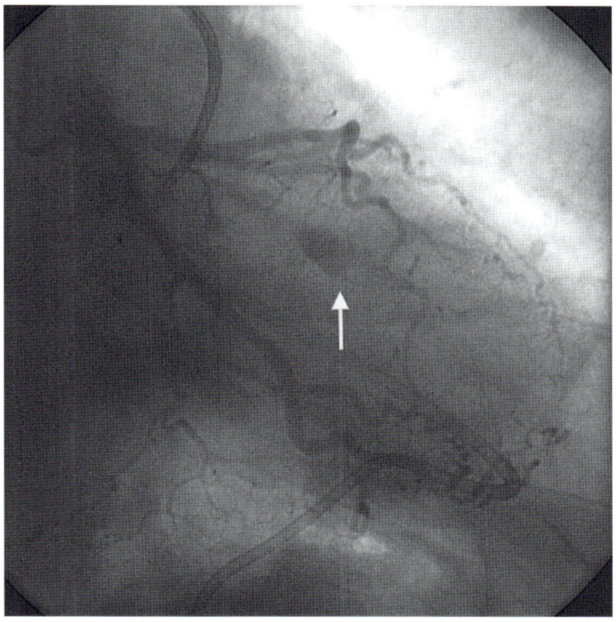

FIGURE 5.19

Right anterior oblique (RAO) caudal view. Repeat coronary angiography after pericardial drainage demonstrating a pericardial stain in the anterior-lateral wall (white arrow). **(LOOP 5.19)**

CASE ANALYSIS

This case illustrates a wire-induced perforation during coronary intervention. Although the perforation was not identified during the procedure, a retrospective evaluation of the angiogram after the OM stent placement did reveal a small localized staining (Figure 5.18, Loop 5.18). The operator overlooked the staining in the remote LAD-diagonal territory while concentrating on the OM stent segment. Clearly, the perforation was small and the accumulation of blood in the pericardium was relatively slow.

Most likely, the perforation was caused by the hydrophilic wire that was used to rewire the diagonal branch during the mini-crush procedure. Hydrophilic wires glide easily into small terminal branches during routine maneuvers if they are not controlled and visualized well at all times. Premature ventricular beats may be the first sign of wire perforation. In general, hydrophilic wires should not be the first choice to canalize nonocclusive stenoses. However, when they are required, they should be exchanged for a nonhydrophilic soft-tip wire. If wire exchange is not possible, the operator should always keep the distal tip of the wire in the field of view and be cognizant of its whereabouts.

LESSONS

- When using hydrophilic guidewires, the operator should always keep the distal tip of the wire in the field of view and be cognizant of its whereabouts at all procedure stages.
- It is good practice to "always" deliberately look for evidence of wire perforation at the end of any PCI procedure because these perforations can be easily missed.
- In patients who have hemodynamic compromise hours after PCI, cardiac tamponade (from wire perforation) should always be suspected as well as stent thrombosis and vascular bleeding.

SUGGESTED READING

Wong CM, Mak GY, Chung DTW. Distal coronary artery perforation resulting from the use of hydrophilic coated guidewire in tortuous vessels. *Cathet Cardiovasc Diag.* 1998;44:93–96.

Gruberg L, Pinnow E, Flood R, et al. Incidence, management, and outcome of coronary artery perforation during percutaneous coronary intervention. *Am J Cardiol.* 2000;86:680–682.

CASE 5.3

Simultaneous Subacute Stent Thrombosis in Two Coronary Arteries

CLINICAL HISTORY AND DIAGNOSTIC TESTING RESULTS

A 55-year-old man with history of hyperlipidemia and smoking was admitted to the hospital with progressive effort angina. Nuclear stress test showed reversible perfusion defects at the anterior, anterior-lateral, and inferior walls. Coronary angiography revealed triple-vessel disease (Figures 5.20, 5.21, and 5.22; Loops 5.20, 5.21, and 5.22) and normal LV function. The benefits and risks of coronary artery bypass grafting (CABG) versus PCI were discussed, and the patient elected to undergo PCI.

PLANNED PROCEDURE

Triple-vessel PCI with drug-eluting stents.

PROCEDURE

Initially, stent implantation was performed in the OM branch (2.5-mm × 8-mm paclitaxel-eluting stent). A second stent was necessary to cover a proximal edge dissection (Figures 5.23 and 5.24, Loops 5.23 and 5.24). The LAD lesions were predilatated with a

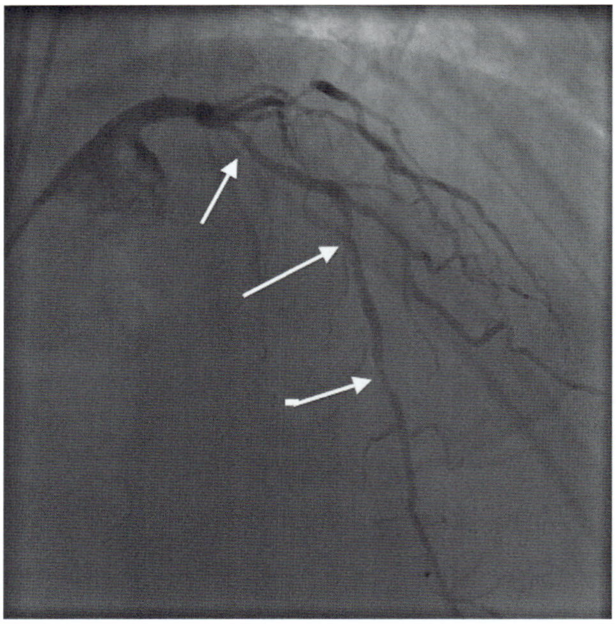

FIGURE 5.21

Anteroposterior (AP) cranial view. Coronary angiography shows multiple sequential lesions in the proximal and mid-LAD (white arrows). **(LOOP 5.21)**

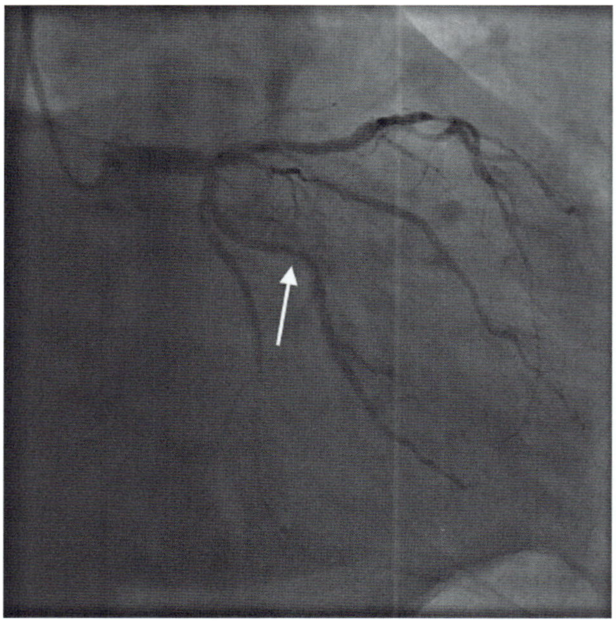

FIGURE 5.20

Right anterior oblique (RAO) caudal view. Coronary angiography shows focal stenosis in the OM branch of the LCX (white arrow). **(LOOP 5.20)**

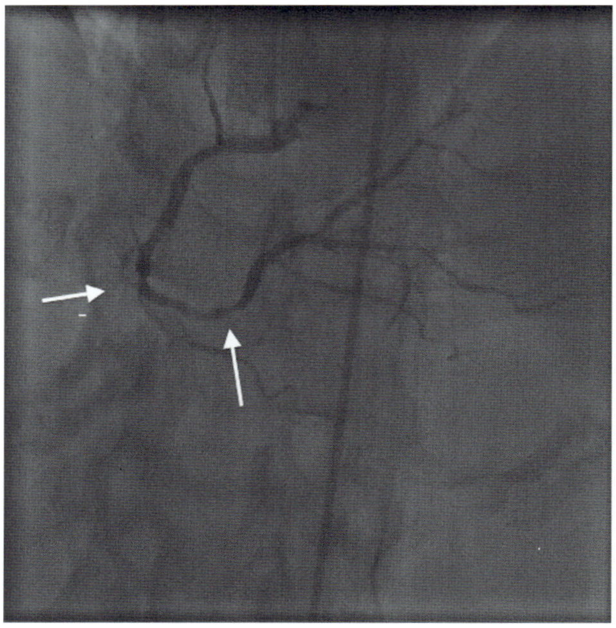

FIGURE 5.22

Anteroposterior (AP) cranial view. Coronary angiography shows tandem lesions in the distal RCA (white arrows). **(LOOP 5.22)**

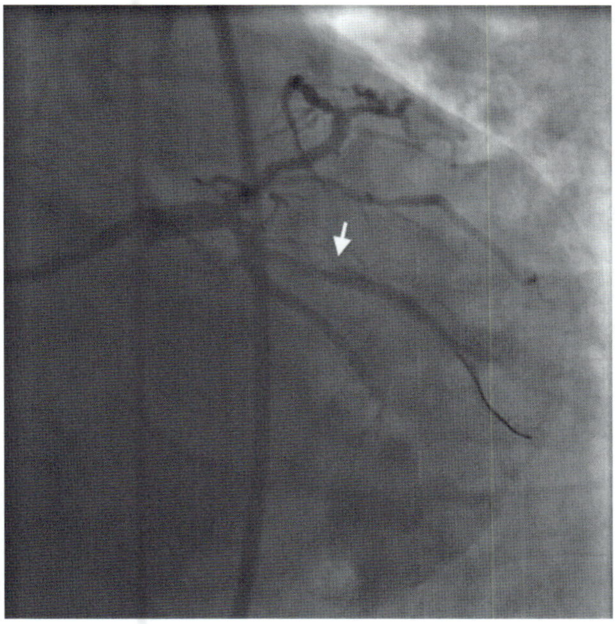

FIGURE 5.23

Residual proximal dissection after stent implantation in the OM branch (white arrow). (LOOP 5.23)

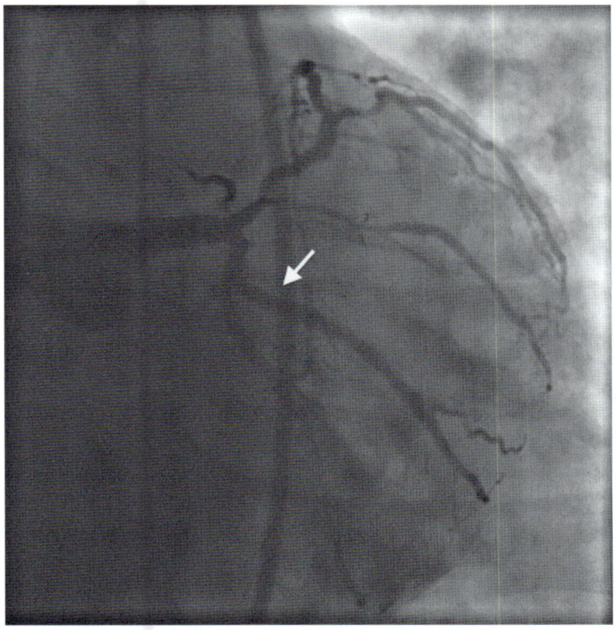

FIGURE 5.24

Coronary angiography (left anterior oblique caudal projection) after stent placement (2.5 × 8 mm) to seal the proximal edge dissection. (LOOP 5.24)

2.5-mm balloon and 3 paclitaxel-eluting stents (2.5 × 16 mm and two 3.0 × 16 mm). They were successfully deployed to cover the diffusely diseased segment with good final results, except for compromise of the diagonal branch (Figure 5.25, Loop 5.25). No intervention

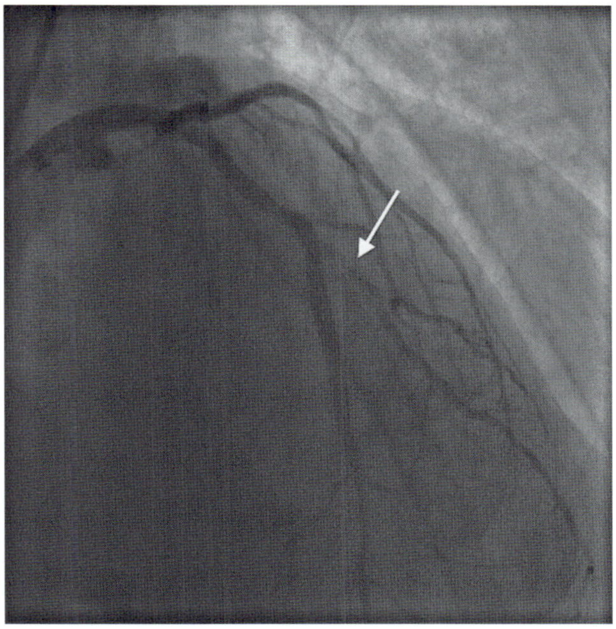

FIGURE 5.25

Coronary angiography (right anterior oblique (RAO) cranial projection) after multiple stent implantation in the mid-LAD. Note the narrowing in the ostium of the diagonal branch (white arrow). (LOOP 5.25)

was performed on the diagonal branch, because the patient was asymptomatic and without ischemic electrocardiogram (ECG) changes. The RCA intervention was deferred and planned as a staged procedure. The patient was discharged home the next day with instructions for dual antiplatelet therapy.

COMPLICATION AND MANAGEMENT

The patient was presented to the emergency department 6 days later with severe chest pain, hypotension (blood pressure = 80/60 mmHg), and extensive anterolateral ST segment elevation. The patient reported that he had been taking clopidogrel since discharge but not aspirin. The patient was brought immediately to the catheterization laboratory for resuscitation with fluids and vasopressors ongoing. Coronary angiography revealed thrombotic occlusions of the LAD and the OM (Figure 5.26, Loop 5.26). IV unfractionated heparin and abciximab were administered. Both the LAD and OM were wired and aspiration thrombectomy was performed, recovering a large amount of thrombus and restoring flow (Figure 5.27, Loop 5.27). Thrombolysis in myocardial infarction grade 3 (TIMI-3) flow was restored after additional aspiration and balloon dilatation but with poor myocardial blush (Figures 5.28 and 5.29, Loops 5.28 and 5.29). The patient sustained a large myocardial infarction (peak CPK = 4,000) and a significant impairment of left ventricular ejection fraction (LVEF = 20%). At follow-up, he remained in congestive heart failure and required heart transplantation one year later.

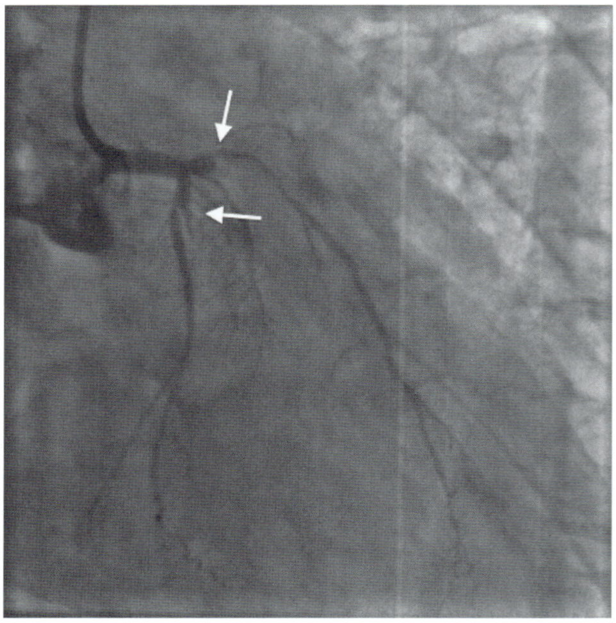

FIGURE 5.26

Coronary angiography (right anterior oblique (RAO) caudal projection) demonstrating thrombotic occlusion of the proximal LAD and the OM branch (white arrows). (LOOP 5.26)

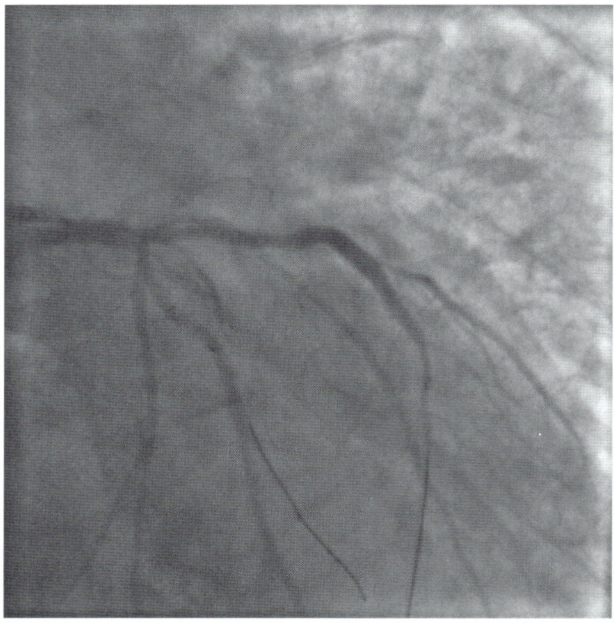

FIGURE 5.27

Coronary angiography (right anterior oblique (RAO) caudal projection) after aspiration thrombectomy of the LAD and LCX with restoration of flow. (LOOP 5.27)

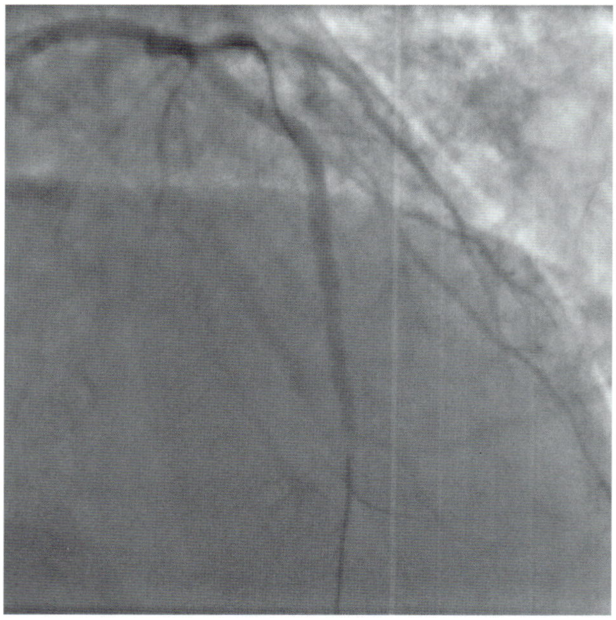

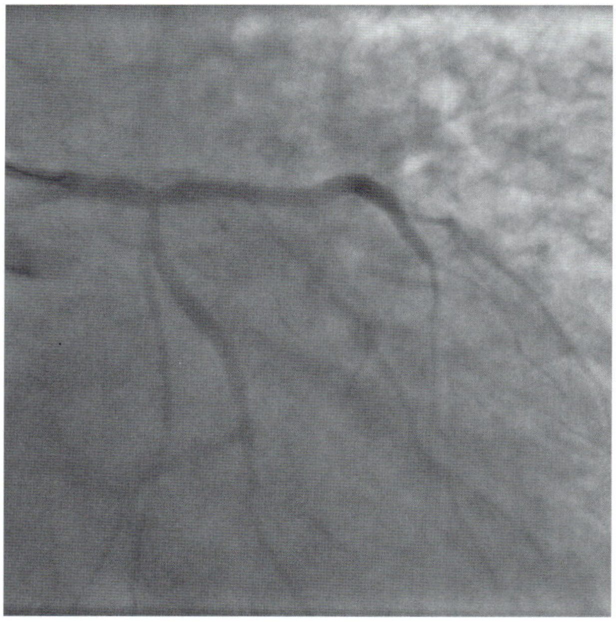

FIGURES 5.28 AND 5.29

Coronary angiography after additional aspiration and balloon dilatations in the LAD and OM. Note that TIMI-3 flow was restored but myocardial blush remained poor. (LOOPS 5.28 AND 5.29)

CASE ANALYSIS

This case illustrates the fatal consequences of simultaneous stent thrombosis in two coronary arteries. Although the primary cause of stent thrombosis in this case might be noncompliance with aspirin therapy, implantation of multiple stents in a vessel with diffuse disease is also a risk factor. Several points are worth highlighting with regard to this patient. First, patient education regarding the importance of compliance with dual antiplatelet therapy is crucial and should be considered part of the treatment; second, in patients undergoing multivessel PCI, the operator should consider and discuss the potential risk of simultaneous stent thrombosis in several vessels; and third, IVUS guidance of coronary stenting should be given serious consideration in patients undergoing multivessel PCI or stenting of diffuse coronary segments to optimize the final results.

LESSONS

- Simultaneous stent thrombosis in 2 vessels is associated with a bad prognosis even with timely and effective revascularization therapy.
- When performing multivessel PCI in patients with high-risk lesions, the risk and consequences of stent thrombosis should be thoroughly considered. All efforts should be made to attain optimal mechanical results and assure compliance with dual antiplatelet therapy.

SUGGESTED READING

Iakovou I, Schmidt T, Bonizzoni E, et al. Incidence, predictors, and outcome of thrombosis after successful implantation of drug-eluting stents. *JAMA*. 2005;293(17):2126–2130.

Jang SW, Kim DB, Kwon BJ, et al. Death caused by simultaneous subacute stent thrombosis of sirolimus-eluting stents in left anterior descending artery and left circumflex artery. *Int J Cardiol*. 2010;140(1):e8-e11.

CASE 5.4

Slow Flow After PCI in a Native Coronary Arterty

CLINICAL HISTORY AND DIAGNOSTIC TESTING RESULTS

A 71-year-old man with history of hypertension, diabetes mellitus, hypercholesterolemia, smoking, and known CAD with prior PCI to the RCA was admitted, with recurrence of class 3 angina pectoris and positive ECG exercise test while on maximal medical therapy. Coronary angiography revealed mid-LAD bifurcation stenosis with ostial involvement of the first and second diagonal branches (Figure 5.30, Loop 5.30). The RCA and LCX were patent, and the LV function was normal.

PLANNED PROCEDURE

PCI of the mid-LAD.

PROCEDURE

The patient was pretreated with clopidogrel (600 mg) and aspirin (325 mg). IV bivalirudin was initiated at the beginning of the procedure (activated clotting time = 420 seconds). An 8-Fr guide catheter was used to engage the left coronary artery. Three soft-tipped coronary wires and two diagonal branches were placed in the LAD . The LAD was interrogated with near-infrared (NIR) spectroscopy, which demonstrated lipid-rich plaque extending to almost 300° of the vessel circumference at the mid-LAD segment (Figure 5.31a). A 2.5- × 15-mm balloon was used to predilate the mid-LAD stenosis.

COMPLICATION AND MANAGEMENT

Coronary angiography after balloon predilation demonstrated TIMI-2 flow (Figure 5.32a, Loop 5.32a). The

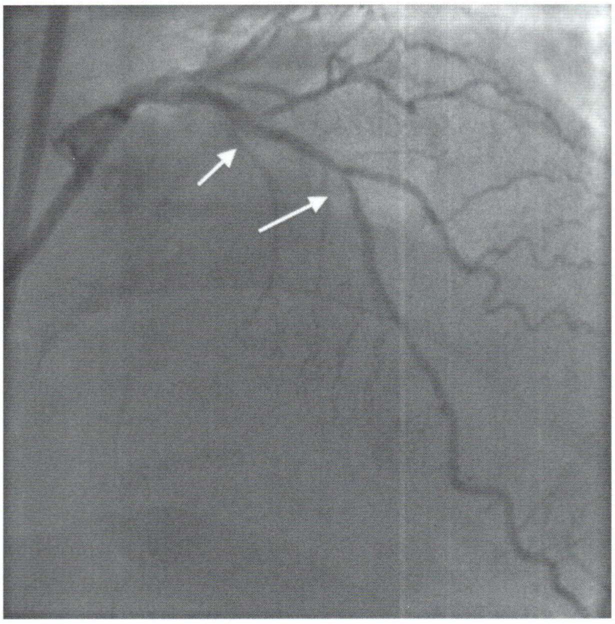

FIGURE 5.30

Coronary angiography (anteroposterior (AP) cranial projection). Note the stenotic mid-LAD segment involving the takeoff of two diagonal branches. **(LOOP 5.30)**

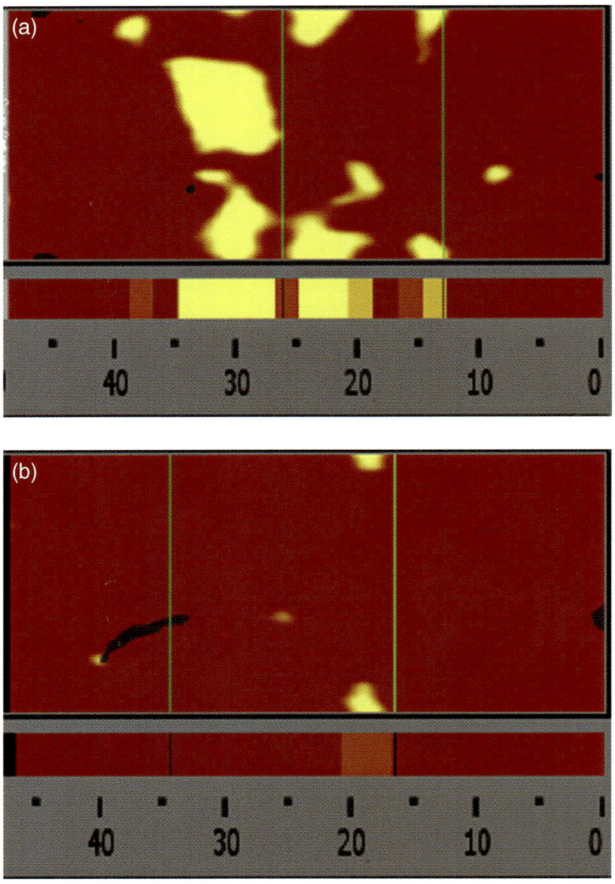

FIGURE 5.31

(a) NIR spectroscopy prior to intervention. Note the lipid-rich plaque extending to almost 300° of the vessel circumference. (b) NIR spectroscopy at the end of the procedure. Note the nearly complete disappearance of the lipid component in this segment.

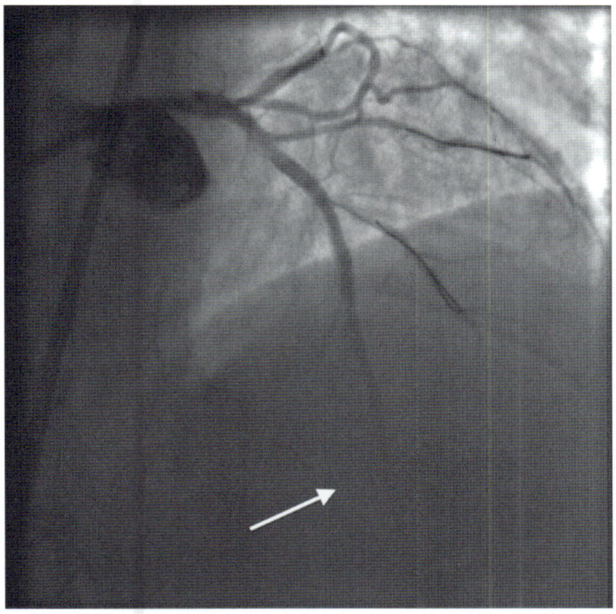

FIGURE 5.32a

Coronary angiography demonstrating slow flow after predilatation of the LAD. (LOOP 5.32a)

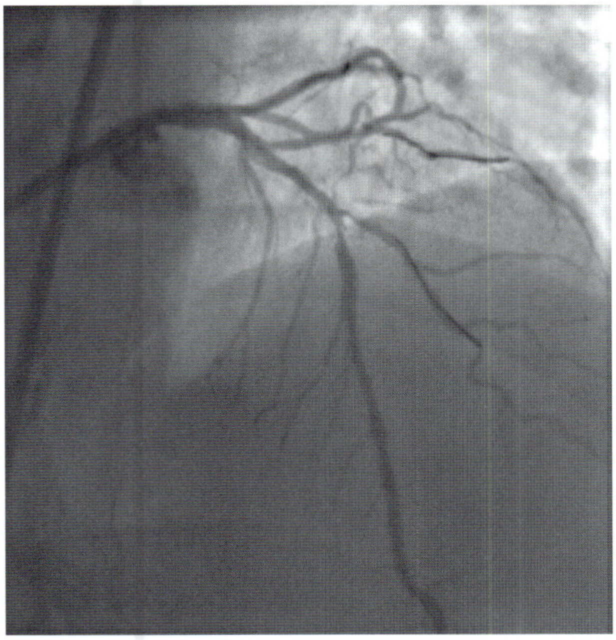

FIGURE 5.32b

Coronary angiography demonstrating flow improvement in the LAD after intracoronary administration of 100 μg of adenosine. (LOOP 5.32b)

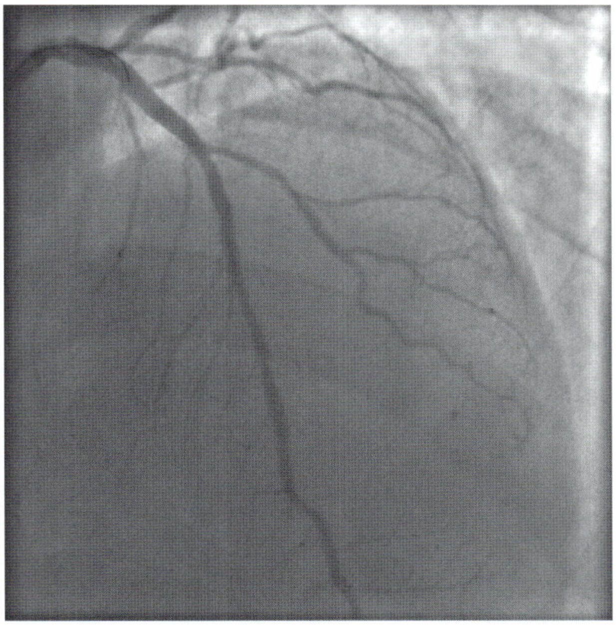

FIGURE 5.33

Final coronary angiography after stent implantation and postdilation. (LOOP 5.33)

patient began to complain of severe chest pain with precipitous drop in blood pressure from 140/80 to 70/30 and 3-mm ST segment elevations in the precordial leads. Administration of IV saline and Neo-Synephrine (200 μg) resulted in blood pressure recovery but no improvement in chest pain, ECG changes, or slow flow. Intracoronary administration of nitroprusside was ineffective as well. Intracoronary administration of 100 μg of adenosine resulted in immediate flow improvement with immediate resolution of symptoms and ECG changes (Figure 5.32, Loop 5.32b). Subsequently, two everolimus-eluting stents (3.0 × 23 mm and 3.5 × 23 mm) were implanted at the mid and proximal LAD and postdilated with final kissing balloon inflation using a balloon in the second diagonal branch. The final angiographic result was good, with no recurrence of chest pain or slow flow (Figure 5.33, Loop 5.33).

CASE ANALYSIS

We did not anticipate slow flow after predilation of the LAD stenosis in this patient because he lacked the typical clinical or angiographic risk factors (such as acute coronary syndrome or thrombotic lesion). Repeat NIR spectroscopy of the LAD at the conclusion of the intervention demonstrated diminution of the lipid signal, indicating that embolization of that material is what might have resulted in slow flow (Figure 5.31b). Distal embolization of disrupted lipid-rich plaque has been proposed as one of the potential causes of unanticipated myocardial injury after balloon dilatation and stenting, which is manifested by the no-reflow phenomenon.

The management of slow or no-reflow phenomenon includes maintenance of effective systemic blood pressure, with vasopressors if necessary, and reversal of the slow flow with administration of intracoronary vasodilators (preferably through a selective infusion catheter or balloon lumen). In our own experience, we find intracoronary nitroprusside more effective than other measures (50–100 μg that can be repeated if the systemic blood pressure permits). In resistant cases, intracoronary administration of high-dose adenosine can be effective, as was demonstrated in this case.

LESSONS

- PCI in native coronary arteries can be associated with slow flow even in patients with stable angina with no visible thrombus. The presumed mechanism is embolization of lipid-laden plaques.
- The mainstay of treatment of slow flow is maintenance of effective systemic blood pressure and selective intracoronary administration of vasodilators.

SUGGESTED READING

Goldstein JA, Grines C, Fischell T, et al. Coronary embolization following balloon dilation of lipid-core plaques. *JACC Cardiovasc Imaging.* 2009;2(12):1420–1424.

Kobatake R, Sato T, Fujiwara Y, et al. Comparison of the effects of nitroprusside versus nicorandil on the slow/no-reflow phenomenon during coronary interventions for acute myocardial infarction. *Heart Vessels.* 2011;26(4):379–384.

Schultz CJ, Serruys PW, van der Ent M, et al. First-in-man clinical use of combined near-infrared spectroscopy and intravascular ultrasound: A potential key to predict distal embolization and no-reflow? *J Am Coll Cardiol.* 2010;56(4):314.

CASE 5.5

IVUS-Induced LMCA Dissection

CLINICAL HISTORY AND DIAGNOSTIC TESTING RESULTS

An 86-year-old woman was admitted with multiple cardiovascular risk factors and known CAD. She was severely symptomatic and unable to walk more than one block without rest. She underwent coronary angiography that showed ulcerated stenosis of the LMCA extending into the LAD (Figure 5.34, Loop 5.34). The patient was referred for PCI of the LMCA after declining CABG surgery.

PLANNED PROCEDURE

PCI of the LMCA.

PROCEDURE

An 8-Fr broad-transition guide catheter was used to engage the left coronary artery. Two soft-tipped coronary wires were placed in the LAD and LCX. IVUS interrogation of the LMCA was performed from both the LAD and LCX to measure the LMCA diameter, evaluate the extension of the lesion into the LAD, and exclude involvement of the ostial LCX. IVUS showed a large ruptured plaque in the LMCA (Figure 5.35, Loop 5.35).

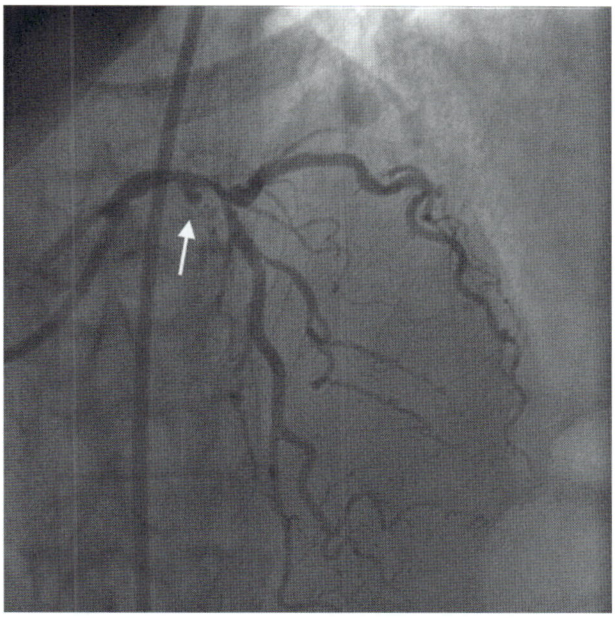

FIGURE 5.34

Coronary angiography demonstrating ulcerated stenosis of the LMCA extending into the LAD. (LOOP 5.34)

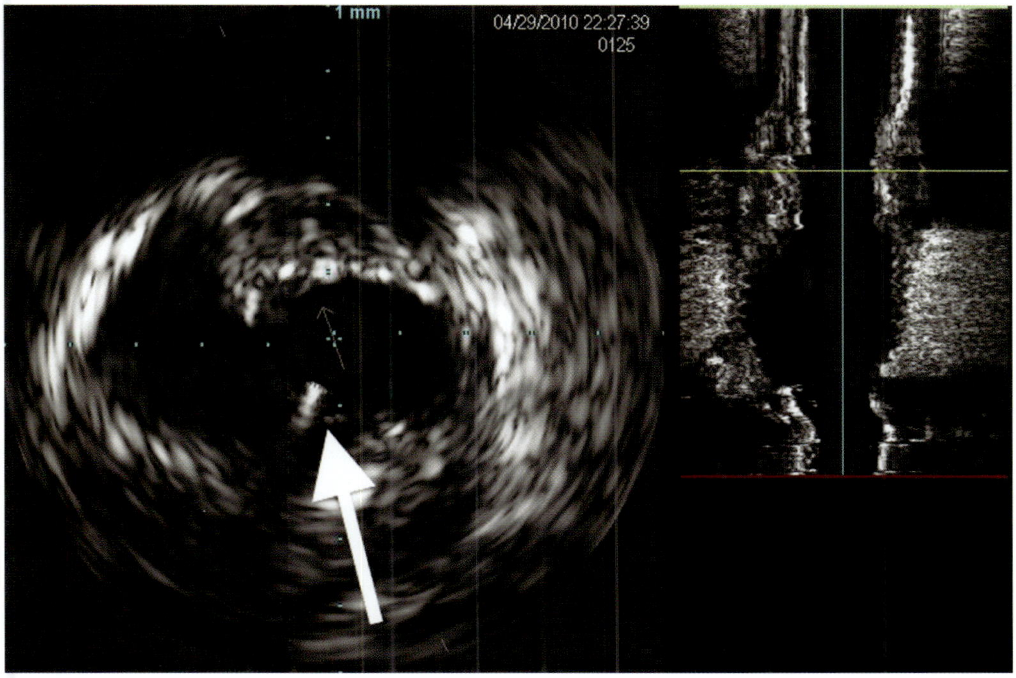

FIGURE 5.35

IVUS assessment of the LMCA. Note the ruptured plaque (white arrow). (LOOP 5.35)

COMPLICATION AND MANAGEMENT

Immediately after IVUS interrogation, the patient developed severe chest pain and ST segment elevation in the anterior leads. Coronary angiography revealed a flow-limiting dissection in the LMCA extending into the LAD (Figure 5.36, Loop 5.36). The LMCA was immediately predilated with a 3-mm balloon and stented with a 3.5- × 23-mm everolimus-eluting stent, jailing the LCX wire. Repeat angiography showed sealing of the dissection in the LMCA and the LAD with TIMI-3 flow but with filling defect in the LCX ostium (Figure 5.37, Loop 5.37). A new wire was used to rewire the LCX, and the previous wire was removed. A 3.5- × 8-mm everolimus-eluting stent was placed at the LCX ostium and postdilated. Final kissing balloon inflation was performed with a 3-mm in the LCX and a 3.5-mm in the LMCA. Finally, the proximal segment of the LMCA stent was dilated with a 4-mm noncompliant balloon. Final angiography showed an excellent result, and the patient was hemodynamically stable and free of symptoms (Figures 5.38 and 5.39, Loops 5.38 and 5.39).

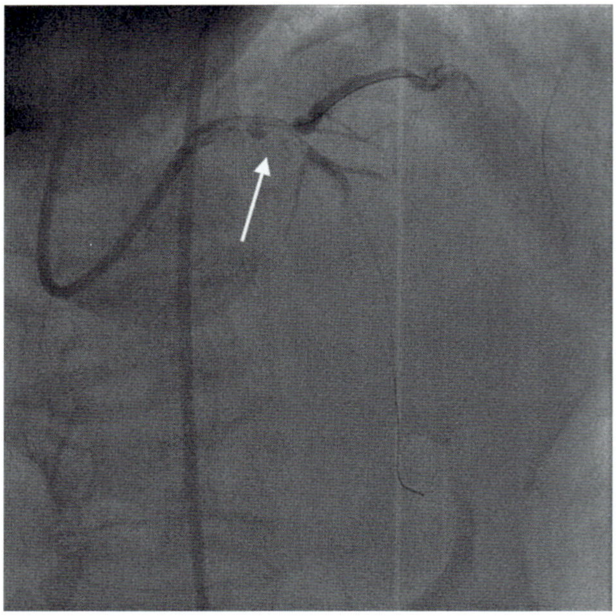

FIGURE 5.36

Coronary angiography after IVUS interrogation of the LMCA. Note the flow-limiting dissection and filling defect in the LMCA extending into the LAD. **(LOOP 5.36)**

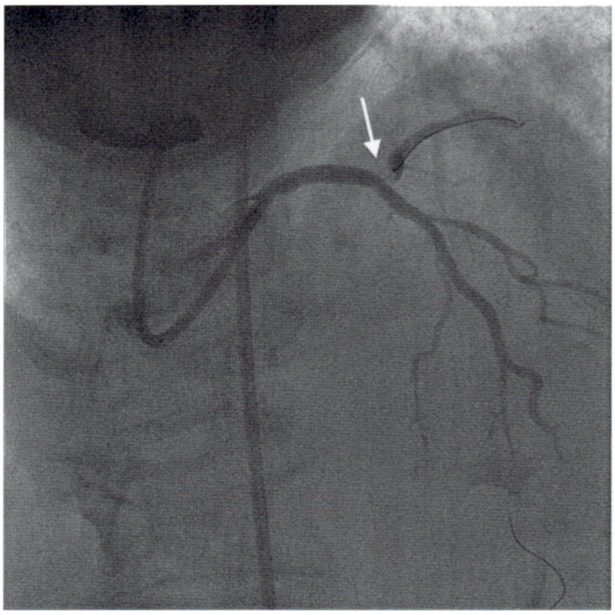

FIGURE 5.37

Coronary angiography after stenting of the LMCA and the ostial LAD. Note the filling defect in the LCX ostium (white arrow). **(LOOP 5.37)**

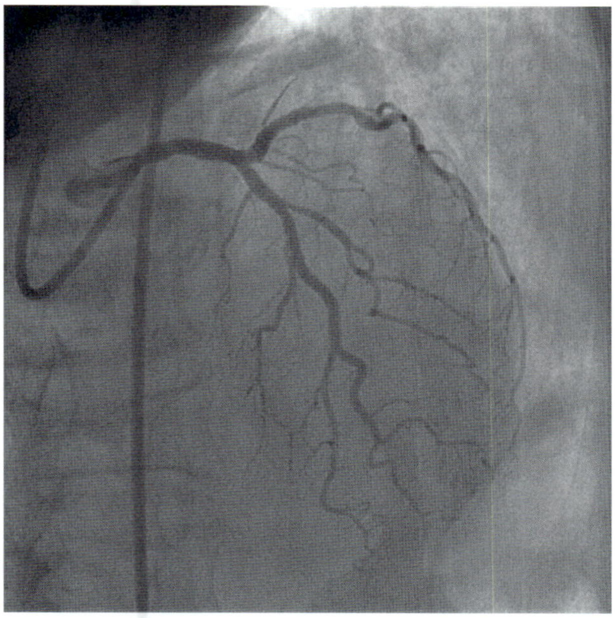

FIGURE 5.38

Final coronary angiography (anteroposterior (AP) cranial projection) after stent placement of the LCX ostium. **(LOOP 5.38)**

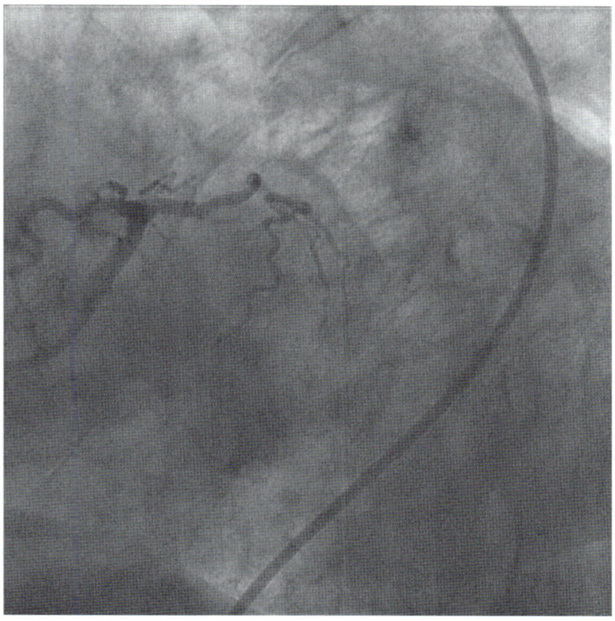

FIGURE 5.39

Final coronary angiography (left anterior oblique caudal projection) after stent placement of the LCX ostium. **(LOOP 5.39)**

CASE ANALYSIS

This case illustrates the risk of dissection while manipulating intracoronary devices through unstable ulcerated lesions. Although IVUS-induced coronary dissections is rare, it can still occur. It is important to remember that if the IVUS catheter encounters resistance as it is advanced, it should not be pushed forcefully.

LESSONS

- Although rare, IVUS interrogation of coronary arteries can be associated with dissection and thrombosis.
- This complication is avoidable by careful IVUS advancement, by adjustment of introduction angle, or by abandoning the attempt if resistance persists.

CASE 5.6

A Guide Catheter–Induced RCA Dissection

CLINICAL HISTORY AND DIAGNOSTIC TESTING RESULTS

A 65-year-old man with multiple cardiovascular risk factors was admitted with chest pain, anterior ST segment depression, and elevated troponin levels. The patient was initially treated with aspirin, clopidogrel, and IV unfractionated heparin. He was brought to the catheterization laboratory within 24 hours of admission. Coronary angiography showed a 75% stenosis of the OM branch (Figure 5.40, Loop 5.40), a 90% stenosis of the mid-RCA with a filling defect (Figure 5.41, Loop 5.41), and patent LAD with normal left ventricular ejection fraction (LVEF).

PLANNED PROCEDURE

PCI of the mid-RCA.

PROCEDURE

The RCA was engaged with a 6-Fr JR 4 guide catheter. Injection of contrast media into the RCA induced an extensive spiral dissection (Figure 5.42, Loop 5.42).

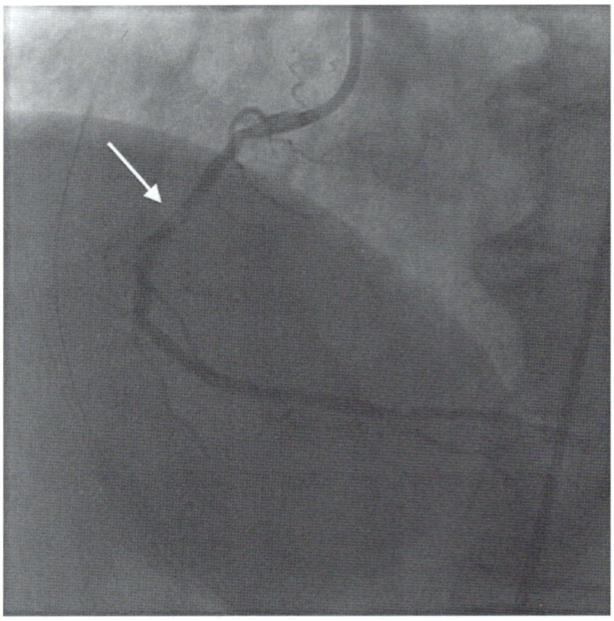

FIGURE 5.41

Baseline coronary angiography (left anterior oblique projection). Note the mid-RCA filling defect (white arrow). **(LOOP 5.41)**

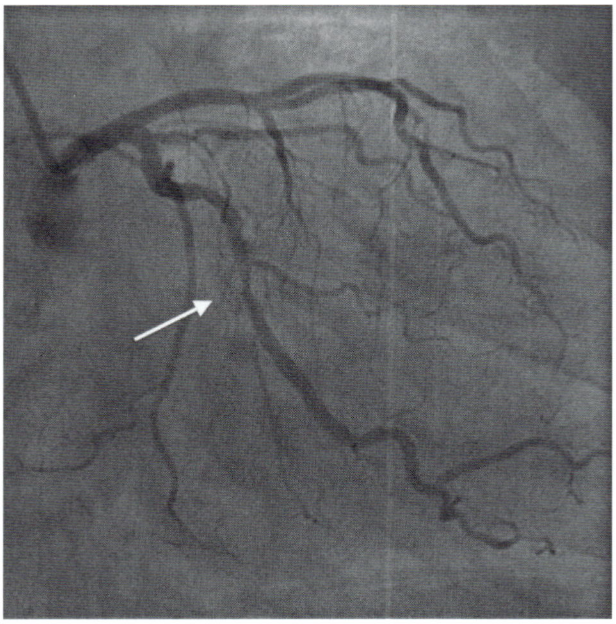

FIGURE 5.40

Baseline coronary angiography (right anterior oblique (RAO) caudal projection). Note the OM branch stenosis (white arrow). **(LOOP 5.40)**

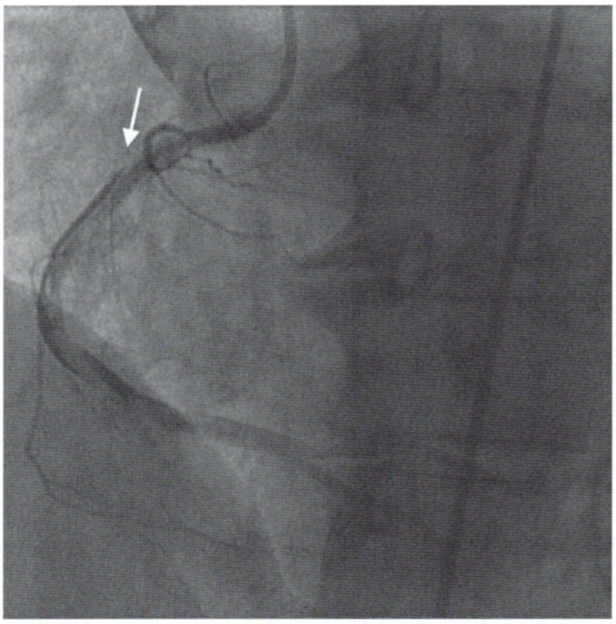

FIGURE 5.42

Coronary angiography after JR4 guide engagement. Note the long spiral dissection of the RCA. **(LOOP 5.42)**

COMPLICATION AND MANAGEMENT

The guide catheter–induced RCA dissection was associated with compromised flow, chest pain, and ST segment elevation in the inferior leads. The operator attempted to wire through the RCA dissection but failed, despite multiple attempts with multiple wires. The patient was referred for urgent CABG surgery to the RCA and OM. Post-CABG, he did well and was discharged home without subsequent events.

CASE ANALYSIS

In this case, the RCA dissection occurred because the operator injected contrast medium while the tip of the guide catheter was embedded against the vessel wall. This complication would have been avoidable if the operator observed the dampening of the pressure waveform and refrained from injecting contrast until the catheter is reoriented to a coaxial position. Once a catheter-induced dissection is observed, it is critical to desist from further dye injections prior to wiring the true lumen because that would lead to further propagation of the dissection.

LESSONS

- Despite significant improvements in guide catheter technology and operator experience, catheter-induced dissection can occur.
- This complication is almost always avoidable if the operator routinely observes the pressure waveform prior to contrast injection.
- Once a catheter-induced dissection is observed, the operator should refrain from injecting contrast until a wire is placed in the distal true lumen because contrast injection will propagate the dissection.

SUGGESTED READING

Wagdi P, Egloff L, Siebenmann R, et al. Catheter-induced dissection of the right coronary ostium and aortic root. *Z Kardiol. 1999*;88(7):526–528. [Article in German]

Taniguchi N, Takahashi A, Sakamoto S. Successful fenestration using a chronic total occlusion-dedicated guidewire in a patient with catheter-induced dissection of the right coronary artery. *J Invasive Cardiol*. 2011;23(2):84–86.

6

Azeem Latib and Antonio Colombo

Coronary Perforations

INTRODUCTION

Coronary artery perforation during percutaneous coronary intervention (PCI) is an infrequent but potentially life-threatening complication (1). It remains one of the most dreaded complications faced in the catheterization laboratory and has repeatedly been shown to be associated with poorer outcomes, particularly myocardial infarction, emergency cardiac bypass surgery, and death (1–4). Fortunately, the incidence of coronary perforation in the general interventional population is low, with a range of 0.1% to 0.5%, and appears to be decreasing over the past 10 years (1–6).

Coronary perforation occurs predominantly as a complication of coronary angioplasty and may range from a self-limiting extravasation of contrast to large vessel rupture with brisk blood extravasation, resulting in cardiac tamponade and hemodynamic compromise. The Ellis classification (Table 6.1) remains the most widely adopted method to angiographically describe coronary perforations (1). This classification also has prognostic importance, with low rates of death occurring in Type 1 perforations, which can usually be managed conservatively, and a high risk of death in Type 3 if not promptly treated. The probable mechanisms of perforation include (*1*) loss of integrity in the vessel wall caused by overstretching of the vessel by a balloon or a stent or by barotrauma from balloon rupture (balloon rupture causes trauma when there is residual air in the balloon or in the system; the compressed air will release energy upon balloon rupture); (*2*) small hole in the arterial wall from a sharp object, such as the tip of a hydrophilic or stiff chronic total occlusion (CTO) guidewire; and (*3*) loss of tissue as a consequence of excessive ablation of tissue by atherectomy, excimer laser, or mechanical thrombectomy devices (5,6).

Clinical situations that carry a particularly high risk of perforation include female gender, older age, calcified and tortuous arteries, bifurcations and angulated lesions, small vessels, acute or chronic occlusions, saphenous vein grafts, and use of atheroablative devices and compliant balloons (2–8). Early diagnosis is based on the careful monitoring of clinical signs, such as puncture-like chest pain during balloon inflation or guidewire advancement, or with resistance to wire and device progression.

The treatment of coronary perforation depends on the cause and size of the perforation, the extent of contrast medium extravasation, and the hemodynamic status of the patient. The management strategy is dictated by the need to stop coronary extravasation and to relieve hemodynamic compromise. The immediate management is always the same, irrespective of the cause of the perforation, and requires a multipronged approach of prolonged balloon inflation, reversal of anticoagulation, maintaining hemodynamic stability, relief of pericardial tamponade, and eventual sealing of the perforation utilizing covered stents or microembolization. A knowledge of materials used to treat complications and a logical treatment algorithm during this often-dramatic complication saves lives. Figure 6.1 summarizes our proposed algorithm for the management of coronary perforations (9).

The management generally differs if the perforation occurred due to vessel rupture or distal guidewire perforation.

Vessel Rupture

Vessel rupture was more often associated with the use of devices in procedures such as atherectomy (directional or rotational) or excimer laser angioplasty, or use of a cutting balloon. However, vessel rupture can also occur at the time of predilatation, stent implantation, or postdilatation. Indeed, a common misconception that needs to be corrected is that stents protect from vessel rupture. It is especially important to avoid using compliant or semicompliant balloons in calcific or fibrotic lesions, or to try to overcome a lesion that cannot be dilated at high pressure using an oversized balloon. The appropriate usage of intravascular ultrasound (IVUS) to evaluate vessel size, lesion morphology, calcification, and the need for atheroablation and strict adherence to the information obtained can be an important tool in reducing the risk of vessel rupture.

TABLE 6.1
Ellis Classification of Coronary Perforations (1).

Type 1	Extraluminal crater without extravasation
Type 2	Pericardial or myocardial blush without contrast jet extravasation
Type 3	Extravasation through frank (>1 mm) perforation
Cavity spilling	Perforation into an anatomic cavity chamber, coronary sinus, etc.
Subtype A	Directed toward the pericardium
Subtype B	Directed toward the myocardium

When coronary perforation occurs, the first step is not to lose control of the situation—in particular, not to lose access of the artery (6). In any risky situation, it remains imperative to deflate the balloon and not remove it until a contrast injection has confirmed the absence of a perforation. In the case of a perforation, immediate balloon inflation at low pressure (with the same balloon that caused the rupture) is the most important step to prevent further extravasation. When possible, prolonged balloon inflation should be attempted either opposing the ruptured vessel wall or crossing over the perforated branch. Unfortunately, perfusion balloons are no longer available for the patients who develop ischemia during balloon inflation. A turning point in the treatment of coronary perforations occurred with the introduction of covered stents (stent grafts), which allow for the percutanenous sealing of the rupture (10,11). There are three balloon-expandable covered stents commercially available in Europe:

1. JOSTENT GraftMaster® (Abbott Laboratories, Abbott Park, IL): stainless steel stent covered with polytetrafluoroethylene (PTFE): wall thickness 0.3 mm; available in sizes 3, 3.5, 4 (6-Fr guiding catheter), 4.5, and 5 (7-Fr guiding catheter). It is bulkier than the other covered stents and the only one presently available in the United States.
2. InSitu Direct-Stent® (Minneapolis, MN) Stent-Graft: stainless steel PTFE-covered stent; wall thickness 0.15 mm and one of the thinnest covered stents available (starting at 1.2-mm crossing profile); available in sizes from 2.5 to 6.0 mm diameter; minimum guiding catheter size is 6 to 7 Fr.
3. Over and Under® (ITGI Medical, Or Akiva, Israel) Pericardium Covered Stent: stainless steel stent covered with equine pericardium (105 μm thickness, highly flexible stent); available in sizes 2.5, 3, 3.5 (6-Fr guiding catheter), and 4 mm (7-Fr guiding catheter). Theoretically, the equine pericardium may be more biocompatible and thus reduces the risk of stent thrombosis.

All these covered stents suffer from similar limitations because they are bulkier than normal stents with reduced flexibility and trackability and because of increased risk of stent thrombosis and restenosis. It is essential not only to ensure sealing of the perforation but also to reduce the risk of stent thrombosis so that the covered stents are deployed at a reasonably high-pressure (14–16 atm), with prolonged balloon inflation to ensure optimal stent expansion.

A major drawback in treating a perforated vessel with a coronary stent graft is the elapsed time between the deflations of the sealing balloon until the final delivery of the covered stent into the lesion site. Thus, we would always recommend the dual-catheter technique for implantation of the covered stent (12). While the sealing balloon is inflated, the guide catheter is withdrawn slightly from the coronary ostia, and a second 7- or 8-Fr guiding catheter from the contralateral femoral artery is used to engage the same coronary ostia, alongside the previous guide. A coronary covered stent graft (or a coil in smaller and distal vessels) is advanced on a new wire through the second guide and placed just proximally to the sealing balloon. The sealing balloon is briefly deflated and withdrawn proximally to allow wire passage, and the coronary covered stent graft is advanced to the site and deployed. Importantly, the first sealing balloon, wire, and guide catheter is retrieved only after gaining adequate seal of the lesion with the covered stent graft.

In cases where sealing of the perforation by conservative measures cannot be achieved, urgent bypass surgery must be performed.

Wire Perforations

These perforations can occur while recanalizing a chronic occlusion or during standard angioplasty. Wire perforations during treatment of chronic occlusions have usually been benign and have been termed "wire exits" rather than perforations. It is important that the operator should not advance a balloon or other device over the incorrectly positioned wire. Distal wire perforations, on the other hand, are more subtle as the operator may not be immediately aware of their occurrence. They most often occur with the use of hydrophilic wires that have been advanced too distally. Indeed, we advise that when using hydrophilic wires, they be left with a loop distally and that the operator always fluoroscopically monitors guidewire position in the distal coronary artery when hydrophilic, tapered, or stiff wires are used. We prefer, whenever possible, exchanging the hydrophilic wire for a regular wire in order to avoid the risk of distal perforation. If distal perforation occurs, the operator can perform distal balloon inflation, coil embolization, or microparticle injection. In cases where distal wire perforation appears to resolve with only prolonged balloon inflation, we recommend close monitoring of the patient for at least 48 hours, as late bleeding and tamponade may sometimes occur. When microcoil embolization is used for distal perforations, it is recommended that the coils are released in as distal a position as possible, commencing deployment within the pericardial space before retreating into the vessel to ensure successful hemostasis. As concerns microparticle embolization, we suggest beginning with 300- to 400-μm particles, increasing to 600- to 700-μm if effective embolization is not obtained (6,13). In rare circumstances, implantation of a PTFE stent to divert the flow into a branch can exclude blood flow to the perforated segment. Surgical ligation remains a therapeutic option if other methods fail.

We are less enthusiastic about the need for and safety of heparin neutralization, especially following implantation of drug-eluting stents. If the operator considers performing prolonged balloon inflation, the safety of using protamine to neutralize the heparin given to the patient becomes questionable. Recently, we have seen three cases of stent thrombosis occurring following neutralization of heparin in the context of treatment of a perforation (see Chapter 9). The use of glycoprotein IIb/IIIa inhibitors or direct thrombin inhibitors poses additional problems regarding the treatment of coronary perforations. Platelet transfusion should be employed for reversal of an abciximab antiplatelet effect. In the presence of normal renal function, infusions of small-molecule glycoprotein IIb/IIIa inhibitors, such as eptifibatide and tirofiban, may be stopped with prompt reversal given their short half-lives (wait a few hours, maybe dialyze).

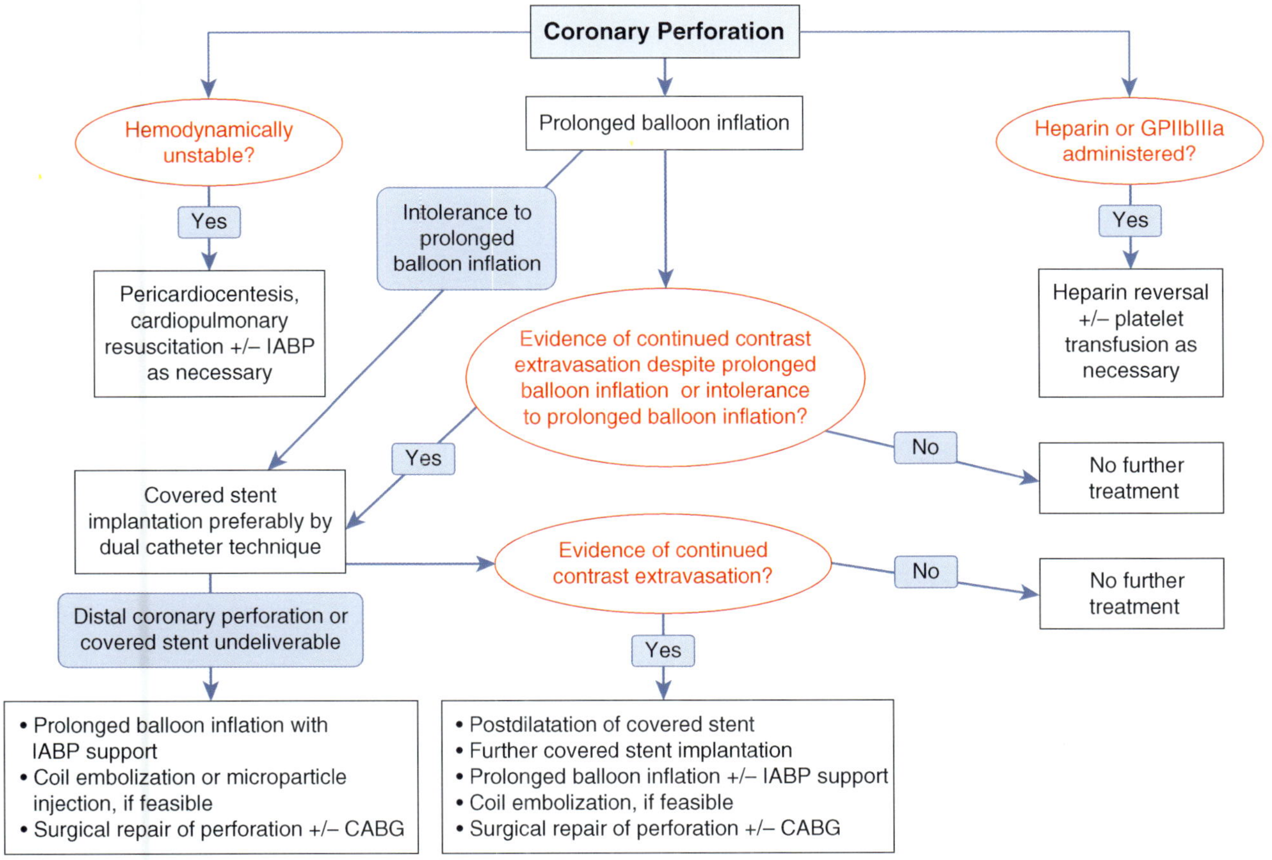

FIGURE 6.1
Coronary perforation.

CASE 6.1

Coronary Rupture Because of High-Pressure Stent Dilation in a Calcified Lesion

CLINICAL HISTORY AND DIAGNOSTIC TESTING RESULTS

An 85-year-old man with a recent admission for an acute coronary syndrome with heart failure treated conservatively. Normal left ventricular function of 54%. The patient presents with angina on minimal effort, and coronary angiography demonstrated critical stenosis of the mid-segment of the codominant right coronary artery (RCA) and proximal-to-middle left anterior descending artery (LAD).

PLANNED PROCEDURE

PCI on LAD with bare-metal stents.

PROCEDURE

The patient had been pretreated with aspirin and clopidogrel, and for the procedure, a bolus and infusion of Bivalirudin was commenced. Baseline angiography of left coronary artery demonstrated long, severe calcific stenosis extending from proximal LAD to mid-LAD (Figures 6.2 and 6.3). A balanced middle weight (BMW) Universal II guidewire (Abbott Vascular Devices, Redwood City, CA) was placed in the distal LAD and in the large septal branch as protection from closure during angioplasty and stenting. The LAD lesion was predilated with a 2.5-mm × 15-mm Maverick percutaneous transluminal coronary angioplasty (PTCA) balloon (Boston Scientific, Natick, MA). The lesion was then stented from distal to proximal with a Genous 3- × 28-mm and 3.5- × 18-mm stents (Figure 6.4). IVUS interrogation showed stent underexpansion. The distal stent was postdilated with a Quantum Maverick 3 × 15 mm at 22 atm, and the overlap zone was postdilated with a Quantum Maverick 3.5 × 12 mm at 22 atm. During postdilatation with the 3.5-mm balloon, the patient complained of stabbing chest pain.

COMPLICATION AND MANAGEMENT

Angiography demonstrated a Grade-3 coronary perforation of the mid-LAD (Figure 6.5). The PTCA balloon that caused the rupture was immediately inflated at the site of the rupture, but despite this, the patient became severely hypotensive. Echocardiography

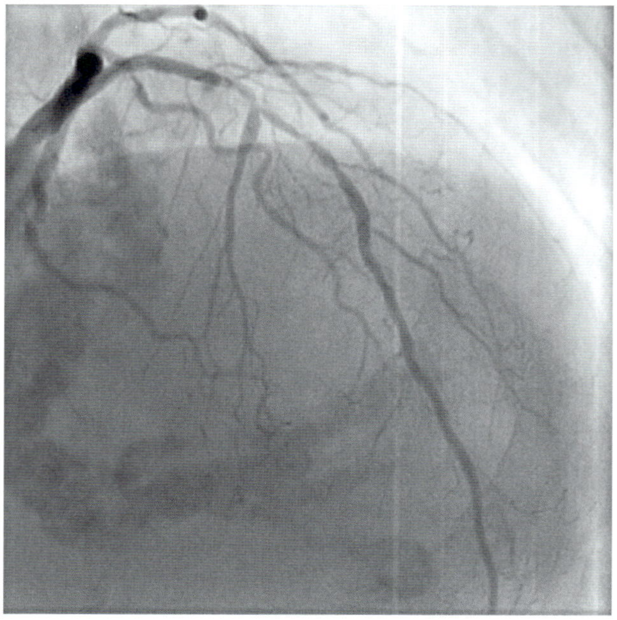

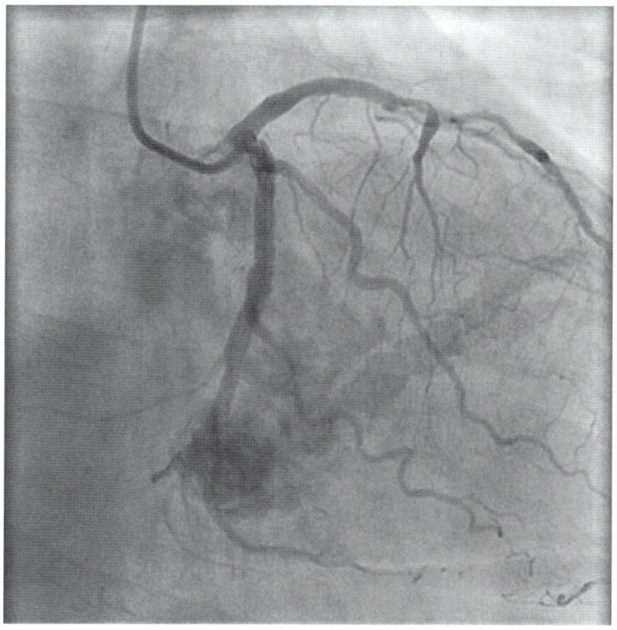

FIGURES 6.2 AND 6.3

Baseline angiography of the left coronary artery demonstrating a long severe calcific stenosis extending from the proximal LAD to mid-LAD. **(LOOPS 6.2 AND 6.3)**

confirmed the presence of a pericardial effusion and cardiac tamponade. Immediate pericardiocentesis was performed via a pigtail catheter placed in the pericardial space, with immediate hemodynamic stability. Repeat angiography demonstrated that the inflated balloon was not sealing the perforation (Figure 6.6). The balloon was then placed more proximally, and repeat angiography confirmed that contrast extravasation no longer occurred (Figure 6.7). A 3- × 19-mm Jostent Graftmaster® PTFE-covered stent was then implanted in the mid-LAD. However, angiography after covered stent placement demonstrated continued contrast extravasation from the rupture site (Figure 6.8). Thus, two more covered stents were implanted (Jostent Graftmaster 3 × 19 mm and InSitu Direct-Stent® 3 × 19 mm, and the covered stents were dilated at 16 atm for at least 30 seconds, especially at the proximal and distal ends. Final angiography confirmed sealing of the perforation without further contrast extravasation (Figure 6.9).

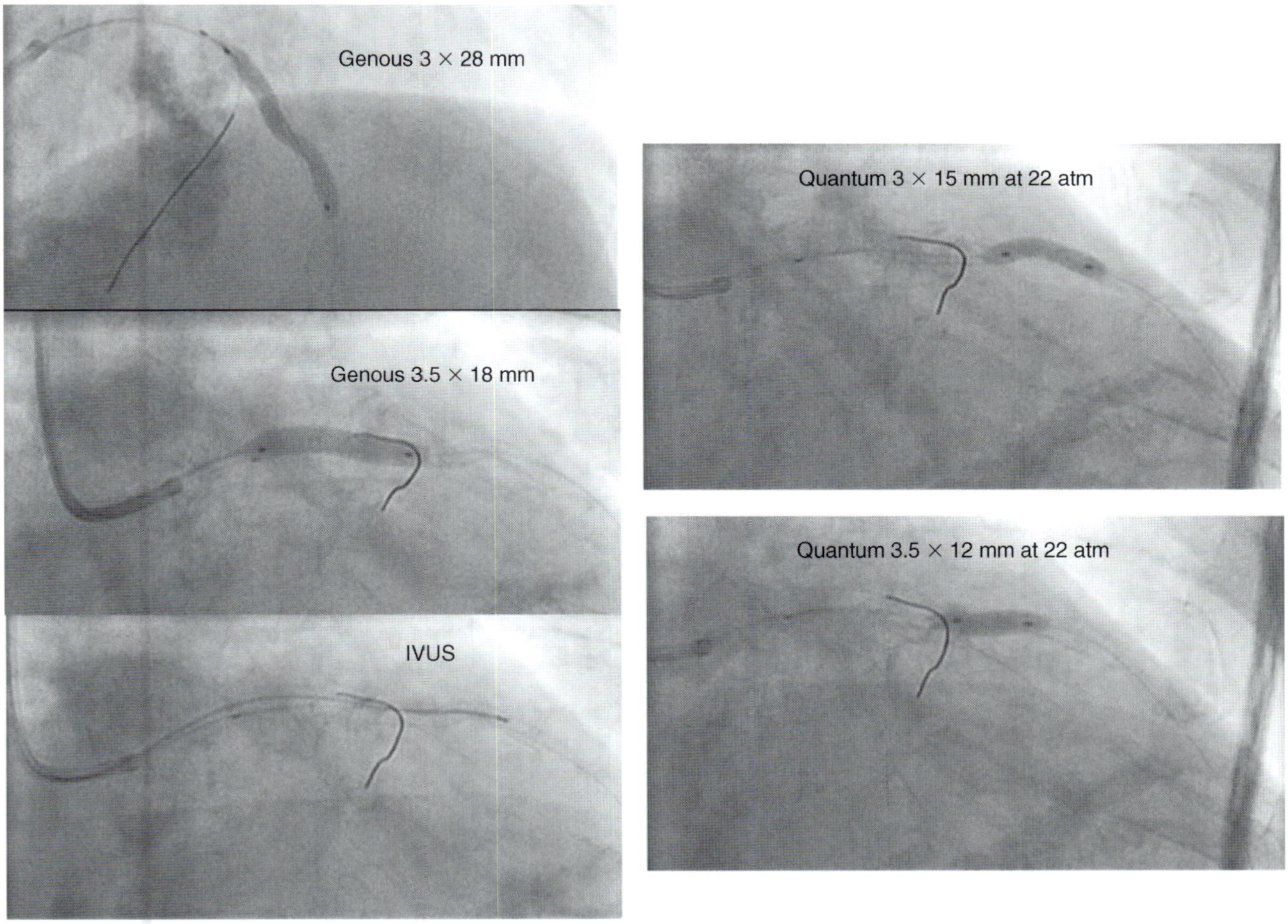

FIGURE 6.4

The LAD was stented from distal to proximal with a Genous 3- × 28-mm and 3.5- × 18-mm stents. IVUS interrogation showed stent underexpansion, and thus the distal stent was postdilated with a Quantum Maverick 3- × 15-mm at 22 atm, and the overlap zone was postdilated with a Quantum Maverick 3.5- × 12-mm at 22 atm.

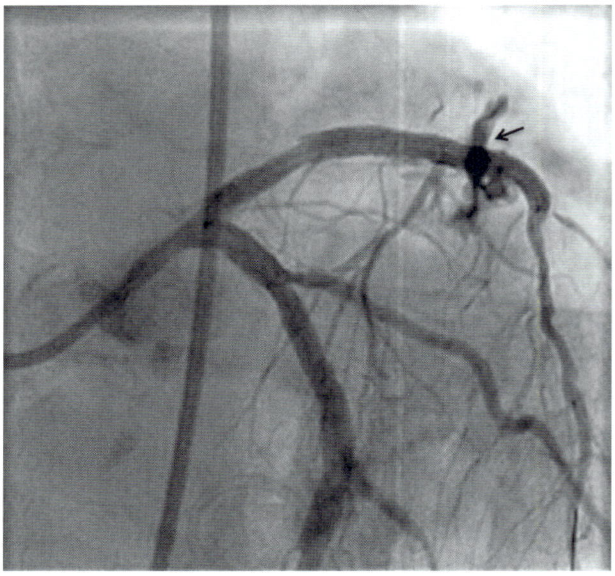

FIGURE 6.5

Angiography demonstrating a Grade 3 coronary perforation (arrow) of the mid-LAD (LOOP 6.5)

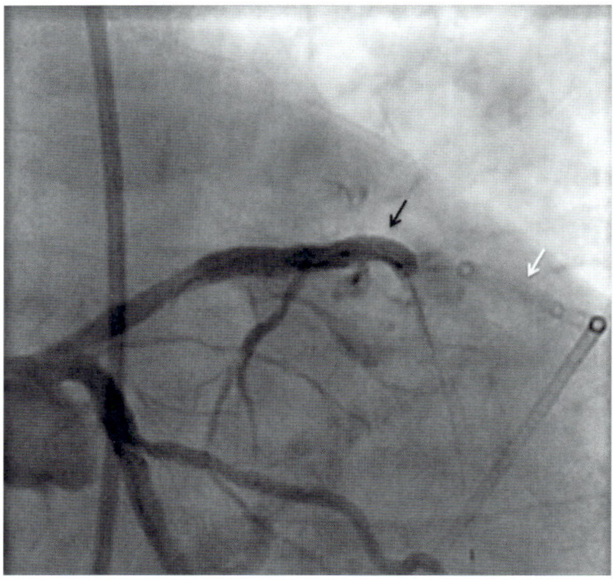

FIGURE 6.7

The balloon was inflated more proximally (black arrow), with resultant sealing of the coronary perforation. A pigtail catheter that was placed in the pericardium for pericardiocentesis is also visible (white arrow). (LOOP 6.7)

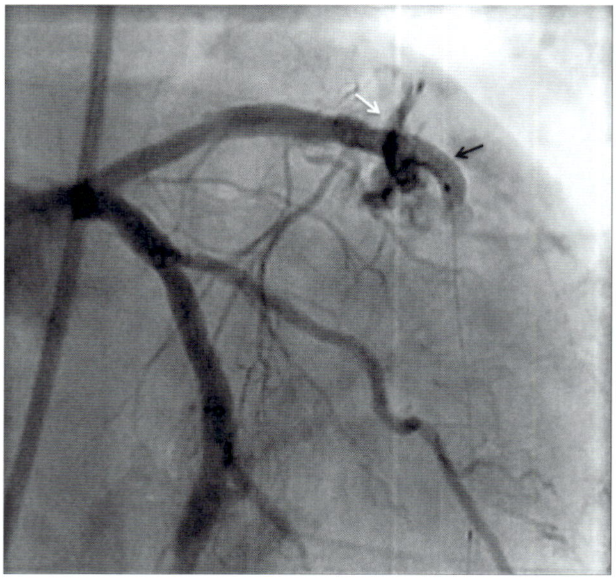

FIGURE 6.6

Angiography demonstrating that balloon inflation (black arrow) was not sealing the perforation (white arrow) (LOOP 6.6)

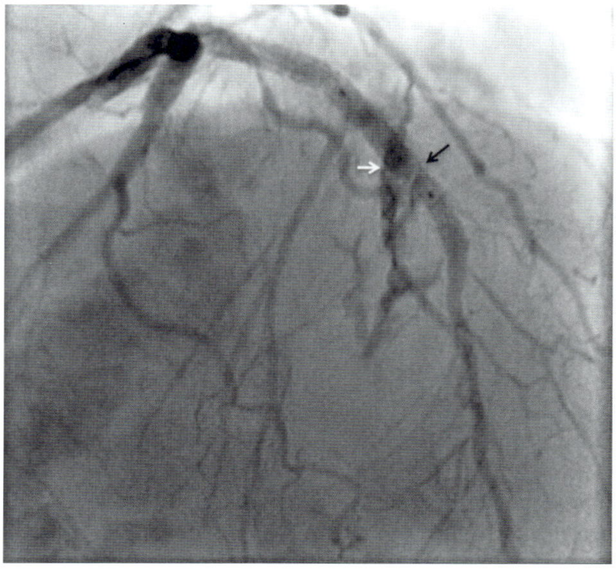

FIGURE 6.8

Angiography performed after implantation of a 3- × 19-mm Jostent Graftmaster® PTFE-covered stent on the mid-LAD (black arrow) showed that contrast extravasation still continued from the perforation site (white arrow). (LOOP 6.8)

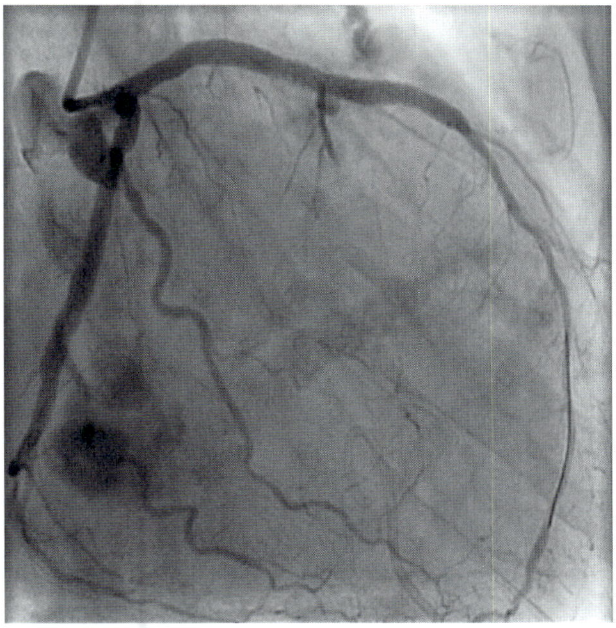

FIGURE 6.9

Final angiography after implantation of two more covered stents (Jostent Graftmaster 3 × 19 mm and InSitu Direct-Stent® 3 × 19 mm) confirmed sealing of the coronary perforation. (LOOP 6.9)

CASE ANALYSIS

The perforation in this case was probably caused by high-pressure postdilatation of a calcified lesion on a bend. Although IVUS was performed and used to determine the diameter of the postdilatation balloon, caution should always be exercised when dilating calcified lesions, especially in elderly patients.

LESSONS

- Caution should be exercised when dealing with an underexpanded stent in a severely calcified lesion. Aggressive balloon sizing, even when guided by accurate IVUS measurements, can result in arterial rupture.
- Immediate balloon inflation with the balloon that caused the vessel rupture is the most important step in ensuring hemodynamic instability. However, it must be ensured that the balloon inflation seals the perforation. If not, more proximal vessel occlusion with its resultant greater ischemia should be considered.
- Knowledge of pericardial drainage is mandatory for every operator performing cardiac interventions.
- Covered stent implantation is usually very effective in sealing perforations. If continued extravasation occurs after covered stent implantation, consider implanting a second covered stent and ensuring adequate high-pressure deployment or postdilatation to properly oppose the stent to the wall and seal the perforation.
- The dual-catheter technique of utilizing a second guiding catheter to implant covered stents or perform embolization, while maintaining sealing of the perforation with balloon inflation, should be the default technique in the percutaneous treatment of severe perforations.

CASE 6.2

Wire-Induced Coronary Perforation

CLINICAL HISTORY AND DIAGNOSTIC TESTING RESULTS

A 56-year-old male smoker with hypertension, abdominal aortic aneurysm repair, bilateral carotid endarterectomy, and previous myocardial infarction presents to us with inducible ischemia on exercise stress test. Coronary angiography demonstrated severe triple-vessel coronary artery disease with a CTO of the RCA and left circumflex artery (LCX), subocclusive stenosis of mid-LAD, and stenosis of proximal ramus intermedius (RI) (Figures 6.10 and 6.11).

PLANNED PROCEDURE

Multivessel PCI and drug-eluting stent implantation.

PROCEDURE

The patient was pretreated with aspirin and clopidogrel and given intravenous unfractionated heparin. As multivessel PCI was planned, a bolus and infusion of tirofiban was also given. The RCA was successfully recanalized, and multiple Taxus paclitaxel-eluting stents (Boston Scientific, Natick, MA) were implanted from the proximal to distal RCA. Subsequently, a Taxus stent was also implanted in the mid-LAD with good angiographic result. The intended strategy was then to recanalize the LCX. An over-the-wire balloon and Athlete Intermediate wire were used, but it was impossible to cross the lesion, and the wire exited from the vessel resulting in contrast extravasation (Figure 6.12).

COMPLICATION AND MANAGEMENT

Angiography demonstrates a Grade-3 coronary perforation caused by a guidewire with extravasation of contrast into the myocardium, resulting in a localized hematoma near the proximally occluded LCX (Figure 6.13). The recanalization attempt of the LCX was abandoned, and tirofiban was stopped. As the patient was stable, the procedure was continued with stenting of the proximal lesion in the RI branch (Figure 6.14) with a Taxus stent (3 × 16 mm at 18 atm). Following successful stenting of the proximal RI branch (not the ostium), an ostial narrowing of the LAD appeared (Figures 6.15 and 6.16). This new finding was not caused by plaque shift because the stent in the RI branch was not placed at its ostium. It thus became evident that the hematoma near the LCX was compressing the ostium of the LAD. A Taxus 3.0- × 24-mm stent was thus placed at the LAD ostium (Figure 6.17). Angiography confirmed a good result at the LAD ostium; however, it was clear that there was continued extravasation from the LCX with an enlarging hematoma (Figure 6.18). We therefore elected to implant a 3.0- × 12-mm PTFE covered stent at the ostium of the RI toward the left main to exclude the very proximal LCX from which the hematoma was originating (Figure 6.19). Immediately after placement of the PTFE stent, there was slow flow in the LAD (Figure 6.20). IVUS confirmed that the compromised flow in LAD was due to protrusion of the PTFE stent into the LAD, causing pinching of the ostium (Figure 6.21). The LAD was reopened by performing kissing-balloon inflation from the left main (LM) to LAD and RI (Figure 6.22). Unfortunately, this was complicated by a linear dissection of the LM (Figure 6.23), which was stented with a Taxus 3.5 × 16 mm at 18 atm, postdilated with a 4-mm noncompliant balloon at 16 atm. Figures 6.24 and 6.25 shows the final angiographic result.

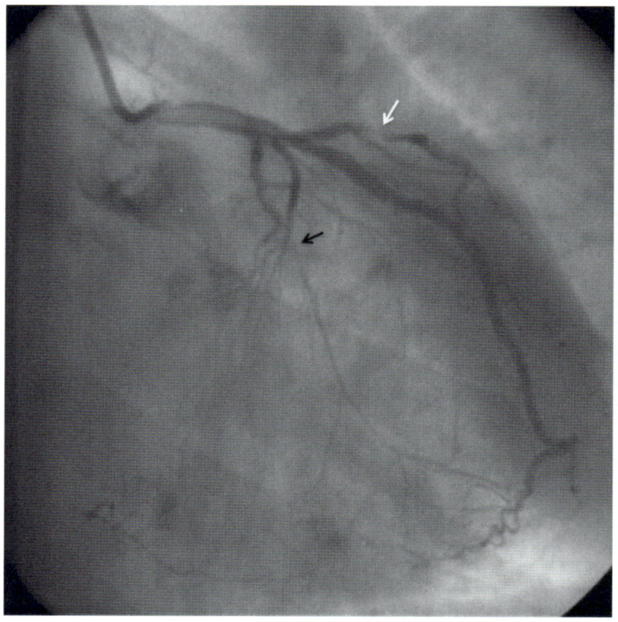

FIGURE 6.10

Caudal projection demonstrating a chronic total occlusion of the proximal LCX (black arrow) and subocclusive stenosis of the mid-LAD (white arrow). (LOOP 6.10)

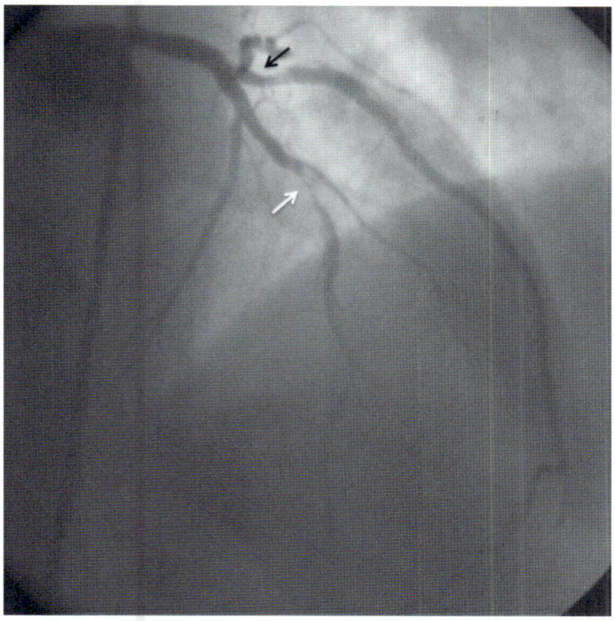

FIGURE 6.11

Cranial projection demonstrating the subocclusive stenosis of the mid-LAD (white arrow) and stenosis of proximal RI (black arrow). (LOOP 6.11)

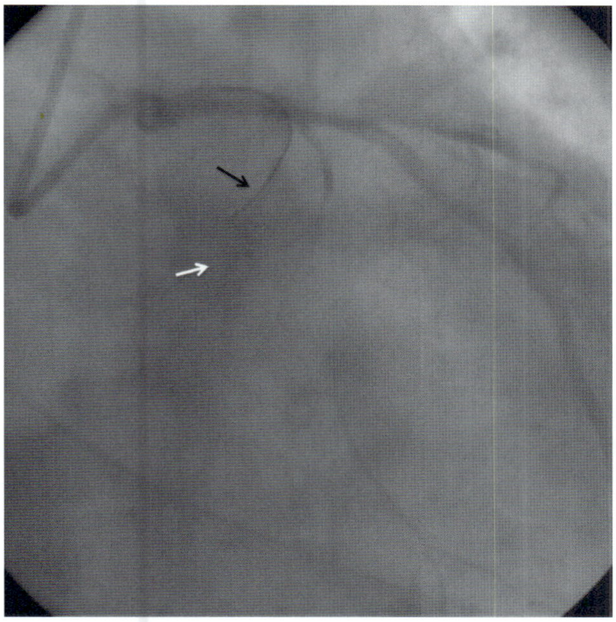

FIGURE 6.12

During recanalization of the LCX occlusion with over-the-wire balloon and Athlete Intermediate wire, the wire exited from the vessel (black arrow) and resulted in contrast extravasation (white arrow). (LOOP 6.12)

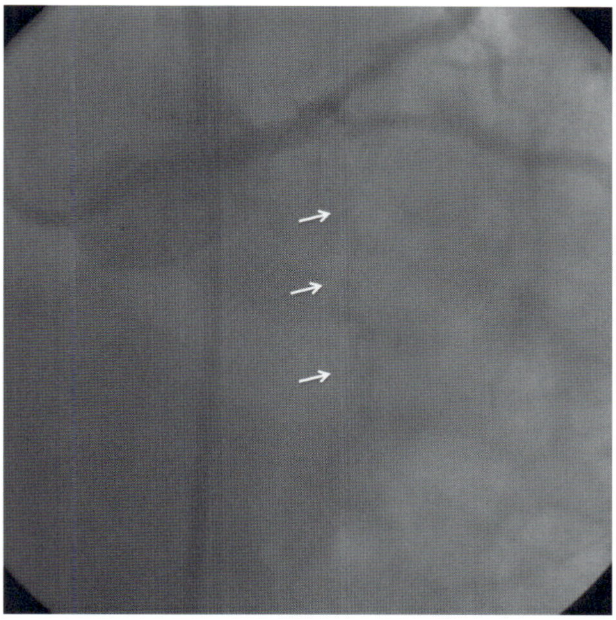

FIGURE 6.13

Grade-3 wire perforation (arrows) with localized hematoma near the proximal LCX. (LOOP 6.13)

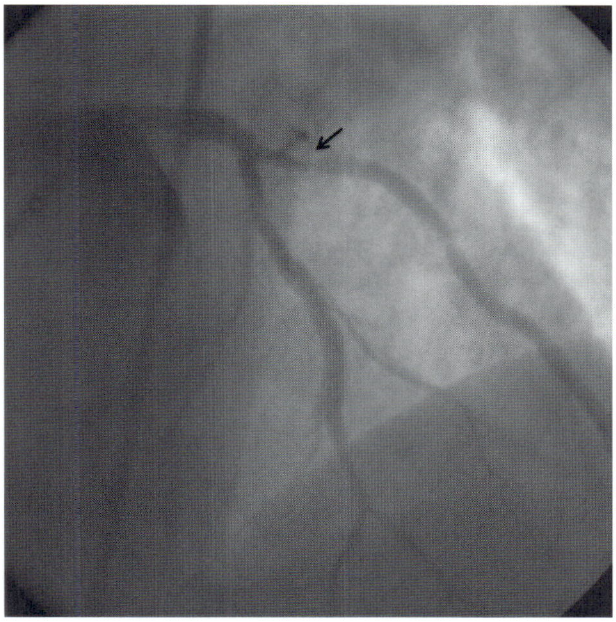

FIGURE 6.14

As the patient remained stable, the operator decided to stent the proximal lesion in the RI branch (arrow) with a Taxus stent (3.0 × 16 mm at 18 atm). (LOOP 6.14)

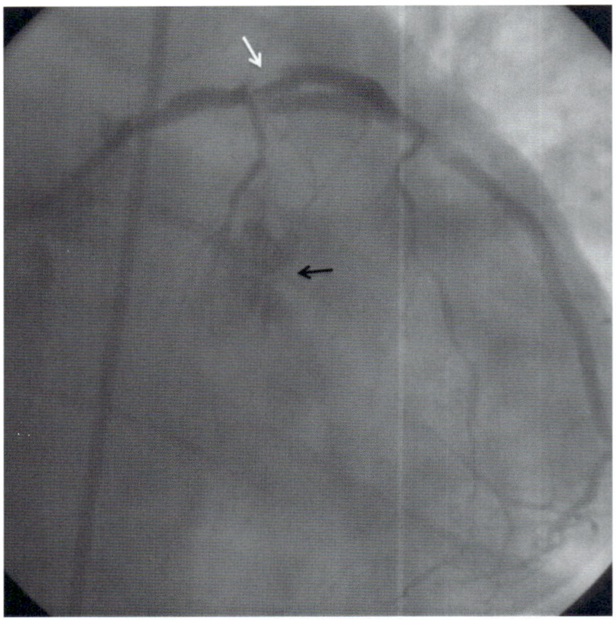

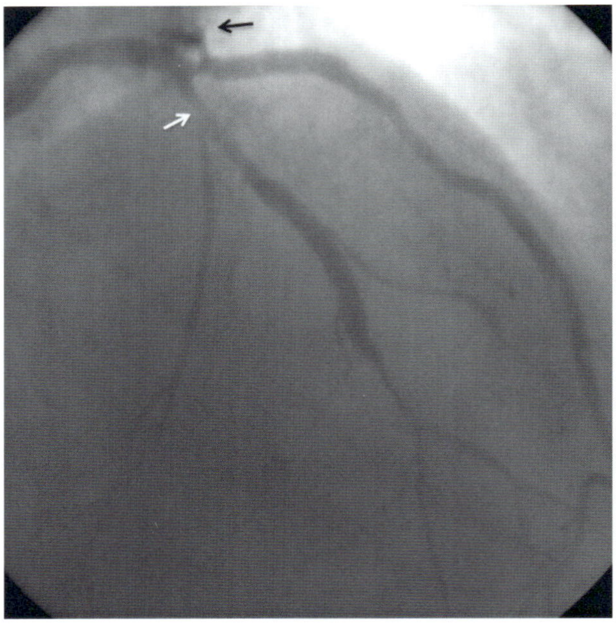

FIGURES 6.15 AND 6.16

Following successful stenting of the proximal RI branch (not the ostium), an ostial narrowing of the LAD appeared (white arrows). Continued extravasation from the LCX wire perforation is also evident (black arrows) (LOOPS 6.15 AND 6.16)

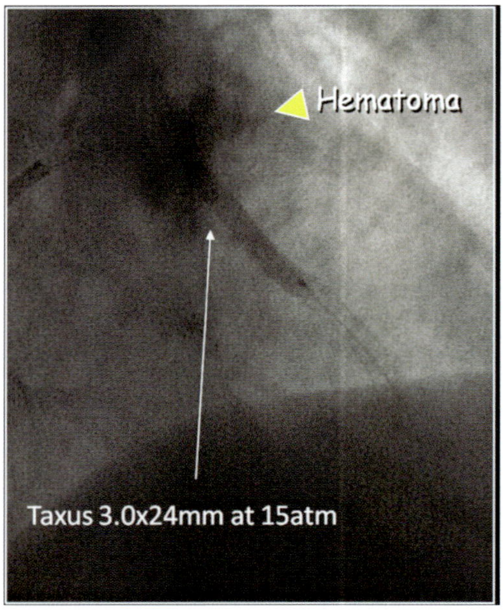

FIGURE 6.17

A hematoma (arrowhead) near the LCX was compressing the LAD ostium, which was stented with a Taxus 3 × 24 mm at 15 atm. (LOOP 6.17)

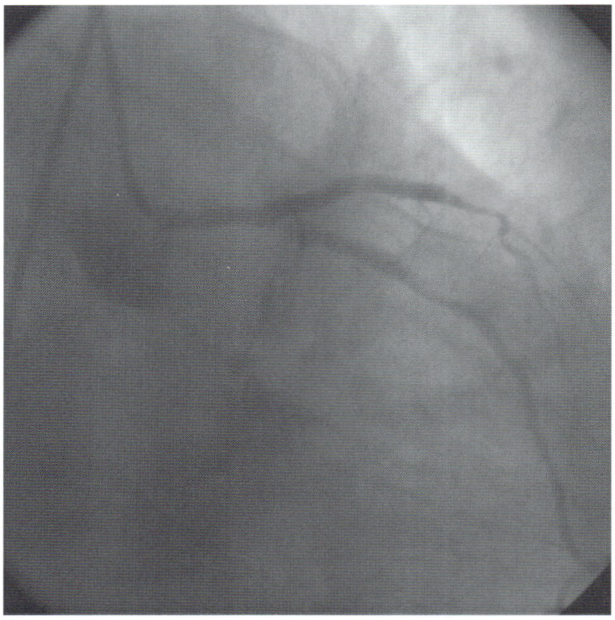

FIGURE 6.18

Angiography demonstrating a good angiographic result at the LAD ostium but continued extravasation from the LCX with an enlarging hematoma. (LOOP 6.18)

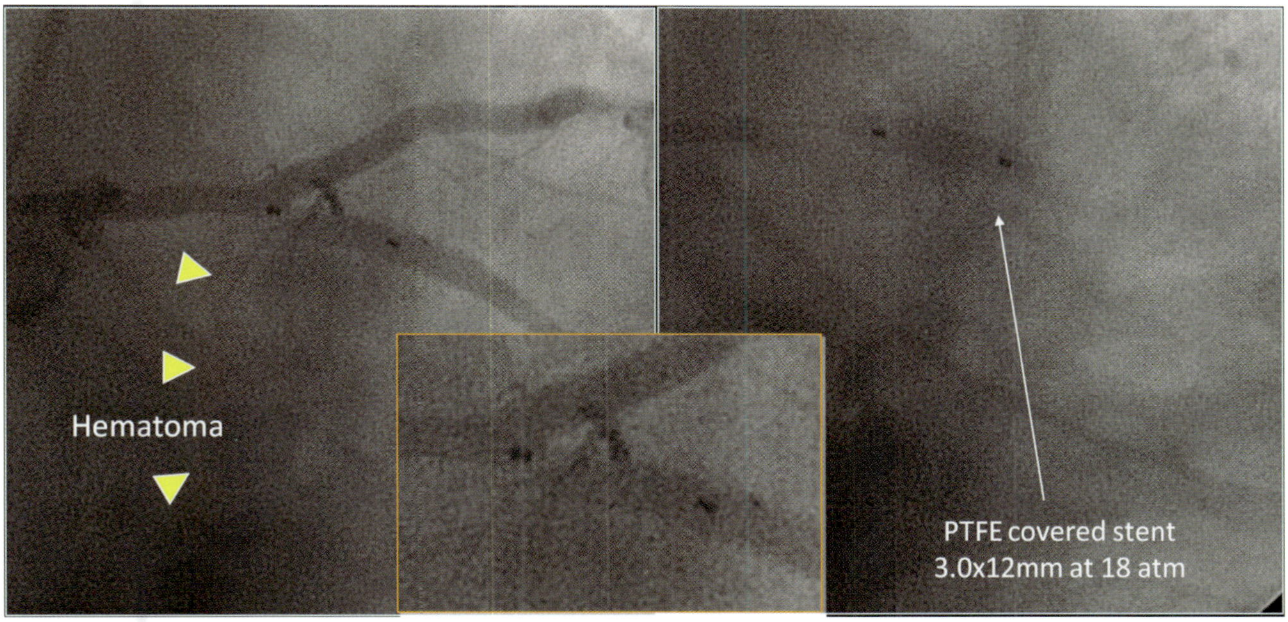

FIGURE 6.19

Implantation a 3 × 12 mm PTFE-covered stent at the ostium of the RI to exclude the very proximal LCX from which the hematoma (yellow arrowheads) was originating. (LOOP 6.19)

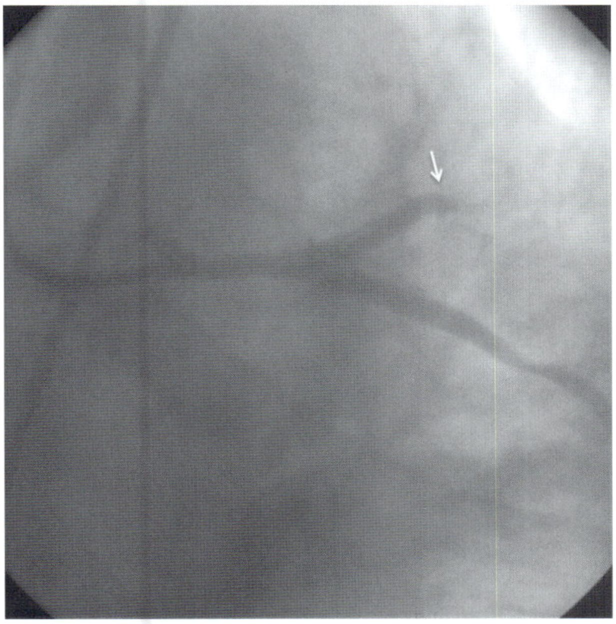

FIGURE 6.20

Slow flow in the LAD (arrow) immediately after placement of the PTFE stent. (LOOP 6.20)

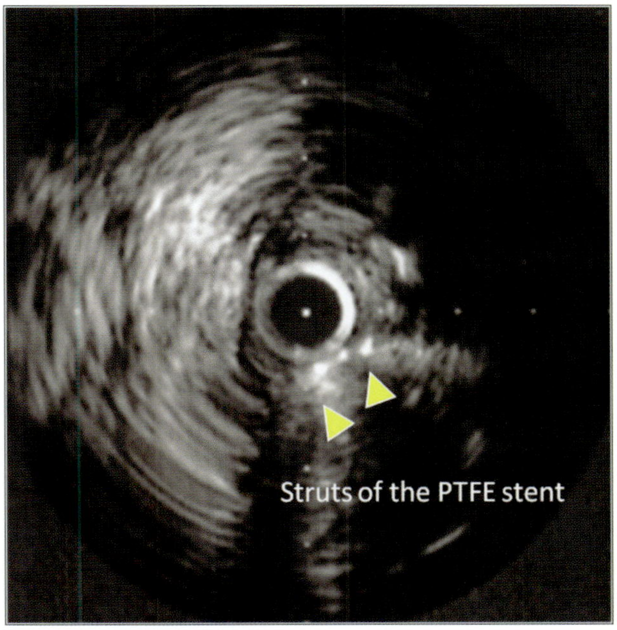

FIGURE 6.21

IVUS interrogation confirmed that the compromised flow in the LAD was due to struts of the PTFE stent (arrowheads) protruding into the ostium of the LAD. (LOOP 6.21)

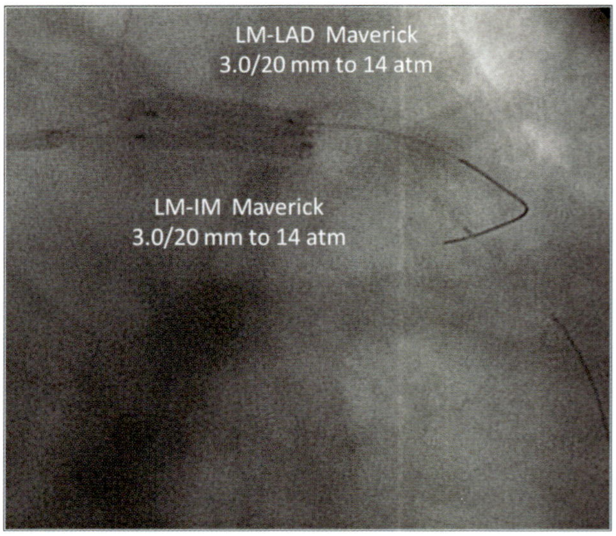

FIGURE 6.22

Kissing-balloon inflation from the LM to LAD and LM to RI. (LOOP 6.22)

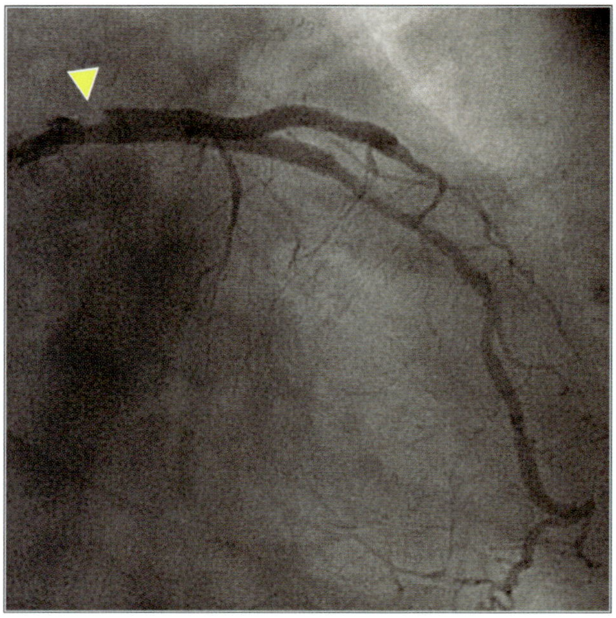

FIGURE 6.23

The kissing-balloon inflation was complicated by a linear dissection of the LM. (LOOP 6.23)

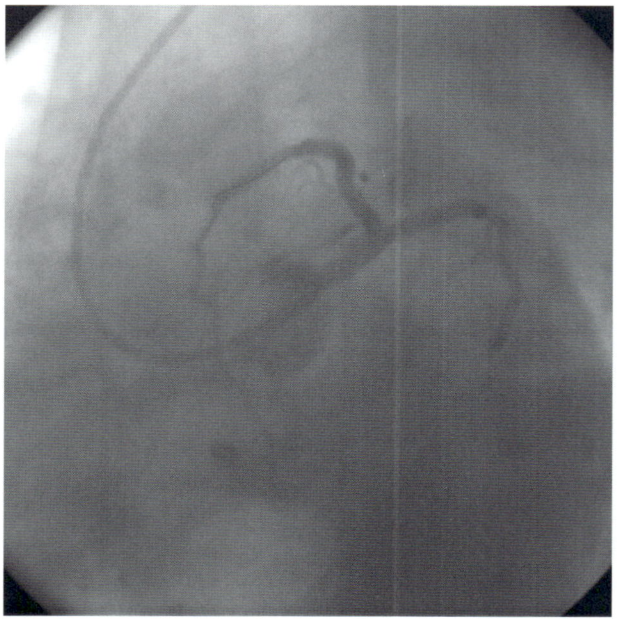

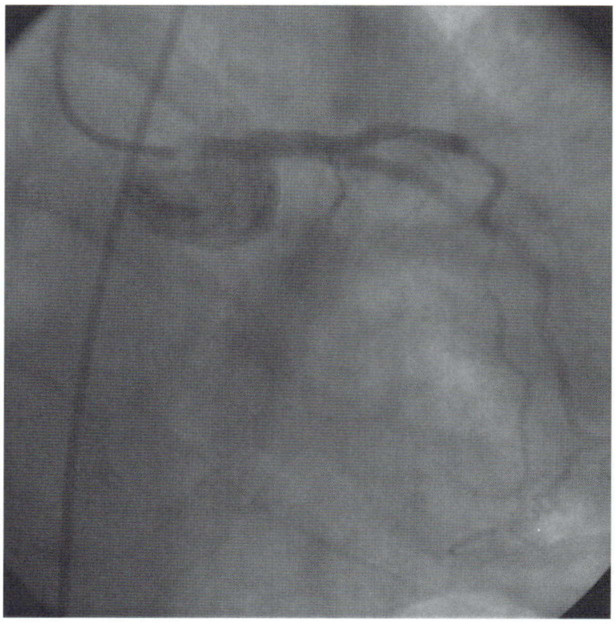

FIGURES 6.24 AND 6.25

Final angiography after stenting of the LM confirming a good result of stenting of the LM, RI, and LAD with complete sealing of the perforation. (LOOPS 6.24 AND 6.25)

CASE ANALYSIS

The perforation in this case was caused by wire exit during CTO recanalization. Wire exits occur mostly without sequelae, but the fact that this patient was on glycoprotein 2b/3a inhibitors probably worsened the perforation and subsequent bleeding. This complication may have been prevented by not administrating glycoprotein 2b/3a inhibitors prior to attempting CTO recanalization. However, the most important mistake in this case was continuing the procedure after the complication had occurred. All subsequent complications could have been avoided by rescheduling PCI on the other lesions.

LESSONS

- Never administer a glycoprotein 2b/3a inhibitor prior to CTO recanalization.
- If a complication occurs during PCI, efforts should be directed at managing the complication. No additional elective interventions should be performed in the same setting.
- Although cardiac tamponade is the immediate concern in the setting of a coronary perforation, the operator should keep in mind the possibility of epicardial hematoma that may compress other vessels or even cardiac chambers.
- One way to seal a distal perforation is to exclude the feeding vessel with a PTFE stent placed in the main vessel toward a side branch.
- When implanting a stent (in particular, a covered stent) at a bifurcation, consider placing a protective standby balloon at the ostium of the other branch.

CASE 6.3

Coronary Perforation Because of False Lumen Dilatation

CLINICAL HISTORY AND DIAGNOSTIC TESTING RESULTS

An 80-year-old woman with known hypertension, dyslipidemia, and chronic renal insufficiency presented with effort-induced angina (CCS III) and strongly positive exercise test. Coronary angiography revealed critical stenosis of ostial and proximal RCA, as well as multiple CTOs of the mid LAD, proximal LCX, and large posterior left (PL) branch. She underwent PCI with implantation of Promus everolimus-eluting stents (Boston Scientific, Natick, MA) on the ostium and proximal RCA a month before the current procedure.

PLANNED PROCEDURE

Recanalization of proximal LCX CTO.

PROCEDURE

The patient had been taking clopidogrel and aspirin since the last procedure and was given an intravenous unfractionated heparin bolus for the current procedure. Baseline angiography showed CTO of the LCX collateralized by ipsilateral and bridging collaterals, with a bifurcation at the distal occlusion site (Figure 6.26). The CTO was approached with a Miracle 3-g guidewire (Asahi Intecc Co Ltd, Nagoya, Japan/Abbott Vascular Devices, Redwood City, CA) with the support of 1.25-mm × 6-mm over-the-wire balloon. The CTO was successfully crossed with the guidewire that was positioned distally in the true lumen of the lower obtuse marginal (OM) branch (Figure 6.27). Predilatation was performed first with the 1.25-mm balloon and then with a 2- × 20-mm semicompliant balloon to a maximum of 12 atm.

COMPLICATION AND MANAGEMENT

Post-predilatation angiography demonstrated a Grade-3 coronary perforation of the proximal segment of the lower OM branch (Figure 6.28). The perforation was contained in the myocardium, as evidenced by the myocardial contrast staining, resulting in an intramural hematoma. Echocardiography confirmed the absence of a pericardial effusion. A BMW Universal II guidewire was then placed in the larger upper OM branch and prolonged balloon inflation was performed with a 2.5- × 30-mm Maverick balloon across the ostium of the perforated branch (Figure 6.29). Angiography showed that extravasation from the lower OM branch was controlled, and thus PCI on the CTO was completed (Figure 6.30). Two (2.5 × 28 and 2.25 × 23 mm) overlapping Cypher sirolimus-eluting stents (Cordis Corp, Johnson & Johnson, Warren, NJ) were implanted from the proximal LCX to the large OM branch, with good angiographic result, but extravasation from the perforation appeared to have increased (Figure 6.31). Although the patient was hemodynamically stable and there was no evidence of pericardial effusion, we were concerned that continued extravasation could result in compression of other cardiac structures. Thus, we recrossed the stent struts and performed prolonged balloon inflation at the perforation site with a 1.5- × 20-mm balloon (Figure 6.32). However, this inflation seemed to worsen the perforation (Figure 6.33). We attempted to deliver a 2.5- × 13-mm covered stent (InSitu Direct-Stent®) to the perforation site, but it did not cross the previously implanted stent in the OM branch. We considered, but opted not to pursue, placing a covered stent across the perforated side branch due to the increased risk of restenosis and stent thrombosis. Alternatively, we introduced a microcatheter into the branch and deployed a 3- × 23-mm Vortex diamond-shaped platinum coil (Boston Scientific, Natick, MA) with complete occlusion of the branch and perforation (Figure 6.34).

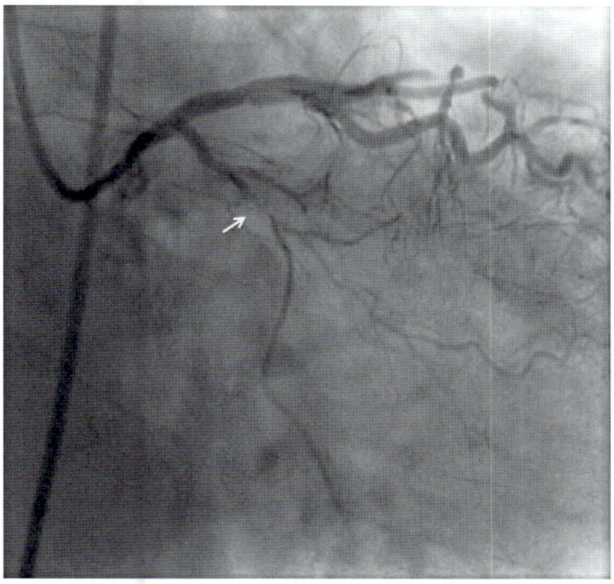

FIGURE 6.26

Baseline angiography demonstrating the target lesion (arrow): A CTO of the LCX collateralized by ipsilateral and bridging collaterals, with a bifurcation at the distal occlusion site. **(LOOP 6.26)**

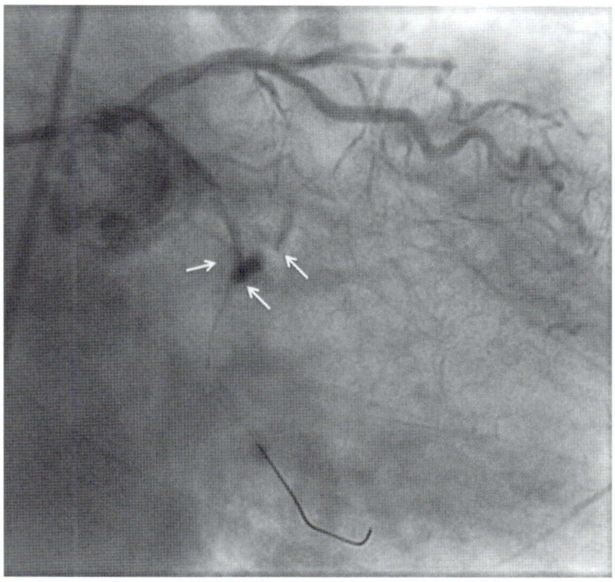

FIGURE 6.28

Angiography after predilatation demonstrated a Grade-3 coronary perforation of the proximal segment of the lower OM branch (arrows). **(LOOP 6.28)**

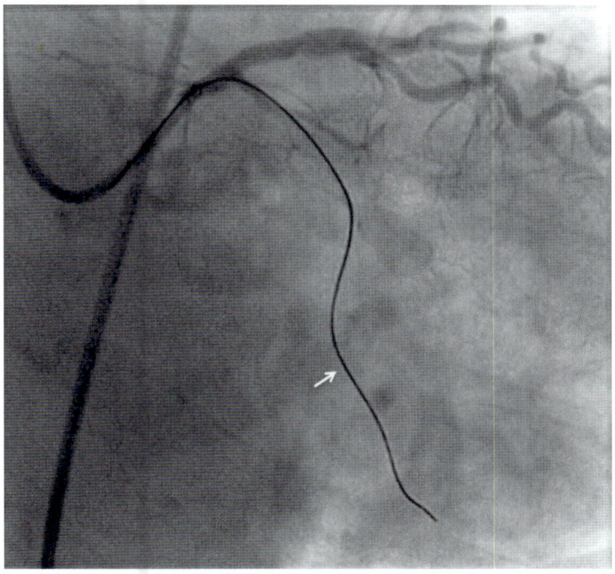

FIGURE 6.27

The CTO was successfully crossed with a Miracle 3-g guidewire, which was placed distally in the true lumen of the lower OM branch (arrow). **(LOOP 6.27)**

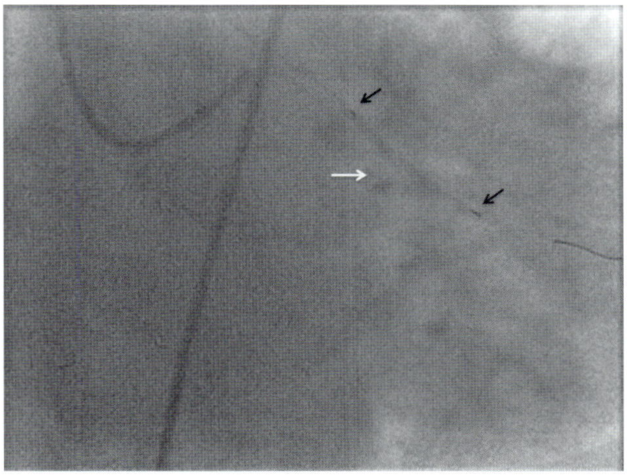

FIGURE 6.29

A guidewire was placed in the larger upper OM branch and prolonged balloon inflation with a 2.5- × 30-mm Maverick balloon (black arrows) was performed across the ostium (white arrow) of the perforated branch. **(LOOP 6.29)**

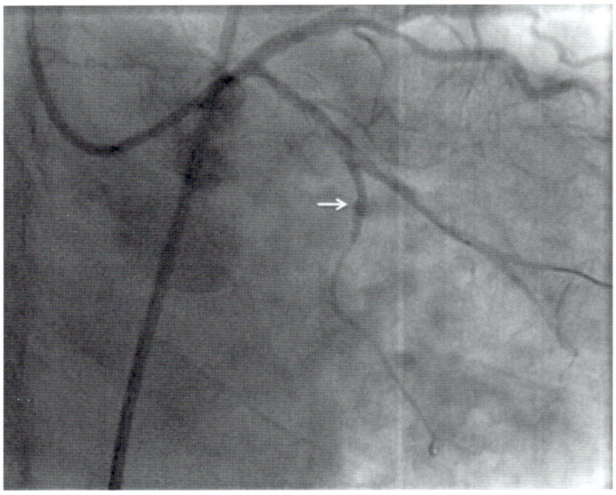

FIGURE 6.30

Angiography after prolonged balloon inflation showed that extravasation from the lower OM branch (arrow) was controlled, and thus PCI was continued (LOOP 6.30)

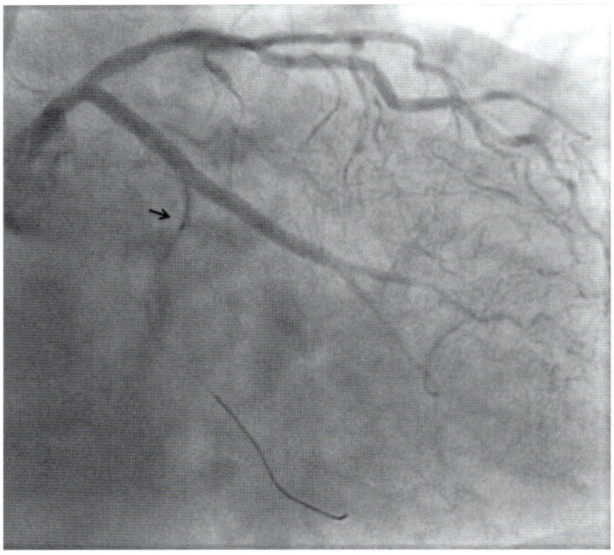

FIGURE 6.32

The stent struts in the upper OM branch were recrossed and prolonged balloon inflation at the perforation site with a 1.5- × 20-mm balloon (arrow) was performed. (LOOP 6.32)

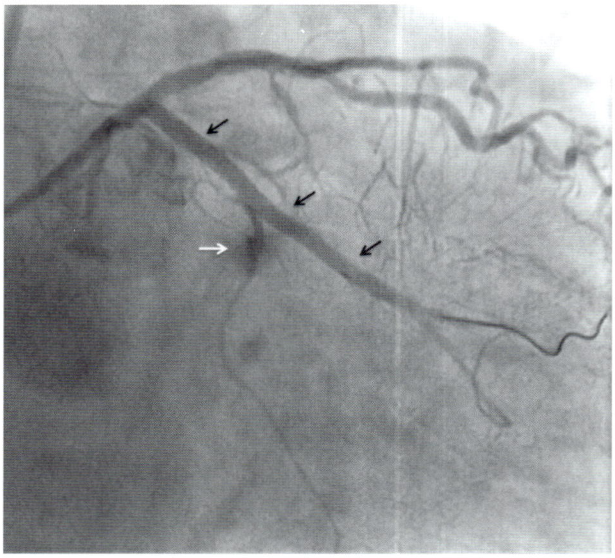

FIGURE 6.31

Two overlapping Cypher (2.5 × 28 mm and 2.25 × 23 mm) stents were implanted from the proximal LCX toward the larger upper OM branch with a good angiographic result (black arrows), but increased extravasation from the lower OM branch also became evident (white arrow). (LOOP 6.31)

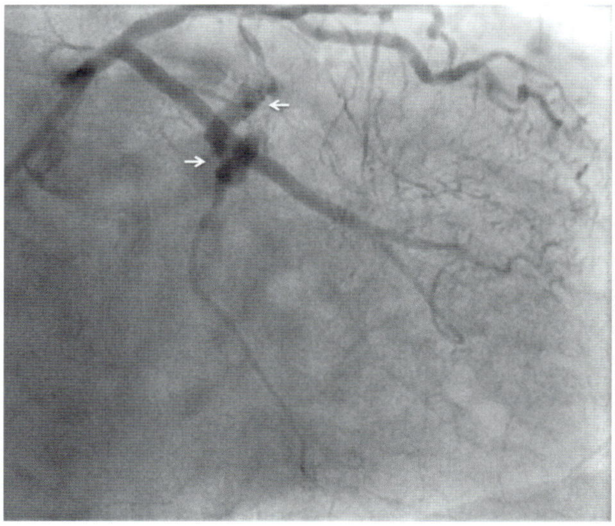

FIGURE 6.33

Balloon inflation did not result in sealing of the perforation but appeared to worsen extravasation from the perforation (arrows). (LOOP 6.33)

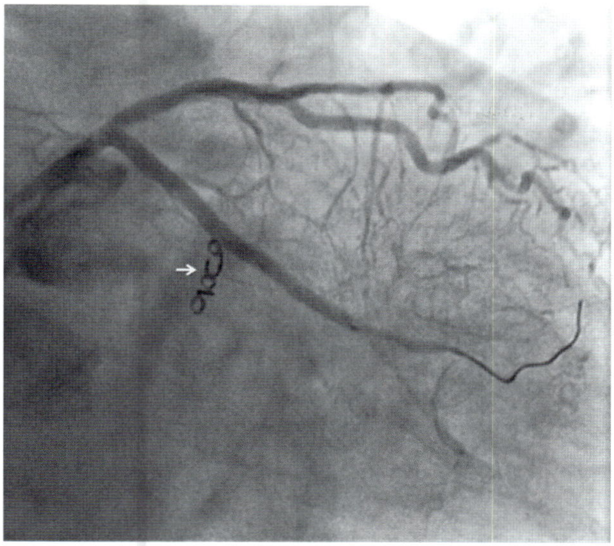

FIGURE 6.34

Coil embolization of the lower OM branch (arrow) resulted in sealing of the perforation. (LOOP 6.34)

CASE ANALYSIS

Balloon dilatation within the false lumen of a recanalized CTO can cause vessel perforation, even if the guidewire is in the distal true lumen. To avoid this complication, we always perform sequential balloon predilatations beginning with undersized balloons, especially when utilizing CTO techniques such as the subintimal tracking and reentry. However, as in this case, even careful predilatation may not prevent a perforation.

LESSONS

- Coil embolization is a valuable technique to occlude perforated vessels when the perforation is located in a distal segment of the vessel or side branch.
- Coil size should be slightly larger than the vessel diameter to prevent dislodgement or migration of the coil.
- Coil embolization is not recommended when the perforation is located in the proximal segment of a vessel.

CASE 6.4

Wire-Induced Coronary Perforation

CLINICAL HISTORY AND DIAGNOSTIC TESTING RESULTS

A 67-year-old man with a history of hypertension and dyslipidemia underwent coronary angiography for exertional angina. Coronary angiography demonstrated critical stenosis of the distal left main coronary artery (LMCA), severe calcific stenosis of the proximal LAD, diffuse disease of mid-LAD, and severe stenosis of the distal RCA extending into the proximal posterior descending artery (PDA) (Figures 6.35 and 6.36).

PLANNED PROCEDURE

Multivessel PCI with drug-eluting stents.

PROCEDURE

The patient was already pretreated with aspirin and clopidogrel, and unfractionated heparin was administered intravenously. An intraaortic balloon pump was electively inserted via the left femoral artery. PCI on the RCA was performed, with implantation of a Cypher 3.5- × 33-mm stent from the distal RCA to the PDA. Subsequently, an 8-Fr XB-4 guiding catheter was utilized to cannulate the left coronary artery. A Whisper guidewire (Abbott Vascular Devices, Redwood City, CA) was placed in the distal LAD, and the LMCA and proximal LAD were predilated. A 3.5- × 33-mm Cypher stent was implanted from the LMCA to LAD (Figure 6.37), with a good angiographic result (Figure 6.38). The stent was postdilated with a 3.5- × 13-mm noncompliant balloon at 20 atm.

COMPLICATION AND MANAGEMENT

Poststent dilatation coronary angiography demonstrated a Grade-3 guidewire perforation of the distal LAD with intramyocardial staining (Figure 6.39). The patient was hemodynamically stable with no evidence of cardiac tamponade on echocardiography. We continued to monitor the patient in the catheterization laboratory for the next 15 to 20 minutes, and he continued to remain stable with no evidence of increase in the size of the perforation or myocardial staining (Figure 6.40). So, we ended the procedure, and the patient was transferred to be monitored in the recovery room. After 15 minutes, the patient became hypotensive and appeared to be in cardiogenic shock. The patient was immediately transferred back to the catheterization laboratory. Echocardiography confirmed

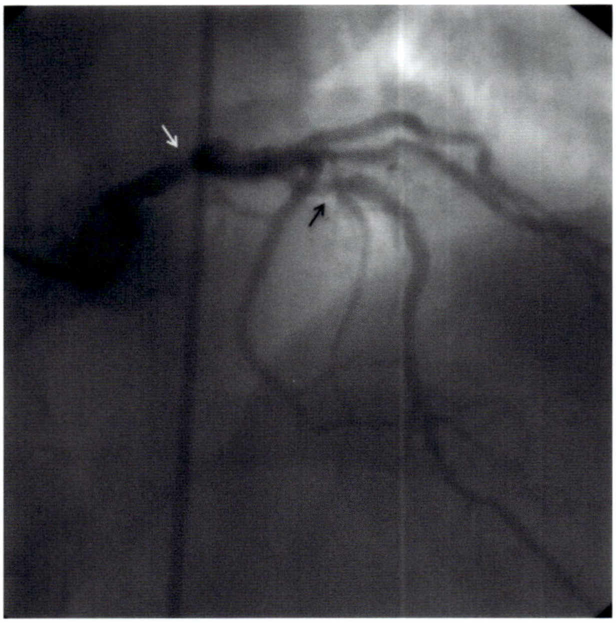

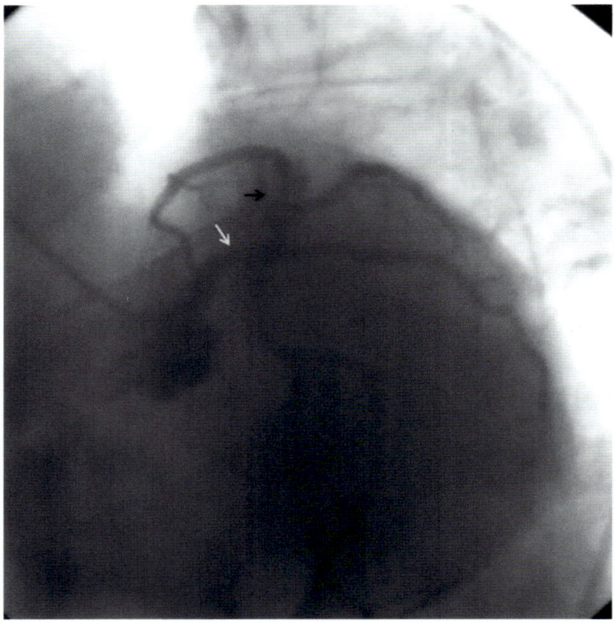

FIGURES 6.35 AND 6.36

Baseline angiography demonstrating a critical stenosis of the distal LMCA (white arrow) and a severe calcific stenosis of the proximal LAD (black arrow). (LOOPS 6.35 AND 6.36)

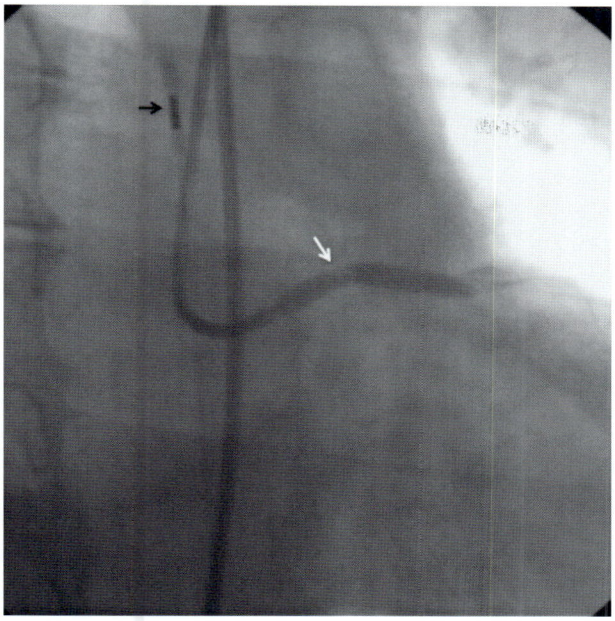

FIGURE 6.37

Implantation of a 3.5- × 33-mm Cypher stent from the LMCA to LAD (white arrow). The intraaortic balloon pump that was placed electively is also visible (black arrow). (LOOP 6.37)

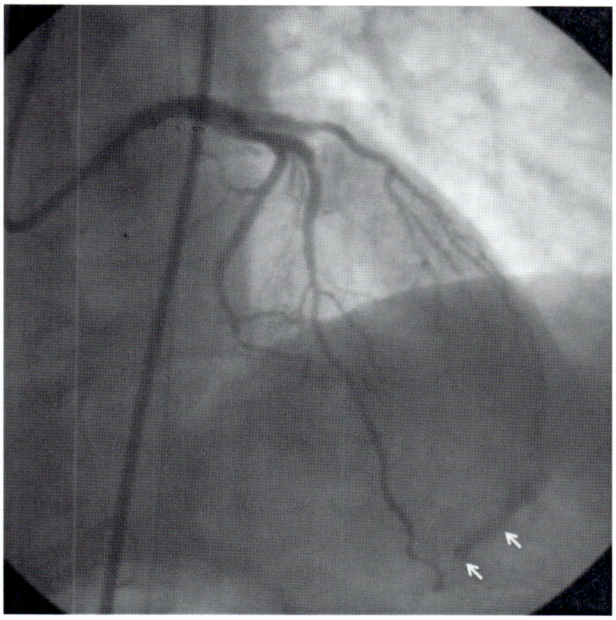

FIGURE 6.39

Angiography demonstrating a Grade-3 guidewire perforation of the distal LAD with intramyocardial staining (arrows). (LOOP 6.39)

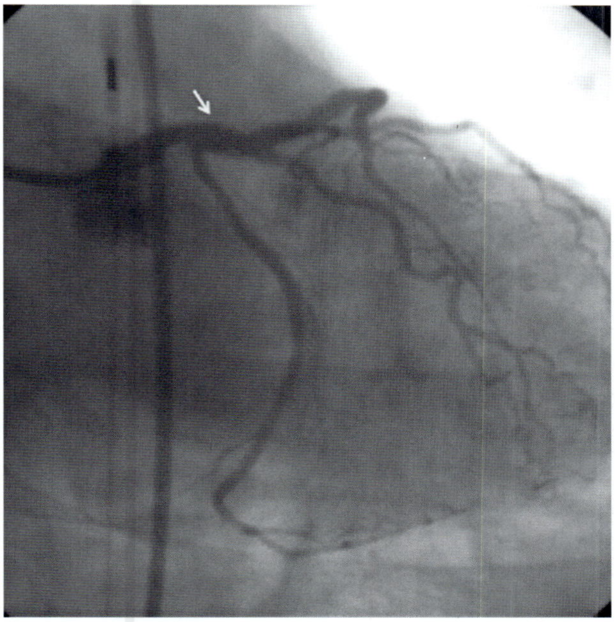

FIGURE 6.38

Angiography confirming good result of LM-LAD stenting (arrow). (LOOP 6.38)

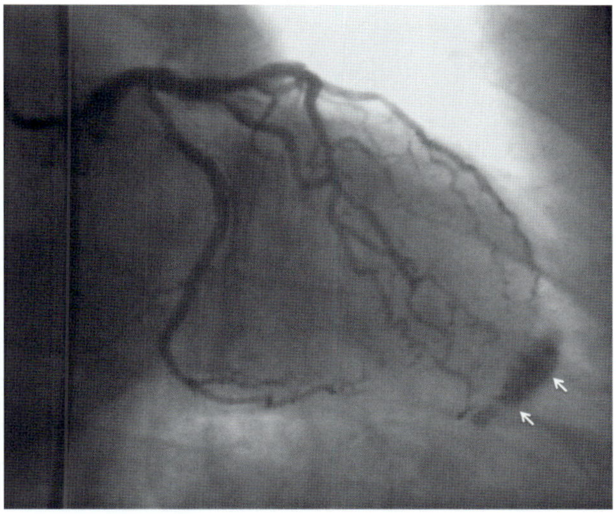

FIGURE 6.40

Angiography performed after 20 minutes of hemodynamic stability confirmed that there was no further contrast extravasation or increase in intramyocardial staining. (LOOP 6.40) a large pericardial effusion with cardiac tamponade. Immediate pericardiocentesis was performed, and 500 cc of frank blood was drained from the pericardium. Coronary angiography showed that the distal perforation had worsened, and contrast was now extravasating into the pericardial space (Figure 6.41). We thought that it would be unlikely that this perforation would resolve with prolonged balloon inflation. We thus decided to perform microparticle embolization of the distal LAD in order to control the perforation. A microcatheter was placed in the distal LAD, and 300 μm polyvinyl alcohol microparticles (Boston Scientific, Natick, MA) were injected into the distal LAD (Figure 6.42). Also, protamine was administered to reverse the anticoagulant effects of heparin and ensure thrombotic occlusion of the embolized distal segment of the LAD. Repeat angiography confirmed occlusion of the distal LAD and sealing of the perforation with slow flow (Figure 6.43). There was evidence of anterior myocardial ischemia after 5 minutes, and the coronary angiogram revealed large filling defects inside the stent (Figure 6.44). We readministered heparin and performed thrombus aspiration and balloon dilatation. After repeated balloon dilatations, coronary angiography confirmed stent patency and absence of distal extravasation (Figure 6.45), and the patient stabilized without evidence of ongoing ischemia.

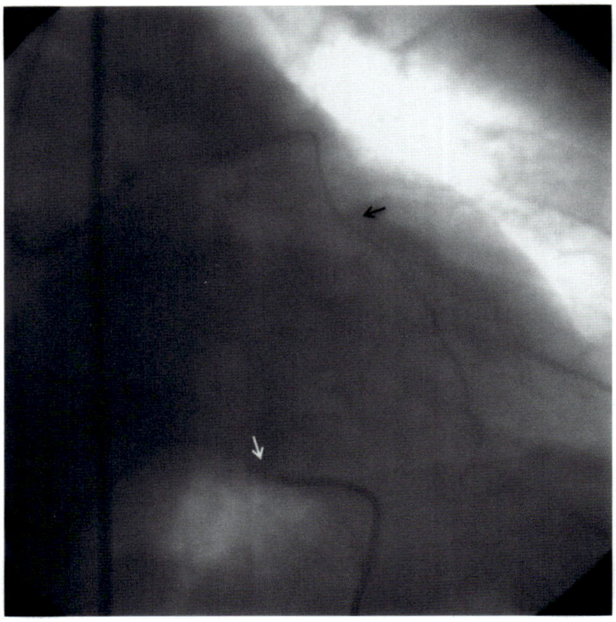

FIGURE 6.42

A microcatheter was placed in the distal LAD and 300-μm polyvinyl alcohol (PVA) microparticles were injected into the distal LAD (black arrow). A pigtail catheter in the pericardium is also visible (white arrow). (LOOP 6.42)

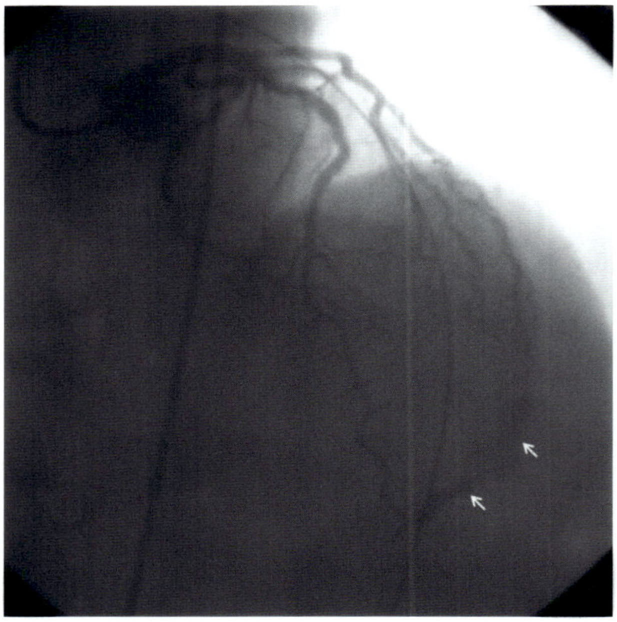

FIGURE 6.41

Angiography performed after the patient underwent pericardiocentesis for cardiac tamponade showed contrast extravasation into the pericardium from the distal wire perforation (arrows). (LOOP 6.41)

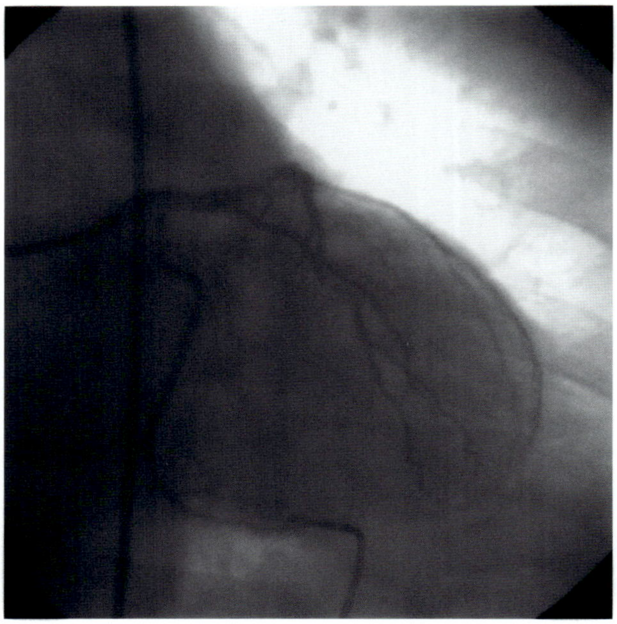

FIGURE 6.43

Angiography performed after microparticle embolization and protamine administration confirmed sealing of the perforation. (LOOP 6.43)

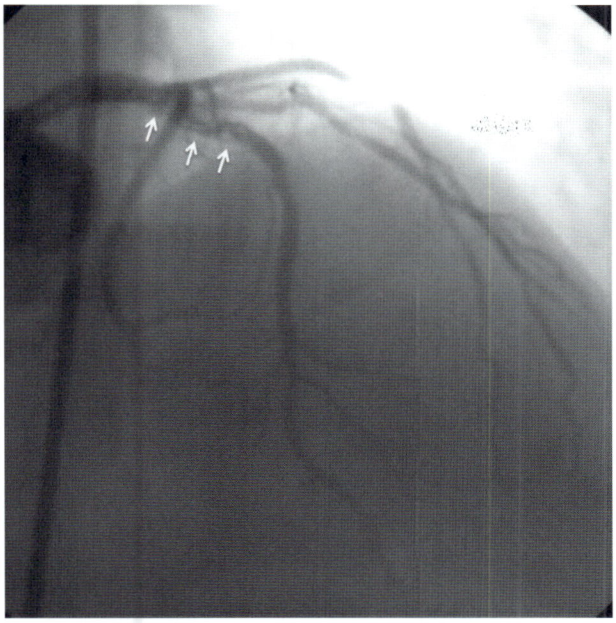

FIGURE 6.44

Multiple in-stent filling defects due to stent thrombosis (arrows). (LOOP 6.44)

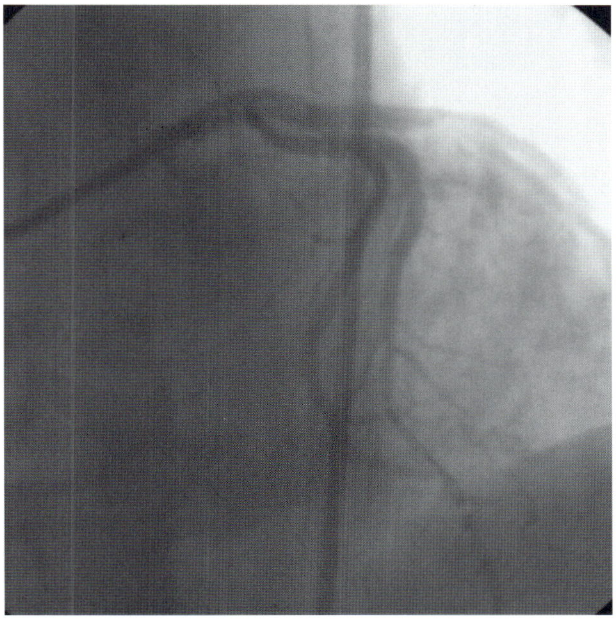

FIGURE 6.45

Final angiography after thrombus aspiration and balloon dilatation showing stent patency and absence of distal extravasation. (LOOP 6.45)

CASE ANALYSIS

The distal perforation in this case was caused by the hydrophilic guidewire (Whisper). This complication could have been prevented by exchanging the hydrophilic guidewire for a floppy guidewire. The second complication of acute drug-eluting stent thrombosis was probably caused by the administration of protamine in the setting of slow flow. In patients who have a Grade-3 coronary perforation after drug-eluting stent implantation, the benefits of reversing heparin versus the risks of stent thrombosis after protamine need to be considered.

LESSONS

- Distal perforations are almost always caused by guidewires.
- Hydrophilic guidewires are the most common coronary guidewires associated with distal vessel perforation. If hydrophilic guidewires are used, the operator should always keep the distal end of the guidewire in the angiographic view, especially when advancing or exchanging devices (using less magnification if necessary) and attempt to leave the hydrophilic wire with a loop distally.
- Wire perforations may present with late cardiac tamponade, and patients should be carefully monitored for 24 to 48 hours after the procedure.
- Microparticle or coil embolization is very effective and sometimes the only percutaneous therapeutic solution in resolving wire perforations.
- Protamine administration can be associated with acute drug-eluting stent thrombosis.

CASE 6.5

Coronary Perforation Because of Aggressive Debulking

CLINICAL HISTORY AND DIAGNOSTIC TESTING RESULTS

A 78-year-old man had hypertension, was an ex-smoker, and had myocardial infarction more than 27 years ago. He underwent coronary artery bypass graft (CABG) with a single sequential saphenous vein graft (SVG) to the OM and PL, and presents now with angina on minimal effort and at rest. Coronary angiography demonstrated a severe calcific stenosis of the distal LM, ostial LCX, and ostial LAD and occlusion at the ostium of the SVG with patency of the jump graft segment between the OM and PL (Figures 6.46 and 6.47).

PLANNED PROCEDURE

PCI and rotational atherectomy of the distal LMCA and ostial LCX.

PROCEDURE

The patient was given a bolus of unfractionated heparin and a bolus and infusion of tirofiban. An 8-Fr XB guide catheter was utilized, and a Rota-floppy guidewire was placed in the LCX. Rotablation with a 1.75-mm burr was then performed on the distal LM and LCX/OM bifurcation (Figure 6.48). Then, balloon dilatation of the LCX/OM bifurcation was performed with an FX Minirail 2.5- × 20-mm balloon (Abbott Vascular Devices, Redwood City, CA) first toward the ostial LCX at 12 atm and then toward the proximal LCX at 14 atm (Figure 6.49).

COMPLICATION AND MANAGEMENT

Angiography performed immediately after FX miniRAIL dilatation demonstrated a Grade-3 perforation of the proximal LCX immediately distal to the bifurcation with the OM (Figure 6.50). Immediate balloon inflation was performed with a Maverick 3.0- × 20-mm balloon toward the OM, thus occluding the LCX and confirming sealing of the perforation (Figure 6.51). Repeat angiography showed continued extravasation of contrast, despite prolonged balloon inflation (Figure 6.52). Thus, a 3- × 19-mm PTFE-covered Jostent was implanted at 18 atm from the proximal LCX toward the OM, excluding the mid-to-distal LCX and sealing the perforation (Figure 6.53). A 3.5- × 18-mm and 3- × 8-mm bare-metal stent was then placed on the ostial LAD and LCX, respectively. Final kissing-balloon inflation was performed with two semicompliant balloons: 3.5- × 20-mm (LAD) and 3- × 20-mm (LCX). Final angiography demonstrated a good result at the LAD and LCX ostium with complete sealing of the perforation (Figure 6.54).

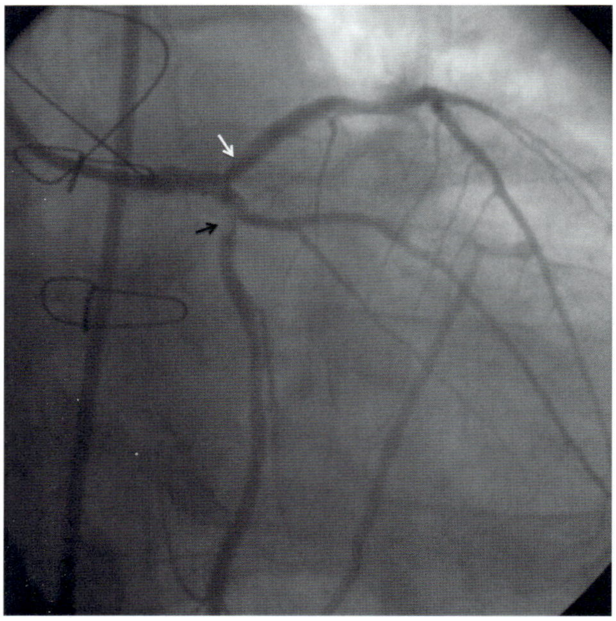

FIGURE 6.46

RAO caudal view showing a severe calcific stenosis of the distal LM, ostial LCX (black arrow), and ostial LAD (white arrow). **(LOOP 6.46)**

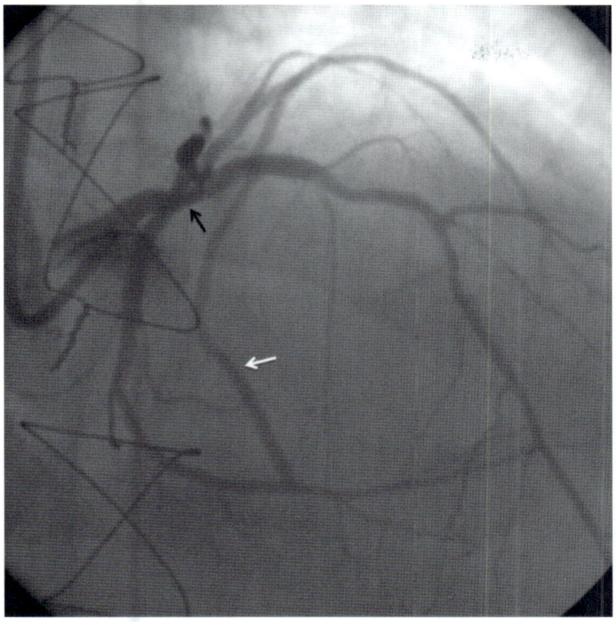

FIGURE 6.47

Cranial view showing stenosis of the distal LM (black arrow) and patency of the jump graft segment between the OM and PL (white arrow). (LOOP 6.47)

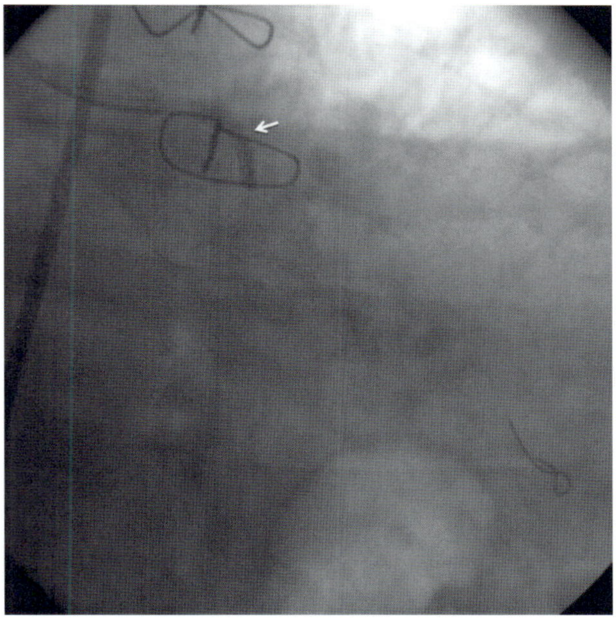

FIGURE 6.49

Balloon dilatation of the proximal LCX with a FX Minirail 2.5- × 20-mm balloon at 14 atm (arrow). (LOOP 6.49)

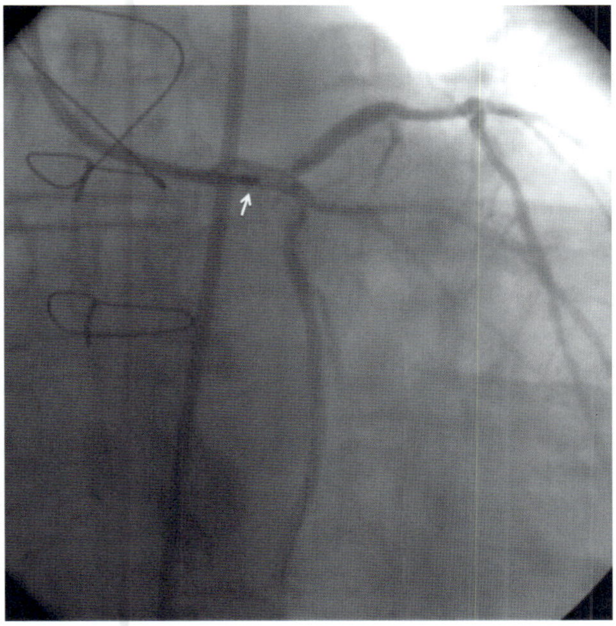

FIGURE 6.48

Rotablation with a 1.75-mm burr (white arrow) performed on the distal LM toward the LCX. (LOOP 6.48)

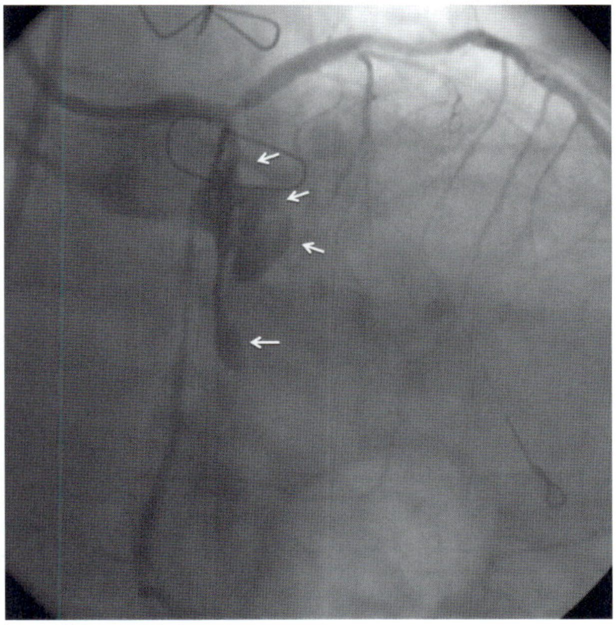

FIGURE 6.50

Grade-3 perforation of the proximal LCX immediately distal to the bifurcation with the OM (arrows). (LOOP 6.50)

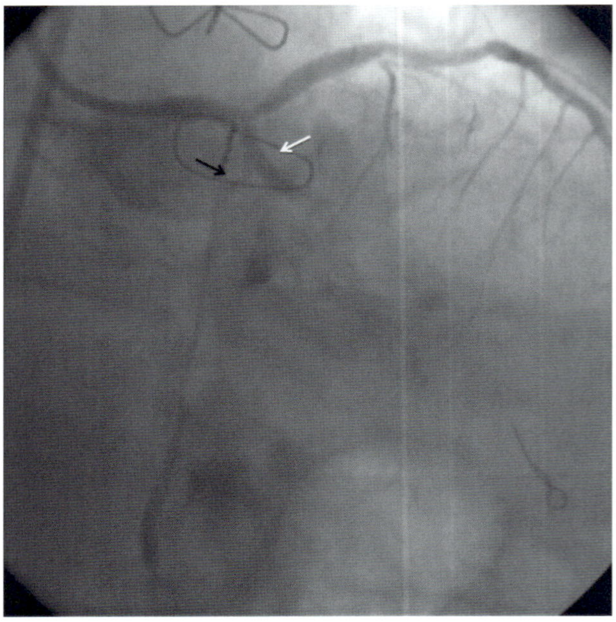

FIGURE 6.51

Balloon inflation with a 3.0- × 20-mm Maverick balloon toward the OM (white arrow), thus occluding the LCX and preventing further extravasation from the perforation (black arrow). (LOOP 6.51)

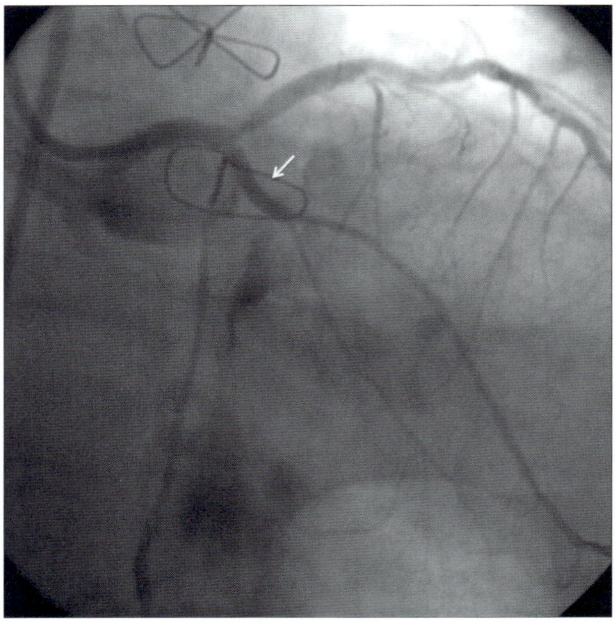

FIGURE 6.53

A 3- × 19-mm PTFE-covered Jostent was implanted from the proximal LCX toward the OM (arrow) to exclude the mid-to-distal LCX and sealing the perforation. (LOOP 6.53)

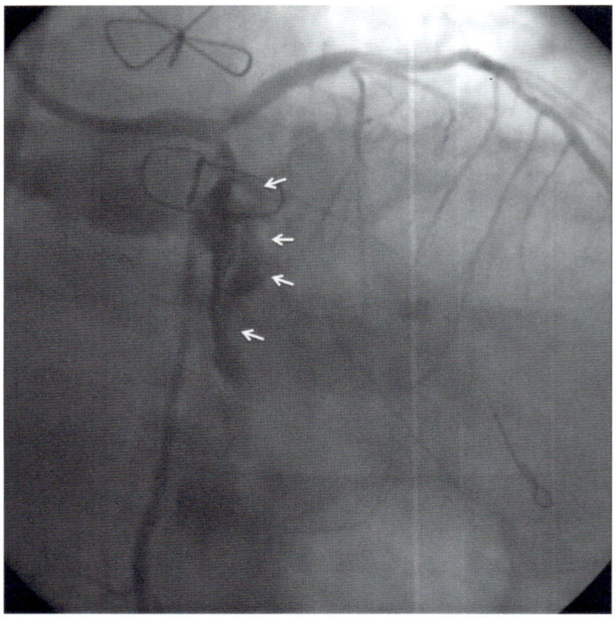

FIGURE 6.52

Repeat angiography after prolonged balloon inflation showing continued extravastion from the perforation site (arrows). (LOOP 6.52)

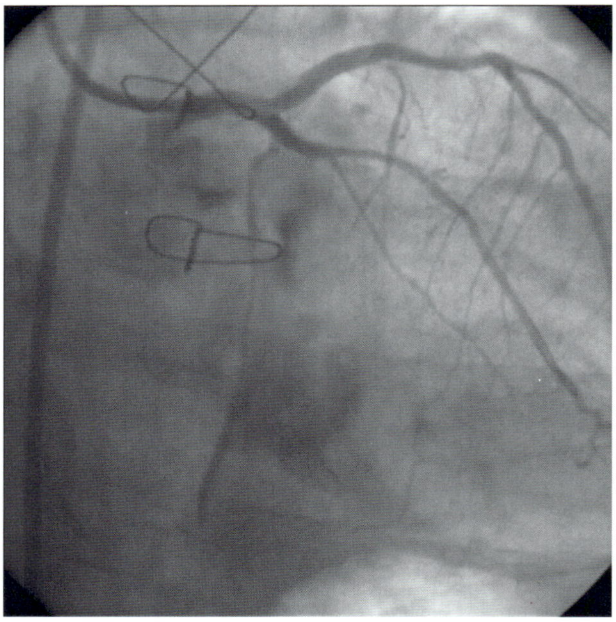

FIGURE 6.54

Final angiography after stent implantation on the LAD and LCX. (LOOP 6.54)

CASE ANALYSIS

The use of a relatively large rotablator burr (1.75 mm) in a calcified lesion on a bend and the use of a second aggressive lesion preparation device (FX Minirail) were probably the factors leading to perforation in this case.

LESSONS

- Calcified, angulated lesions involving a bifurcation in elderly patients are high-risk lesions for coronary perforation.
- In calcified lesions on a bend, it may be more appropriate to start rotational atherectomy with a smaller burr and then increase the size of the burr if necessary.
- Aggressive dilatation should probably be avoided after aggressive rotational atherectomy.
- In perforations involving smaller side branches that do not resolve with prolonged balloon inflation and where it is not possible to deliver a covered stent; excluding the branch using a covered stent placed across the ostium is a valid alternative to sealing the perforation. This technique is generally preferred in smaller side branches that will not result in significant ischemia if occluded. However, this technique can also be used as a stabilizing procedure for larger side branches and then soon after bypassing the occluded vessel.

References

1. Ellis SG, Ajluni S, Arnold AZ, Popma JJ, Bittl JA, Eigler NL, Cowley MJ, Raymond RE, Safian RD, Whitlow PL. Increased coronary perforation in the new device era. Incidence, classification, management, and outcome. *Circulation*. 1994;90(6):2725–2730.
2. Fasseas P, Orford JL, Panetta CJ, Bell MR, Denktas AE, Lennon RJ, Holmes DR, Berger PB. Incidence, correlates, management, and clinical outcome of coronary perforation: analysis of 16,298 procedures. *Am Heart J*. 2004;147(1):140–145.
3. Javaid A, Buch AN, Satler LF, Kent KM, Suddath WO, Lindsay J Jr., Pichard AD, Waksman R. Management and outcomes of coronary artery perforation during percutaneous coronary intervention. *Am J Cardiol*. 2006;98(7):911–914.
4. Stankovic G, Orlic D, Corvaja N, Airoldi F, Chieffo A, Spanos V, Montorfano M, Carlino M, Finci L, Sangiorgi G, Colombo A. Incidence, predictors, in-hospital, and late outcomes of coronary artery perforations. *Am J Cardiol*. 2004;93(2):213–216.
5. Schiele F, Meneveau N. Coronary perforation: incidence, predictive factors, management, and prevention. In: Eeckhout E, Carlier S, Lerman A, Kern M, eds. *Handbook of Complications during Percutaneous Cardiovascular Interventions*: Informa Healthcare; 2007:111–124.
6. Stankovic G, Colombo A. Acute coronary dissection, occlusion, and perforation during percutaneous coronary intervention: surgical, percutaneous, or medical management. In: Martinez EE, Lemos PA, Ong ATL, Serruys PW, eds. *Common Clinical Dilemmas in Percutaneous Coronary Interventions*. London: Informa Healthcare;2007:225–232.
7. Gunning MG, Williams IL, Jewitt DE, Shah AM, Wainwright RJ, Thomas MR. Coronary artery perforation during percutaneous intervention: incidence and outcome. *Heart*. 2002;88(5):495–498.
8. Witzke CF, Martin-Herrero F, Clarke SC, Pomerantzev E, Palacios IF. The changing pattern of coronary perforation during percutaneous coronary intervention in the new device era. *J Invasive Cardiol*. 2004;16(6):257–301.
9. Al-Lamee R, Ielasi A, Latib A, Godino C, Ferraro M, Mussardo M, Arioli F, Carlino M, Montorfano M, Chieffo A, Colombo A. Incidence, predictors, management, immediate and long term outcomes following grade III coronary perforation *JACC Cardiovasc Interv*. 2010;4:96–97.
10. Briguori C, Nishida T, Anzuini A, Di Mario C, Grube E, Colombo A. Emergency polytetrafluoroethylene-covered stent implantation to treat coronary ruptures. *Circulation*. 2000;102(25):3028–3031.
11. Lansky AJ, Yang YM, Khan Y, Costa RA, Pietras C, Tsuchiya Y, Cristea E, Collins M, Mehran R, Dangas GD, Moses JW, Leon MB, Stone GW. Treatment of coronary artery perforations complicating percutaneous coronary intervention with a polytetrafluoroethylene-covered stent graft. *Am J Cardiol*. 2006;98(3):370–374.
12. Ben-Gal Y, Weisz G, Collins MB, Genereux P, Dangas GD, Teirstein PS, Singh VP, Rabbani LE, Kodali SK, Sherman W, Leon MB, Moses JW. Dual catheter technique for the treatment of severe coronary artery perforations. *Catheter Cardiovasc Interv*. 2010;75(5):708–712.
13. Godino C, Sharp AS, Carlino M, Colombo A. Crossing CTOs-the tips, tricks, and specialist kit that can mean the difference between success and failure. *Catheter Cardiovasc Interv*. 2009;74(7):1019–1046.

7

Shilesh Nandish and Steven R. Bailey

Abrupt Coronary Occlusion, Slow Flow, and No Reflow

INTRODUCTION

Abrupt occlusion and no reflow are categorized by diminished, static, or absent flow in the epicardial arteries. This may be due to arterial trauma, such as a dissection or intramural hematoma, thrombus at the lesion site resulting in embolization, either macroscopic or microscopic, or the release of vasoactive substances in the distal vessel causing endothelial swelling and closing arterioles.

Abrupt coronary occlusion is associated with several risk elements that can be categorized as either angiographic factors or predisposing clinical conditions. Angiographic factors include intraluminal thrombus, complex Type B or C lesions, ostial right coronary artery disease, saphenous vein grafts (SVG), and subtotal occlusions. Predisposing clinical conditions include non-ST elevation myocardial infarction (NSTEMI) and unstable angina, advanced age (>80 years), diabetes, and female gender.

The no-reflow phenomenon is the inability to reperfuse a portion of the myocardium after reestablishment of patency with percutaneous treatment of a stenosis or a previously occluded epicardial coronary artery. This is most commonly seen in the setting of high thrombus burden, such as that occurs during primary percutaneous coronary intervention (PCI) for a ST elevation myocardial infarction (STEMI) or SVG interventions. No-reflow phenomenon may be present even if the epicardial coronary artery is fully patent with normal thrombolysis in myocardial infarction stage 3 (TIMI-3) flow at coronary angiography.

No reflow occurs in 0.6% to 2% of all coronary interventions, and this has been primarily associated, as noted above, with treatment of thrombotic lesions (STEMI, NSTEMI, SVGs), atherectomy procedures, and intervention of high plaque volume lesions.

The occurrence of persistent no-reflow is an angiographic marker for worse short-term and late clinical outcomes, including increased postprocedure myocardial infarction and mortality. Patients who are older, with poor left ventricular ejection fraction (LVEF), congestive heart failure (CHF), multivessel disease, unstable angina, and multivessel disease are at increased risk of mortality if this major complication occurs. Suggested approach to acute vessel closure is presented in Flowchart 7.1.

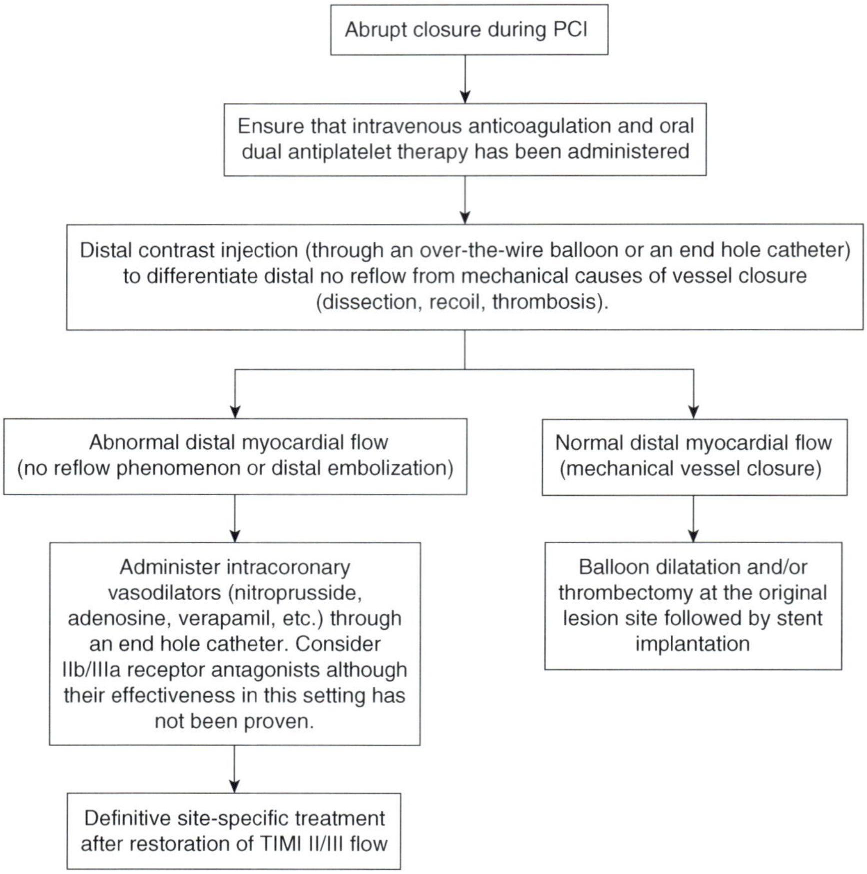

FLOWCHART 7.1
The clinical approach to the evaluation of abrupt closure.

CASE 7.1

Slow Flow After PTCA in a Diffusely Diseased Vessel

CLINICAL HISTORY AND DIAGNOSTIC TESTING RESULTS

A 57-year-old woman with diabetes, hypertension, dyslipidemia, and atherosclerotic heart disease with prior two-vessel coronary artery bypass graft (CABG) followed by PCI to her left circumflex artery (LCX) and obtuse marginal (OM) was admitted previously with NSTEMI. Coronary angiography revealed native three-vessel disease with occluded middle left anterior descending artery (mid-LAD), multiple serial 80%–90% stenoses in the right coronary artery (RCA) and 80% stenosis in the mid-LCX proximal to previously placed stents, with an additional 70% stenosis distally. Graft angiography revealed a patent left internal mammary artery (LIMA) graft to LAD. However, her other SVGs were occluded and were not seen to fill even on aortic root angiography.

Outpatient gated myocardial perfusion single photon emission computed tomography (SPECT) at rest and stress showed anteroseptal, septal, inferior, and lateral wall ischemia, which was consistent with multivessel disease with LVEF of 36% and transient ischemic dilatation of 1.4 with stress.

After 2 months, she returned for planned PCI of her RCA due to intermittent Class-3 exertional angina, despite being on optimum medical therapy. Her physical examination was unremarkable, and laboratory data were within normal limits.

PLANNED PROCEDURE

Plain old balloon angioplasty (POBA) and stent of middle and distal RCA.

PROCEDURE

Patient was pretreated with acetylsalicylic acid (ASA) and reloaded with Plavix 300 mg the evening before the procedure. A 6-Fr JR4 guide catheter was used to selectively engage the RCA. Angiography revealed a subtotal RCA occlusion with long serial stenoses involving the proximal, middle, and distal segments (Figure 7.1). A 0.014-inch × 300-cm Asahi soft guidewire was used to cross the lesions, and the distal wire tip was placed in a posterior descending artery branch. An intravascular intrasound (IVUS) catheter could not be advanced across the lesion. Following this, the entire vessel was predilated with a 2-mm × 30-mm balloon at 6 atm, sequentially (Figure 7.2).

COMPLICATION AND MANAGEMENT

After percutaneous transluminal coronary angioplasty (PTCA) there was no reflow due to dissection in proximal segment with chest pain and inferior ST elevation (Figure 7.3). Distal RCA flow was reestablished with repeat PTCA in the proximal/middle segments and administration of intracoronary adenosine and nitroprusside delivered distally through an over the wire balloon (Figure 7.4). Despite pharmacologic therapy, flow remained limited, and evaluation of the angiogram demonstrated the presence of proximal and distal coronary dissections (Figure 7.5). The RCA was treated with overlapping stents. An Endeavor 2.5- × 30-mm drug-eluting stent (DES) was placed distally at 16 atm, a Resolute 3- × 38-mm in the mid-segment at 18 atm, followed by a second Resolute 3- × 38-mm stent in the proximal segment to the ostium at 20 atm for a total of three stents placed and dilation of the overlap segments (Figure 7.6). Poststent, there was excellent angiographic results with TIMI 3 flow and good myocardial perfusion (Figure 7.7). A small right ventricular (RV) branch was jailed, with loss of flow with an unsuccessful attempt to recross with a 0.014-inch × 185-cm Kinetix guidewire.

Poststent, IVUS with Volcano Eagle Eye catheter revealed good apposition of the stent to the vessel wall, and no dissection or thrombus was noted.

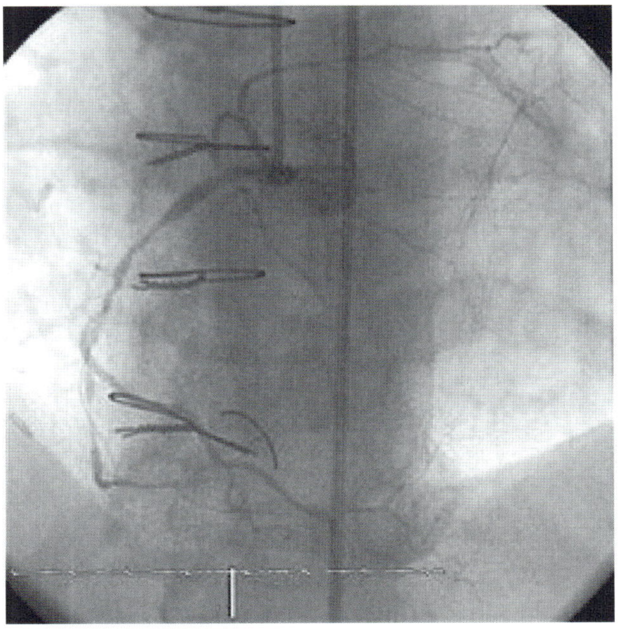

FIGURE 7.1
Base coronary angiography of the RCA.

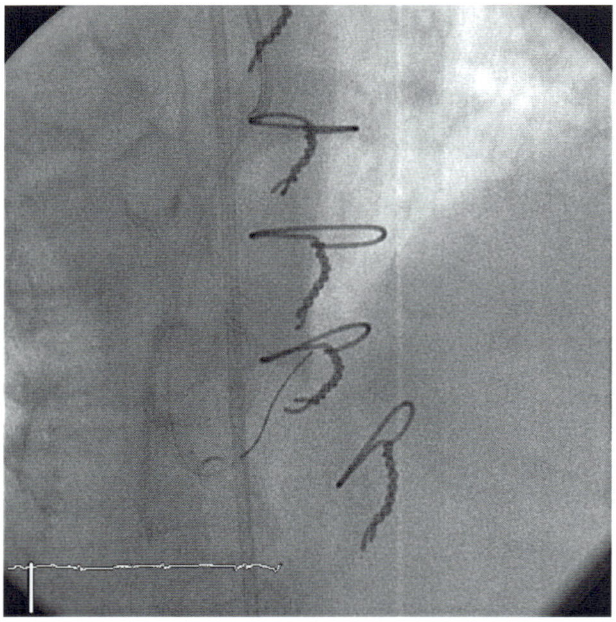

FIGURE 7.2
RCA dissection after balloon predilatation.

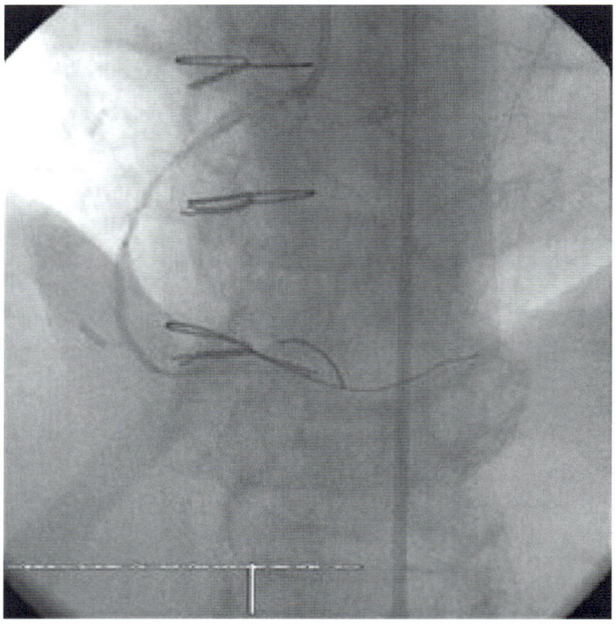

FIGURE 7.4
Post-IC nitroprusside and balloon angioplasty.

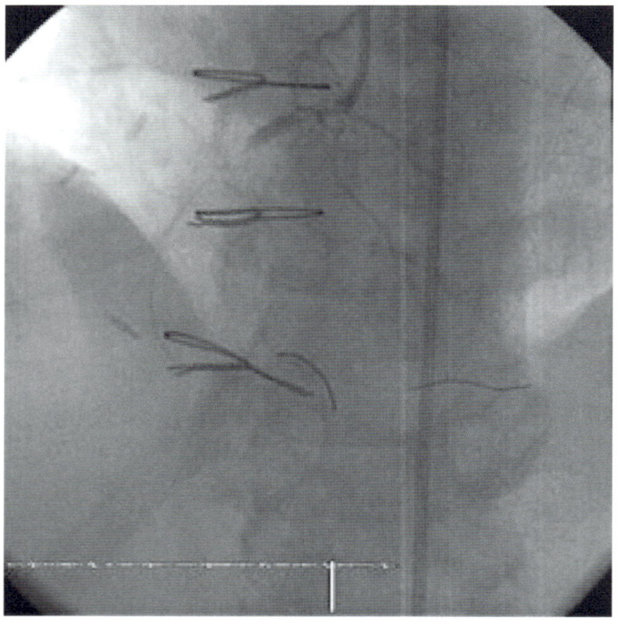

FIGURE 7.3
No reflow.

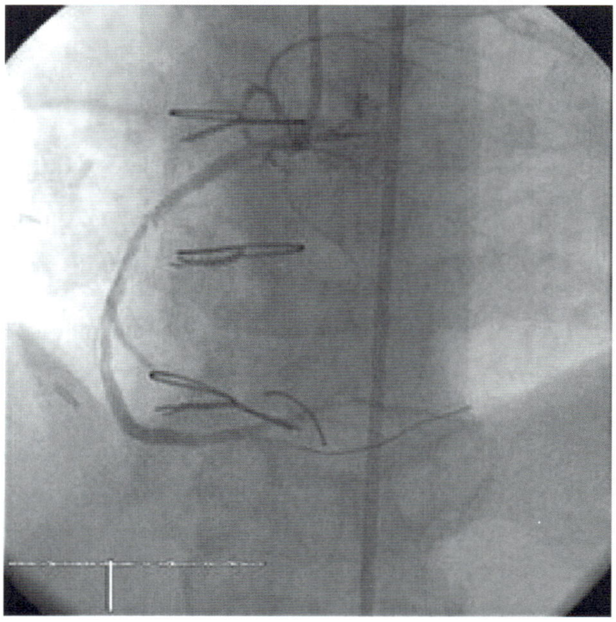

FIGURE 7.5
Distal stent implantation.

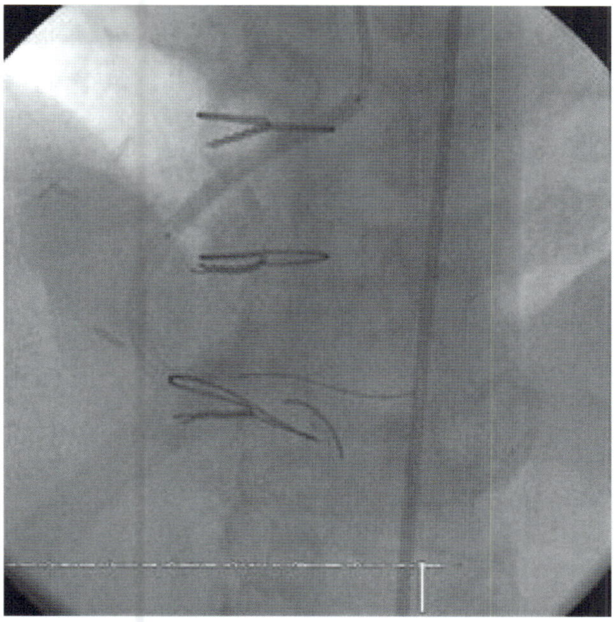

FIGURE 7.6
Proximal stent implantation.

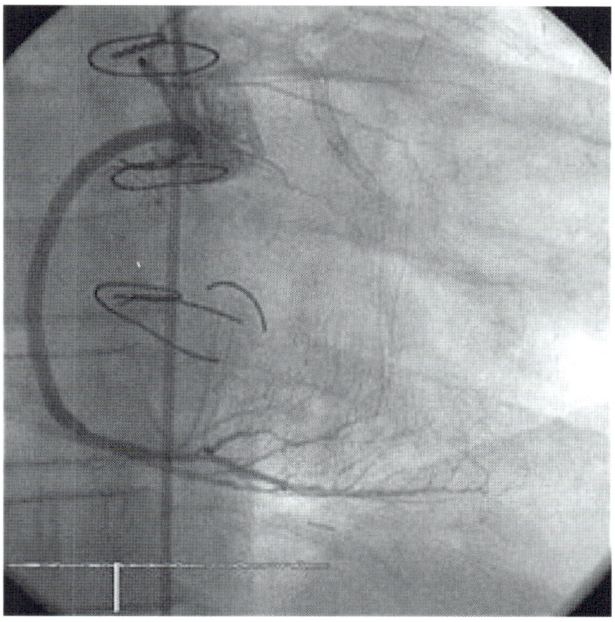

FIGURE 7.7
Final coronary angiography.

CASE ANALYSIS

Small vessels having diffuse disease with unstable clinical presentations are at risk for dissection and thrombus formation. Anticipation of thrombus formation due to low flow states and restoration of optimal vessel flow is critical to resolution of the myocardial ischemia.

LESSONS

Vessel preparation to allow stent placement along with appropriate pharmacologic treatments to improve the microcirculation is important in allowing optimal therapy. When treatment of a small vessel with diffuse disease with vasoactive agents failed to improve the flow, a search for other etiologies confirmed the presence of flow-limiting dissections that required stent placement for definitive therapy.

SUGGESTED READING

Metz JA, Mooney MR, Walter PD, et al. Significance of edge tears in coronary stenting: initial observations from the STRUT registry [abstract]. *Circulation*. 1995;92:I-546.

Uren NG, Schwarzacher SP, Metz JA, et al, for the POST Registry. Intravascular ultrasound prediction of stent thrombosis: insights from the POST registry [abstract]. *J Am Coll Cardiol*. 1997;29:60A.

Sheris, SJ, Canos MR, Weissman Nj. Natural history of intravascular ultrasound-detected edge dissections from coronary stent deployment. *Am Heart J*. 2000;139(1 Pt 1):59–63.

CASE 7.2

LIMA PTCA Complicated With Downstream Dissection

CLINICAL HISTORY AND DIAGNOSTIC TESTING RESULTS

A 63-year-old woman with hypertension, diabetes mellitus, dyslipidemia, and prior stroke with no significant residual deficits, who underwent three-vessel CABG in 1999, presented for evaluation for progressive dyspnea on exertion and chest pain. Echocardiogram revealed depressed left ventricular (LV) systolic function with ejection fraction of 35%. Dobutamine stress echo revealed multizone ischemia in the LAD and RCA distribution.

She then underwent coronary angiography, which revealed patent left main, and severe three-vessel disease of her native coronaries. Vein graft to her first obtuse marginal branch was patent, but the vein graft to the second obtuse marginal branch was occluded. LIMA graft to her LAD had a significant kinking, with stenosis in the mid-segment, and appeared to be adherent to the chest wall.

In view of her symptoms and abnormal dobutamine stress echo, a decision was made to intervene on this lesion after extensive discussion with the patient, cardiothoracic surgery team, and referring cardiologist.

PLANNED PROCEDURE

POBA and provisional stent of LIMA.

PROCEDURE

The patient was preloaded with Plavix 300 mg the evening before the procedure.

A 6-Fr LIMA guide catheter was advanced to the LIMA ostium. A balanced middle weight (BMW) wire was advanced across kinked segment of the mid-body of the LIMA and the wire tip placed in the distal native LAD. Initial angioplasty with 2.5- × 12-mm Maverick balloon resulted in distal shift of the kink and intimal dissection (Figure 7.8).

A Promus 2.5- × 18-mm DES was deployed at the dissected segment at 9 atm (Figure 7.9). Follow-up angiography revealed complete coverage of the dissection segment; however, there was a new high-grade kinking or dissection noted distal to the stent, which was then covered with a 2.5- × 12-mm Promus DES at 7 atm (Figures 7.10 and 7.11).

Final angiography demonstrated no residual dissection, 0% residual kink/stenosis, and TIMI 3 flow (Figure 7.12). The patient tolerated the procedure well and was transferred to the floor in stable condition.

COMPLICATION

Dissection of LIMA requiring mechanical scaffolding using a stent.

MANAGEMENT

Follow-up cineangiography revealed a contained distal edge dissection, and this was treated with a second PROMUS 3- × 12-mm drug-eluting stent (DES) at 14 atm, overlapping with the proximal stent. Final angiography after removal of all devices and guidewire revealed excellent angiographic results with 0% residual stenosis and TIMI 3 flow. The patient tolerated the procedure well and was transferred to the floor in stable condition.

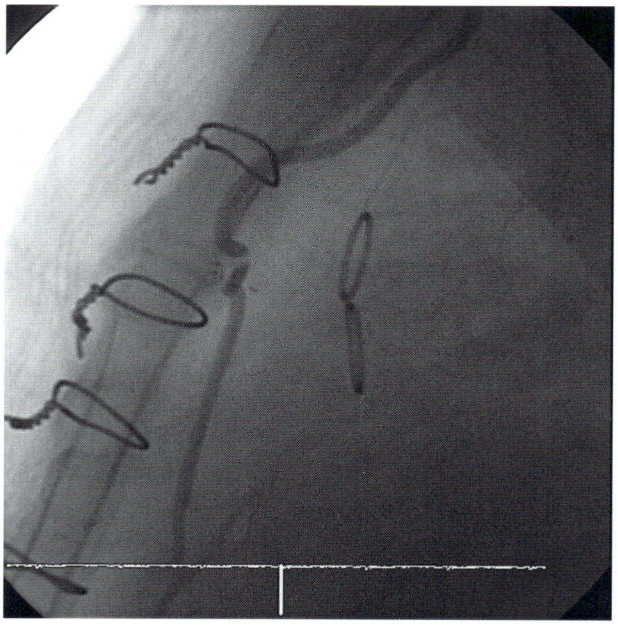

FIGURE 7.8

Baseline coronary angiography. (LOOP 7.8)

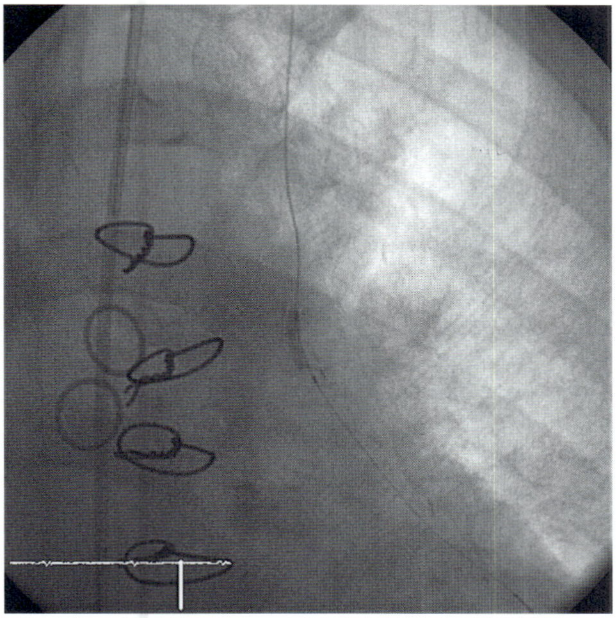

FIGURE 7.9
PTCA of LIMA. (LOOP 7.9)

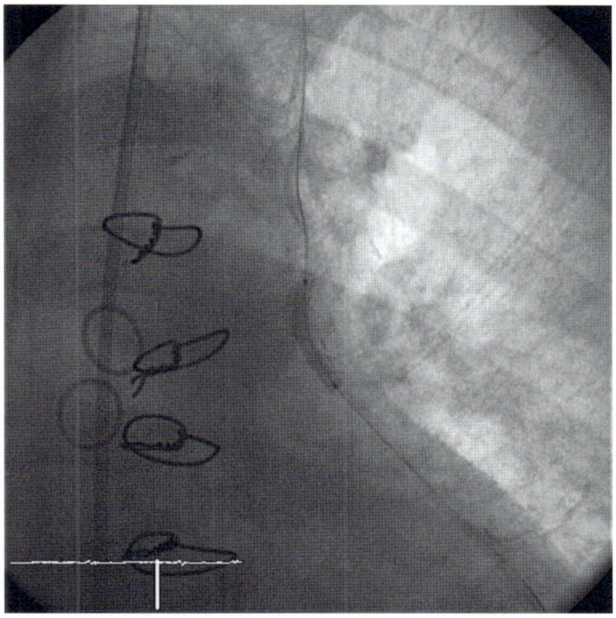

FIGURE 7.11
Second stent implantation in LIMA. (LOOP 7.11)

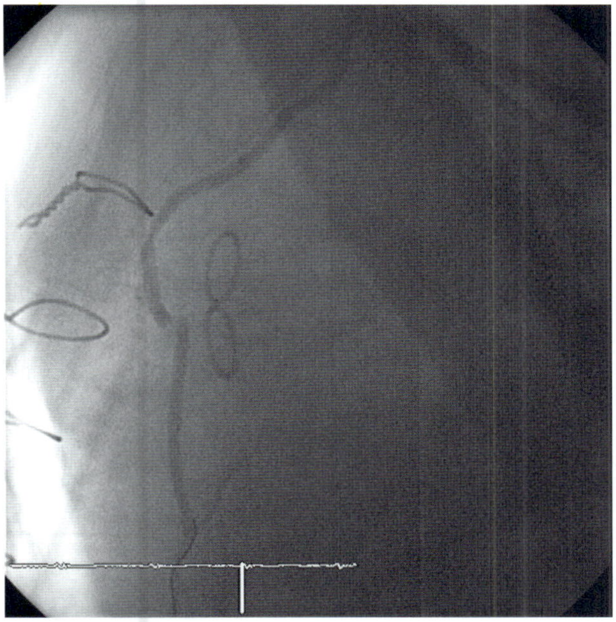

FIGURE 7.10
Poststent-1 implant angiogram. (LOOP 7.10)

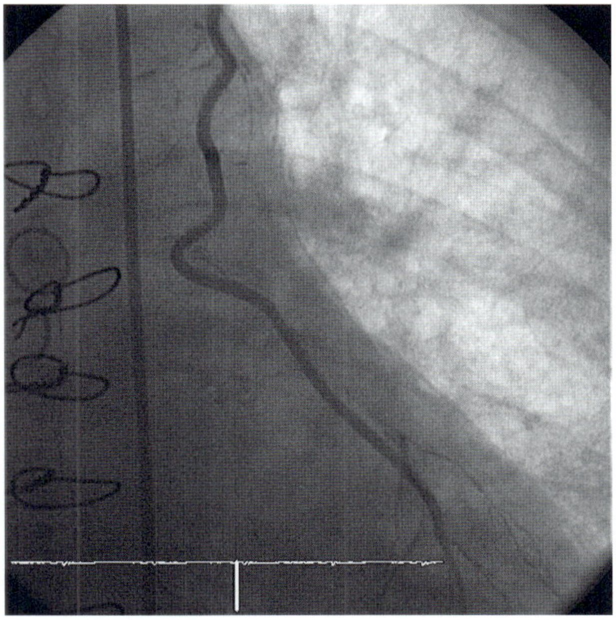

FIGURE 7.12
Final angiogram after second stent distal dissection. (LOOP 7.12)

CASE ANALYSIS

Diseased small vessels were at increased risk for edge dissection, particularly in high-pressure implantations. Anticipation of and evaluation for edge dissection are critical to avoiding a late complication. Careful evaluation of the postimplantation angiogram and/or the use of IVUS are particularly important when treating small vessels.

LESSONS

Vessel sizing and plaque composition are important to assess prior to and after stent deployment. Even stable lesions can be converted to unstable lesions with stent implantation. Other considerations include dilatation of lesions on a bend and the fixation of a vessel segment by "kink transfer," where a new lesion is formed due to wire and vessel interactions.

SUGGESTED READING

Alfonso F, Hernández R, Bañuelos C, et al. Initial results and long-term clinical and angiographic outcome of coronary stenting in women. *Am J Cardiol.* 2000;86(12): 1380-1383.

Köckeritz U, Reynen K, and Knaut M, et al. Results of angioplasty (with or without stent) at the site of a narrowed coronary anastomosis of the left internal mammary artery graft or via the internal mammary artery. *Am J Cardiol.* 2004;93(12):1531–1533.

Angle JF, Matsumoto AH, McGraw JK. Percutaneous angioplasty and stenting of left subclavian artery stenosis in patients with left internal mammary-coronary bypass grafts: clinical experience and long-term follow-up. *Vasc Endovascular Surg.* 2003;37(2):89–97.

CASE 7.3

Stent Thrombosis Presenting as Stent Restenosis

CLINICAL HISTORY AND DIAGNOSTIC TESTING RESULTS

A 71-year-old man presented with history of hypertension, dyslipidemia, and coronary artery disease, with prior DES to his proximal and distal LAD in 2006, followed by a DES to his mid-LAD in 2007 was admitted with stable angina following a markedly abnormal nuclear imaging study. He was on optimum medical therapy with ASA, 81 mg/d; Plavix, 75 mg/d; Metoprolol, 50 mg po bid; and a statin. He was compliant with his medications and had not missed any Plavix dose. He was hemodynamically stable, and his physical exam was unremarkable, except for a S4 on cardiac auscultation. A routine myocardial perfusion imaging study performed by his primary-care physician demonstrated a large area of ischemia in the LAD territory, with new decreased LVEF.

The patient was taken to the cath lab, and a diagnostic coronary angiogram (Figure 7.13) revealed high-grade mid-LAD lesion within the previously placed mid-LAD stent.

PLANNED PROCEDURE

POBA and stent of mid-LAD.

PROCEDURE

Patient was treated overnight with hydration and ASA, reloaded with Plavix 300 mg, and started on 150 mg Plavix per day.

After unfractionated heparin was administered, a 6-Fr JL4 guide catheter was used to successfully engage the left main coronary artery, and a baseline angiogram was performed demonstrating TIMI 2 flow (Figure 7.13). A 0.014-inch × 300-cm Asahi soft guidewire was used to cross the 99% instent mid-LAD lesion, and the wire tip was positioned in the distal LAD. Passage of the wire resulted in no distal flow beyond the lesion (Figure 7.14). Activated coagulation time (ACT) was confirmed to be greater than 250 seconds. The patient did not have chest pressure but did demonstrate <1-mm ST segment elevation on the monitor. Dilatation of the in-stent stenosis (Figure 7.15) resulted in restoration of flow. A stent was deployed inside the original stent (Figure 7.16) with restitution of TIMI 3 flow at the completion of the procedure as seen in Figure 7.17.

COMPLICATION AND MANAGEMENT

No reflow resulting from initial wire passage across a subtotally occluded LAD stenosis. Aspiration thrombectomy was performed with Pronto V3 thrombectomy catheter. No thrombus was aspirated, and the epicardial flow was not improved. This was followed by the administration of intracoronary nitroglycerine, nicardipine, and abciximab. Subsequent PTCA of the lesion demonstrated improved flow and was followed by placement of a Xience V DES. Final angiography revealed <10% residual stenosis and TIMI 3 flow in the LAD. The patient was continued on abciximab for 6 hours postprocedure. The patient tolerated the procedure well without postprocedure troponin rise or EKG changes.

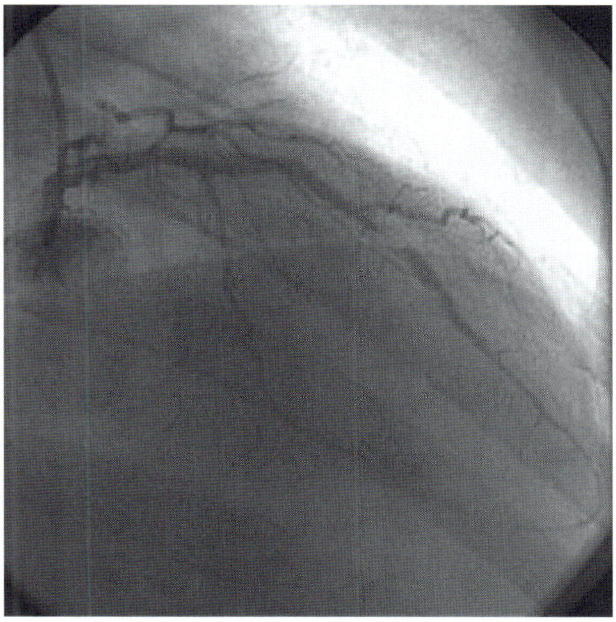

FIGURE 7.13
Baseline coronary angiography. (LOOP 7.13)

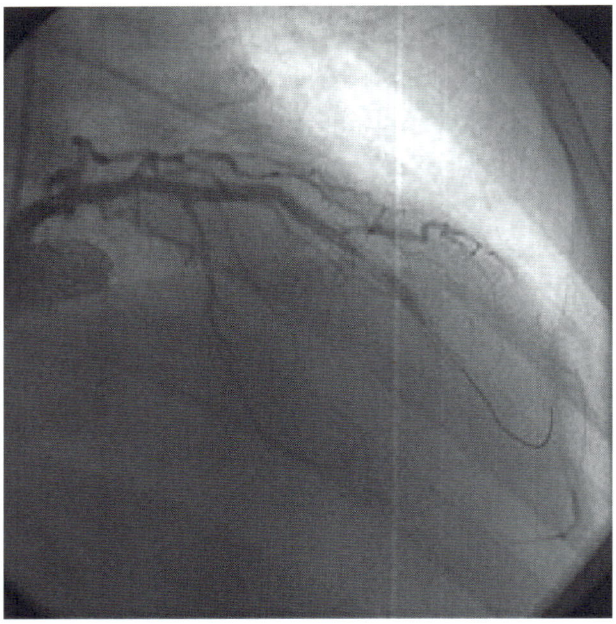

FIGURE 7.14
Guidewire across the lesion. (LOOP 7.14)

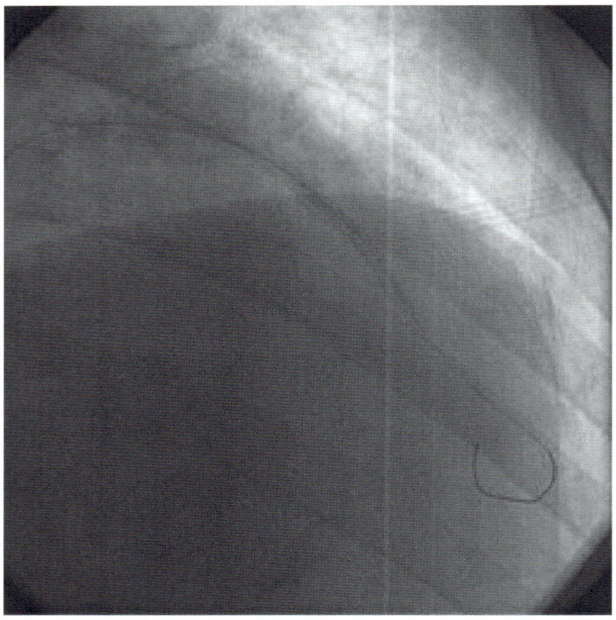

FIGURE 7.15
PTCA of lesion. (LOOP 7.15)

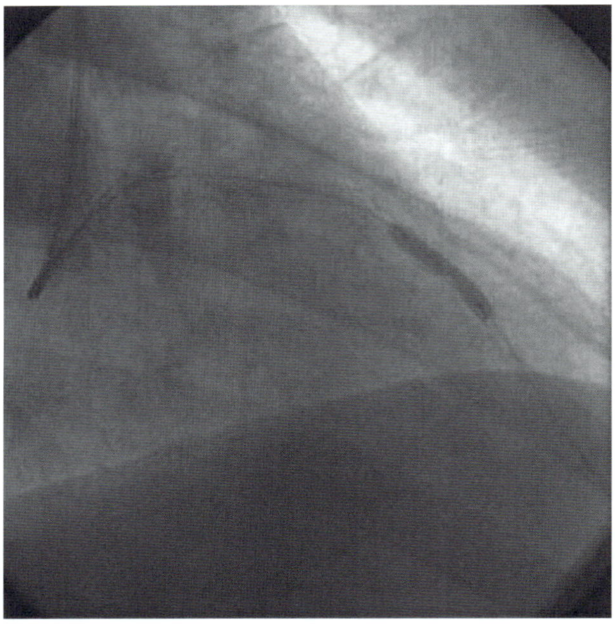

FIGURE 7.16
Stent of in-stent lesion. (LOOP 7.16)

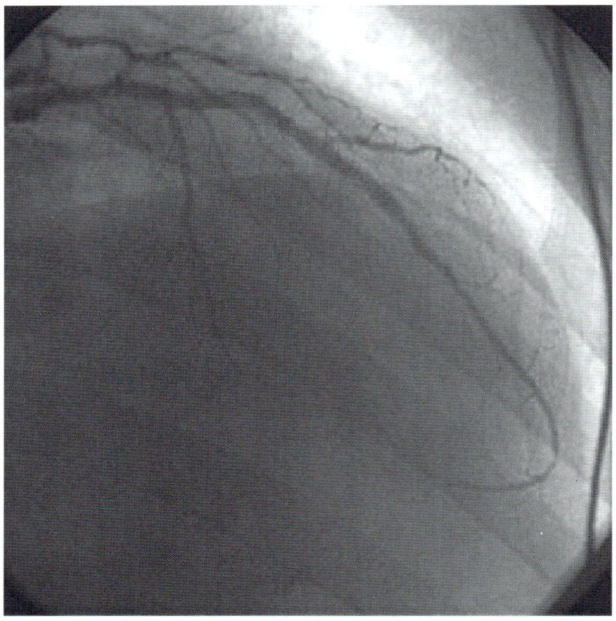

FIGURE 7.17
Final angiogram. (LOOP 7.17)

CASE ANALYSIS

Late stent thrombosis occurred in an asymptomatic patient discovered during a nuclear imaging study. The diagnosis of a tight stenosis occurring within a DES must include not only neointimal hyperplasia but also thrombus formation.

LESSONS

In patients who present with instent stenosis of a DES, consider the possibility of thrombus. If this seems likely, pretreatment with a glycoprotein IIb/IIIa inhibitor may improve clinical outcomes.

SUGGESTED READING

Holmes DR Jr, Kereiakes DJ, Garg S, et al. Stent thrombosis *J Am Coll Cardiol.* 2010;56:1357–1365.

Vaknin-Assa H, Assali A, Lev El, et al. Failure of drug eluting stents presented as definite stent thrombosis. *Catheter Cardiovasc Interv.* 2010;76:1,93–97.

Lemesle G, Bouallal R, and Sudre A, et al. Thrombus aspiration for the treatment of definite stent thrombosis. *Arch Cardiovasc Dis.* 2010;103(1):33–38. Epub 2010 Jan 15.

8

Azeem Latib and Antonio Colombo

Trapped Devices in the Coronary Arteries

INTRODUCTION

Loss or entrapment of a device in the coronary tree is one of the more distressing complications of percutaneous coronary interventions (PCI), probably because it occurs rarely and thus many operators may not be familiar with retrieval equipment and techniques. Fortunately, the incidence of device loss during PCI appears to have decreased in recent years, most likely due to technological improvements in equipment design and the almost universal use of premounted stents (1). Devices that can dislodge, brake, embolize, or become trapped in the coronary tree include stents, coronary guidewires, balloons, intravascular ultrasound (IVUS) catheters, distal protection devices, and rotablator burrs. The most common is stent loss or embolization, which, in the year 2000, was estimated to have an incidence of 1.2% (2). However, in a recently published, large, single-center experience of 11,773 procedures over a 10-year period from 1994 to 2004, the incidence of stent loss was reported to be 0.32% (1). Dislodgement of a stent may result in systemic embolization and cause cerebrovascular events, whereas intracoronary embolization is associated with an increased risk of coronary thrombosis and myocardial infarction. Knowledge of the percutaneous management of this rare complication can avoid bail-out cardiac surgery and serious complications, such as stroke, myocardial infarction, vessel perforation, and death (2).

In this chapter, we will specifically address the problem of stent loss as stents are the most frequent to become trapped in a coronary artery. However, the techniques described here can be applied to any trapped or embolized interventional material. Stent loss is more likely to occur in lesions with severe calcification, that are located on a bend, or that have significant proximal angulation, or in attempts to pass distally through a stent. Direct stenting may also be associated with a higher risk of stent loss, presumably due to the increased resistance to stent advancement through an undilated lesion. The dislodgement does not occur when trying to cross the lesion; the stent is stripped off when trying to pull back the stent delivery system that will not advance further.

REMOVAL OF EMBOLIZED MATERIAL FROM THE CORONARY SYSTEM

The golden rule when a problem with defective equipment arises in the coronary tree is not to lose the guidewire position in the distal vessel as this makes a broad variety of retrieval methods possible. A second rule to keep in mind is to avoid applying continuous and strong pull on the trapped device as this action will only secure the device more tightly. The next rule is to bring the embolized material safely to the iliac artery, where further manipulations can be performed without any major risk because of the larger arterial size and because peripheral embolization is usually not associated with serious clinical sequelae. If retrieval of a stent appears challenging or not possible, another potential technique is to deploy the stent in the area where it has embolized or in an inconsequential location if the wire is still within the stent (1, 2). However, if the wire has been inadvertently retracted from the stent, another option is to crush the underexpanded stent against the vessel wall with another stent. The most commonly used techniques for removal of embolized material from the coronary artery are as follows.

Small-Balloon Technique (1–5)

This is usually the primary approach for removing a lost stent because this technique does not require specific material and is usually the simplest to perform. A low-profile 1.25- to 1.5-mm angioplasty balloon is advanced through and beyond the lost stent (provided the wire has been maintained in the stent), the balloon is inflated distally to the stent, and the balloon together with the lost stent is gently withdrawn out of the coronary artery toward the guiding catheter. If the guiding catheter is maintained coaxially and the stent has not been deformed, it is sometimes possible to withdraw the balloon and stent directly into the guiding catheter. However, this is often not possible and thus when the stent is secured between the balloon and guiding catheter, the entire system is withdrawn to the iliac artery and removed through the arterial sheath. This small-balloon technique can also be used to advance the embolized stent and deploy it at the lesion or another location. This technique cannot be used if the wire position through the embolized stent is lost.

Loop Snare Technique

This technique can be used to retrieve lost stents or embolized fragments of other devices. The loop snare essentially consists of a catheter that contains a movable wire with a loop. The loop is manipulated under fluoroscopic guidance to encircle the embolized device. Once the loop is in the right position, it is closed, thus trapping the device between the wire and catheter. Then, by maintaining continuous traction, the entire system with embolized device is withdrawn. The correct technique when the snare encircles the device is to tighten the loop by advancing the transport catheter and not by pulling on the loop. Indeed, withdrawing the ends of the wire to capture the embolized material can cause disengagements with the loop slipping off the device, especially when trying to snare fragments of catheters or guidewires (2). When the embolized device is secured by the snare, the entire system can be withdrawn as a whole to the iliac artery and retrieved through the femoral sheath. The loop snare is commercially available (Amplatz GooseNeck snare; ev3, Plymouth, MN) or a makeshift snare can also be prepared in the catheterization laboratory using an exchange-length guidewire and microcatheter or diagnostic multipurpose catheter. Handmade devices may be suitable for peripheral usage but can be traumatic if employed in the coronary tree. The Amplatz GooseNeck snare consists of a 4-Fr catheter that tapers to a 2.3-Fr tip that contains a nitinol snare loop of varying diameters that is angulated at 90° to the shaft axis. The right angle of the loop facilitates grasping of the target object.

This technique can be utilized irrespective of whether the guidewire is still inside the embolized device and is the preferred technique in cases of inadvertent loss of guidewire position. However, if the embolized fragment is quite distal in the coronary tree, it may be impossible to retrieve it safely with a loop snare. If the wire is still inside the stent or fragmented device, then access to the device is facilitated, and free movement is limited to the longitudinal axis of the wire. The loop of the snare should be passed over the angioplasty wire encircling it and then advanced to the coronary ostium. If there is difficulty positioning the snare, a second wire should be placed beside the original wire. The second wire can be used either as a rail on which the snare device can be moved without shifting the position of the lost stent or to deliver a microcatheter distally, through which a loop snare can be placed and pulled from a distal to proximal direction in order to capture the distal end of the embolized device (6). On the other hand, if the stent or embolized material is free (i.e., not on an angioplasty wire), then snaring the device can be challenging and depends on correct alignment of the loop to the free end of the target fragment. The free end usually pulsates and can sometimes be identified under careful fluoroscopic evaluation. The snare should then be positioned with its plane at right angles to the estimated plane of the embolized material. If correctly positioned in relation to the target fragment, the snare should be seen as a straight line or a closed loop on fluoroscopy, confirming its vertical plane in relation to the fragment or stent (2). If the loop snare is parallel to the plane of the embolized material, ensnarement is impossible. As a general rule, the snaring should be done on the more proximal extremity of the device rather than in the mid- or distal segment.

Two-Wire Technique (7, 8)

The two-wire technique can only be performed if the original guidewire is still through the stent. It involves twisting a second wire around the stent or distally around the first wire in order to mingle the wires, which will trap the dislodged stent when the guidewires are pulled back. This technique can be performed by manipulating a second wire through the struts of the dislodged stent or by simply placing the second wire distally to the stent (less effective). However, it is essential that the second wire not pass through the central lumen of the lost stent. The two wires are then bound together outside the guiding catheter by placing the wires within a single torquing device, which is then rotated clockwise 15 to 20 times until the wires are observed twisting together near the proximal end of the stent. Then both wires are pulled together slowly. An important sign that the stent has been properly trapped between the twisted wires is that the guiding catheter should engage deeper into the ostium during withdrawal of the two wires. If the second wire went through the central lumen of the stent or the wires are not sufficiently twisted together, both wires could easily be pulled out at this stage, leaving the free stent behind. The stent twisted between the two wires and the guiding catheter are pulled out gently as a single unit and brought to the level of the iliac artery, where it can be removed by conventional methods after the wires are untwisted.

REMOVAL OF EMBOLIZED MATERIAL FROM THE ILIAC VESSELS

Embolized material from the coronary artery should always be brought to the level of the iliac artery where further manipulations can be performed without the risk of cerebrovascular complications. The aim is to remove the embolized material through the vascular sheath without the need for vascular cut-down. It may sometimes be necessary to upsize the sheath in order to recover safely the embolized device. The options for removing the embolized material from the iliac vessels are as follows.

Retraction of the Stent Into the Guiding Catheter

This should always be performed at the level of the iliac artery because of the risk of dislodgement. Usually, the stent can be retracted into the guiding catheter only if there is excellent coaxial alignment, which can sometimes be facilitated by retracting the guiding catheter into the arterial sheath in order to straighten its tip.

Removal of Material With a Gooseneck Snare

The snare can be placed from the ipsilateral or contralateral femoral artery and, if possible, should be tightened at the distal end of the embolized material. By snaring the distal part, rather than proximal part, it is easier to manipulate into the tip of the femoral sheath.

Removal of Material With an Alligator Forceps or Cardiac Bioptome (9–11)

These devices can be used to grasp materials and retrieve them. However, they are limited by the difficulty in grasping small materials and the risk of endovascular trauma during manipulation.

If a dislodged stent is removed from the coronary artery into the iliac vessels but cannot be removed through the femoral sheath, the stent could be crushed against the arterial wall using a peripheral stent (12). Distal stent embolization into a small peripheral arterial branch may be left untreated because the distally embolized stents appear to have a benign clinical course. Indeed, in a study by Alfonso et al (13), none of the eight patients with distal stent embolization had any clinical sequelae during 6 months of follow-up.

A good knowledge of these retrieval techniques and the material available in the catheterization laboratory to deal with these complications is essential and can result in retrieval success in as high as 86% of patients (1). If all retrieval efforts fail and crushing or deployment is not desirable, then surgical removal should be considered.

TRAPPED ROTABLATOR BURR

Although we have concentrated predominantly on dislodged stents and embolized material in this chapter, a working knowledge of managing an entrapped rotablator burr is essential. An entrapped rotablator burr is a rare complication but is extremely disconcerting for the operator, and for the patient, when it occurs. It is usually related to the burr getting stuck in the lesion itself (because of a diffuse, heavy calcified angled narrowing) or just distal to the lesion due to the "Kokesi" effect. The Kokesi is a Japanese wooden doll whose head is bulb shaped and is larger than the hole on the body to which it is attached. The head is attached to the body by rotating the head and forcing it through the hole and is thus prevented from coming back through the hole given its bulb shape. Similarly, the rotating burr slips pass a lesion without forward ablation but cannot be withdrawn because the burr is larger than the hole (14). We suggest the following for removing an entrapped burr:

1. Gently apply manual traction with care to prevent vessel laceration and deep engagement of the guiding catheter, especially when the burr is stuck in the left coronary system as the guiding catheter may dissect the left main. Increasing the burr speed before retrying manual traction is also sometimes helpful.
2. Insert a second wire distal to the trapped burr and inflate a low-profile balloon along the side of the burr to create a space between the lesion and burr, allowing for retraction of the burr. If there is insufficient space within the guiding catheter to insert another wire (e.g., 1.5-mm burr in 6-Fr guide), we suggest the dual-catheter technique for inserting another wire (i.e., utilize a second guiding catheter from another access site).
3. Retract the distal wire against the burr. The distal diameter of the rotawire is 0.014 inch, whereas that of the shaft is 0.009 inch. The operator can now use the wire to gain additional traction on the burr and should withdraw both the wire and burr together during this maneuver.
4. Disassemble the rotablator apparatus to expose the burr shaft and advance a loop snare just proximal to the burr. This snare can provide direct traction on the burr during withdrawal.

If the burr is successfully recovered, the operator should be prepared to deal with any ensuing complication, such as no reflow, vessel laceration, or perforation. If all the above maneuvers are unsuccessful in retrieving the burr, urgent surgical intervention would be required.

CONCLUSIONS

Entrapment of interventional devices in the coronary tree is a rare but technically challenging complication with potentially detrimental consequences for the patient either from the trapped device itself or from efforts to retrieve it. These devices can be retrieved in the majority of cases using a variety of techniques as described above. The selection of a specific technique depends on the patient's clinical condition, operator's experience, and availability of retrieval equipment in the catheterization laboratory. In the case of dislodged stents, deploying or crushing the stent in the coronary artery may be a safe alternative to retrieval.

CASE 8.1

Dislodged Stent in the Mid Right Coronary Artery

CLINICAL HISTORY AND DIAGNOSTIC TESTING RESULTS

A 72-year-old woman had a history of hypertension, hypercholesterolemia, Type 2 diabetes mellitus, and triple-vessel coronary artery disease. She recently underwent PCI with bare-metal stent implantation of the distal right coronary artery (RCA) and proximal posterior descending artery (PDA), followed 3 months later by drug-eluting stent implantation of the distal RCA toward the posterolateral (PL) branch. She continued to have angina with evidence of inferolateral ischemia on stress perfusion imaging. Baseline angiography demonstrated patent stents on the RCA, a large bifurcating PL branch with a severe stenosis of the midsegment and distal occlusion (Figures 8.1 and 8.2).

PLANNED PROCEDURE

PCI and recanalization of chronic total occlusion (CTO) of PL branch.

PROCEDURE

Despite the use of multiple dedicated CTO guidewires, it was not possible to recanalize the distal PL branch. Thus, it was decided to treat only the lesion in the midsegment of the PL branch, which was predilated with a 2.5- × 12-mm semicompliant balloon. The operator then attempted to stent the lesion with a 3- × 18-mm Xience V stent (Abbott Vascular, Abbott Park, IL) but was unable to cross the lesion (Figure 8.3). There was considerable friction and resistance when trying to remove the stent delivery system.

COMPLICATION AND MANAGEMENT

As the stent was being retrieved, it slipped off the balloon and was dislodged in the mid-RCA. The operator unfortunately also lost the guidewire position that was within the stent, thus leaving a free stent within the mid-RCA (Figure 8.4). A floppy guidewire was placed distally parallel to the dislodged stent. The operator decided not to attempt stent retrieval due to the distal location of the dislodged stent, its oblique position in the coronary artery, the marked calcification of the vessel, and the loss of the original wire position. Instead, it was decided that a simpler option would be to crush the underexpanded stent with another stent. A 4- × 24-mm Promus Element (Boston Scientific, Natick, MA) was implanted in the mid-RCA crushing the dislodged stent against the wall (Figure 8.5). The stent was postdilated with a noncompliant balloon, with a good final angiographic result and no evidence of obstruction to coronary flow (Figure 8.6).

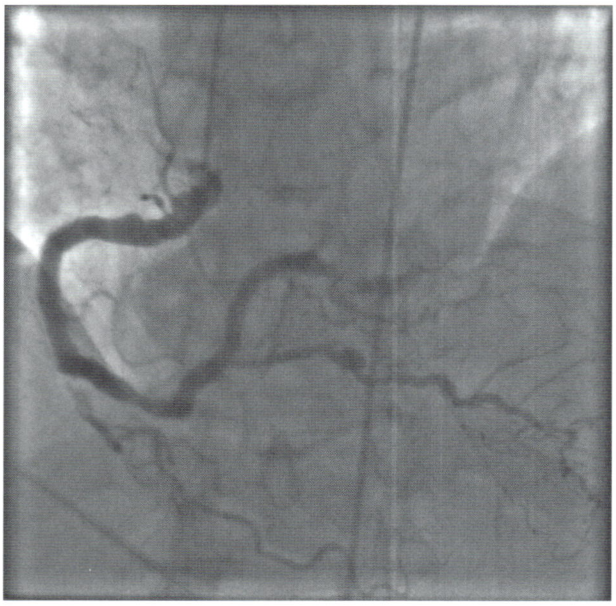

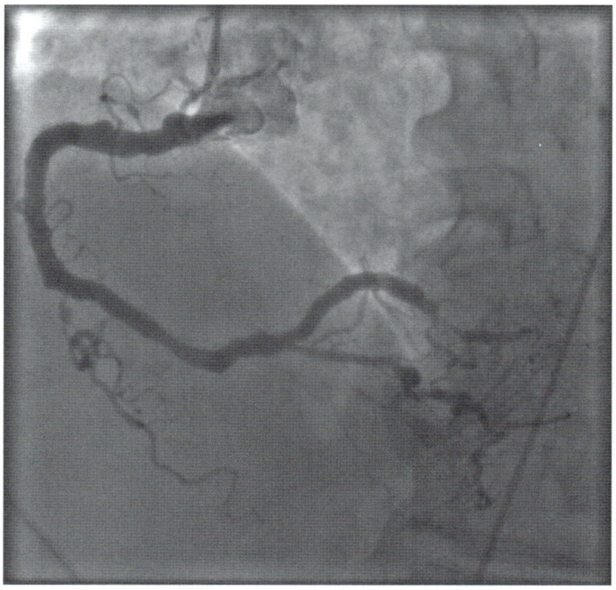

FIGURES 8.1 AND 8.2

Baseline angiography demonstrating patent stents in the RCA, a large bifurcating PL branch with a severe stenosis of the midsegment and distal occlusion. **(LOOPS 8.1 AND 8.2)**

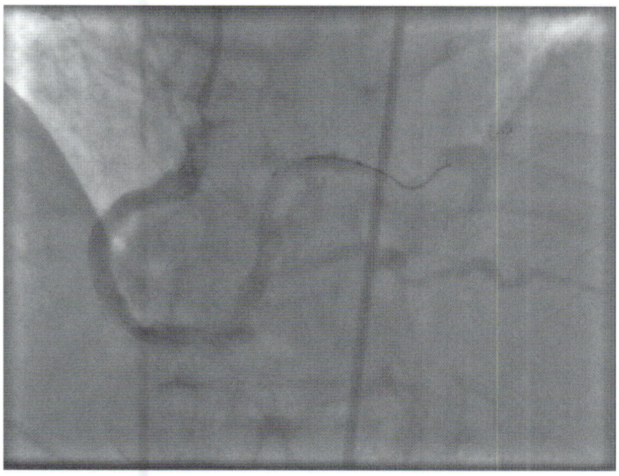

FIGURE 8.3

Despite predilatation, a 3- × 18-mm stent could not be delivered to the lesion. (LOOP 8.3)

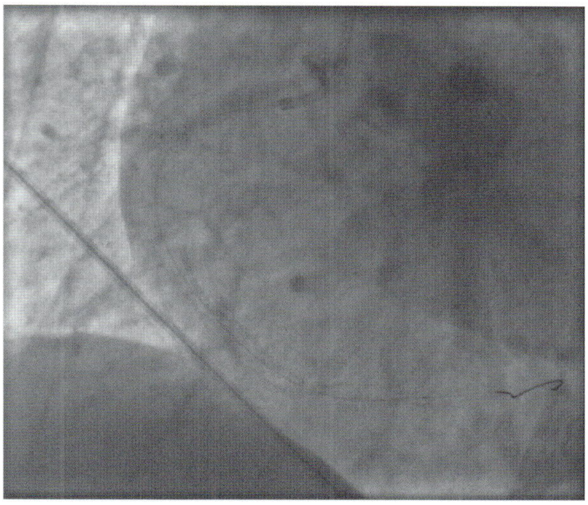

FIGURE 8.4

Note the dislodged stent in the mid-RCA without a guidewire. (LOOP 8.4)

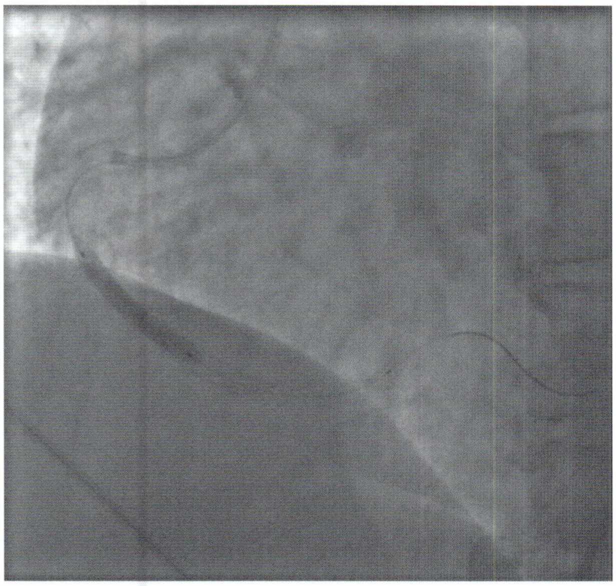

FIGURE 8.5

Note deployment of a 4- × 24-mm Promus Element stent at the site of the dislodged stent, which was crushed against the vessel wall. (LOOP 8.5)

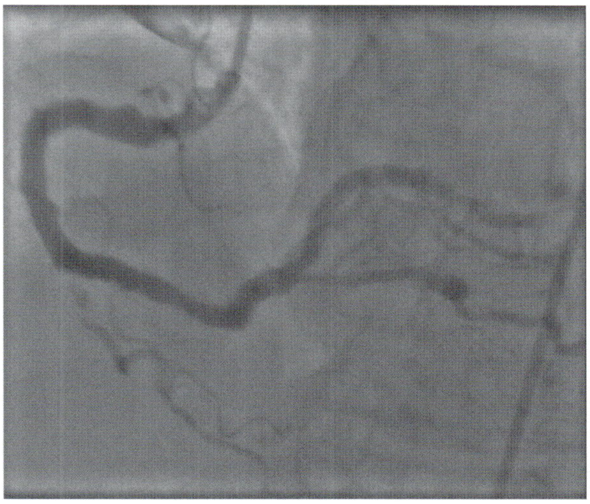

FIGURE 8.6

Final coronary angiography. (LOOP 8.6)

CASE ANALYSIS

Care should always been taken when trying to retrieve a stent that would not pass from a tortuous and calcified vessel. In this case, retrieval was made difficult by the fact that guidewire within the stent was lost.

LESSONS

- Maintaining the guidewire position through a dislodged stent, or fragmented or embolized device, is essential for successful retrieval.
- In some cases, deployment of a dislodged stent in an inconsequential location or crushing the stent against the vessel wall with another stent may be the simplest and safest option.
- When crushing an underexpanded stent with another stent, it is essential to ensure good stent apposition and IVUS should be considered to confirm stent apposition and expansion.

CASE 8.2

Dislodged Stent in the Left Main Coronary Artery Ostium

CLINICAL HISTORY AND DIAGNOSTIC TESTING RESULTS

A 78-year-old woman had a history of hypertension, dyslipidemia, and multiple revascularization procedures for triple-vessel coronary artery disease. Six years ago, the patient underwent coronary artery bypass grafting, including left internal mammary artery to left anterior descending artery (LAD) and saphenous vein graft (SVG) to PDA; 4 years ago, she underwent bare-metal stent implantation in the middle and distal left circumflex artery (LCX) followed by Cypher (Cordis Corp, Johnson & Johnson, Warren, NJ) implantation in the left main coronary artery toward the LAD and LCX, After a recent admission for an acute coronary syndrome that was treated conservatively, she was admitted for coronary angiography because of ongoing effort-induced angina. Baseline angiography demonstrated patent stents in the left main, LAD, and LCX; CTO of the mid-LAD; and a critical stenosis of the distal LCX (Figures 8.7 and 8.8).

PLANNED PROCEDURE

PCI with DES implantation in the distal LCX.

PROCEDURE

A floppy guidewire was passed into the distal LCX and the target lesion predilated with a 2.5- × 20-mm balloon. We attempted to implant a 2.5- × 20-mm Endeavor stent (Medtronic, Minneapolis, MN) in the distal LCX, but the stent would not pass through the previous stent in the distal left main and proximal LCX. While trying to retrieve the stent, it slipped off the delivery system and was dislodged in the left main coronary artery with partial protrusion from the left main ostium (Figure 8.9).

COMPLICATION AND MANAGEMENT

We attempted to retrieve the dislodged stent in the left main artery with the small-balloon technique, but the balloon would not pass through the dislodged stent

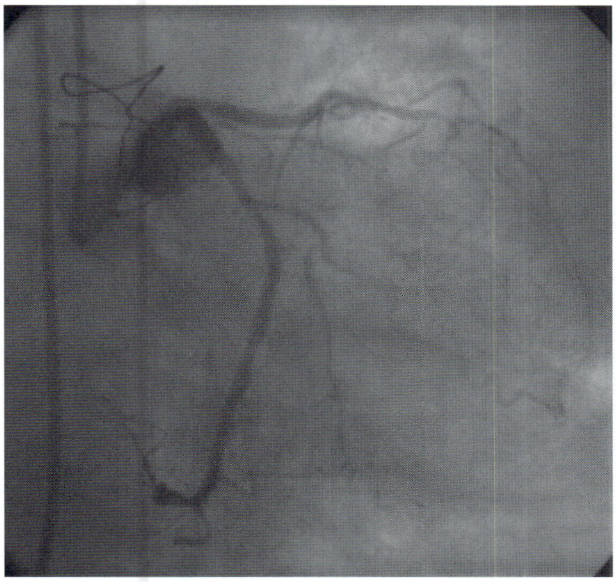

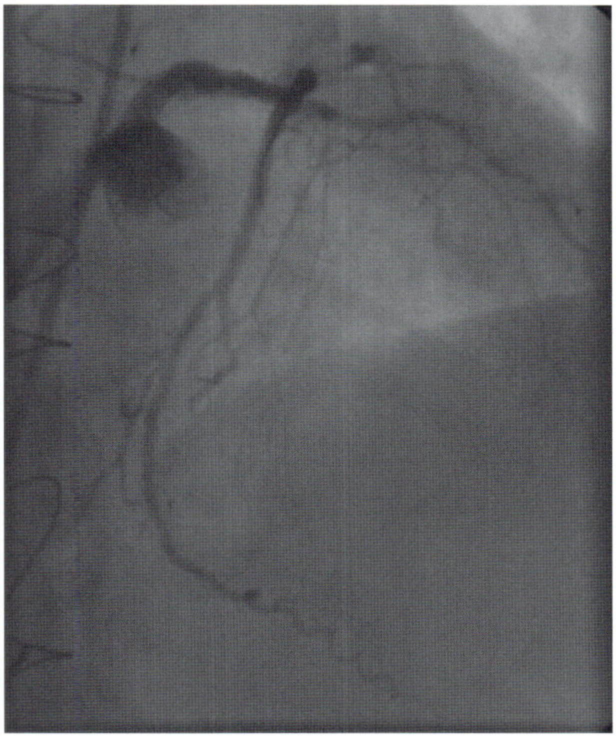

FIGURES 8.7 AND 8.8

Baseline coronary angiography demonstrating patent stents in the left main, LAD, and LCX arteries; a CTO of the mid-LAD; and a critical stenosis of the distal LCX. **(LOOPS 8.7 AND 8.8)**

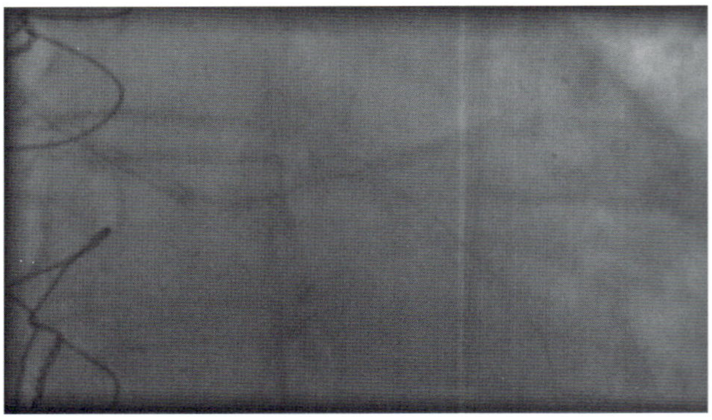

FIGURE 8.9

A noncontrast image showing the dislodged stent protruding from the left main coronary artery ostium. (LOOP 8.9)

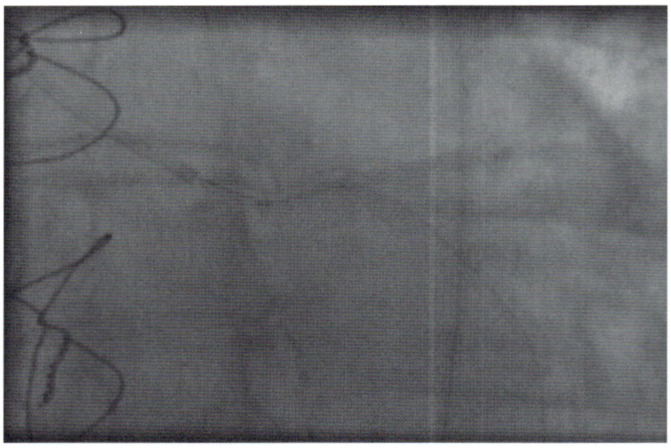

FIGURE 8.10

An attempt to retrieve the stent with the small-balloon technique was unsuccessful as the balloon could not pass through the stent. (LOOP 8.10)

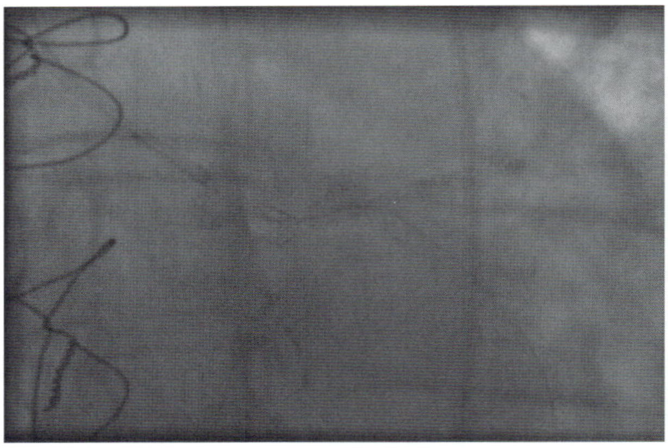

FIGURE 8.11

A noncontrast image demonstrating the Amplatz GooseNeck snare being advanced to retrieve the dislodged stent. (LOOP 8.11)

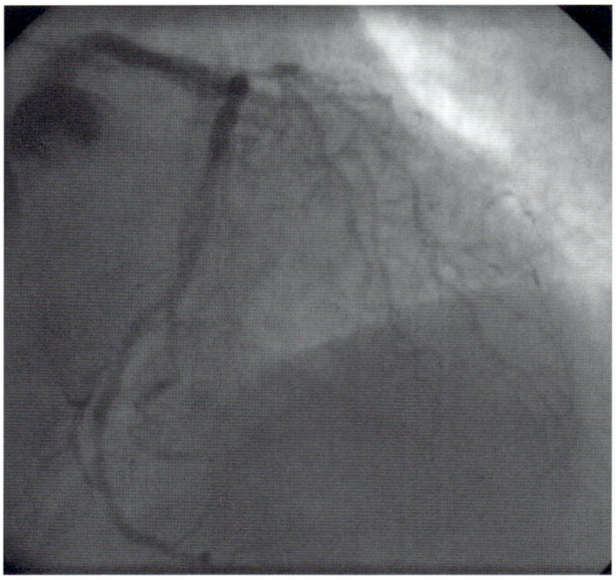

FIGURE 8.12

Final coronary angiography. (LOOP 8.12)

(Figure 8.10). It was also not possible to implant it in this position because it was protruding into the aorta. Thus, an Amplatz GooseNeck snare (ev3, Plymouth, MN) was advanced over the wire that passed through the dislodged stent; the stent was snared and removed from the coronary artery (Figure 8.11) via the femoral sheath. The final result was good without any evidence of dissection (Figure 8.12).

CASE ANALYSIS

Passing a stent through previously implanted stents can often be very difficult, and there is a risk that the stent may get entrapped within the struts of the previously implanted stent. In these cases, the stent can be dislodged when trying to retrieve the delivery system. When trying to pass a stent through previously implanted stents, if the stent does not advance, it is important not to force the stent forward but consider balloon dilatation of the stents, a buddy wire or buddy balloon, or a child-in-mother device such as the Guideliner (Vascular Solutions Inc, Minneapolis, MN).

LESSONS

- This case demonstrates the importance of maintaining wire access through the dislodged stent, which gives the operator a wide range of options to retrieve the stent.
- Balloon-assisted retrieval is effective only if the operator is able to pass a small balloon through the dislodged stent.
- When performing the loop snare technique, it is essential to be sure that the loop encircles the dislodged stent and to perform the snaring by advancing the delivery catheter rather than pulling on the snare.

CASE 8.3

Broken IVUS Catheter Tip in the Proximal LAD

CLINICAL HISTORY AND DIAGNOSTIC TESTING RESULTS

An 80-year-old man with exertional angina and anterior wall ischemia on stress perfusion imaging was admitted for coronary angiography. Baseline coronary angiography demonstrated a stenosis of the proximal LAD (Figures 8.13 and 8.14).

PLANNED PROCEDURE

PCI on the proximal LAD.

PROCEDURE

A 7-Fr JL guiding catheter was used, and the lesion was crossed with a Rinato guidewire (Asahi Intec, Santa Ana, California). Preprocedural IVUS was attempted with the Boston Atlantis Pro2 catheter (Boston Scientific, Natick, MA), but the IVUS catheter could not be advanced through the lesion.

COMPLICATION AND MANAGEMENT

While removing the IVUS catheter, it was noted that the radiopaque marker remained in the LAD (i.e., the tip of the IVUS catheter was broken off) (Figure 8.15). An attempt to snare the proximal end of the broken IVUS catheter tip with a loop snare failed because it was not visible on fluoroscopy (Figure 8.16). In order to create more room to snare the catheter tip, the lesion was dilated with a 3-mm balloon, which unfortunately caused the fragment to embolize more distally in the LAD. An attempt to entangle the broken catheter tip with the twisting two-wire technique also failed (Figure 8.17). The catheter tip was in the distal LAD, where manipulation with a snare would be difficult and where there was a greater risk of losing the wire position through the tip. A 2.0- × 15-mm balloon was inflated at 4 atm distal to the catheter tip and pulled back like a Fogarty catheter. This successfully moved the catheter fragment as far as the mid-LAD (Figure 8.18). The balloon was then replaced with a larger 3.0-mm balloon, and the same maneuver was repeated to retrieve the catheter tip, which was not possible as the fragment was stuck at the tip of the guiding catheter (Figure 8.19). As this point, we thought it will be extremely difficult to snare the proximal end of the catheter, so the alternative approach would be to snare the broken catheter fragment by moving the loop snare from distal to proximal (Figure 8.20, Loop 8.20). A microcatheter was advanced into the distal LAD over the buddy wire, which was then removed

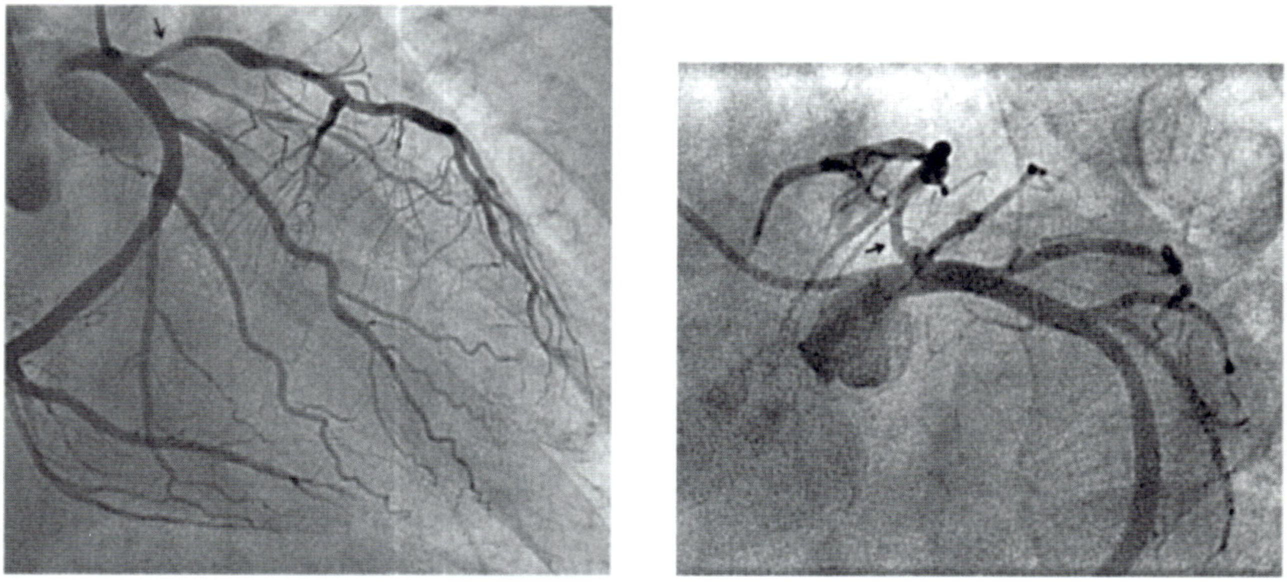

FIGURES 8.13 AND 8.14

Baseline coronary angiography demonstrated a stenosis of the proximal LAD (arrow).

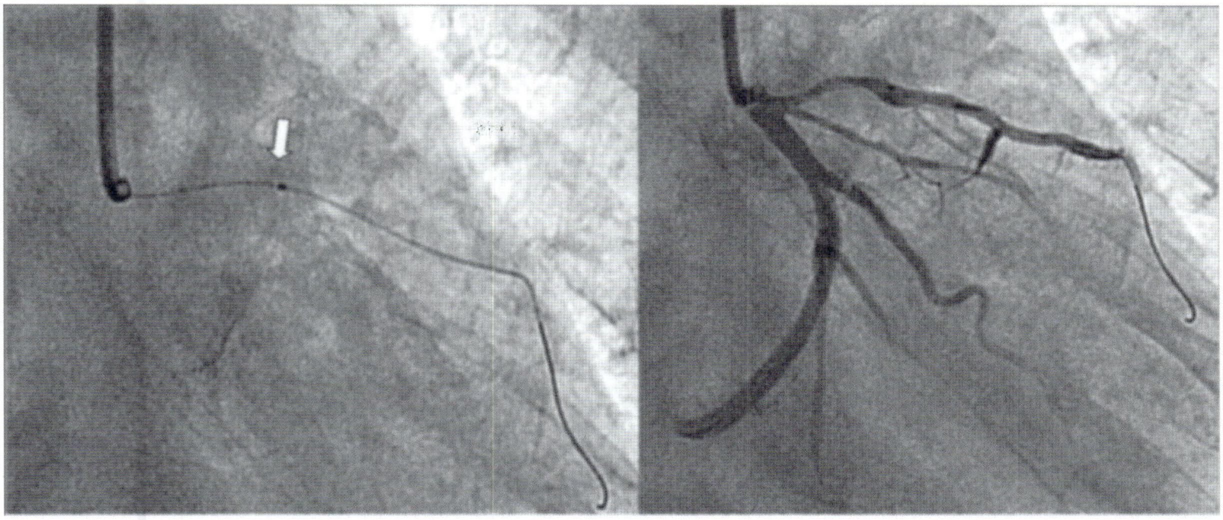

FIGURE 8.15
A broken tip of the IVUS catheter trapped in the proximal LAD (arrow).

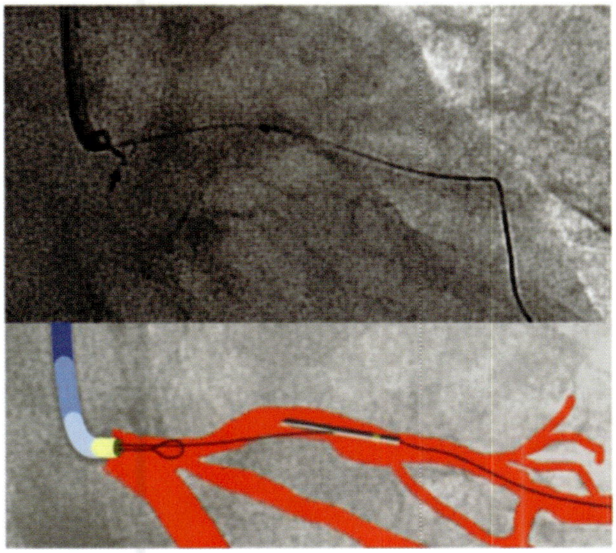

FIGURE 8.16
An attempt to snare the proximal end of the IVUS catheter, with a gooseneck was unsuccessful (arrow).

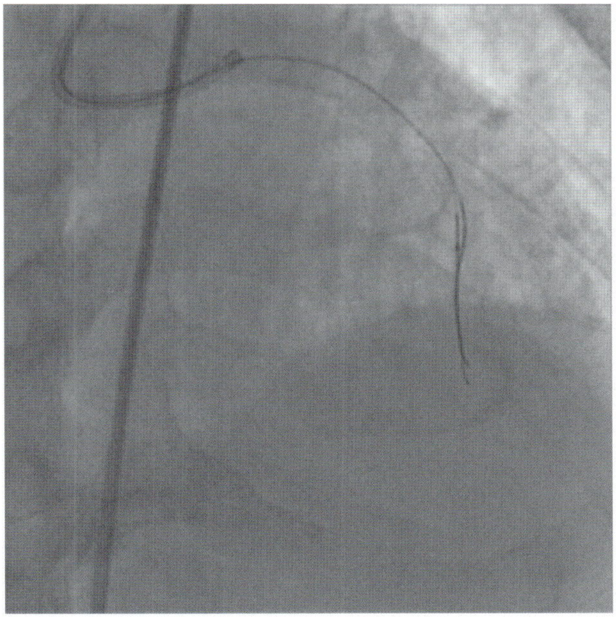

FIGURE 8.17
An attempt to snare the broken fragment by twisting two guidewires around it was also unsuccessful. (LOOP 8.17)

and replaced with a loop snare. The guidewire within the IVUS catheter tip was then manipulated into the loop (Figure 8.21). The loop snare was then pulled from distal to proximal until it encircled the broken catheter fragment (Figure 8.22). The loop snare was tightened and the IVUS catheter tip successfully retrieved into the guiding catheter (Figures 8.23 and 8.24). The lesion was then stented with a 3.5- × 13-mm sirolimus-eluting stent with a good final angiographic result (Figure 8.25).

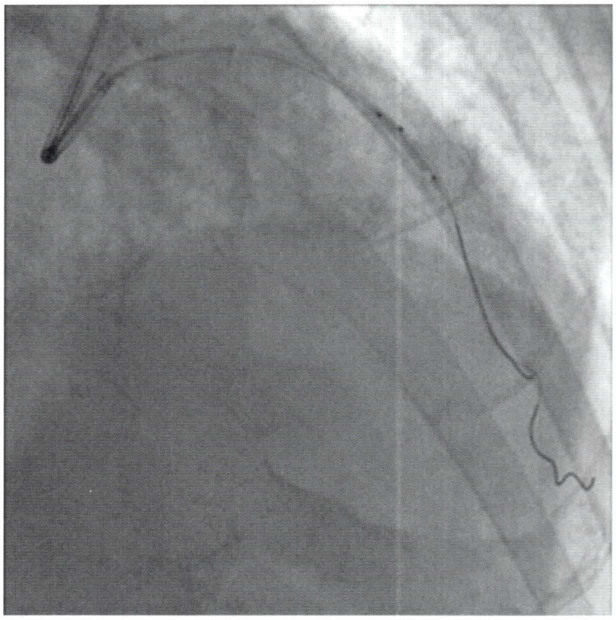

FIGURE 8.18

A 2.0- × 15-mm balloon was inflated at low pressure distal to the catheter tip and pulled back like a Fogarty catheter, successfully moving the catheter fragment more proximally. (LOOP 8.18)

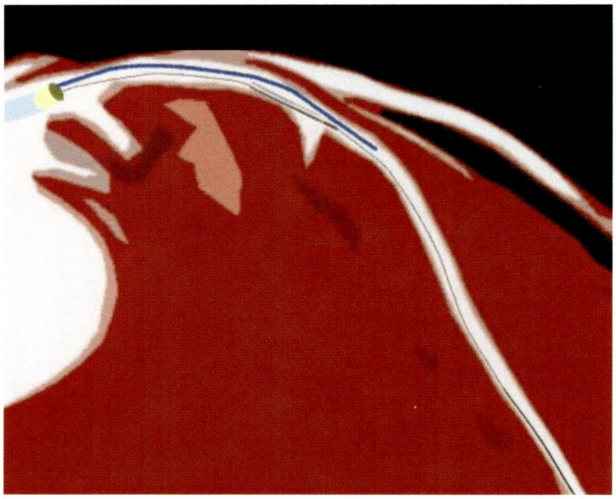

FIGURE 8.20

An animation demonstrating the technique of snaring the broken IVUS catheter tip by using a buddy wire. (LOOP 8.20)

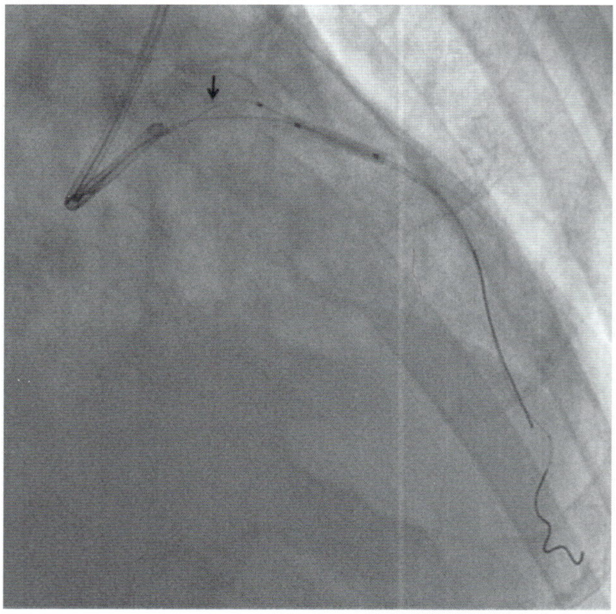

FIGURE 8.19

An attempt to remove the catheter tip from the mid-LAD with a larger balloon and the same maneuver was unsuccessful, as the fragment could not be pulled into the guiding catheter (arrow). (LOOP 8.19)

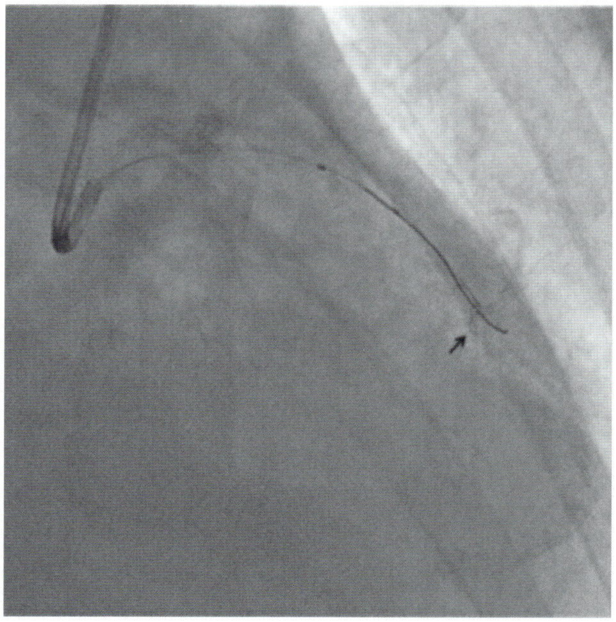

FIGURE 8.21

An angiogram demonstrating the application of the animation shown in Loop 8.20. The loop snare was placed in the distal LAD via a microcatheter. Then the guidewire within the broken catheter tip was manipulated into the loop (arrow). (LOOP 8.21)

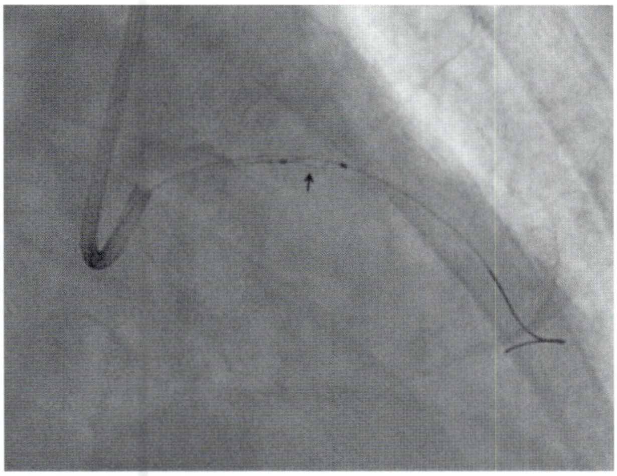

FIGURE 8.22
The loop snare was pulled from distal to proximal until it encircled the catheter fragment (arrow). (LOOP 8.22)

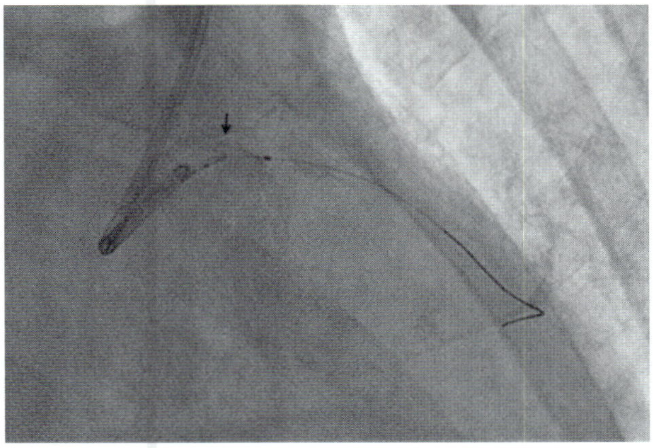

FIGURE 8.23
The loop snare was tightened around the broken catheter tip (arrow) and retrieved into the guiding catheter. (LOOP 8.23)

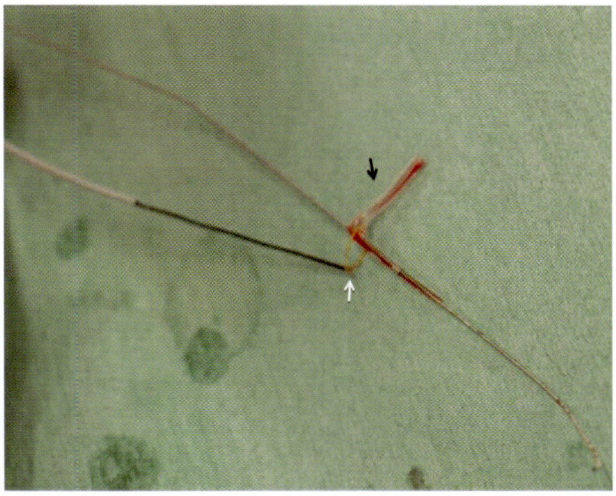

FIGURE 8.24
Photograph of the broken IVUS catheter tip (black arrow) and loop snare (white arrow) after removal from the patient.

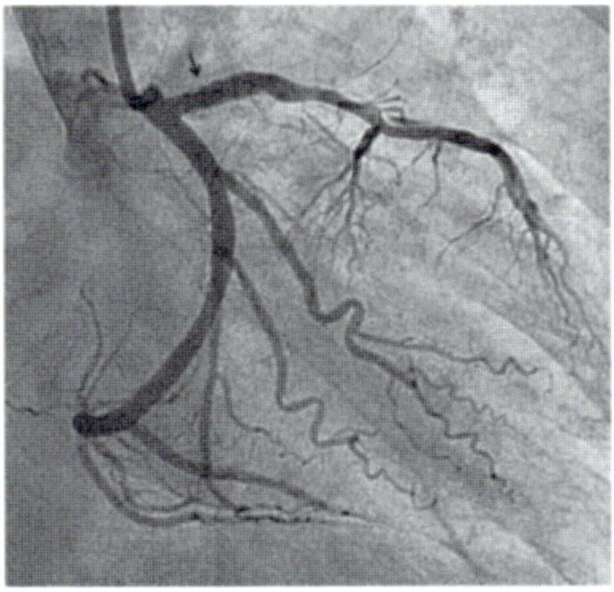

FIGURE 8.25
Final angiographic result after stent implantation on the proximal LAD (arrow).

CASE ANALYSIS

While advancing catheters with very short monorail segment, such as the IVUS catheter, through tortuous or severely calcified segments, care should be taken that these catheters do not become entrapped. Interestingly, in this case, the operator did not feel resistance while withdrawing the IVUS catheter. If marked resistance was felt, the catheter would not be pulled aggressively as it might break or dissect the artery. In these cases, one might consider dilating the lesion even with an undersized balloon in order to create more space and facilitate catheter retrieval.

*This case was presented at the Joint Interventional Meeting 2010 by Dr Atsushi Funatsu, MD and reprinted from Funatus A et al. *J Invas Cardiol.* 2010; 22:E197-E200, with permission from HMP Communications.

LESSONS

- This case once again reinforces the concept that the most important lesson when a device becomes entrapped or fragmented in the coronary tree is not to lose the original guidewire position.
- When part of a catheter or balloon fragments in the coronary tree, it may be difficult to snare the device from the proximal end, which is often not visible on angiography, and may have an oblique or eccentric position with the tip against the vessel wall.
- As in this case, often multiple techniques need to be attempted before an embolized fragment can be successfully retrieved.
- Inflating a small balloon at low pressure distal to an embolized fragment can be used as a Fogarty catheter to pull the fragment proximally. However, this should be performed carefully and stopped if resistance is encountered as this technique could result in vessel dissection or perforation.
- Utilizing a microcatheter to place a loop snare distal to the embolized fragment and pulling the snare from distal to proximal is an effective technique to retrieve intracoronary foreign bodies.

CASE 8.4

Entrapped Rotational Atherectomy Burr in the Proximal LAD

CLINICAL HISTORY AND DIAGNOSTIC TESTING RESULTS

A 77-year-old man had a history of hypertension, dyslipidemia, Type 2 diabetes mellitus, and chronic renal failure requiring hemodialysis. He presented with a non-ST-elevation myocardial infarction (MI) and underwent coronary angiography, which demonstrated a severe calcific and angulated stenosis of the proximal-to-mid-LAD (Figures 8.26 and 8.27).

PLANNED PROCEDURE

PCI with drug-eluting stent implantation in the LAD.

PROCEDURE

Two floppy guidewires were placed in the LAD and large first diagonal branch (Figure 8.28). All attempts at crossing the lesion with a balloon (even a 1.5-mm balloon) were unsuccessful. Thus, it was decided to perform rotational atherectomy. A rota floppy wire was placed in the distal LAD, and rotablation with a 1.25-mm burr was performed on the proximal LAD (Figure 8.29). Rotablation was successfully performed on the proximal segment of the lesion, but when the burr was advanced to the distal part of the lesion, it became entrapped.

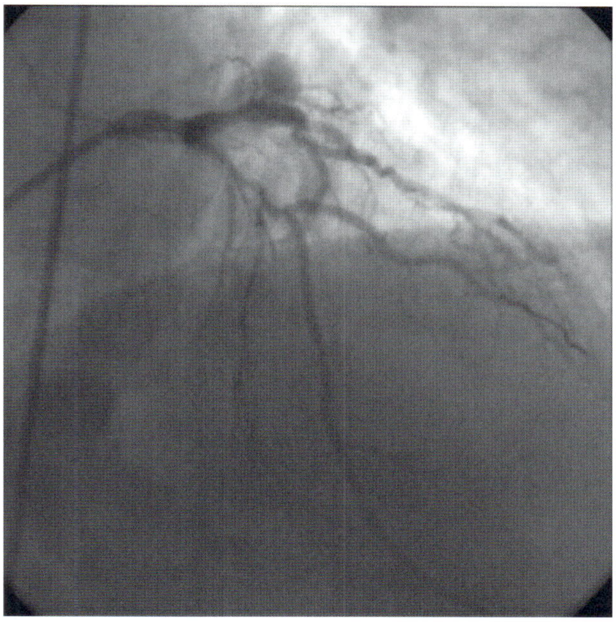

FIGURE 8.28

Two floppy guidewires were placed in the LAD and first diagonal branch. **(LOOP 8.28)**

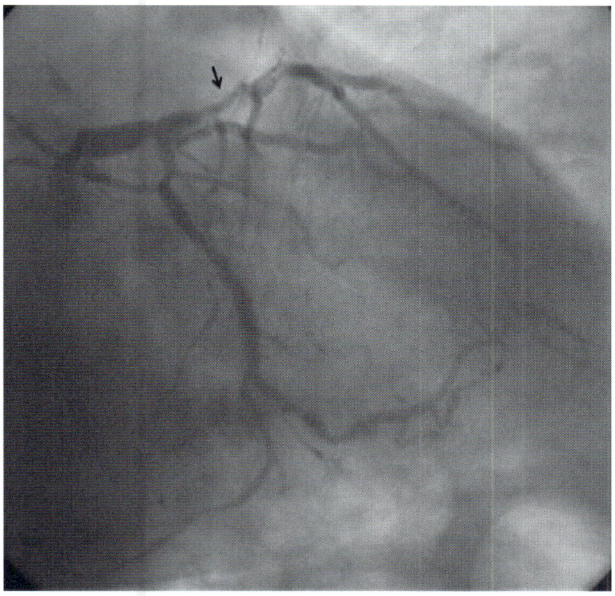

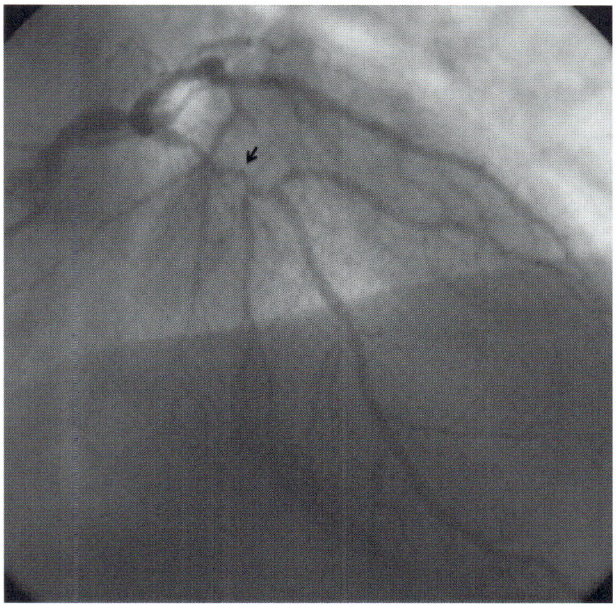

FIGURES 8.26 AND 8.27

Baseline coronary angiography demonstrating a severe calcific and angulated stenosis of the proximal-to-mid-LAD. **(LOOPS 8.26 AND 8.27)**

TABLE 8.1

Therapeutic Options in the Management of Embolized Material.

No treatment for peripherally embolized small stents
Nonretrieval of a stent or broken guidewire:
Deployment of the embolized stent in inconsequential locations if wire still inside the stent
Crushing the stent or guidewire against the vessel wall with another stent
Small-balloon technique: inflating a small balloon distally and withdrawing balloon together with lost stent
Removal of embolized material with a loop snare
Two-wire technique: removal of stent by intertwining two wires
Device retrieval in aorta or peripheral arteries with a myocardial biopsy forceps, biliary forceps, Cook fragment retriever, or basket retrieval device.

Source: Adapted from Farah et al (2).

COMPLICATION AND MANAGEMENT

The rotablator burr could not be removed even with vigorous pulling and deep engagement of the guiding catheter. Thus, a second guiding catheter was placed via the contralateral groin, and a floppy guidewire was successfully manipulated next to the trapped burr and into the large diagonal branch (Figure 8.30). A 1.25-mm, followed by 2-mm, balloon was successfully advanced next to the burr and inflated in order to create more space between the burr and the vessel wall. This maneuver was successful in freeing the burr, which was removed without complication. Also, it was now possible to cross and dilate the lesion with a balloon. Two overlapping Endeavor Resolute stents (Medtronic, Minneapolis, MN) were implanted in the mid- (2.5 × 13 mm) and proximal (3 × 22 mm) LAD. The final angiographic result was excellent (Figures 8.31 and 8.32).

CASE ANALYSIS

Burr entrapment is more common in long calcified and angulated lesions, where the burr becomes entrapped within or distal (Kokesi effect) to the lesion. This complication may have been prevented by using a 1.5-mm burr, which would not have passed the lesion without some degree of plaque ablation.

LESSONS

- When performing rotational atherectomy, it is essential to choose the correct burr size, as an undersized burr is more likely to become entrapped.
- Optimal rotational atherectomy technique is also important in preventing burr entrapment. It is important to perform rotablation with a "pecking motion," and with long lesions, it is important to ablate the proximal segment adequately before advancing the burr.
- If an entrapped burr cannot be removed with vigorous pulling, passing the entrapped burr with a guidewire and performing balloon dilatation next to the burr can be successful in releasing the burr.

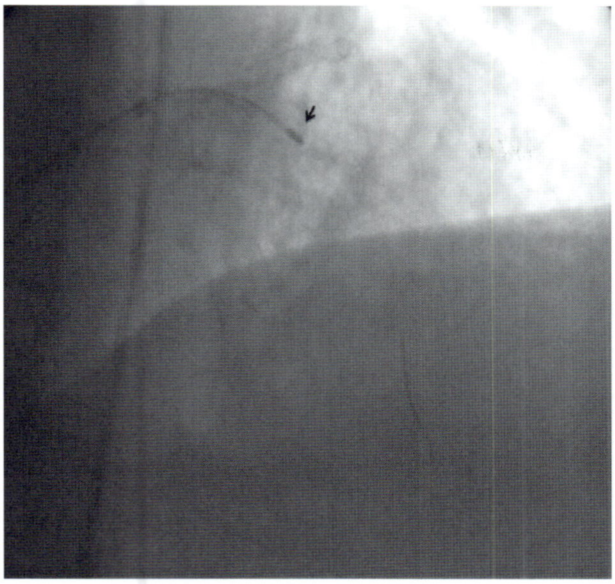

FIGURE 8.29

A rota floppy wire was placed in the distal LAD, and rotablation with a 1.25-mm burr (arrow) was performed on the proximal LAD. **(LOOP 8.29)**

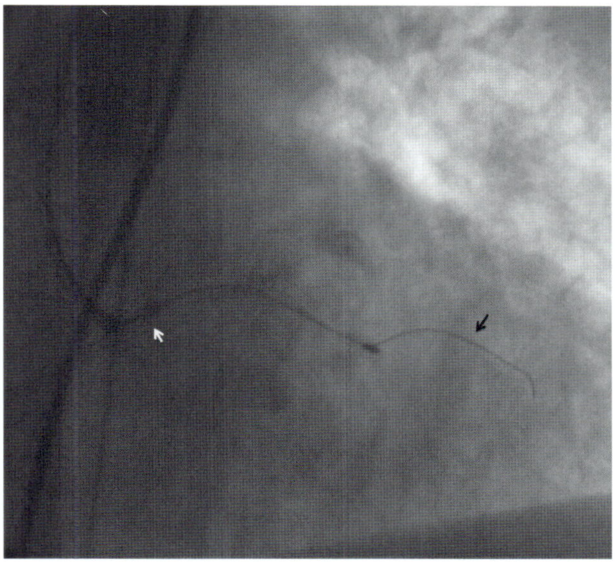

FIGURE 8.30

A second floppy guidewire was manipulated into the large diagonal branch (black arrow) next to the trapped burr (the wire was advanced through a second guide catheter from the contralateral groin). **(LOOP 8.30)**

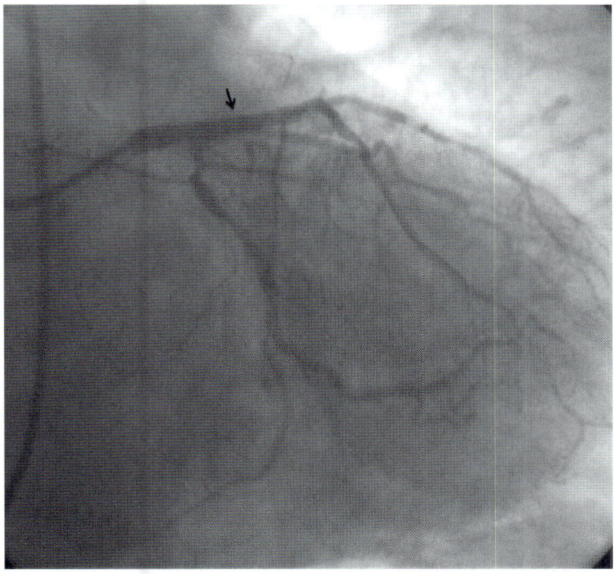

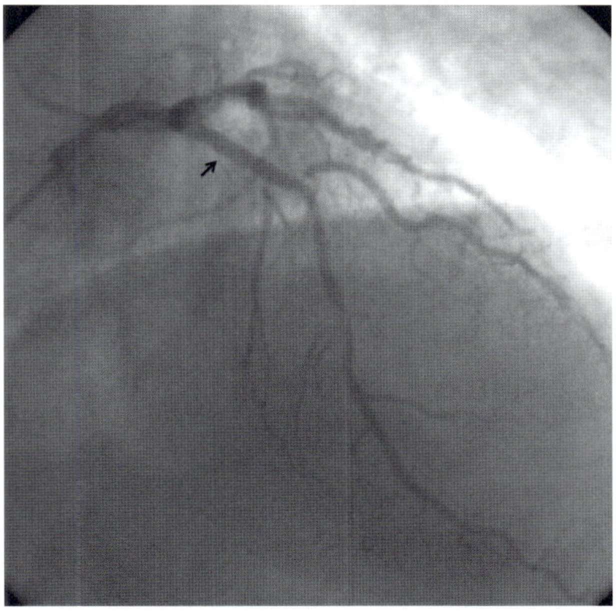

FIGURES 8.31 AND 8.32

Final angiographic result after the entrapped burr was retrieved and the lesion dilated with a balloon and stented (arrow). **(LOOPS 8.31 AND 8.32)**

References

1. Brilakis ES, Best PJ, Elesber AA, et al. Incidence, retrieval methods, and outcomes of stent loss during percutaneous coronary intervention: a large single-center experience. *Catheter Cardiovasc Interv.* 2005;66:333–340.
2. Farah B, Fajadet J, Marco J. Management of stent loss and foreign body retrieval. In: Eeckhout E, Carlier S, Lerman A, Kern M, eds. *Handbook of Complications during Percutaneous Cardiovascular Interventions.* London, UK: Informa Healthcare; 2007:103–109.
3. Cishek MB, Laslett L, Gershony G. Balloon catheter retrieval of dislodged coronary artery stents: a novel technique. *Cathet Cardiovasc Diagn.* 1995;34:350–352.
4. Eggebrecht H, Haude M, von Birgelen C, et al. Nonsurgical retrieval of embolized coronary stents. *Catheter Cardiovasc Interv.* 2000;51:432–440.
5. Qiao S, Gao R, Chen J, et al. Successful retrieval of intracoronary lost balloon-mounted stent using a small balloon. *Chin Med. J* (Engl) 2000;113:93–94.
6. Funatsu A, Kobayashi T, Nakamura S. Successful retrieval of a broken intravascular ultrasound catheter tip in the coronary artery. *J Invasive Cardiol.* 2010; 22:E197-E200.
7. Wong PH. Retrieval of undeployed intracoronary Palmaz-Schatz stents. *Cathet Cardiovasc Diagn.* 1995; 35:218–223.
8. Veldhuijzen FL, Bonnier HJ, Michels HR, el Gamal MI, van Gelder BM. Retrieval of undeployed stents from the right coronary artery: report of two cases. *Cathet Cardiovasc Diagn.* 1993;30:245–248.
9. Berder V, Bedossa M, Gras D, Paillard F, Le Breton H, Pony JC. Retrieval of a lost coronary stent from the descending aorta using a PTCA balloon and biopsy forceps. *Cathet Cardiovasc Diagn.* 1993;28:351–353.
10. Foster-Smith KW, Garratt KN, Higano ST, Holmes DR Jr. Retrieval techniques for managing flexible intracoronary stent misplacement. *Cathet Cardiovasc Diagn.* 1993;30:63–68.
11. Eeckhout E, Stauffer JC, Goy JJ. Retrieval of a migrated coronary stent by means of an alligator forceps catheter. *Cathet Cardiovasc Diagn.* 1993;30:166–168.
12. Meisel SR, DiLeo J, Rajakaruna M, Pace B, Frankel R, Shani J. A technique to retrieve stents dislodged in the coronary artery followed by fixation in the iliac artery by means of balloon angioplasty and peripheral stent deployment. *Catheter Cardiovasc Interv.* 2000;49:77–81.
13. Alfonso F, Martinez D, Hernandez R, et al. Stent embolization during intracoronary stenting. *Am J Cardiol.* 1996;78:833–835.
14. Tierstein PS, Gollapudi RR, Price MJ. Calcified and undilatable lesions. In: Colombo A, Stankovic G, eds. *Problem Oriented Approaches in Interventional Cardiology.* London, UK: Informa Healthcare; 2007:79–86.

9

Alfonso Ielasi, Azeem Latib, and Antonio Colombo

Stent Thrombosis

INTRODUCTION

Although coronary stents have undoubtedly improved the safety and efficacy of percutaneous coronary interventions (PCIs), their introduction have created a new complication, namely stent thrombosis (ST). The frequency of ST has declined from 6% to 24% in the early days (1) (due to suboptimal implantation technique and lack of antiplatelet therapy) to about 1% after the introduction of dual antiplatelet therapy (DAT) with aspirin and thienopyridines and improvement in stent implantation technique (2). ST, irrespective of whether in a drug-eluting stent (DES) or bare-metal stent (BMS), usually results in myocardial infarction (MI) or death (60% to 87% with BMS and 66% to 100% with DES) (3,4). In addition, patients suffering from ST are at significant risk of recurrent thrombotic stent occlusion (16% –18%) (5), recurrent MI, and death for up to 3 years (3,6).

The Academic Research Consortium (ARC) has developed a standardized definition of ST, incorporating timing and diagnostic certainty (7). Although ARC's definition added uniformity, it remains an imperfect balance of sensitivity and specificity; "definite" ST is highly specific but likely underestimates true frequency, whereas "possible" ST, although more sensitive, lacks diagnostic certainty. It is important to recognize that there is an intrinsic risk to overestimate ST, even with the frequently accepted definition of probable ST; any plaque rupture causing MI in the stented vessel will fall in to such a definition.

ST is a multifactorial phenomenon associated with patient, lesion, and procedure- or device-related characteristics, as well as compliance with, or resistance to antiplatelet agents. Early ST has been generally viewed as a problem originating from procedural factors, whereas late ST appears to be more associated with multiple variables, particularly related to the interaction between the device and the arterial wall. Because of the multifactorial etiology of ST, strategies aimed at its prevention should be multimodal as well. Although preventive strategies are of central importance to reduce the incidence of ST, this complication can still occur, despite the best efforts to prevent it. Thus, the principal objective must be to obtain early effective reperfusion, which will be the focus of this chapter. It is important to note that thrombus quality in a setting of ST differs from that in patients presenting with an acute MI due to thrombotic occlusion of a nonstented coronary artery (8). In the case of ST, the thrombus is almost totally composed of platelets and contains a poor amount of fibrin. This fact may explain the poor efficacy of thrombolysis to obtain effective reperfusion in this setting. The recommendations we suggest for the management of ST are as follows:

1. Acute administration of glycoprotein IIb–IIIa should be mandatory (even with an intracoronary bolus injection), considering the thrombus burden in ST. Their use is associated with a reperfusion success rate of 90% when associated with PCI and with a decrease in recurrent thrombotic events after a successfully treated ST (9).
2. Proceed to emergent PCI of the target lesion with the goal of obtaining optimal results without repeat stent implantation, if possible. Prolonged balloon inflations (1–2 minutes) with a slightly oversized balloon inflated at low–medium pressure are preferable. The implantation of another stent during PCI for ST should be avoided unless clearly required as a bailout option to manage dissections, plaque, or thrombus shift outside the previously implanted stent and previously untreated adjacent atherosclerotic disease (6).
3. Intravascular ultrasound (IVUS) should be mandatory to identify and correct potential index procedure-related factors (i.e., incomplete stent apposition or suboptimal stent expansion) that could have contributed to ST.
4. Mechanical aspiration devices should be considered on a case-by-case basis. Thrombus aspiration is particularly helpful in the presence of large thrombus burden.
5. If slow or no reflow occurs, selective intracoronary administration of adenosine (30–50 μg) or nitroprusside (80 μg) should be considered. The dosage of these agents can be increased progressively, and

multiple injections are often required. In hypotensive patients, intracoronary pressor agents (adrenaline 50–200 μg) should be considered to allow for the administration of a higher dose of intracoronary vasodilators.

6. Lastly, if ST occurs in a patient who was compliant with DAT (aspirin and clopidogrel), serious consideration should be given to replace clopidogrel with a more potent antiplatelet agent, such as prasugrel or ticagrelor. In addition, lifetime administration of DAT should be considered in patients who are at low bleeding risk and who sustained ST in the absence of identifiable procedural-related factors.

CASE 9.1

Acute ST After Primary PCI

CLINICAL HISTORY AND DIAGNOSTIC TESTING RESULTS

A 56-year-old woman with hypertension, dyslipidemia, and a family history of coronary artery disease was admitted with an anterior ST-elevation MI. The patient underwent immediate coronary angiography, which showed a thrombotic occlusion of the proximal left anterior descending artery (LAD) (Figure 9.1).

PLANNED PROCEDURE

PCI of the proximal LAD.

PROCEDURE

The patient was given intravenous aspirin, a loading dose of 300 mg of clopidogrel, intravenous bivalirudin bolus, and infusion. The LAD occlusion was recanalized with a floppy guidewire, and a second floppy guidewire was placed in the diagonal branch (Figure 9.2). A 3- × 28-mm Taxus (Boston Scientific, Natick, MA) stent was directly implanted in the proximal LAD at 14 atm, which resulted in good angiographic result and progressive ST segment normalization (Figure 9.3).

COMPLICATION AND MANAGEMENT

Shortly following stent implantation, anterior ST segment elevation reappeared, and repeat angiography

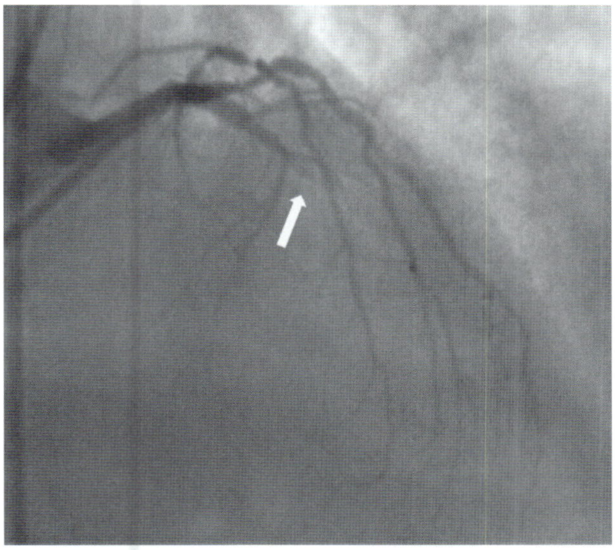

FIGURE 9.1

Thrombotic occlusion of the proximal LAD (arrow). (LOOP 9.1)

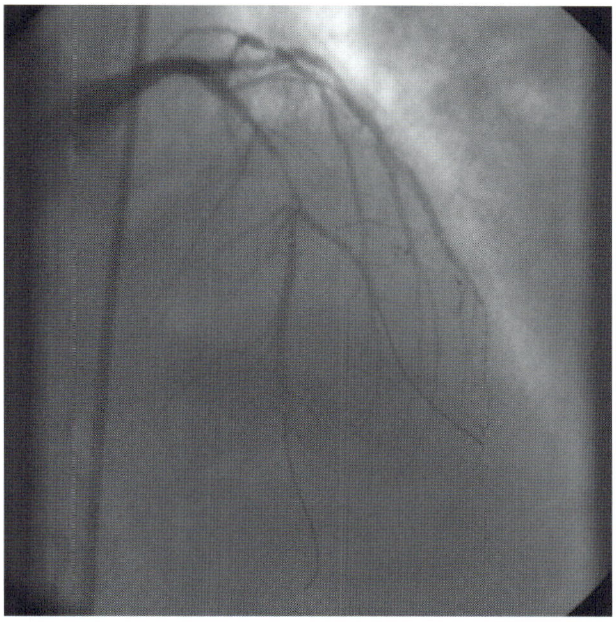

FIGURE 9.2

Recanalization of the acute thrombotic occlusion with floppy guidewires placed in the distal LAD and in the D1 branch. (LOOP 9.2)

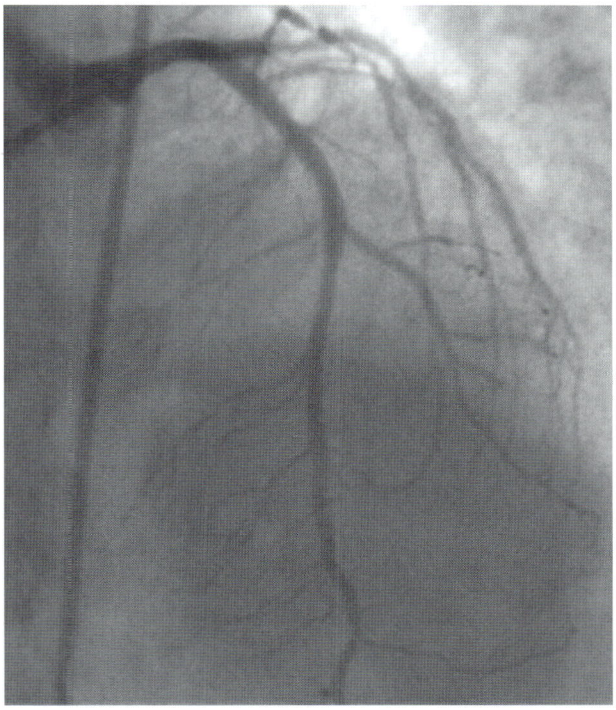

FIGURE 9.3

Excellent angiographic result after direct stenting of the proximal LAD. (LOOP 9.3)

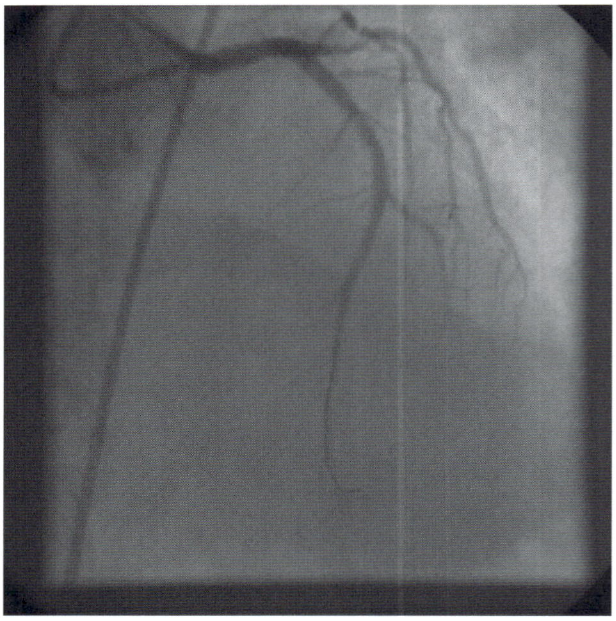

FIGURE 9.4

Note the intrastent filling defects in the proximal LAD. (LOOP 9.4)

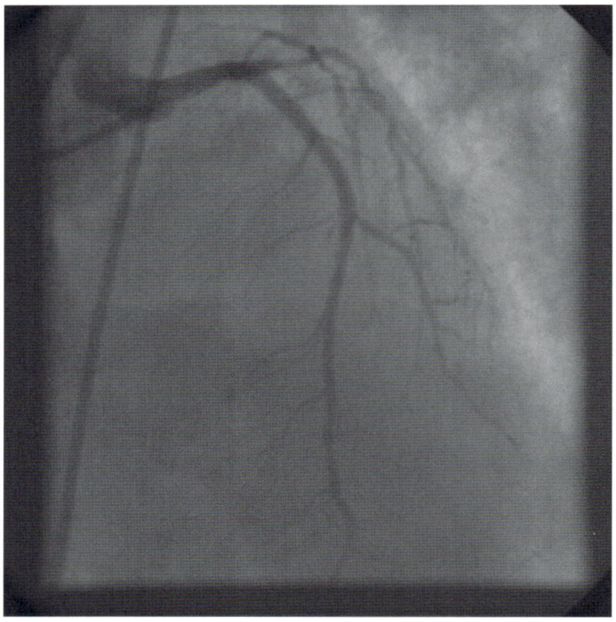

FIGURE 9.5

Final coronary angiography demonstrating TIMI-3 flow. (LOOP 9.5)

showed intrastent thrombosis (Figure 9.4). An intracoronary bolus and intravenous infusion of abciximab were administered and multiple inflations were performed inside the stent with a 3.5- × 20-mm noncompliant balloon, obtaining a good final angiographic result (Figure 9.5). IVUS was then performed to assure stent apposition and expansion.

CASE ANALYSIS

Although the exact cause of acute ST in this case cannot be determined with certainty, stent implantation in a thrombotic milieu is a risk factor for ST, particularly in the absence of optimal antiplatelet activity. In the HORIZONS-AMI trial, intravenous bivalirudin, compared with intravenous heparin and glycoprotein IIb/IIIa antagonists, was associated with excess ST. In our own experience, we have observed intraprocedural ST in patients who received only intravenous bivalirudin in ST elevation myocardial infarction (STEMI) patients. In this setting, the loading dose of clopidogrel is usually given <90 minutes before primary PCI, and maximal inhibition of platelet aggregation is not guaranteed. Faster acting and more potent antiplatelet agents are indicated in patients undergoing primary PCI, who have not been well prepared with thienopyridines. On this basis, we now administer a 60-mg loading dose of prasugrel (often on the catheterization table) in patients undergoing primary PCI in STEMI. This strategy should reduce the risk of intraprocedural or acute ST due to insufficient platelet inhibition.

LESSONS

- In patients undergoing primary PCI for STEMI, maximal platelet inhibition is fundamental to reduce the risk of ischemic events.
- In patients undergoing primary PCI for STEMI, the use of intravenous bivalirudin without IIb/IIIa antagonists has been associated with excess incidence of ST.
- Always consider administering intravenous or intracoronary IIb/IIIa in patients presenting with ST, particularly if they were noncompliant with, or have not received, adequate oral antiplatelet therapy.

CASE 9.2

Acute ST After Administration of Intravenous Protamine

CLINICAL HISTORY AND DIAGNOSTIC TESTING RESULTS

A 68-year-old woman with history of hypertension and hyperlipidemia was admitted for unstable angina. Coronary angiography demonstrated a stenosis of the proximal left circumflex artery (LCX) with chronic total occlusions (CTOs) of the proximal LAD and middle right coronary artery (mid-RCA). Left ventricular function was normal (EF, 60%) (Figures 9.6 and 9.7).

PLANNED PROCEDURE

Recanalization of the LAD, CTO, and DES implantation in the proximal LCX.

PROCEDURE

Intravenous unfractionated heparin was administered (8,000 units). A 6-Fr XB 3.5 guiding catheter (Cordis, a Johnson and Johnson Company, Warren, NJ) was used to engage the left main coronary artery. A BMW Universal II guidewire (Abbott Vascular Devices, Redwood City, CA) was placed in the distal

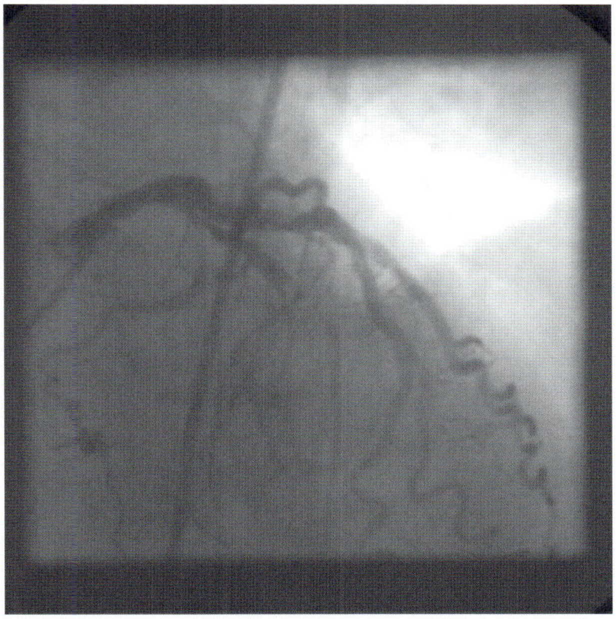

FIGURE 9.7
Baseline coronary angiography (cranial view) showing CTO of the proximal LAD. (LOOP 9.7)

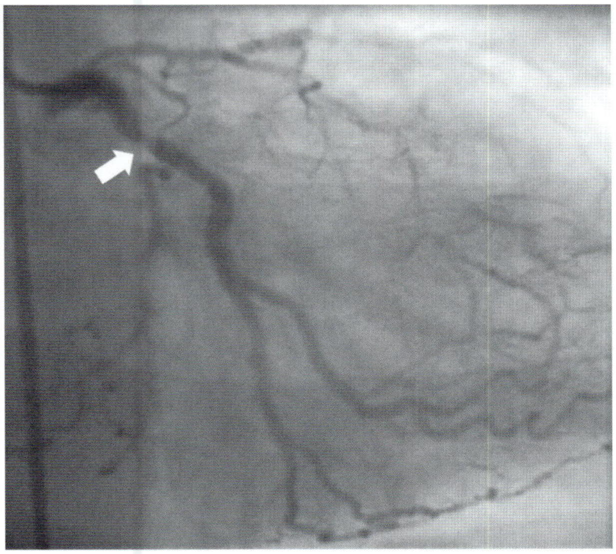

FIGURE 9.6
Baseline coronary angiography (RAO view) showing a focal stenosis of the proximal LCX (arrow). (LOOP 9.6)

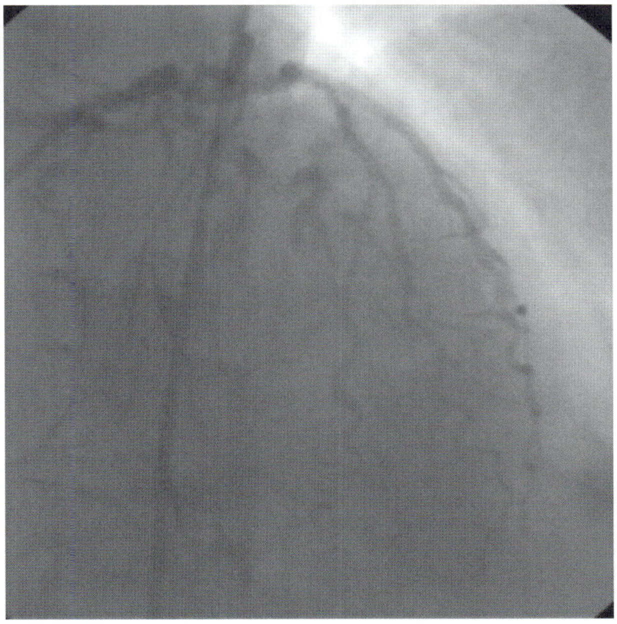

FIGURE 9.8
Coronary angiography showing a perforation with intramyocardial hematoma in the mid-LAD. (LOOP 9.8)

LCX, and a 3.5- × 13-mm Cypher stent (Cordis, a Johnson and Johnson Company, Warren, NJ) was implanted in the proximal LCX without predilatation. The stent was postdilated with a 4- × 8-mm Quantum Maverick (Boston Scientific, Natick, MA) noncompliant balloon at 26 atm. During attempts to recanalize the totally occluded LAD with a hydrophilic wire (Pilot 50, Abbott Vascular Devices, Redwood City, CA), a perforation leading to intramyocardial hematoma was observed (Figure 9.8). The operator administered 50 mg of intravenous protamine. A few minutes later, the patient complained of severe chest pain, developed hypotension, and had a full cardiac arrest.

COMPLICATION AND MANAGEMENT

Immediate coronary angiography showed an occluded proximal LCX at the stent site (ST) (Figure 9.9). Cardiopulmonary resuscitation was initiated with manual chest compression, intravenous vasopressors, and percutaneous cardiopulmonary support system. A balanced middle weight (BMW) Universal II guidewire was used to recanalize the occluded LCX artery, and balloon dilatation of the occluded segment was performed using a Quantum Maverick noncompliant balloon (4 × 8 mm at 16 atm). Despite successful reopening of the occluded LCX (Figure 9.10) and the other supportive measures, the patient died.

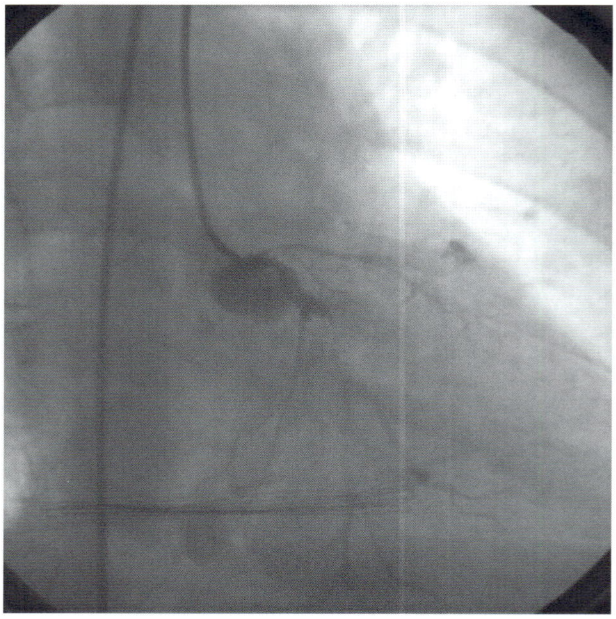

FIGURE 9.9

Coronary angiography after cardiac arrest (following protamine administration) demonstrating an occluded stent in the proximal LCX. (LOOP 9.9)

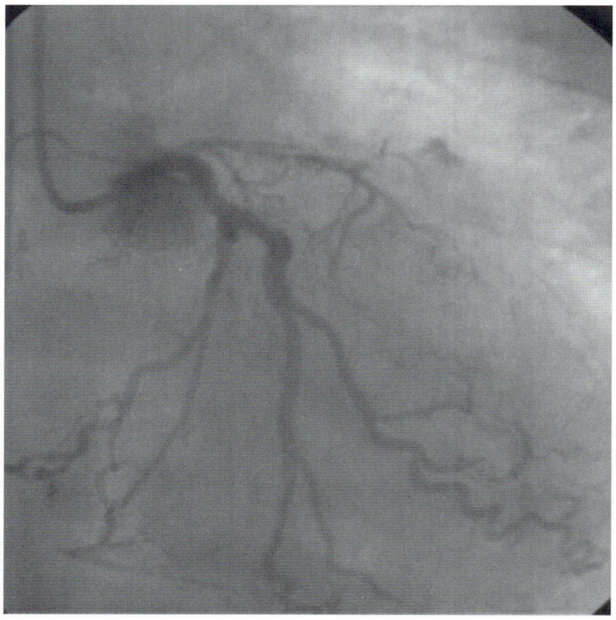

FIGURE 9.10

Coronary angiography showing recanalization of the proximal LCX stent. (LOOP 9.10)

CASE ANALYSIS

In this case, there are two decision points that may have contributed to the unfortunate outcome: (*1*) The decision to recanalize the LAD CTO in the same setting of stenting the only remaining vessel (LCX), and (*2*) the administration of protamine in the setting of acute stent implantation. We have experienced three cases of acute DES thrombosis occurring soon after protamine administration. After this experience, we try not to administer protamine immediately after DES implantation, unless life-threatening bleeding occurs.

LESSONS

- In patients undergoing PCI of a single remaining vessel, elective CTO recanalization of other vessels should be deferred for at least 4 weeks.
- In the event of vessel perforation, after stent implantation, all remedies to obtain hemostasis should be exhausted before administration of protamine (it should only be used as a last resort).
- Despite the tremendous progress in PCI strategies, ST still carries a poor prognosis.

SUGGESTED READING

Cosgrave J, Qasim A, Latib A, Aranzulla TC, Colombo A. Protamine usage following implantation of drug-eluting stents: a word of caution. *Catheter Cardiovasc Interv.* 2008;71(7):913–914.

CASE 9.3

Subacute ST Due to Suboptimal Initial Stent Implantation

CLINICAL HISTORY AND DIAGNOSTIC TESTING RESULTS

A 49-year-old man with prior acute inferolateral MI (2 weeks ago) status post BMS implantation in the proximal LCX presented with new onset unstable angina. Coronary angiography showed patent proximal LCX stent, known occluded RCA and proximal LAD stenosis, and new subocclusive stenosis in the distal LCX (was not significant 2 weeks ago) (Figures 9.11 and 9.12).

PLANNED PROCEDURE

DES implantation in the distal LCX lesion.

PROCEDURE

The patient was already taking aspirin and clopidogrel after his initial stent implantation, 2 weeks earlier. A bolus of intravenous unfractionated heparin was administered. A balance guidewire was placed in the distal LCX, and lesion predilatation was performed using a 2.5- ×12-mm Maverick (Boston Scientific, Natick, Massachusetts) semicompliant balloon at 12 atm. Subsequently, two Promus Element stents (2.5 × 16 mm and 2.5 × 12 mm) (Boston Scientific, Natick, MA) were implanted from middle to distal LCX. Following stent implantation, coronary angiography showed a type A dissection at the distal edge of the stent (Figures 9.13 and 9.14). However, the operator decided not to implant another stent due to the nonflow-limiting nature of the dissection. The patient was discharged the day after the procedure, and DAT was recommended for 12 months.

COMPLICATION AND MANAGEMENT

Three weeks later, the patient was readmitted with recurrent unstable angina associated with ST segment depression in the posterolateral leads, despite adherence to DAT. Coronary angiography showed occlusion of the distal LCX at the site of the Promus stent (ST) (Figure 9.15). A floppy guidewire failed to recanalize the occluded segment. Subsequently, a Fielder FC guidewire (Asahi Intecc Co Ltd, Nagoya, Japan/Abbott Vascular Devices, Redwood City, CA) in an over-the-wire balloon was used to recanalize the thrombotic lesion (Figure 9.16). Sequential dilatations with noncompliant balloons of increasing diameter (2.0 × 12 mm; 2.5 × 12 mm) were performed instent and at the distal stent edge, restoring thrombolysis in myocardial infarction grade 2 (TIMI-2) flow with residual intraluminal defects (Figure 9.17). IVUS interrogation showed a dissection at the distal stent edge (Figure 9.18), underexpansion of the

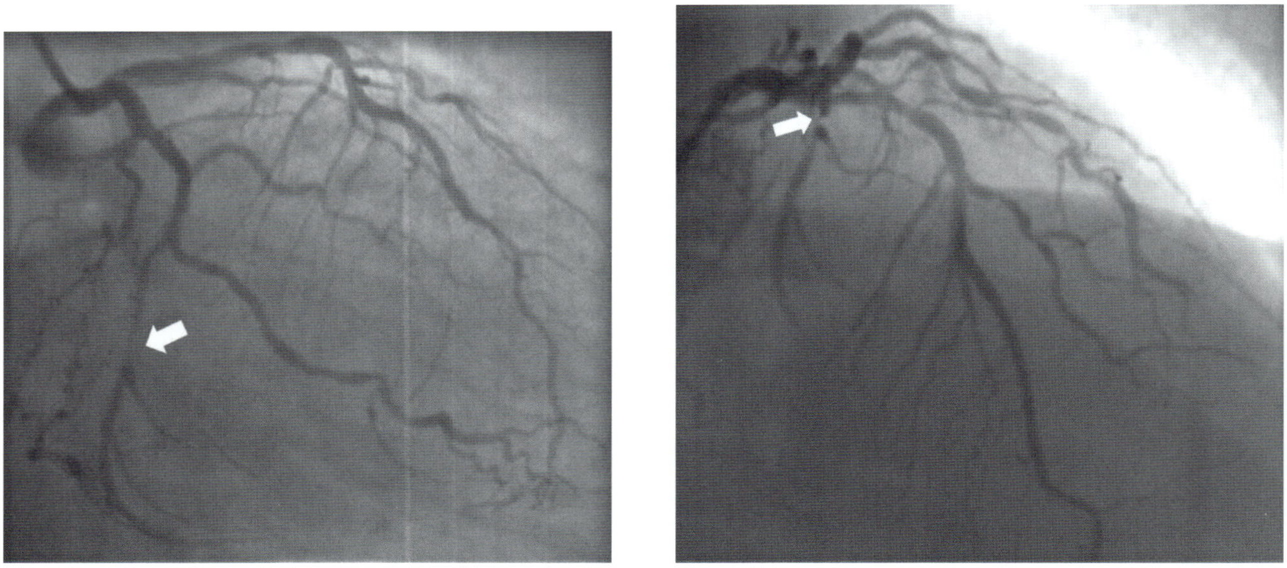

FIGURES 9.11 AND 9.12

Baseline coronary angiography showing patent proximal LCX BMS and subocclusive stenosis of the distal LCX (arrow). (LOOPS 9.11 AND 9.12)

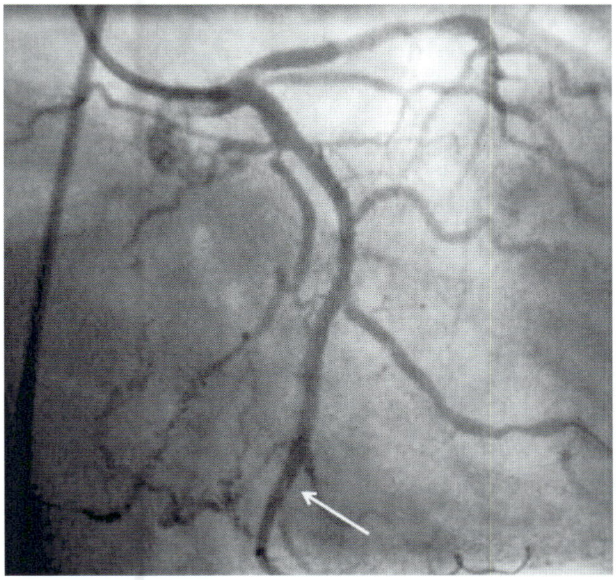

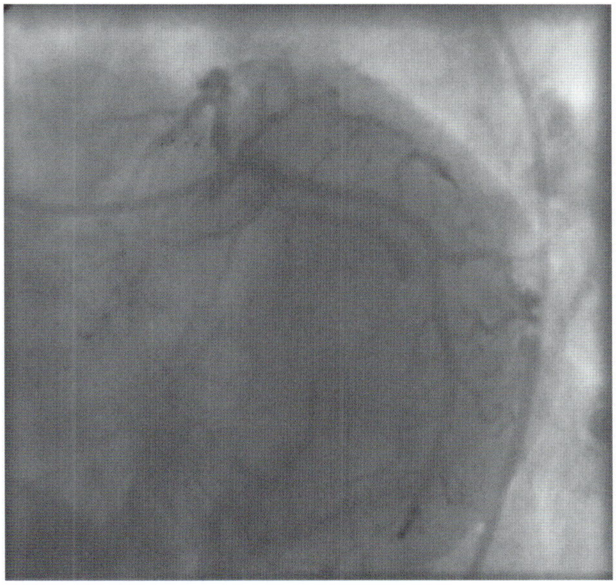

FIGURES 9.13 AND 9.14

Coronary angiography after implantation of the distal LCX stents. Note the type A dissection at the distal edge of the newly implanted stents (arrow). **(LOOPS 9.13 AND 9.14)**

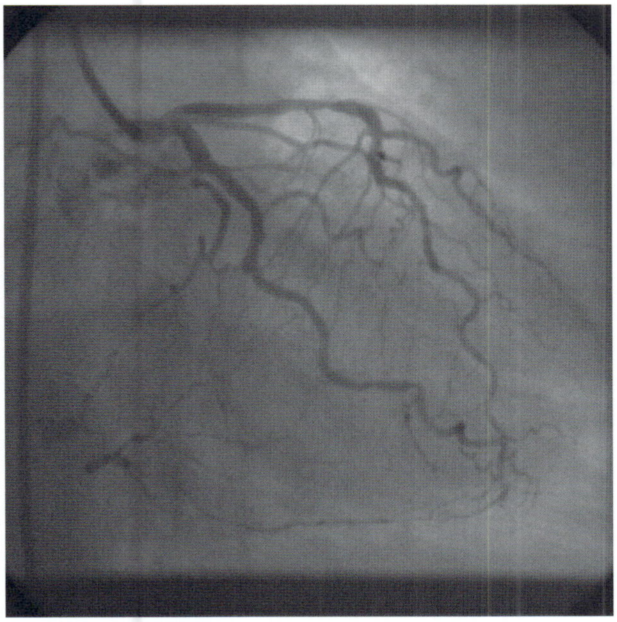

FIGURE 9.15

Coronary angiography performed 3 weeks later for unstable angina. Note the distal LCX occlusion (subacute ST). **(LOOP 9.15)**

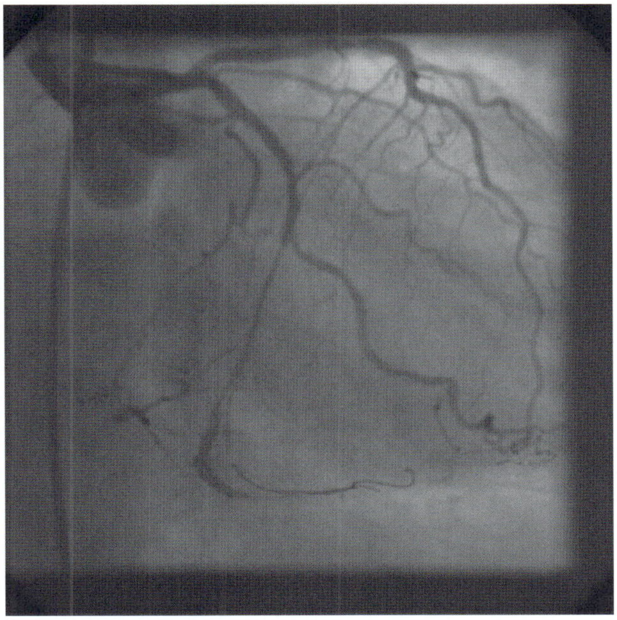

FIGURE 9.16

Coronary angiography after wire recanalization of the distal LCX. **(LOOP 9.16)**

Promus 2.5-mm stents (as the media-to-media diameter was 3.5 × 3.09 mm) (Figure 9.19), and significant stenosis at the proximal stent edge. Two 3- × 18-mm Endeavor Resolute (Medtronic Vascular, Santa Rosa, CA) stents were implanted proximally and distally to the Promus stents. IVUS-guided postdilatation was performed using a 3.5- × 12-mm and 3.0- × 12-mm noncompliant balloons on the mid and distal LCX, obtaining a good final angiographic result (Figure 9.20).

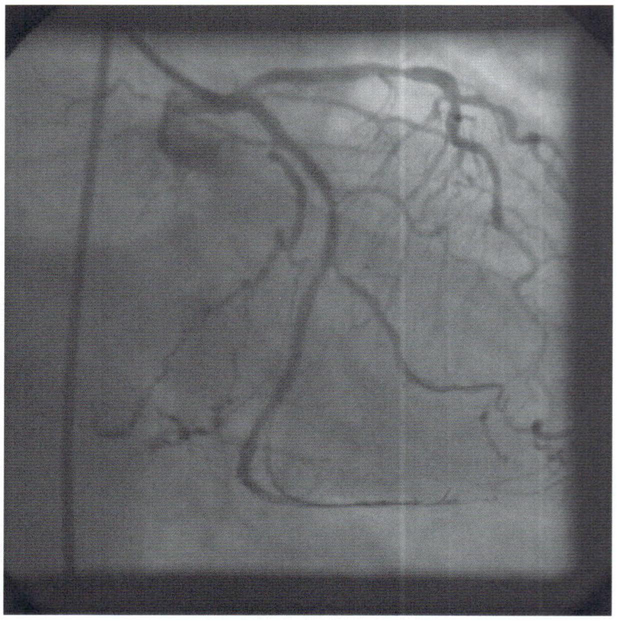

FIGURE 9.17

Coronary angiography after balloon angioplasty of the thrombosed stents. Note the TIMI-2 flow with residual intraluminal defects. (LOOP 9.17)

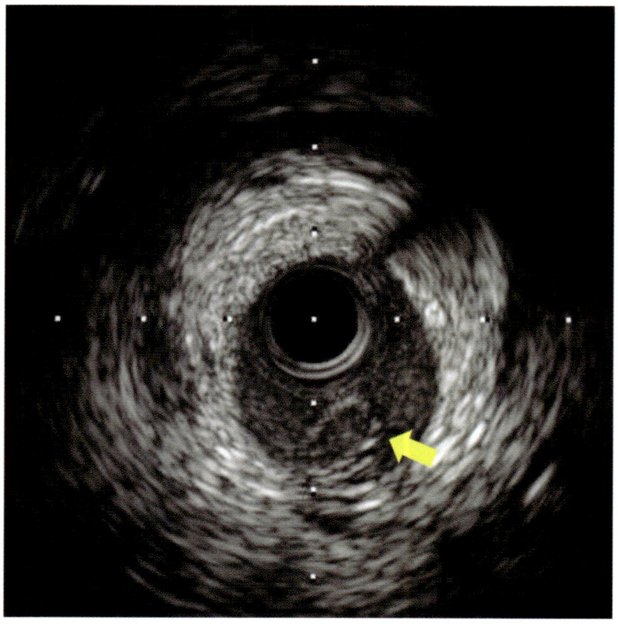

FIGURE 9.18

IVUS image demonstrating a dissection at the distal stent edge (arrow). (LOOP 9.18)

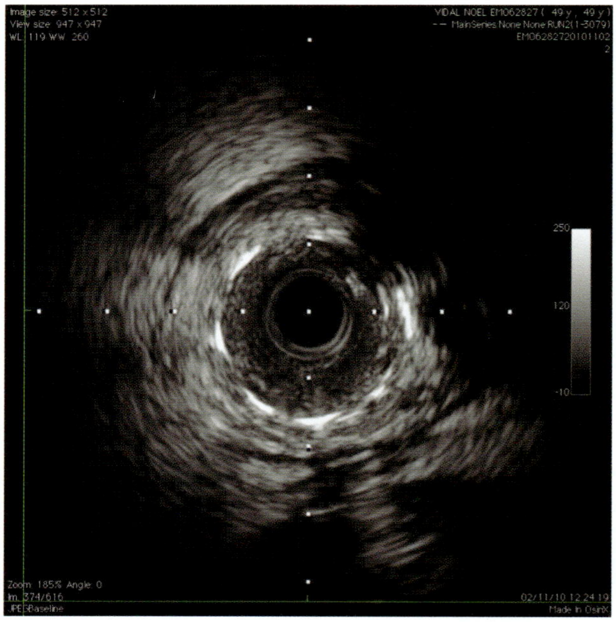

FIGURE 9.19

IVUS image demonstrating underexpansion of the Promus stent. (LOOP 9.19)

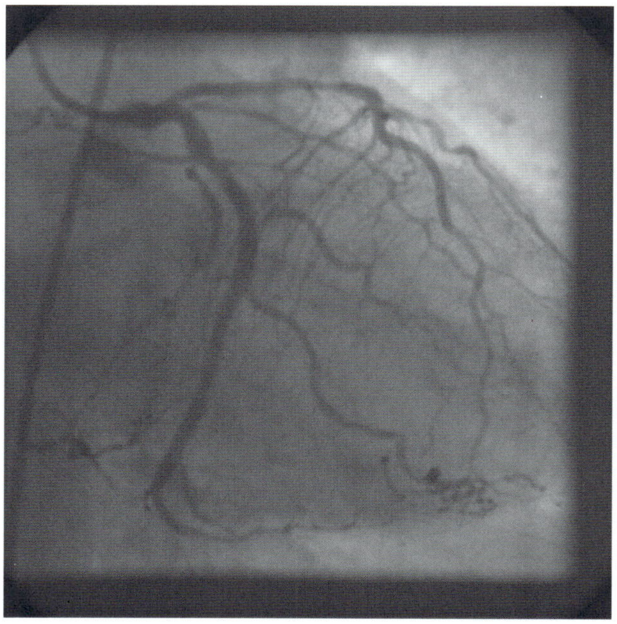

FIGURE 9.20

Final coronary angiography after implantation of two Endeavor Resolute stents and IVUS-guided postdilation. (LOOP 9.20)

CASE ANALYSIS

In this case, subacute ST occurred as a result of suboptimal initial stent implantation. At the time of ST, IVUS interrogation showed residual distal dissection, underexpanded stents, and residual lesion proximal to the stents. During the initial stent implantation procedure, the operator did not perform IVUS or stent postdilation due to satisfactory angiographic appearance, despite the presence of small distal edge dissection. Although it is difficult to ascertain whether the distal edge dissection was a contributor to ST, it is a probability that should not be ignored. We think that every effort should be made to seal dissections at the inflow and outflow of stents with either prolonged balloon inflations or deploying another stent.

LESSONS

- Subacute ST is often associated with suboptimal stent deployment.
- Residual dissections after DES implantation can be associated with adverse clinical outcome.
- IVUS interrogation at the time of ST is invaluable in detecting treatable causes of ST.

SUGGESTED READING

Biondi-Zoccai G, Agostoni P, Sangiorgi G, et al. Incidence, predictors, and outcomes of coronary dissections left untreated after drug-eluting stent implantation. *Eur Heart Journal.* 2006;27:540–546.

Fujii K, Carlier SG, Mintz GS, et al. Stent underexpansion and residual reference segment stenosis are related to stent thrombosis after sirolimus-eluting stent implantation: an intravascular ultrasound study. *J Am Coll Cardiol.* 2005;45:995–998.

CASE 9.4

Late ST Due to Interruption of DAT

CLINICAL HISTORY AND DIAGNOSTIC TESTING RESULTS

A 65-year-old woman with history of transient ischemic attacks (TIAs), known two-vessel coronary artery disease (CAD) status post-PCI to mid RCA (with BMS) and ostial LAD and LCX (with drug-eluting stent [DES]) 10 months ago, was admitted for exertional angina. Coronary angiography revealed instent restenosis (ISR) of the mid-RCA BMS. The RCA ISR was treated by implantation of 3.0- × 12-mm Taxus (Boston Scientific, Natick, MA) stent. The patient was prescribed 12 months of DAT. Five months after DES implantation in the mid-RCA, the patient was readmitted for congestive heart failure and new onset atrial fibrillation. Echocardiography revealed severe mitral regurgitation associated with severe tricuspid regurgitation and normal left ventricular systolic function (EF, 55%).

PLANNED PROCEDURE

Surgical repair of the mitral and tricuspid valves 5 months after DES implantation.

PROCEDURE

DAT was stopped 5 days before surgical intervention. Diagnostic coronary angiography that was performed 4 days prior to valve surgery confirmed patency of all stents and no new obstructive disease (Figures 9.21 and 9.22).

COMPLICATION AND MANAGEMENT

One day prior to the surgical procedure, the patient complained of acute chest pain associated with inferior ST elevation. Emergent coronary angiography showed ST in the mid-RCA (Figure 9.23). A floppy wire was used to recanalize the occlusion. Intracoronary abciximab was administered, and manual thrombectomy with a Diver catheter (Invatec, Roncadelle/Brescia, Italy) was performed (Figure 9.24). Subsequently, balloon angioplasty with a 3- × 15-mm semicompliant balloon (Maverick) was performed with an excellent final result and TIMI-3 flow (Figure 9.25).

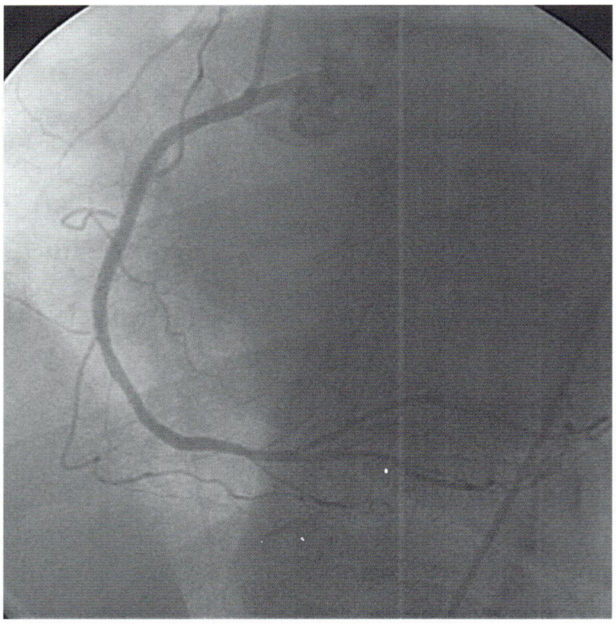

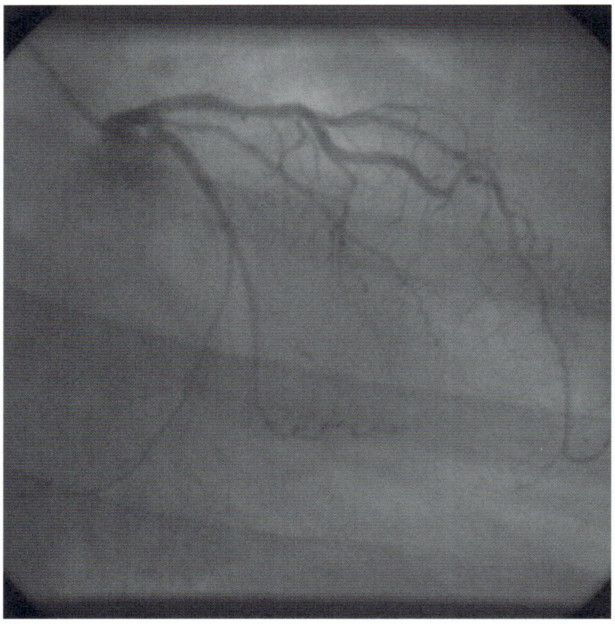

FIGURES 9.21 AND 9.22

Diagnostic coronary angiogram performed 4 days prior to valve surgery, showing patency of the DES previously implanted on the RCA, LAD, and LCX. **(LOOPS 9.21 AND 9.22)**

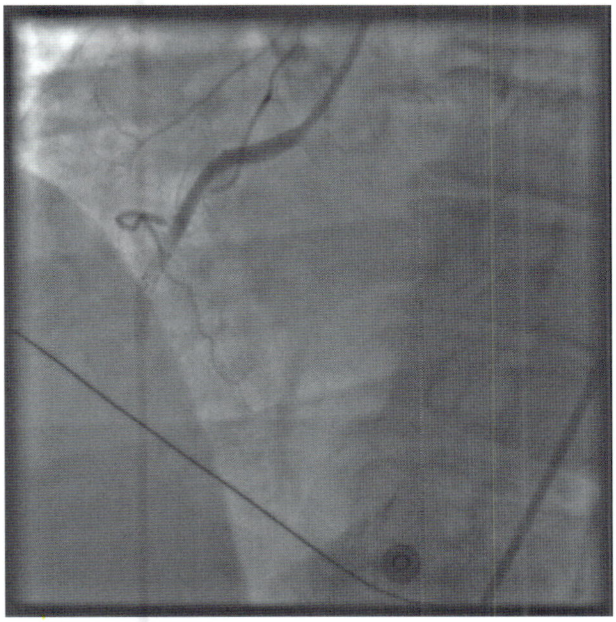

FIGURE 9.23

Emergency coronary angiography performed 1 day prior to the surgical procedure for inferior ST elevation MI, demonstrating ST in the mid-RCA. **(LOOP 9.23)**

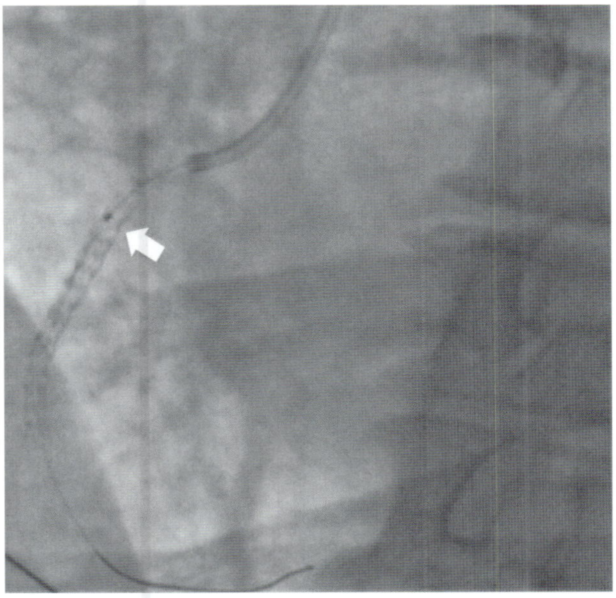

FIGURE 9.24

Manual thrombectomy performed after floppy wire placement in the distal RCA and intracoronary injection of abciximab (arrow). **(LOOP 9.24)**

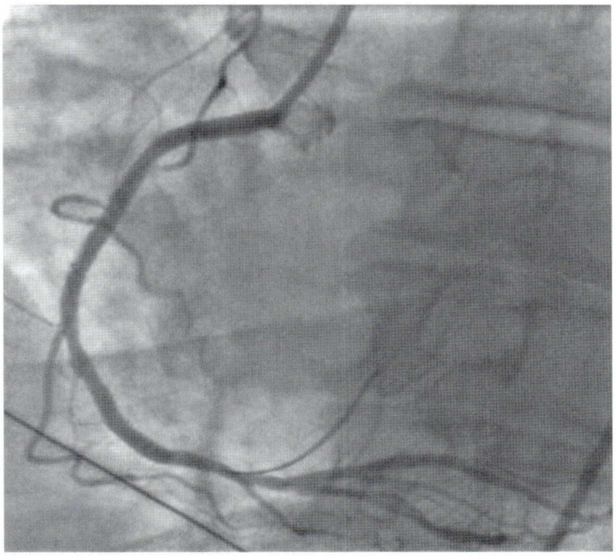

FIGURE 9.25

Final angiographic result after balloon angioplasty only using a semicompliant (3.5 × 12 mm) balloon. **(LOOP 9.25)**

CASE ANALYSIS

In this case, the occurrence of late ST was a result of two decisions: (*1*) The decision to perform elective surgery prior to 6 months after DES implantation, and (*2*) discontinuation of DAT 5 days prior to surgery without antiplatelet protection. One would wonder whether it would have been possible to delay the valve surgery several months and manage the patient medically in the interim. Premature discontinuation of DAT (<6 months from the procedure) is an independent predictor of DES thrombosis. Although discontinuation of DAT was necessary in this case, glycoprotein IIb/IIIa inhibitors should have been used as a bridge therapy prior to valve surgery. Although rigorous studies are lacking, bridging with tirofiban or eptifibatide should be started within 2 to 3 days after stopping oral antiplatelets and continued until 6 to 12 hours prior to surgery.

LESSONS

- All elective surgical procedures should be delayed by at least 6 months and ideally 12 months after DES placement.
- If surgery cannot be delayed and DAT must be interrupted, "bridge" therapy with a short half-life glycoprotein IIb/IIIa inhibitor (i.e., eptifibatide or tirofiban) should be strongly considered.

SUGGESTED READING

Abualsaud A, Eisenberg M. Perioperative management of patients with drug-eluting stents. *J Am Coll Coll Intv.* 2010;3:131–142.
Windecker S, Meier B. Late coronary stent thrombosis. *Circulation.* 2007;116:1952–1965.

CASE 9.5

Very Late Stent Thrombosis (ST)

CLINICAL HISTORY AND DIAGNOSTIC TESTING RESULTS

A 63-year-old female ex-smoker with history of idiopathic recurrent pericarditis on chronic steroid therapy and known CAD status post-BMS implantation on the second diagonal (D2) branch 1-year prior, presents with stable angina (CCS III) and a positive stress test with anterior ischemia. Coronary angiography showed a stenosis of the mid-LAD at the level of the bifurcation with D2, which also had moderate intimal hyperplasia at the ostium (Figure 9.26).

PLANNED PROCEDURE:

Reverse crush stenting of the LAD-D2 bifurcation.

PROCEDURE

Patient underwent successful reverse crush stenting of the LAD-D2 bifurcation optimized with a two-step final kissing balloon inflation (A 3.5- × 20-mm Taxus stent at the mid distal LAD crushed with a 2.75- × 28-mm Taxus stent from the proximal LAD toward D2) (Figure 9.27). Final results were optimal by IVUS and angiography (Figure 9.28). Sixteen months later, the patient presented with recurrent angina. Coronary angiography demonstrated severe stenosis of the distal apical segment of the LAD and the proximal segment of D1, and patent LAD/D2 bifurcation stents (Figures 9.29 and 9.30). The patient underwent successful PCI with implantation of a 2.25- × 18-mm Cypher stent (Cordis, a Johnson and Johnson Company, Warren, NJ) in the distal LAD and a 2.5- × 18-mm Cypher stent in the proximal D1 (Figure 9.31). The patient was placed on DAT for 12 months.

COMPLICATION AND MANAGEMENT

Five years later, the patient was admitted to another hospital with acute chest pain and ECG evidence of an acute anterolateral MI associated with cardiogenic shock. Clopidogrel had been discontinued 3 years ago after the patient had taken DAT for 24 months after the last DES implantation. After an intraarterial balloon pump (IABP) was placed, coronary angiography showed thrombotic subtotal occlusion (very late ST) of the mid-LAD stent, with extension to the D1 and D2 stents (Figure 9.32). A floppy guidewire was used to recanalize the LAD, and manual aspiration was performed on the LAD stent following IIb/IIIa administration (abciximab [ReoPro]) with only limited improvement (Figure 9.33). A guidewire was then placed in D2, and multiple inflations were performed in the mid and proximal segments with a 2.5- × 15-mm semicompliant balloon. Multiple inflations were also performed in the mid-LAD with a 3.5- ×12-mm noncompliant balloon and in the distal LAD using a 2.5- × 15-mm semicompliant balloon. Finally, D1 was also recanalized with a floppy guidewire, and several balloon inflations were performed. Despite all these maneuvers, thrombolysis in myocardial infarction grade 3 (TIMI-3) flow was never attained (Figure 9.34), and the patient died in the catheterization laboratory.

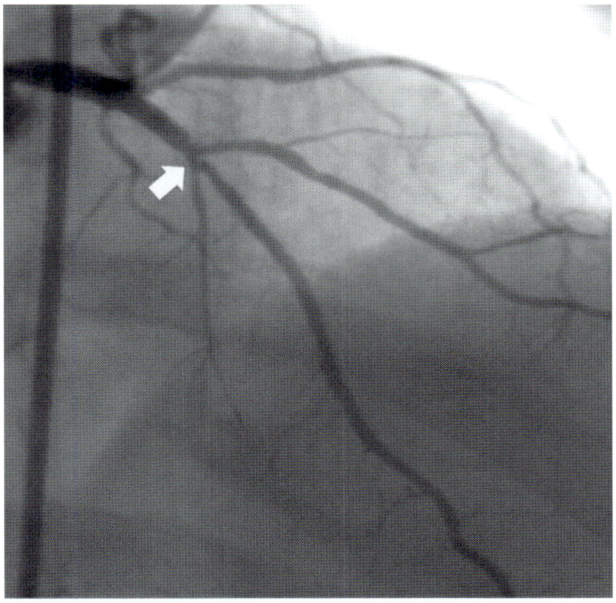

FIGURE 9.26

Coronary angiogram showing stenosis of the mid-LAD at the level of the bifurcation with D2 (arrow), which also had moderate intimal hyperplasia at the ostium. **(LOOP 9.26)**

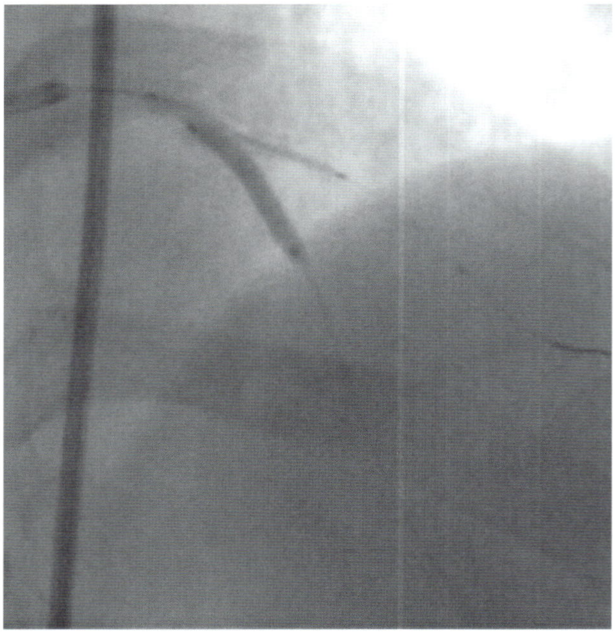

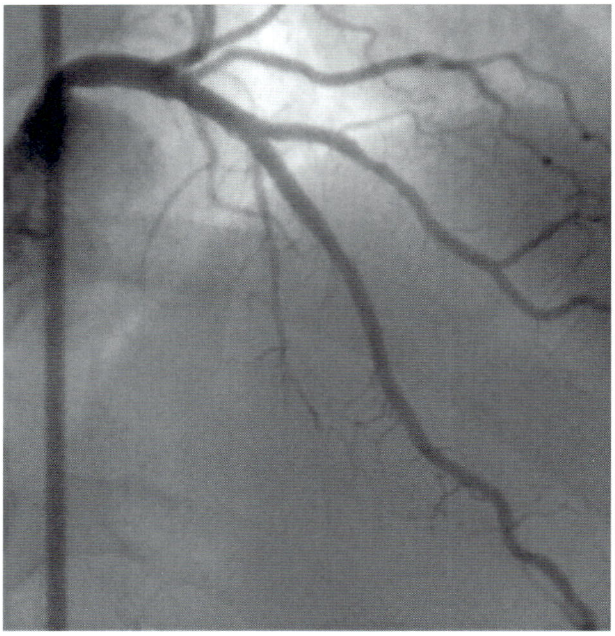

FIGURES 9.27 AND 9.28

Reverse crush stenting of the LAD-D2 bifurcation (Taxus 3.5 × 20 mm at the mid-distal LAD crushed with a Taxus 2.75 × 28 mm from the proximal LAD toward D2) optimized with a two-step final kissing balloon inflation. **(LOOPS 9.27 AND 9.28)**

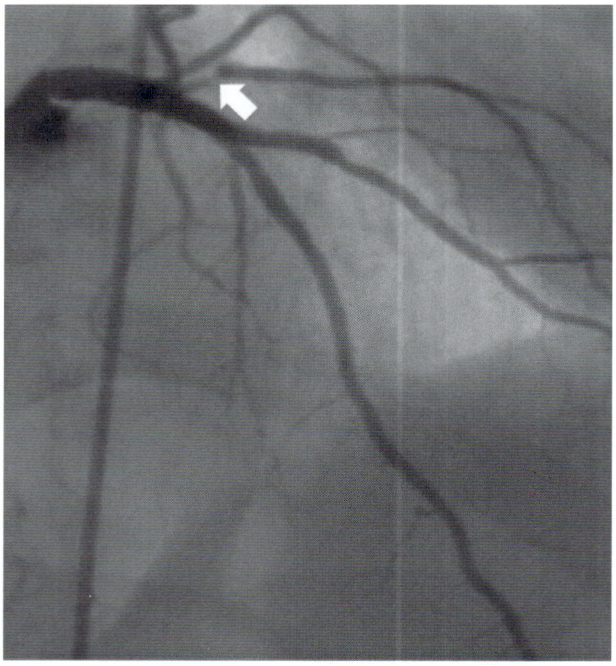

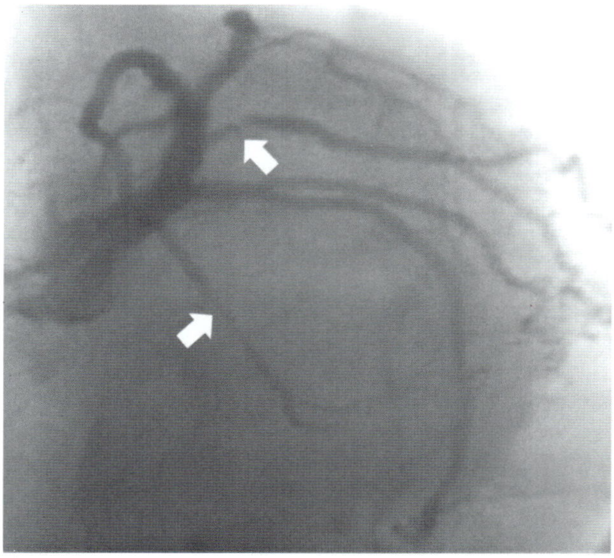

FIGURES 9.29 AND 9.30

Ischemic-driven follow-up coronary angiography demonstrating patency of LAD/D2 bifurcation stents and severe stenosis of the proximal segment of D1 and of the distal apical segment of the LAD. **(LOOPS 9.29 AND 9.30)**

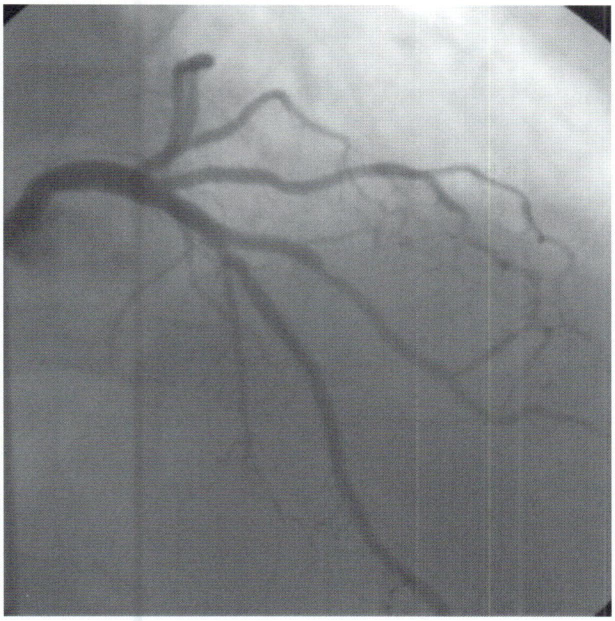

FIGURE 9.31

Final angiography after implantation of Cypher stents implanted on the distal LAD (2.25 × 18 mm) and proximal D1 (2.5 × 18 mm). **(LOOP 9.31)**

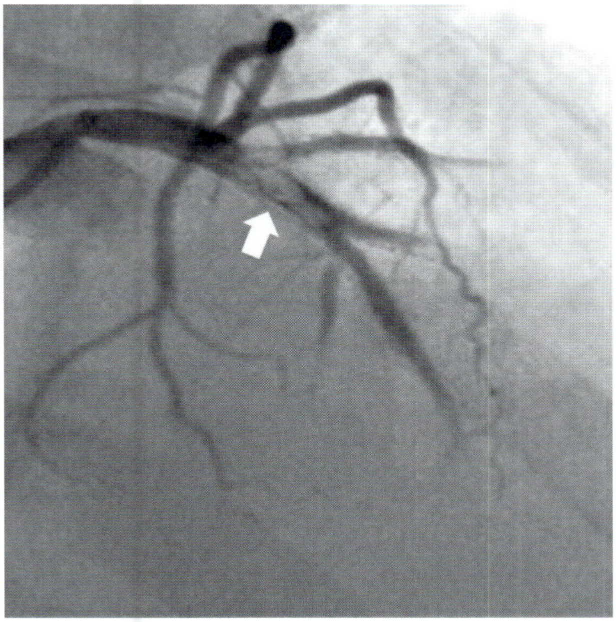

FIGURE 9.32

Emergent coronary angiography performed 5 years later in the setting of an acute anterior MI showing thrombotic occlusion of the mid-LAD stent (arrow) with extension to the D1 and D2 stents. **(LOOP 9.32)**

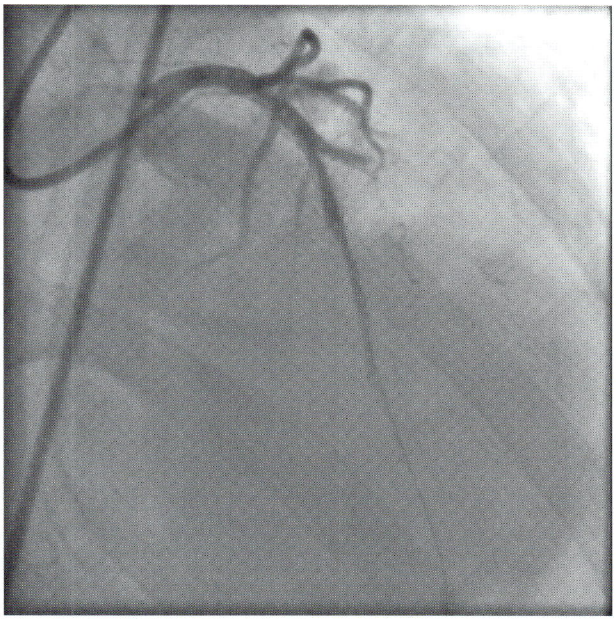

FIGURE 9.33

Recanalization of the LAD followed by manual aspiration and glycoprotein IIb/IIIa administration resulted in only limited improvement. **(LOOP 9.33)**

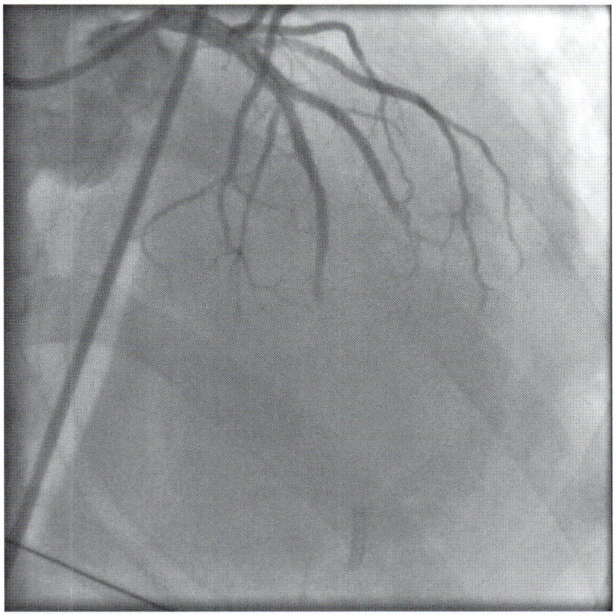

FIGURE 9.34

Final TIMI flow (<3) despite multiple maneuvers (multiple balloon inflations on mid-LAD, prox D2 and D1 recanalization). **(LOOP 9.34)**

CASE ANALYSIS

Although very late ST is a rare event, it can be lethal. The causes of very late ST remain unknown. Although some argue that indefinite DAT may prevent late and very late ST, this remains unproven. In this specific case, the patient was not taking DAT for 3 years when the ST occurred. We do not know what factors triggered this event or whether DAT if continued would have prevented it. Although rigorous studies regarding best strategies to treat ST are lacking, anecdotal experience supports the value of thrombectomy and glycoprotein IIb/IIIa inhibitors. In this case, manual aspiration had limited success in removing the thrombus. It is unclear whether rheolytic thrombectomy could have been more effective because of the large thrombus burden.

LESSONS

- The triggers and preventive measures of very late ST remain unknown.
- Bifurcation lesions treated with DES implantation are a known risk factor for ST and thus optimization of the final result is essential to reduce the risk of this complication.
- Glycoprotein IIb/IIIa receptor antagonists and thrombectomy are essential tools for treatment of ST.
- Rheolytic thrombectomy may be a better option than manual aspiration for removal of a very large clot burden.

SUGGESTED READING

Baran KW, Lasala JM, Cox DA, et al. ARRIVE Investigators. A clinical risk score for the prediction of very late stent thrombosis in drug-eluting stent patients. *EuroIntervention*. 2011;6(8):949–954.

Jung HJ, Sir JJ, Lee HK, Kang YK, Song BG, Choi SK. Very late thrombosis of sirolimus-eluting stent despite dual antiplatelet therapy for 4 years in a patient with lung cancer. *Minerva Cardioangiol*. 2011;59(1):113–116.

References

1. Serruys PW, Strauss BH, Beatt KJ, et al. Angiographic follow-up after placement of a self-expanding coronary-artery stent. *N Engl J Med.* 1991;324(1):13–17.
2. Colombo A, Hall P, Nakamura S, et al. Intracoronary stenting without anticoagulation accomplished with intravascular ultrasound guidance. *Circulation.* 1995;91(6):1676–1688.
3. Daemen J, Wenaweser P, Tsuchida K, et al. Early and late coronary stent thrombosis of sirolimus-eluting and paclitaxel-eluting stents in routine clinical practice: Data from a large two-institutional cohort study. *Lancet.* 2007;369(9562):667–678.
4. Cutlip DE, Baim DS, Ho KK, et al. Stent thrombosis in the modern era: A pooled analysis of multicenter coronary stent clinical trials. *Circulation.* 2001;103(15):1967–1971.
5. van Werkum JW, Heestermans AA, de Korte FI, et al. Long-term clinical outcome after a first angiographically confirmed coronary stent thrombosis: An analysis of 431 cases. *Circulation.* 2009;119(6):828–834.
6. Burzotta F, Parma A, Pristipino C, et al. Angiographic and clinical outcome of invasively managed patients with thrombosed coronary bare metal or drug-eluting stents: The OPTIMIST study. *Eur Heart J.* 2008;29(24):3011–3021.
7. Cutlip DE, Windecker S, Mehran R, et al. Clinical end points in coronary stent trials: A case for standardized definitions. *Circulation.* 2007;115(17):2344–2351.
8. Jeong MH, Owen WG, Staab ME, et al. Porcine model of stent thrombosis: Platelets are the primary component of acute stent closure. *Cathet Cardiovasc Diagn.* 1996;38(1):38–43.
9. Wenaweser P, Rey C, Eberli FR, et al. Stent thrombosis following bare-metal stent implantation: Success of emergency percutaneous coronary intervention and predictors of adverse outcome. *Eur Heart J.* 2005;26(12):1180–1187.

II

COMPLICATIONS OF VALVULAR AND STRUCTURAL HEART DISEASE INTERVENTIONS

10

Dabit Arzamendi and Igor Palacios

Complications of Mitral Valvuloplasty

INTRODUCTION

Rheumatic heart disease has been shown to be the most prevalent cause of mitral stenosis (MS). Although the rheumatic process may affect all cardiac valves, the mitral valve is involved most frequently, and the stenosis occurs from leaflet thickening, commissural fusion, and chordal shortening. MS is most commonly found in the United States among patients who have emigrated from areas where rheumatic fever is still endemic, and approximately 1,500 mitral valvuloplasties are performed every year (1).

Percutaneous mitral valvuloplasty (PMV) produces good immediate hemodynamic results with clinical improvement in the majority of patients and with a low rate of complications (2). However, the incidence of complications and procedural failures is related to operator's experience. The first step to reduce complications related to PMV is to know the indications (Figure 10.1) and contraindications of the procedure (Table 10.1) and to obtain a good-quality echocardiographic assessment of the mitral valve. Different echocardiographic scores have been used to predict the PMV results. The Wilkins score grades each of the following components of mitral apparatus from 1 to 4: leaflet mobility, thickness, calcification, and impairment of subvalvular apparatus (3). The Padial score grades the leaflets thickening (each separately), the commissural calcification, and the subvalvular disease from 1 to 4 (4). Patients with a Wilkins score < 8, Padial < 10, and less-than-moderate regurgitation have better outcomes. Thus, in patients with higher scores, a surgical approach is advisable; however, in patients with serious comorbidities for surgery, PMV may still provide benefit.

Once the patient has been properly evaluated and considered suitable for PMV, a transesophageal echocardiography (TEE) should be performed prior to the procedure to detect thrombus in the left atrium. If thrombus is found, PMV should be postponed and the patient should be started on warfarin for 3 to 6 months, and a new TEE should be repeated to confirm the disappearance of the clot. The rate of periprocedural stroke has been estimated between 0% and 4% (5–16), and this can be avoided with TEE evaluation, gentle manipulation of the wire or balloons, and proper anticoagulation during the procedure.

There are three main steps during the PMV: vascular access, transseptal puncture, and balloon valvuloplasty. Vascular access complications range between 1% and 1.4%. Some operators suggest preclosing the vein with a Perclose device; however, experience is limited. Transseptal puncture is the most crucial step in PMV. Major complications with regard to the Brockenbrough puncture are related to penetration of the needle into the adjacent structure (ascending aorta and the pericardial space). The most common serious complication is hemopericardium, with an incidence of 0% to 2.0%. (5–16). Several maneuvers can be used to minimize the risk of perforation. First, the spatial relationship of the ascending aorta and its surrounding structures should be known, and this could be achieved by positioning a pigtail catheter in the noncoronary sinus. Second, it is essential to know the movements of the Mullins sheath and the Brockenbrough needle to get into the left atrium through the septum. Initially, the needle and the sheath are positioned horizontally and pointing to the patient's left; the entire system is then rotated clockwise until the needle flange arrow is positioned at 4 o'clock. Under fluoroscopy, the entire system is then withdrawn across three sequential landmark "bumps," or leftward movements of the needle: (*1*) as it enters the superior vena cava/right atrium junction, (*2*) as it moves over the ascending aorta, where the tactile sensation of aortic pulsations aids in localization, and (*3*) as it passes over the limbus to fall into the fossa ovalis. On a lateral view, the correct position for puncture is posterior and inferior to the aorta (marked by the pigtail catheter). Successful penetration of the septum is heralded by a change from right atrial to left atrial pressure waveform. After successful interatrial puncture, the entire system is rotated counterclockwise to 3 o'clock and carefully advanced under fluoroscopic and hemodynamic guidance until it is certain that the dilator lies within the left atrium. Septal puncture can also be performed under TEE or intracardiac

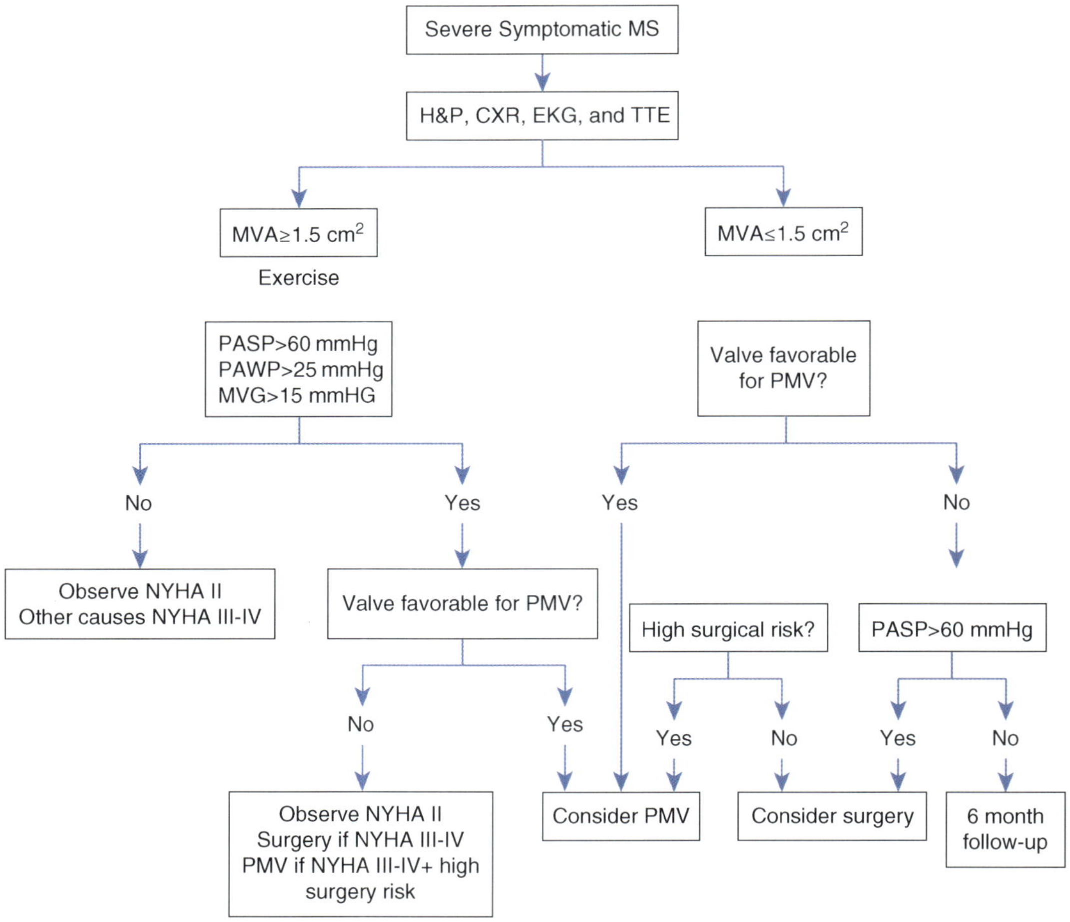

FIGURE 10.1

Indications of percutaneous mitral valvuloplasty (PMV) in patients with severe mitral stenosis. Adapted from Bonow et al (permission from the American Heart Association). MS, mitral stenosis; H&P, history and physical exam; CXR, chest x-ray; EKG, electrocardiogram; TTE, transthoracic echocardiogram; MVA, mitral valve area; PASP, pulmonary artery systolic pressure; PAWP, pulmonary artery wedge pressure; MVG, mitral valve gradient.

TABLE 10.1

Contraindications to PMV.

Persistent left atrial or left atrial appendage thrombus.
Obstruction of the inferior vena cava (e.g., by tumor, thrombus, therapeutic ligation, or filter placement).
Systemic anticoagulation.
Bleeding diathesis.
Anatomic deformity, such as severe kyphoscoliosis or patients with previous pneumonectomy resulting in severe rotation of the heart.
More than moderate mitral regurgitation.
Massive or bicommissural calcification.
Severe concomitant aortic valve disease.
Severe organic tricuspid stenosis or severe functional regurgitation withenlarged annulus.
Severe concomitant coronary artery disease requiring by-pass surgery.

echocardiography (ICE) guidance. A pericardiocentesis kit should be always available in the room during the procedure. In rare occasions, urgent surgery might be needed for ventricular perforation intractable to treatment by pericardiocentesis.

Antegrade PMV can be accomplished using single- or double-balloon techniques. Although the double-balloon technique is effective, it is more technically demanding and requires longer procedural times, which may lead to complications. The wire positioning in the apex of the left ventricle might induce perforation leading to cardiac tamponade. PMV using a single Inoue balloon yields equivalent efficacy when compared with the double-balloon technique and with lower procedural risks. The selection of the appropriate balloon size is essential to achieve a good result with minimal mitral regurgitation. To avoid injury to the mitral valve apparatus, stepwise dilatation technique under echocardiographic guidance appears to be the most efficient. If a significant increase of the mitral regurgitation (MR), a tearing at noncommissural part, or an excessive tearing of the commissures is observed, the procedure should be stopped. Severe MR is relatively rare, with a frequency of 1.4% to 9.4% (6,10). Although MR may be tolerated well, it more often requires elective surgical intervention. Iatrogenic left-to-right shunt may persist after the procedure with a frequency of 10% to 90%, depending on the detection technique. These shunts are usually small and without clinical consequences. In our experience, only 0.1% of cases require percutaneous closure (2).

Finally, procedural mortality ranges from 0% to 3%, main causes of death being left ventricular perforation or the poor general condition of the patient (Table 10.2) (5–16).

TABLE 10.2
Complications of PMV.

	N	MEAN AGE (YEAR)	TECHNIQUE	TAMPONADE (%)	EMBOLIC EVENTS (%)	SEVERE MR (%)	DEATH (%)
Arora (5)	4850	27	SB/DB/MV	0.2	0.1	1.4	0.2
Chen (6)	4832	37	SB	0.8	0.5	1.4	0.1
Iung (7)	2773	47	SB/DB	0.2	0.4	4.1	0.4
Joseph (8)	2361	31–33	SB/DB	0.6–0.8	0.3–0.6	2.4–2.6	0.4–0.8
Neumayer (9)	1123	57	SB	0.9	0.9	6	0.4
Palacios (10)	879	55	SB/DB	1	1.8	9.4	0.6
National Heart, Lung, Blood Institute Registry	738	54	SB/DB				
n<25				6	4	4	2
25≤n≤100				4	2	3	1
n≥100 (11)				2	1	3	0.3
Ben Farhart (12)	654	33	SB/DB	0.6	1.5	4.6	0.5
Hernandez (13)	620	53	SB	0.6	–	4	0.5
Fawzy (14)	551	31	SB	0.7	0.5	1.6	–
Meneveau (15)	532	54	SB/DB	1.1	–	3.9	0.2
Stefanadis (16)	441	44	SB/DB	0	0	3.4	0.2

DB, double balloon; SB, single balloon; MV, mechanical valvulotome.

CASE 10.1

Severe Mitral Regurgitation After Percutaneous Mitral Valvuloplasty

CLINICAL HISTORY AND DIAGNOSTIC TESTING RESULTS

A 57-year-old woman presented with symptomatic severe mitral stenosis in New York Heart Association (NYHA) functional class III. TEE showed no thrombus, mild mitral regurgitation, and 8/16 Wilkins score. Hemodynamic study showed a mean mitral gradient of 11 mmHg, mitral valve area of 0.66 cm^2 and pulmonary systolic pressure of 57 mmHg. There was no obstructive coronary artery disease (CAD).

PLANNED PROCEDURE

Percutaneous mitral valvuloplasty with the Inoue balloon (Toray Group, Japan).

PROCEDURE

The procedure was performed via a femoral approach with a 9-Fr sheath in the vein and a 5-Fr sheath in the artery. Transseptal catheterization was performed via a standard Brockenbrough procedure using anteroposterior views. After septal puncture, 5,000 IU of unfractionated heparin was administered. Simultaneous left atrial and left ventricular pressures were measured before the valvuloplasty (Figure 10.2). In addition, a left ventriculogram was done to assure there was no significant regurgitation (Figure 10.3).

The Inoue wire was advanced to the left atrium through the Mullins sheath, and the septum was dilated with the dilator. Maximum Inoue balloon volume was chosen following "height (in cm) / 10 + 10" equation: 160 cm / 10 + 10 = 26 mm. The balloon was advanced through the interatrial septum into the left atrium. Two balloon inflations at 26 and 28 mm were performed (Figure 10.4). After the last inflation, the patient had sudden pulmonary edema and hypotension.

COMPLICATION AND MANAGEMENT

Immediate hemodynamic assessment showed equalization of pressures between the left atrium and left ventricle (Figure 10.5), and left ventriculography showed massive mitral regurgitation (Figure 10.6). The patient went into shock and required immediate intubation, intraaortic balloon pump placement, nitroprusside infusion, and immediate transfer to the operation room. An intraoperative TEE showed paracommissural tear of the valve (Figure 10.7), which required valve replacement using a 23-mm ON-x mechanical valve.

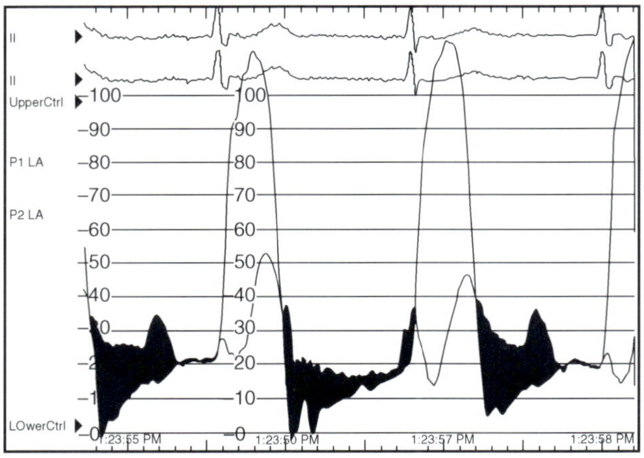

FIGURE 10.2

Simultaneous left atrial and left ventricular pressures revealing a severe mitral stenosis (mean gradient 11 mmHg). A prominet V wave is observed.

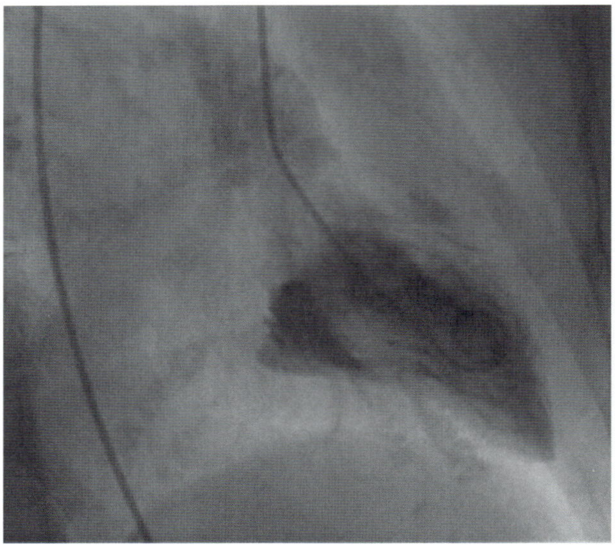

FIGURE 10.3

Left ventriculogram prior to mitral valvuloplasty. No significant mitral regurgitation is observed despite the prominet V waves. **(LOOP 10.3)**

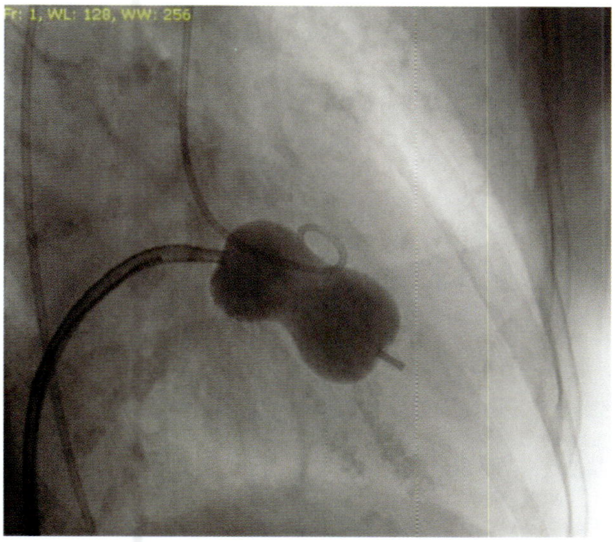

FIGURE 10.4
Full inflation of the 28-mm Inoue balloon.

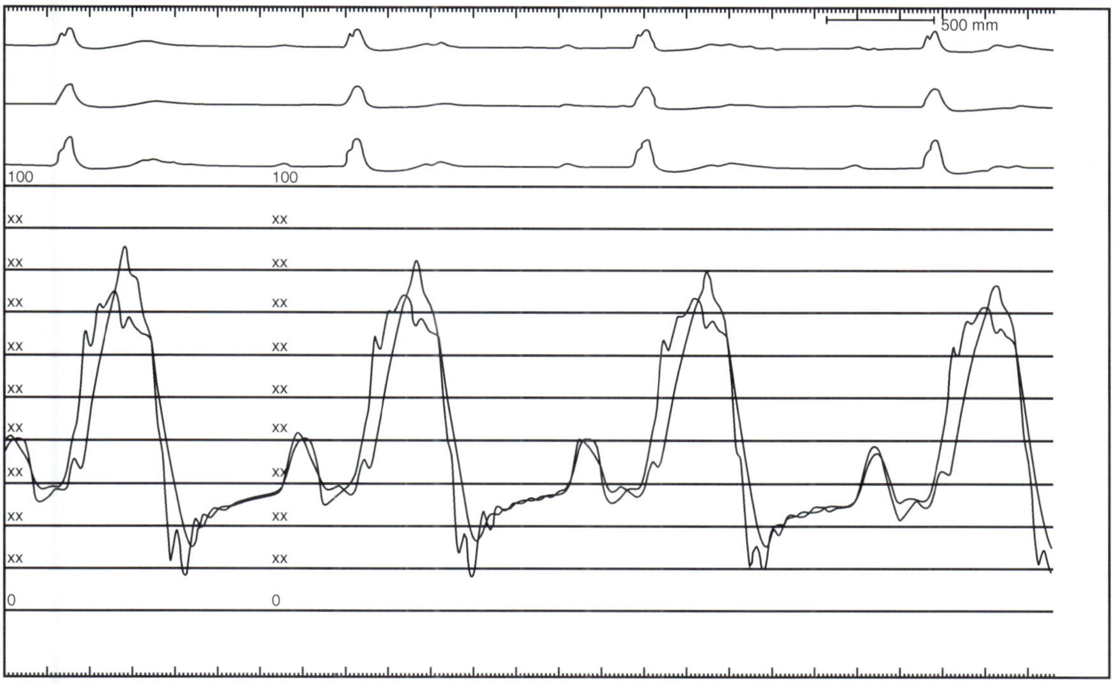

FIGURE 10.5
Simultaneous left atrial and left ventricular pressures revealing equalization of pressures between the two chambers, suggesting a massive mitral regurgitation.

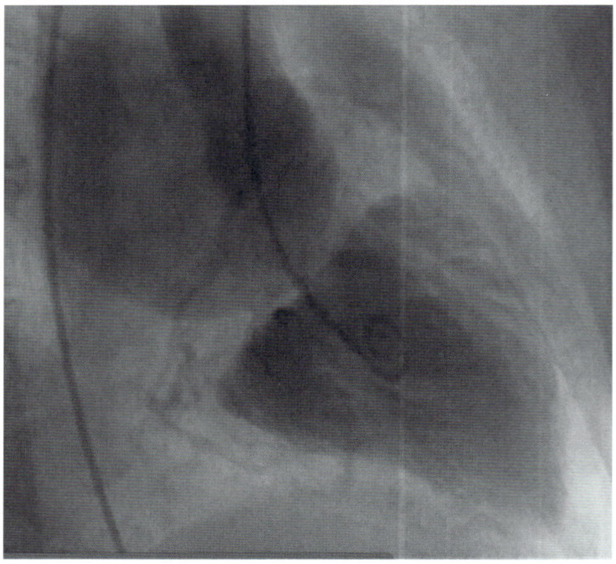

FIGURE 10.6

Left ventriculogram after the second inflation of the Inoue balloon showing a complete feeling of the left atrium and pulmonary veins during the systole suggestive of Grade 4 mitral regurgitation. **(LOOP 10.6)**

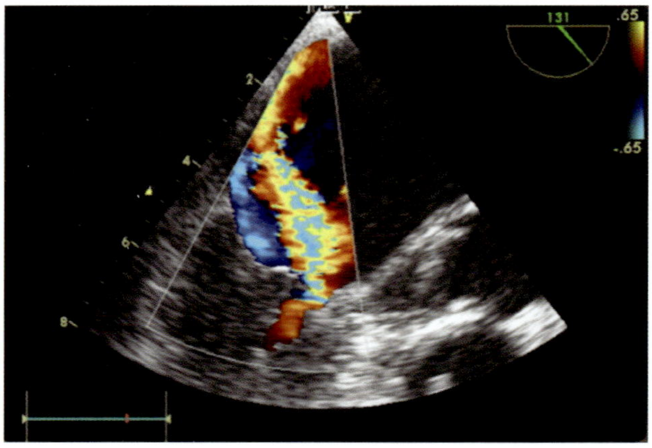

FIGURE 10.7

Transesophageal echocardiogram during the surgery revealed a severe mitral regurgitation due to a posterior paracommissural tearing.

CASE ANALYSIS

This complication occurred because of oversizing of the Inoue balloon. The first inflation was performed using the largest balloon size (26 mm) according to patient's height. Upsizing the balloon by 2 mm without echocardiographic confirmation of the results after the first inflation should not have been done.

LESSONS

- The stepwise dilation technique under TTE guidance between inflations is necessary to avoid the complete tearing and the subsequent severe MR during PMV, especially in those cases where the mitral valve area is severely reduced and the commissures are severely calcified.
- Inoue balloon oversizing beyond the height-based formula should be avoided.

SUGGESTED READING

Complications and mortality of percutaneous balloon mitral commissurotomy. A report from the National Heart, Lung, and Blood Institute Balloon Valvuloplasty Registry. *Circulation.* 1992;85:2014–2024.

Nobuyoshi M, Arita T, Shirai S, et al. Percutaneous balloon mitral valvuloplasty: A review. *Circulation.* 2009;119: e211–e219.

CASE 10.2

Pulmonary Artery Perforation After Transseptal Puncture for Percutaneous Mitral Valvuloplasty

CLINICAL HISTORY AND DIAGNOSTIC TESTING RESULTS

A 70-year-old man presented with symptomatic severe mitral stenosis and atrial fibrillation in NYHA functional class 2. Patient had previous aortic valve replacement in 1995 for severe aortic stenosis. TEE showed no left atrial thrombus, mild mitral regurgitation, and 8/16 Wilkins score. Mitral mean gradient was 12 mmHg, mitral valve area was 1.2 cm^2, and left ventricular ejection fraction was normal. There was no evidence of obstructive CAD.

PLANNED PROCEDURE

Percutaneous mitral valvuloplasty with the Inoue balloon.

PROCEDURE

The procedure was performed via a femoral approach with an 8-Fr sheath in the vein and a 6-Fr sheath in the artery. A 6-Fr pigtail catheter was advanced retrogradely into the noncoronary cusp. Transseptal puncture was performed with the Brockenbrough needle under fluoroscopic and hemodynamic guidance in the anteroposterior and lateral views.

Pressure tracing and contrast injection showed pulmonary artery perforation. TTE did not show any evidence of pericardial effusion or tamponade. The patient remained thermodynamically stable, and the decision was made to stop the procedure.

COMPLICATION AND MANAGEMENT

The complication in this case was pulmonary artery perforation during transseptal puncture. A chest CT scan demonstrated mediastinal hemorrhagic collection extending from the inferior aspect of the right pulmonary artery (RPA) and tracking posterior to the left atrium, representing a contained rupture/pseudoaneurysm (Figure 10.8). Subsequent pulmonary angiography showed a posteroinferior leak in the right pulmonary artery, with extravasation of contrast into the LA and the free space (Figures 10.9 and 10.10).

A follow-up chest CT scan was performed 24 hours later, which showed a middle mediastinal hemorrhagic collection (5.5 × 6.5 × 4.6 cm) that communicates with the RPA and the roof of the left atrium. This collection was bounded anteriorly by the left atrium, posteriorly by the trachea, superiorly by the RPA/PA, and inferiorly by the descending aorta (Figures 10.11, 10.12, and 10.13).

The patient was referred to surgery. The injuries to the right pulmonary artery and left atrium were repaired, and the mitral valve was replaced by a 29-mm St. Jude mechanical valve.

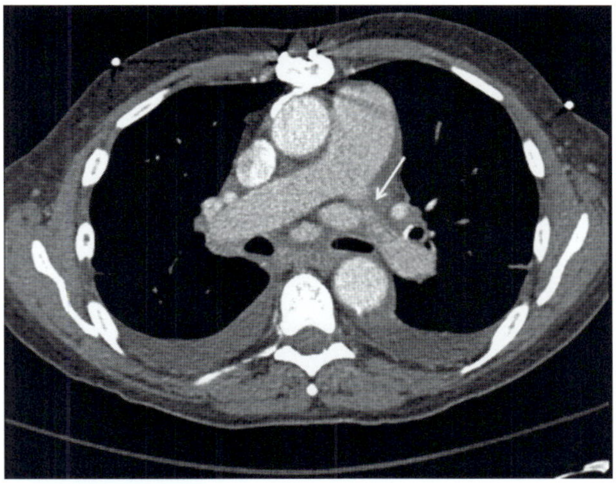

FIGURE 10.8
Chest CT scan revealing a mediastinal hemorrhagic collection extending from the inferior aspect of the right pulmonary artery (RPA) and tracking posterior to the left atrium, representing a contained rupture/pseudoaneurysm (white arrow).

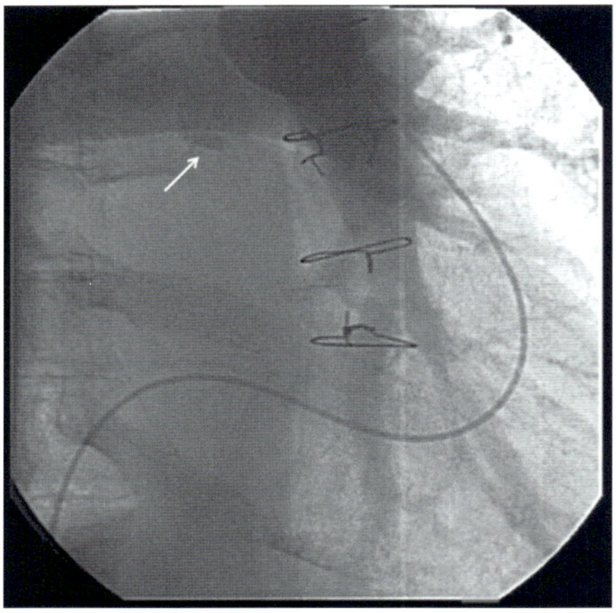

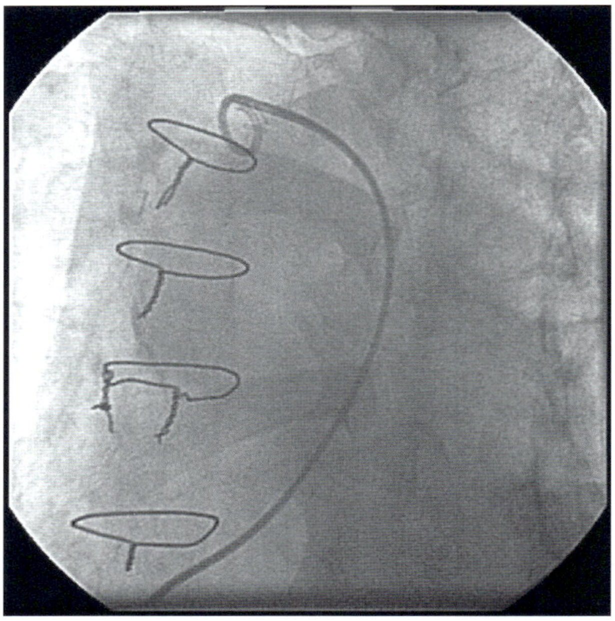

FIGURE 10.9 AND 10.10

Pulmonary angiography revealing a posteroinferior leak in the right pulmonary artery. **(LOOPS 10.9 AND 10.10)**

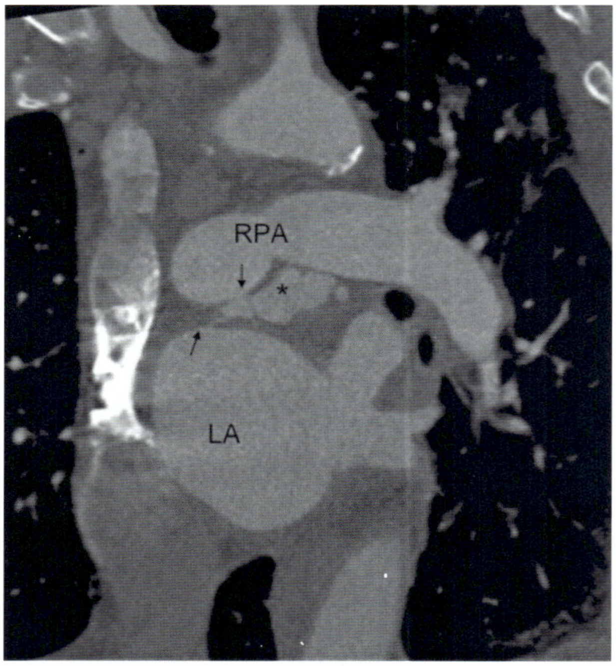

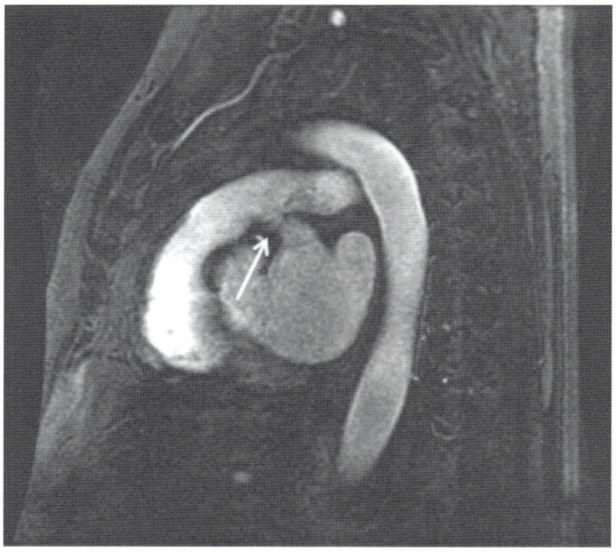

FIGURE 10.11 AND 10.12

Chest CT scan showing the coronal (left) and sagital views (right) of a mediastinal hemorrhagic collection (*) that communicates with the right pulmonary artery (RPA) and the roof of the left atrium (LA).

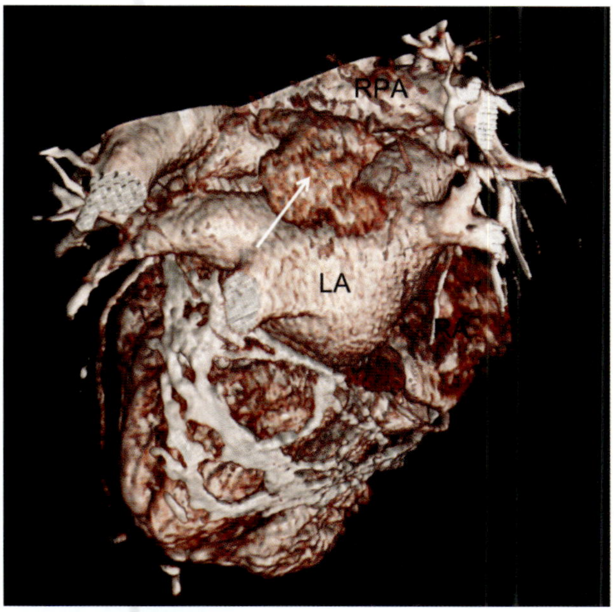

FIGURE 10.13
Chest CT scan 3D reconstruction revealing an hemorrhagic collection of 5.5 × 6.5 × 4.6 cm communicating the RPA and LA.

CASE ANALYSIS

In this case, the transseptal puncture was complicated with right pulmonary artery perforation through the roof of the left atrium. This complication occurred despite using a marker pigtail in the aortic root and biplanar fluoroscopy. After the needle crossed the septum, it was advanced deeply toward the left atrial roof without proper counterclockwise rotation toward the left atrium cavity and away from the left atrium roof.

LESSONS

- Defining anatomic landmarks and fluoroscopic views is important, but not sufficient, to prevent inadvertent puncture of periinteratria septal structures.
- Introduction of a 0.014-inch coronary wire through the transseptal needle as it enters the LA and positioning it in the left upper pulmonary vein can prevent LA roof damage.
- ICE or TEE guidance of transseptal puncture and needle position can reduce the likelihood of inadvertent collateral damage.

SUGGESTED READING

Kronzon I, Glassman E, Cohen M, Winer H. Use of two-dimensional echocardiography during transseptal cardiac catheterization. *J Am Coll Cardiol.* 1984;4:425–428.

Roelke M, Smith AJ, Palacios IF. The technique and safety of transseptal left heart catheterization: the Massachusetts General Hospital experience with 1,279 procedures. *Cathet Cardiovasc Diagn.* 1994;32:332–339.

References

1. Carabello BA. Modern management of mitral stenosis. *Circulation.* 2005;112(3):432–437.
2. Palacios I, Block PC, Brandi S, et al. Percutaneous balloon valvotomy for patients with severe mitral stenosis. *Circulation.* 1987;75(4):778–784.
3. Wilkins GT, Weyman AE, Abascal VM, et al. Percutaneous balloon dilatation of the mitral valve: An analysis of echocardiographic variables related to outcome and the mechanism of dilatation. *Br Heart J.* 1988;60(4):299–308.
4. Padial LR, Freitas N, Sagie A, et al. Echocardiography can predict which patients will develop severe mitral regurgitation after percutaneous mitral valvulotomy. *J Am Coll Cardiol.* 1996;27(5):1225–1231.
5. Arora R, Kalra GS, Singh S, et al. Percutaneous transvenous mitral commissurotomy: immediate and long-term follow-up results. *Catheter Cardiovasc Interv.* 2002;55(4):450–156.
6. Chen CR, Cheng TO. Percutaneous balloon mitral valvuloplasty by the Inoue technique: a multicenter study of 4832 patients in China. *Am Heart J.* 1995;129(6):1197–1203.
7. Iung B, Nicoud-Houel A, Fondard O, et al. Temporal trends in percutaneous mitral commissurotomy over a 15-year period. *Eur Heart J.* 2004;25(8):701–707.
8. Joseph G, Chandy S, George P, et al. Evaluation of a simplified transseptal mitral valvuloplasty technique using over-the-wire single balloons and complementary femoral and jugular venous approaches in 1,407 consecutive patients. *J Invasive Cardiol.* 2005;17(3):132–138.
9. Neumayer U, Schmidt HK, Fassbender D, et al. Early (three-month) results of percutaneous mitral valvotomy with the Inoue balloon in 1,123 consecutive patients comparing various age groups. *Am J Cardiol.* 2002;90(2):190–193.
10. Palacios IF, Sanchez PL, Harrell LC, et al. Which patients benefit from percutaneous mitral balloon valvuloplasty? Prevalvuloplasty and postvalvuloplasty variables that predict long-term outcome. *Circulation.* 2002;105(12):1465–1471.
11. Complications and mortality of percutaneous balloon mitral commissurotomy. A report from the National Heart, Lung, and Blood Institute Balloon Valvuloplasty Registry. *Circulation.* 1992;85(6):2014–2024.
12. Ben-Farhat M, Betbout F, Gamra H, et al. Predictors of long-term event-free survival and of freedom from restenosis after percutaneous balloon mitral commissurotomy. *Am Heart J.* 2001;142(6):1072–1079.
13. Hernandez R, Banuelos C, Alfonso F, et al. Long-term clinical and echocardiographic follow-up after percutaneous mitral valvuloplasty with the Inoue balloon. *Circulation.* 1999;99(12):1580–1586.
14. Fawzy ME, Shoukri M, Al Buraiki J, et al. Seventeen years' clinical and echocardiographic follow up of mitral balloon valvuloplasty in 520 patients, and predictors of long-term outcome. *J Heart Valve Dis.* 2007;16(5):454–460.
15. Meneveau N, Schiele F, Seronde MF, et al. Predictors of event-free survival after percutaneous mitral commissurotomy. *Heart.* 1998;80(4):359–364.
16. Stefanadis CI, Stratos CG, Lambrou SG, et al. Retrograde nontransseptal balloon mitral valvuloplasty: immediate results and intermediate long-term outcome in 441 cases—A multicenter experience. *J Am Coll Cardiol.* 1998;32(4):1009–1016.

11

Andrea Pacchioni, Dimitrios Nikas, Carlo Penzo, Salvatore Saccà, Luca Favero, Gianpaolo Pasquetto, Francesco Versaci, and Bernhard Reimers

Complications of Transcatheter Aortic Valve Implantation

INTRODUCTION

Transcatheter aortic valve implantation (TAVI) is increasingly being used as a therapeutic option for patients with severe aortic stenosis who are ineligible or at high risk for surgery. Despite the tremendous added value of these procedures, they remain highly complex and can be associated with severe complications at every step of the procedure. These complications include vascular complications, improper prosthesis positioning, coronary obstruction, cardiac perforation, stroke, mitral valve injury, annular and root rupture, heart block, renal failure, and structural valve failure.

CASE 11.1

Improper CoreValve Prosthesis Positioning, Coronary Occlusion, and Iliac Artery Avulsion

CLINICAL HISTORY AND DIAGNOSTIC TESTING RESULTS

A 70-year-old woman with known severe aortic stenosis was admitted to the hospital for worsening heart failure. She had a history of rheumatoid arthritis on steroid therapy for 20 years, hypertension, ischemic cardiomyopathy, and coronary artery disease (CAD) with prior percutaneous coronary intervention (PCI) to the left anterior descending artery (LAD), left circumflex artery (LCX), and right coronary artery (RCA). A recent echo evaluation demonstrated a mean aortic gradient of 54 mmHg, aortic valve area of 0.71 cm^2, thickened and hypomobile aortic valve cusps, moderate aortic regurgitation, mild mitral regurgitation, and preserved left ventricular ejection fraction. Cardiac surgeons at three different hospitals refused to perform surgical aortic valve replacement. The patient was being treated with intravenous diuretics, with limited improvement in her clinical status.

PLANNED PROCEDURE

TAVI with the CoreValve (Medtronic).

PROCEDURE

Prior to TAVI, ascending aorta and aorto-ilio-femoral angiography was performed (Figure 11.1). A 26-mm CoreValve prosthesis was chosen based on the aortic annulus measurements. The right common femoral artery was accessed (correct puncture site confirmed with contrast injection), (Figure 11.2), a 10-Fr Prostar (Abbott Vascular, Abbott Park, IL) was deployed, and a 10-Fr introducer sheath was introduced. A contralateral arterial femoral access was also obtained; a pigtail catheter was introduced to the aortic root, and a temporary pacemaker was placed. After systemic heparinization, the left ventricle (LV) was canalized per standard technique, and a preshaped Amplatz superstiff wire was introduced through a pigtail catheter. The 10-Fr sheath was then exchanged for an 18-Fr sheath, and balloon valvuloplasty was performed with single-balloon inflation (NuMed, AB Medica, Italy) during pacing (200 bpm). Subsequently, the CoreValve was advanced and positioned across the aortic valve and deployment commenced as per standard technique (Figure 11.3).

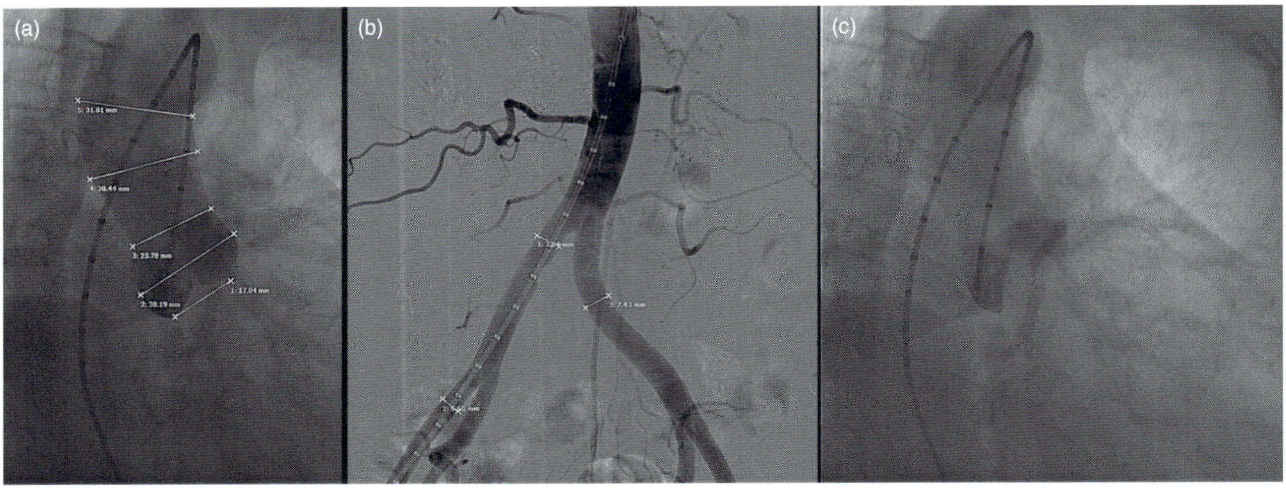

FIGURE 11.1
(a) Ascending aorta angiography, (b) aorto-ilio-femoral angiography, and (c) aortic cusp angiography to determine the distance between the coronary ostia and the aortic annulus plane.

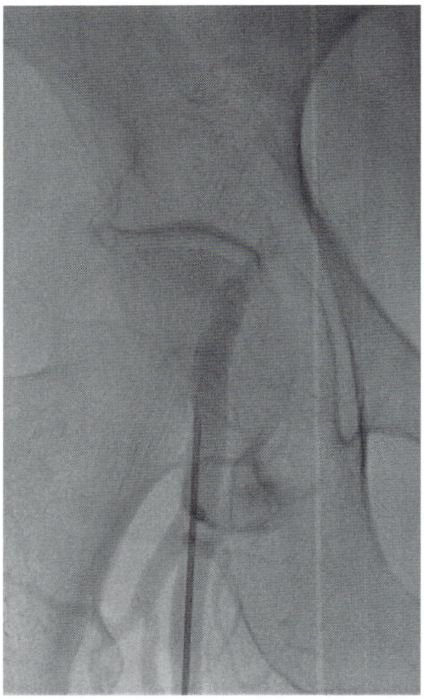

FIGURE 11.2
Contrast injection through the puncture needle to assess femoral puncture site prior to sheath placement.

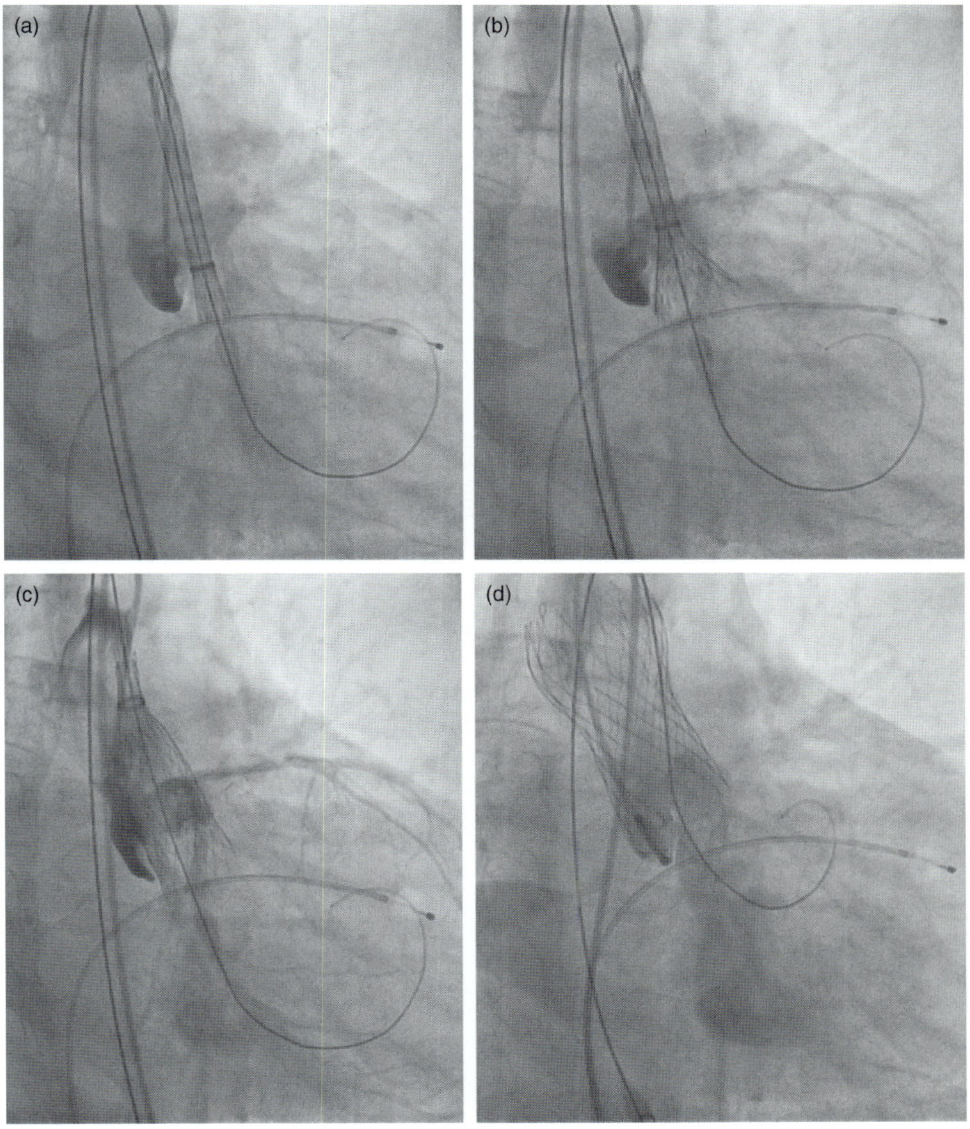

FIGURE 11.3
(a) Positioning of the CoreValve prosthesis across the dilated aortic valve. (b, c) Deployment of the CoreValve with multiple contrast injections in order to assess position. (d) Final deployment position of the Corevalve. Note the upward slippage of the prosthesis.

COMPLICATION 1 AND MANAGEMENT

At the end of deployment, the prosthesis migrated into the ascendenig aorta (Figure 11.4). This resulted in severe aortic regurgitation and subsequent cardiac arrest, requiring CPR and vasopressor administration. During the resuscitation efforts, a second prosthesis was prepared and deployed within 8 minutes of initial prosthesis migration. The patient recovered almost immediately after successful prosthesis deployment (Figure 11.5).

CASE ANALYSIS Complication 1

CoreValve prosthesis migration/malpositioning can result from the following: *(1)* incomplete valve detachment from the delivery catheter before retrieval; *(2)* during removal of delivery catheter, the distal olive may get caught on the prosthesis and cause inadvertent migration; and *(3)* the absence of leaflet calcifications may increase the possibility of prosthesis slippage. Both the Edwards-Sapien and the CoreValve prostheses can migrate or be malpositioned. While the balloon-expandable prosthesis cannot be repositioned, the CoreValve prosthesis position can be adjusted before final release.

Incorrect positioning, undersizing, or underexpansion of the prosthesis can cause moderate or severe paravalvular aortic regurgitation, which is likely to manifest immediately. Diagnosis is suspected by observing the pressure waveform and is confirmed by aortography or echocardiography. Paravalvular leak from prosthesis underexpansion can be addressed by a more aggressive second balloon dilatation, whereas a paravalvular leak due to prosthesis malposition requires implantation of a second prosthesis.

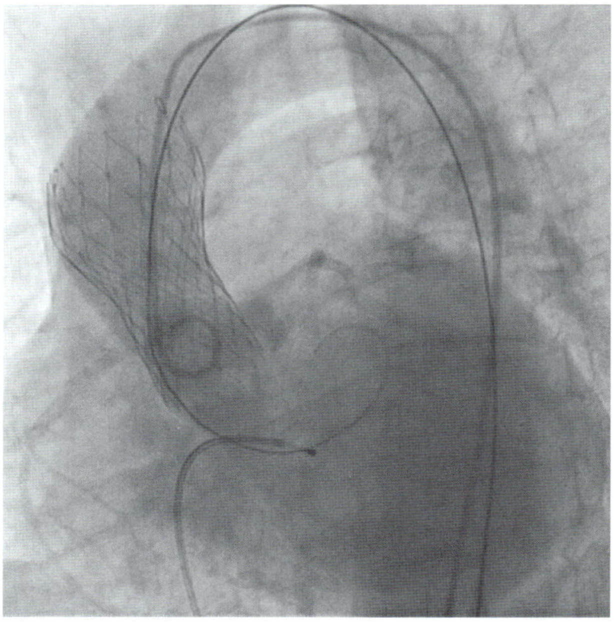

FIGURE 11.4
Further slippage of the CoreValve into the aortic root and massive aortic regurgitation.

LESSONS Complication 1

- Multiple contrast injections are needed during valve deployment for adequate positioning. The CoreValve prosthesis requires significant skill to adjust for the downward/backward motion of the delivery system during deployment.
- Sudden hemodynamic compromise after prosthesis deployment should trigger suspicion for severe aortic regurgitation.
- When severe aortic paravalvular regurgitation occurs after improper prosthesis, positioning a "valve-in-valve" implantation is feasible and effective.

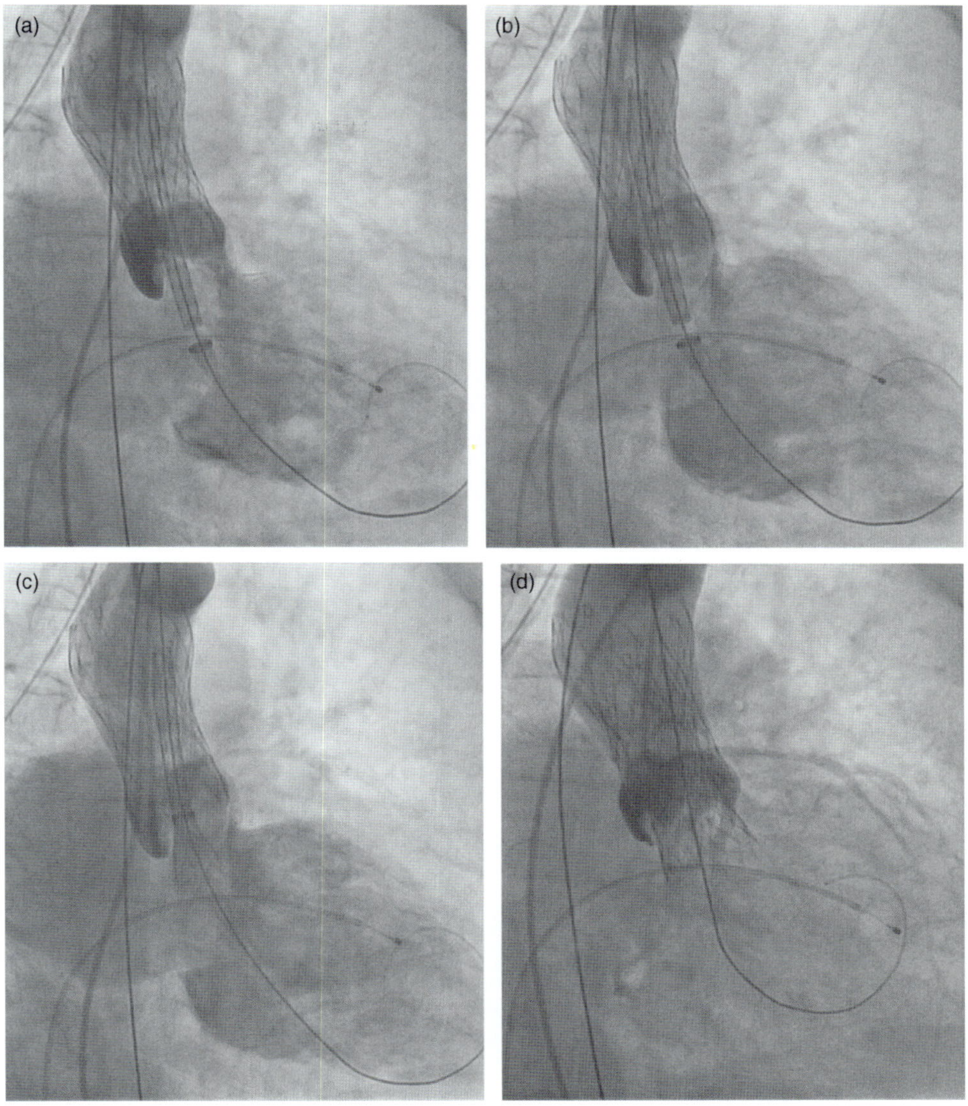

FIGURE 11.5

(a) Positioning of the second CoreValve prosthesis across the aortic native valve. (b, c) Deployment of the CoreValve with multiple contrast injections in order to assess position. (d) Deployment and release of the CoreValve in the proper position.

COMPLICATION 2 AND MANAGEMENT

Five minutes after resolution of the severe aortic regurgitation with the "valve-in-valve" implantation, the patient complained of chest pain with progressive ST segment elevation and another cardiac arrest ensued. CPR was initiated and coronary angiography performed, demonstrating subtotal occlusion of the left main coronary artery (Figure 11.6). An XB 3.5 guiding catheter was used to engage the left main coronary artery (LMCA), and a 0.014-inch coronary guidewire was introduced without difficulty. Balloon angioplasty of the LMCA through the sinus into the aorta (opening the cusps of the first CoreValve implant) was performed. This was followed by implantation of 4.5-mm × 23-mm bare metal stent from left main through the sinus (i.e., through the two valves) into the aorta (Figure 11.7). The clinical status of the patient stabilized with resolution of ST segment elevation.

CASE ANALYSIS — Complication 2

It is estimated that coronary occlusion occur in 0.4% to 4.1% of TAVI procedures. In general, risk factors for this complication include (a) anatomic factors, such as distance between the coronary ostia and the aortic annulus (< 10–12 mm), presence of bulky calcifications in the aortic cusps, and narrow root with shallow sinuses of Valsalva, and (b) procedural factors, such as valve misplacement or emboli.

In our case example, the valve cusps of the first malpositioned prosthesis occluded the left coronary ostium. This complication could have been avoided by retrieval of the misplaced valve into the ascending aorta using a gooseneck catheter. However, the hemodynamic condition of the patient did not allow time for this.

This complication can be avoided by careful patient selection with regard to the above risk factors, as well as aortic root angiography during balloon valvuloplasty. A double arterial access is advisable: cannulation and wiring of left main with guiding catheter via radial access allows the completion of the procedure, being ready to face the complication if occurs.

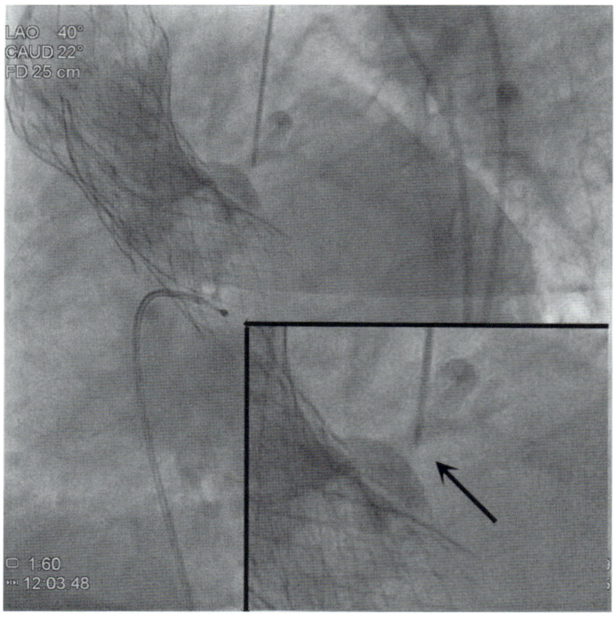

FIGURE 11.6
Subocclusion of left main coronary artery (arrow, in the box) after the valve-in-valve deployment. The occlusion probably occurred as a result of displacement of the leaflets of the first CoreValve.

LESSONS — Complication 2

- In cases of malpositioned CoreValve at the level of the coronary ostia, all attempts should be made to retrieve the prosthesis to a higher level in the ascending aorta.
- Consider anatomical preprocedural features that can contraindicate the procedure.
- If there is potential of left main occlusion, wire it!

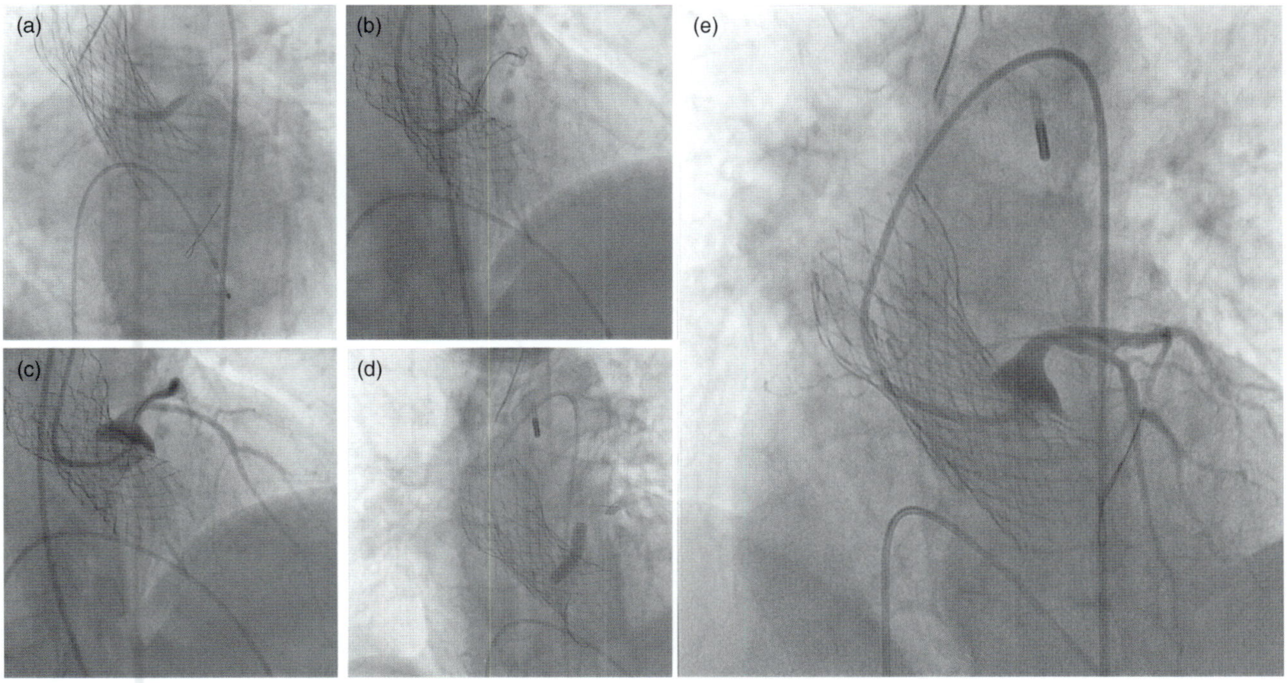

FIGURE 11.7
(a–c) Wiring and balloon dilatation of the left main coronary artery (3.5 mm and 4 mm × 20 mm at 14 mm), (d) deployment and postdilation of a bare metal stent (4.5 × 23 mm), and (e) final result.

COMPLICATION 3 AND MANAGEMENT

During removal of the 18-Fr sheath, the patiet had hemodynamic collapse. Aorto-iliac angiography through the contralateral access site showed right external iliac artery rupture (Figure 11.8). A 28-mm aortic occlusion balloon was advanced through the left common femoral artery and inflated in the distal aorta. A second left common femoral arterial access was obtained few centimeters above the first sheath and a 7-Fr crossover sheath (Destination 45 cm, Terumo, Japan) was advanced to the right common iliac artery. Through this sheath, two Fluency stent grafts (8 mm × 80 mm and 10 mm × 60 mm) and two Jostent graft masters (6–12 mm × 48 mm and 5 mm × 19 mm, Abbott, IL) were deployed in the iliac artery, however, without achieving complete vessel sealing (Figure 11.9 and 11.10). Despite immediate blood transfusions and transfer to the surgical suite for open surgery, the patient died of hemorrhagic shock.

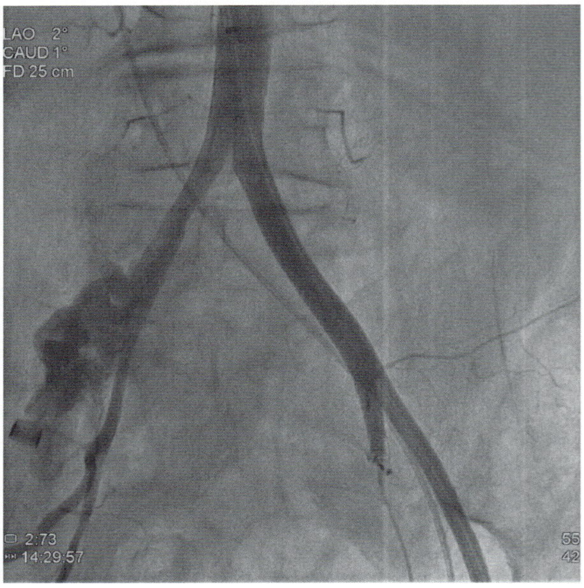

FIGURE 11.8
External iliac artery avulsion with dramatic hemorrhage associated with sudden hemodynamic collapse.

CASE ANALYSIS **Complication 3**

In this case, arterial rupture occurred because the external iliac artery diameter was 5.5 mm (below the minimum required diameter of 6 mm to accommodate an 18-Fr sheath). Although an artery of 5 to 6 mm can occasionally accommodate an 18-Fr sheath, if it is nontortuous and noncalcified, it is not always predictable, as demonstrated in this case. Also, what contributed to vessel avulsion is forced sheath removal despite encountering resistance. Resistance to sheath removal is a sign that the sheath has adhered to the vessel wall because of size mismatch and prolonged procedure time. When this occurs, the operator should stop attempting sheath withdrawal, alert a vascular surgeon to stand by for possible surgical intervention, and place an 8-Fr crossover sheath from the contralateral side to the ipsilateral common iliac artery. Through this sheath, a 0.035-inch guidewire can be advanced through the lumen of the ipsilateral prosthesis sheath, and an appropriately sized balloon can be placed in the common iliac artery. Then gentle attempts to remove the sheath can be made with contrast injections from the contralateral sheath to exclude vessel perforation. If vessel perforation is observed, the balloon in the common iliac artery is immediately inflated to obtain proximal occlusion and stop the bleeding. At this point, a decision is made whether to place stent graft or perform surgical intervention to seal the perforation.

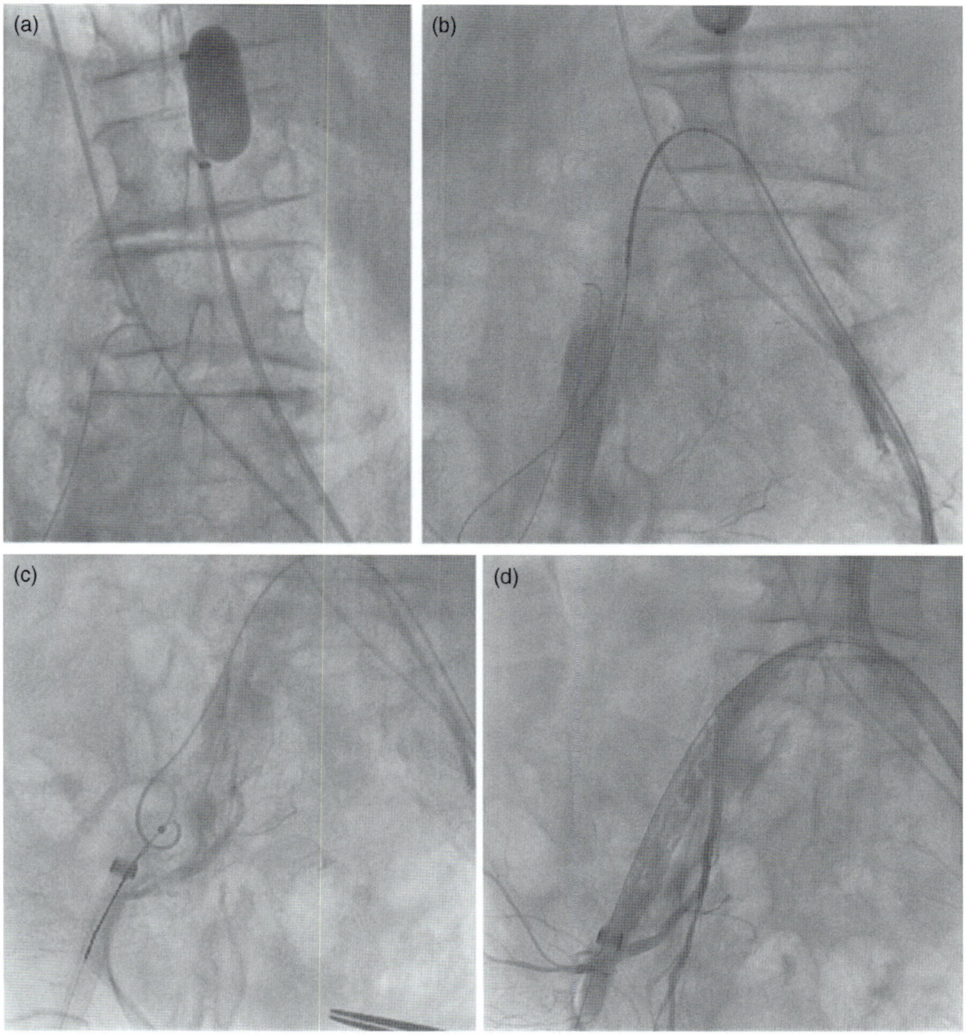

FIGURE 11.9

(a) Deployment of an occlusive balloon in the distal abdominal aorta. (b) Placement of a 0.035-inch guidewire and pigtail catheter with crossover technique. (c–d) Externalization of the 0.035-inch guidewire through the 18-Fr sheath with a gooseneck snare.

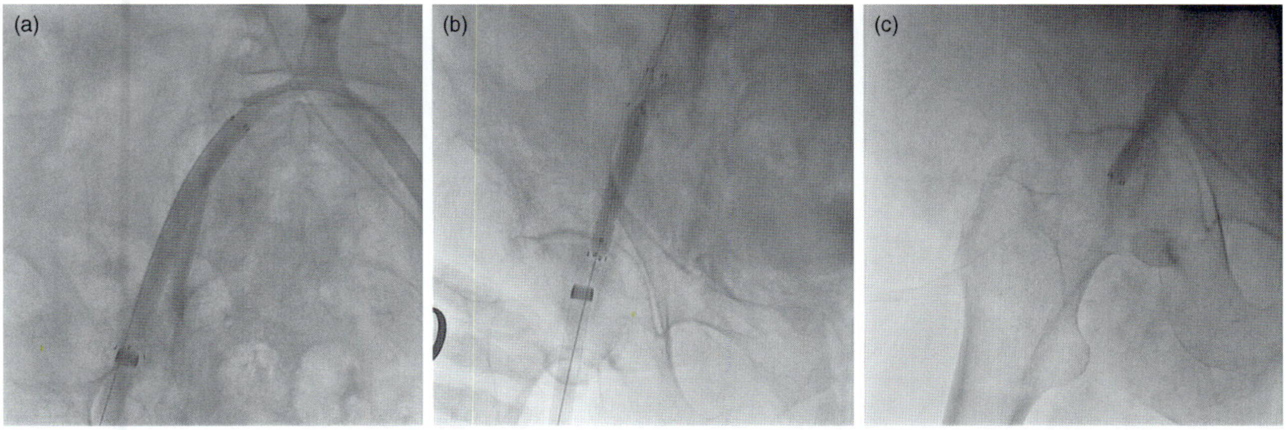

FIGURE 11.10

(a–c) Deployment of several covered stent grafts (Fluency and Jostent grafts) in the common and external iliac artery without achieving complete seal.

LESSONS **Complication 3**

- Selection of proper patient is the most important factor in preventing vascular complications with TAVI. Particular attention should be paid to vessel diameter, presence and extent of calcifications, and vessel tortousity.
- Routine placement of a 0.014- or 0.018-inch guidewire in the ipsilateral superficial femoral artery (at the side of the prosthesis insertion) from the contralateral access site prior to prosthesis sheath placement is an important technique to facilitate prompt vessel occlusion in case of iliac perforation.
- When resistance is encountered during removal of the prosthesis sheath, attempts to remove the sheath should be stopped. The operator should ensure that he or she has adequate endovascular or surgical bailout technique ready in case sheath removal results in vessel perforation.

SUGGESTED READING

Detaint D, Lepage L, Himbert D, et al. Determinants of significant paravalvular regurgitation after transcatheter aortic valve implantation. Impact of device and annulus discongruence. *J Am Coll Cardiol Intv.* 2009;2:821–827.

Kapadia SR, Svensson L, Tuzcu EM. Successful percutaneous management of left main trunk occlusion during percutaneous aortic valve replacement. *Catheter Cardiovasc Interv.* 2009;73:966–972.

Rodes-Cabau J, Dumont E, Doyle D. "Valve-in-valve" for the treatment of paravalvular leaks following transcatheter aortic valve implantation. *Cather Cardovasc Interv.* 2009;74:1116–1119.

Sharp ASP, Michev I, Maisano F, et al. A new technique for vascular access management in transcatheter aortic valve implantation. *Catheter Cardiovasc Interv.* 2010;75(5):784–793.

Stabile E, Sorropago G, Cioppa A, et al. Acute left main obstructions following TAVI. *EuroIntervention.* 2010;6:100–105.

Ussia GP, Mulè M, Tamburino C. The valve-in-valve technique: transcatheter treatment of aortic bioprothesis malposition. *Catheter Cardiovasc Interv.* 2009;73:713–716.

Webb JG. Coronary obstruction due to transcatheter valve implantation *Catheter Cardiovasc Interv.* 2009;73:973.

CASE 11.2

Embolization of an Edward Sapien Valve to the Left Ventricle and Left Ventricular Rupture

CLINICAL HISTORY AND DIAGNOSTIC TESTING RESULTS

A 63-year-old woman with severe aortic regurgitation and congestive heart failure (New York Heart Association grade III) was sent to us by a cardiac surgeon to perform coronary angiography and aortography prior to surgical intervention. There was no evidence of coronary artery disease (CAD), but she had a porcelain aorta. Subsequently, three cardiac surgeons refused to operate. The patient was then referred to us for consideration of "off-label" compassionate Transcatheter aortic valve implantation (TAVI). The patient underwent transesophageal echocardiography (TEE) and chest computed tomography (CT) scan that showed an aortic annulus diameter of 24 mm and 26 to 27 mm. There were very little calcifications at the aortic annulus (Figure 11.11).

PLANNED PROCEDURE

TAVI with a 26-mm Edwards Sapien valve.

PROCEDURE

The TAVI procedure was performed per standard technique. After bilateral common femoral artery sheath insertion (the TAVI sheath in the right commom femoral artery [CFA], usual systemic heparinization was administered and a transvenous temporary pacemaker placed. An Amplatz superstiff wire was placed in the left ventrical (LV) and balloon valvuloplasty performed with a 25-mm balloon to confirm stable position and complete valve sealing during contrast injection (Figure 11.12). Then a 26-mm Edwards Sapien valve was implanted per standard technique.

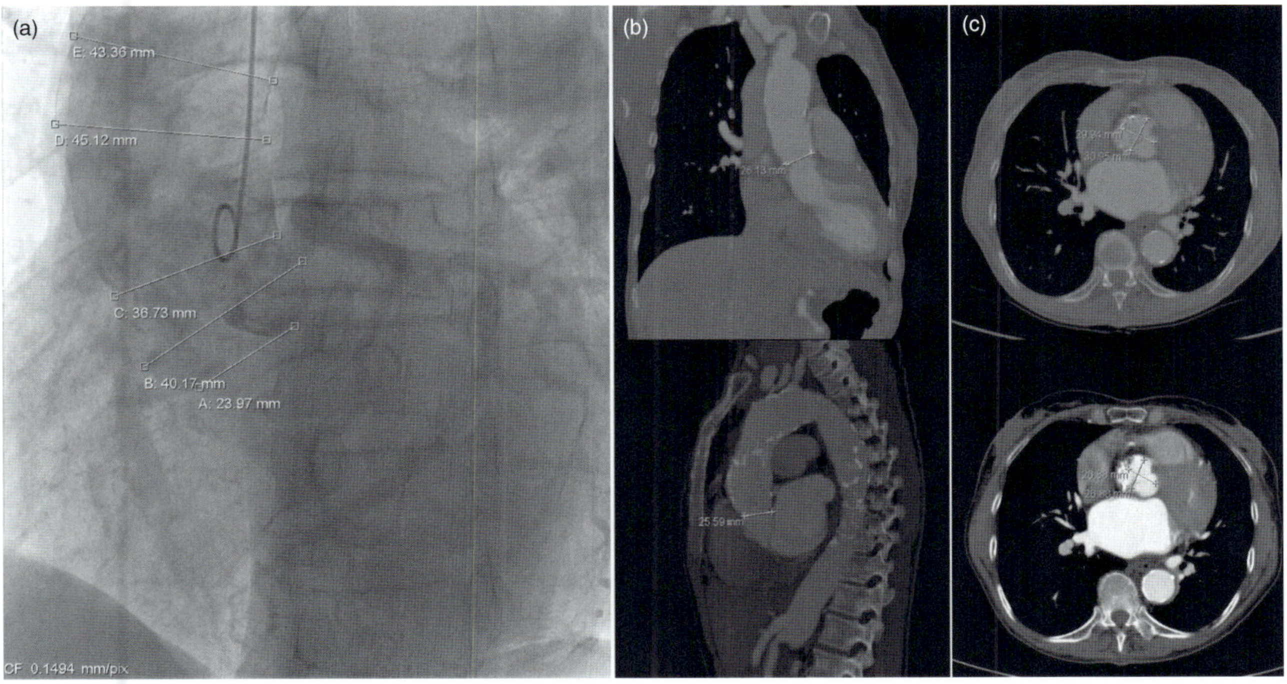

FIGURE 11.11

(a) Diagnostic angiography of the aortic root and ascending aorta. (b–c) Multiple cuts of chest CT scan with contrast to assess the aortic annulus diameter.

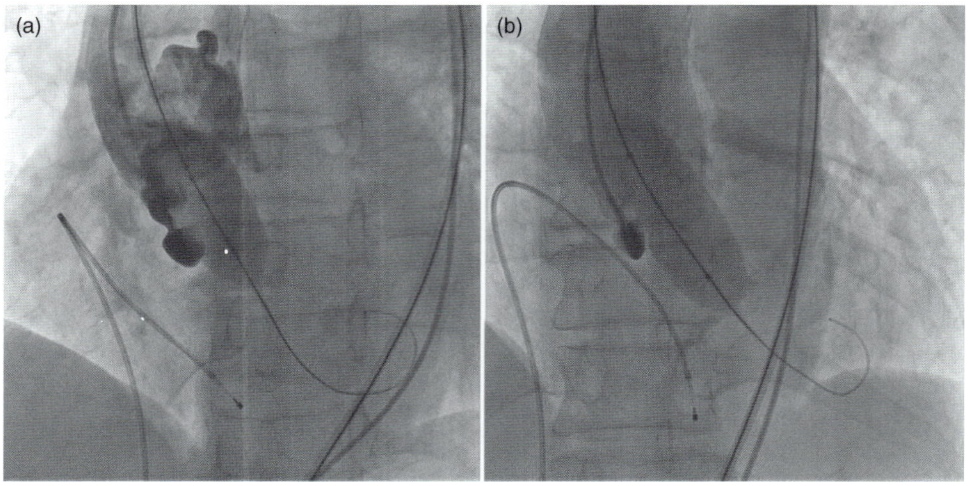

FIGURE 11.12

Diagnostic angiography of the aortic root during balloon valvuloplasty to assess whether the contrast enters the left ventricle, (a) with 22-mm balloon, and (b) with 25-mm balloon.

COMPLICATION AND MANAGEMENT

The Edwards Sapien valve migrated into the left ventricle immediately after its deployment (Figure 11.13). We attempted to retrieve the prosthesis by inflating the valvuloplasty balloon distal to the valve and toward the ascending aorta, but this was not successful, neither were the attempts to snare the prosthesis with a bent 0.035-inch wire (Figure 11.14). Finally, we were successful in retrieving the prosthesis using a 5-Fr Simmons catheter (Terumo, Tokyo, Japan), and the valve was repositioned and deployed successfully in the abdominal aorta just above the renal arteries (Figure 11.15). Consequently, a 29-mm CoreValve was prepared and delivered across the native aortic valve, but by mistake, the deployment catheter was retrieved before complete detachment of the prosthesis, which led to migration of the CoreValve to the ascending aorta (Figure 11.16). A third valve, a 29-mm CoreValve prosthesis, was finally successfully deployed with resolution of aortic regurgitation (Figure 11.17). After transfer to the intensive care unit, the patient had sudden hypotension with evidence of cardiac tamponade. Immediate pericardiocentesis was performed and the patient underwent subsequent surgical exploration that revealed small tear in the LV apex that was successfully repaired. The patient was extubated the day after surgery and discharged home 7 days later in stable condition. At 6 months follow-up, the patient had only mild aortic regurgitation, and she had minimal dyspnea on exertion.

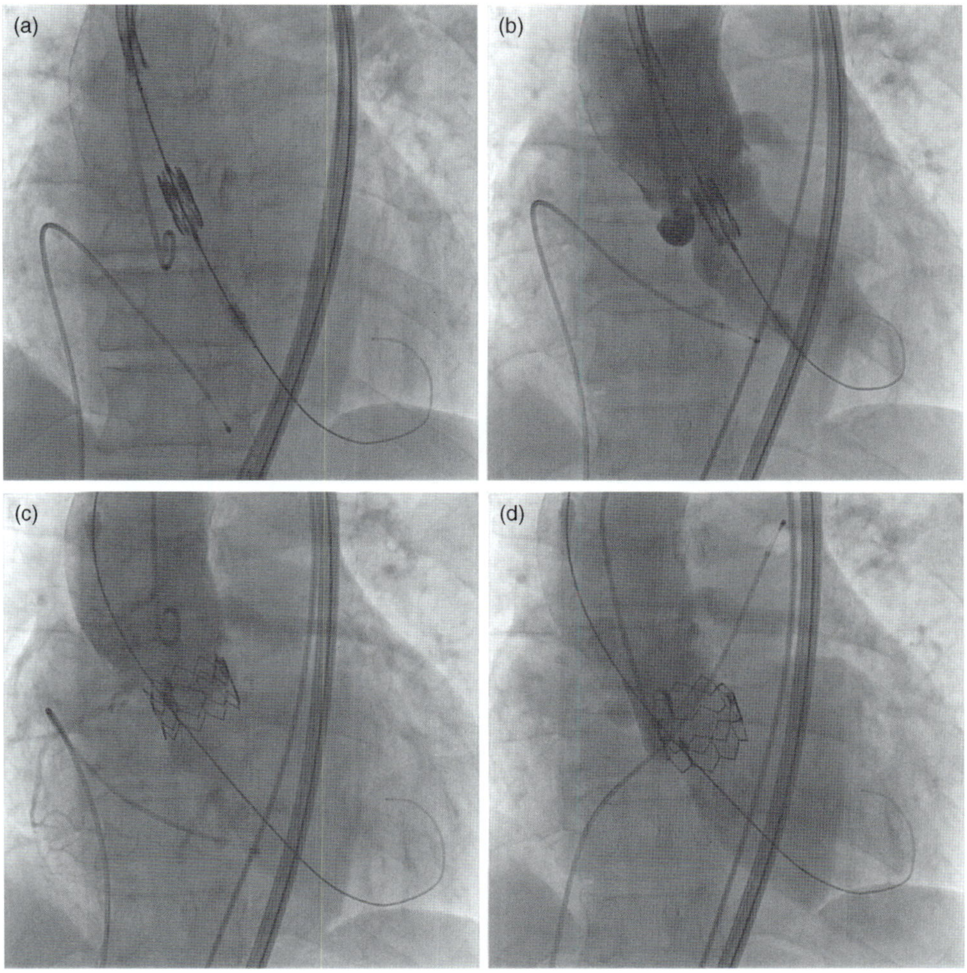

FIGURE 11.13

(a, b) A 26-mm Edwards Sapien valve advancement and positioning at the level of the aortic annulus. (c, d) Valve deployment and migration into the left ventricle.

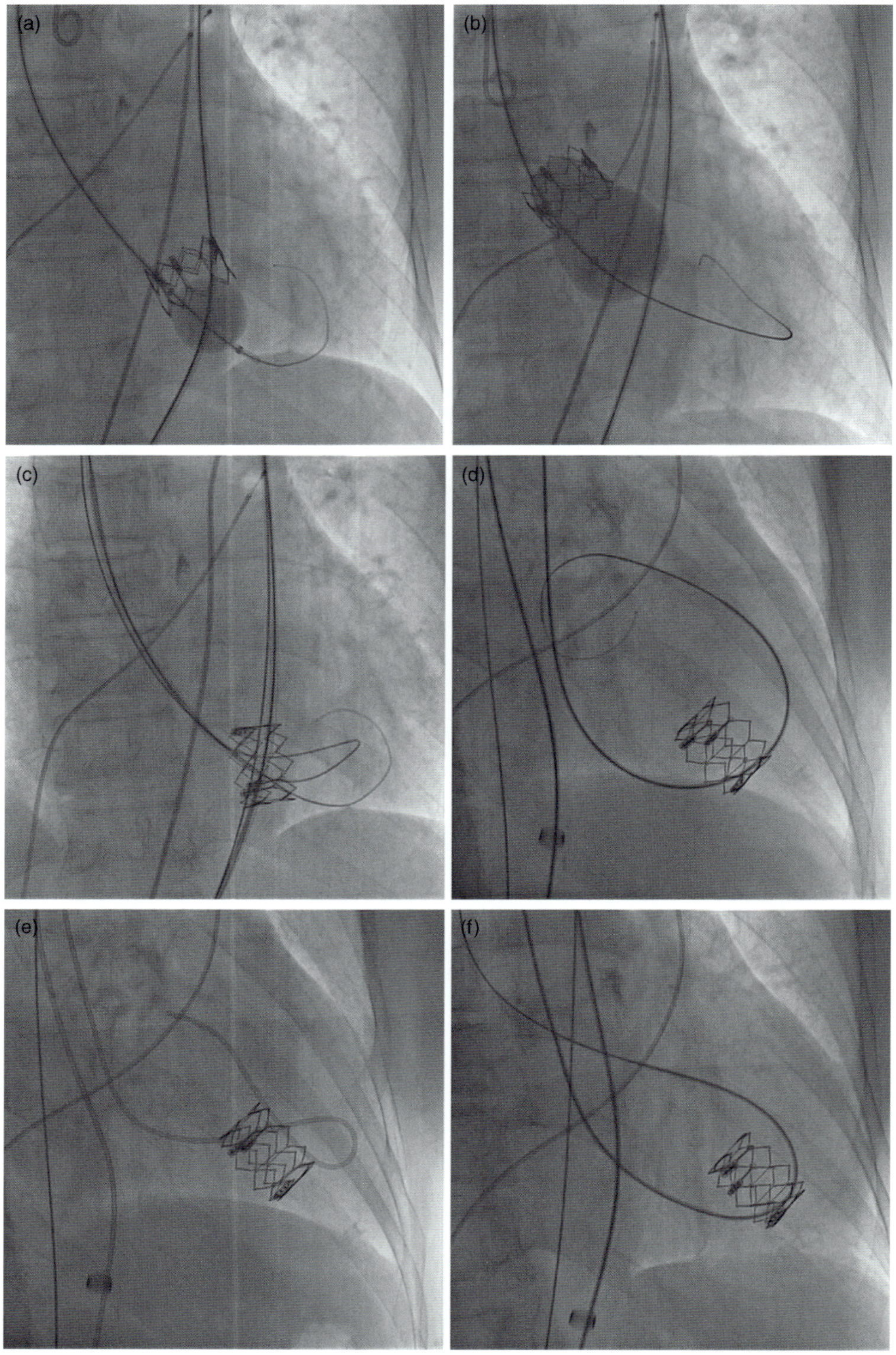

FIGURE 11.14

(a, b) A failed attempt to recover the embolized prosthesis by inflating a balloon distal to the valve and retrieving it back toward the annulus aortic balloon. (c) A failed attempt to use a 0.035-inch wire as a gooseneck to retrieve the valve. (d) A 5-Fr Simmons catheter advanced over a super stiff guidewire. (e) The Simmons catheter alone did not have sufficient support to retrieve the prosthesis. (f) A 0.035-inch Terumo soft wire was inserted in the Simmons catheter and advanced into ascending aorta. The catheter was subsequently advanced over the wire into ascending aorta. Finally a goose neck easily snared the wired Simmons catheter, enabling the system to retrieve the valve to the descending thoracic aorta.

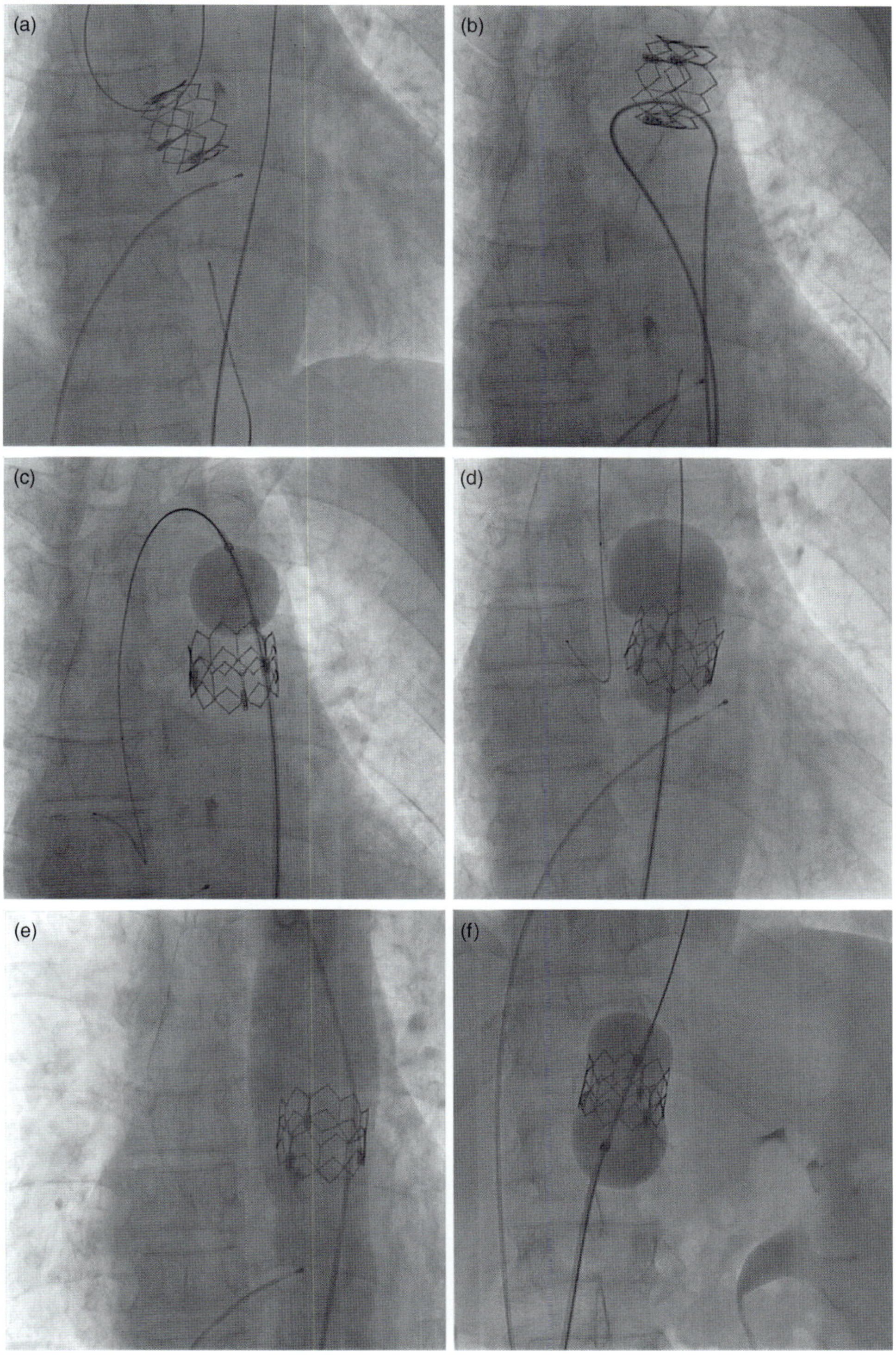

FIGURE 11.15
(a, b) The prosthesis, snared by the wired Simmons catheter, was retrieved to the descending thoracic aorta and then to the abdominal aorta. (c-d) The coaxial position of the prosthesis was maintained as it was moved down using an aortic balloon inflated proximally. (e, f) The prosthesis was deployed in the abdominal aorta.

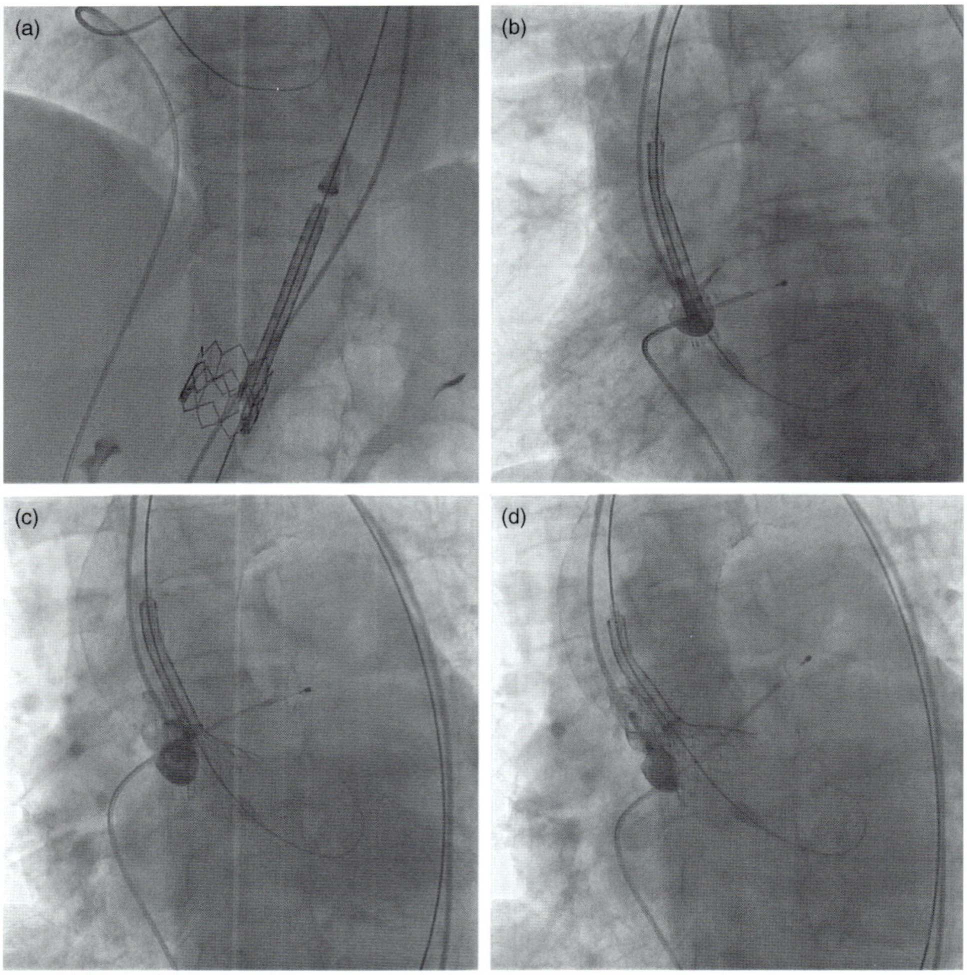

FIGURE 11.16
(a, b) A 29-mm CoreValve was advanced through the Edwards Sapien prosthesis in the abdominal aorta and positioned across the native aortic valve. (c–d) The CoreValve was deployed using multiple contrast injections to visualize positioning, however, the prosthesis was inadvertently pulled back to the ascending aorta as the deployment catheter was pulled back before detaching the valve. Subsequently, the prosthesis was retrieved to the descending thoracic aorta, where it was deployed (Figure not available).

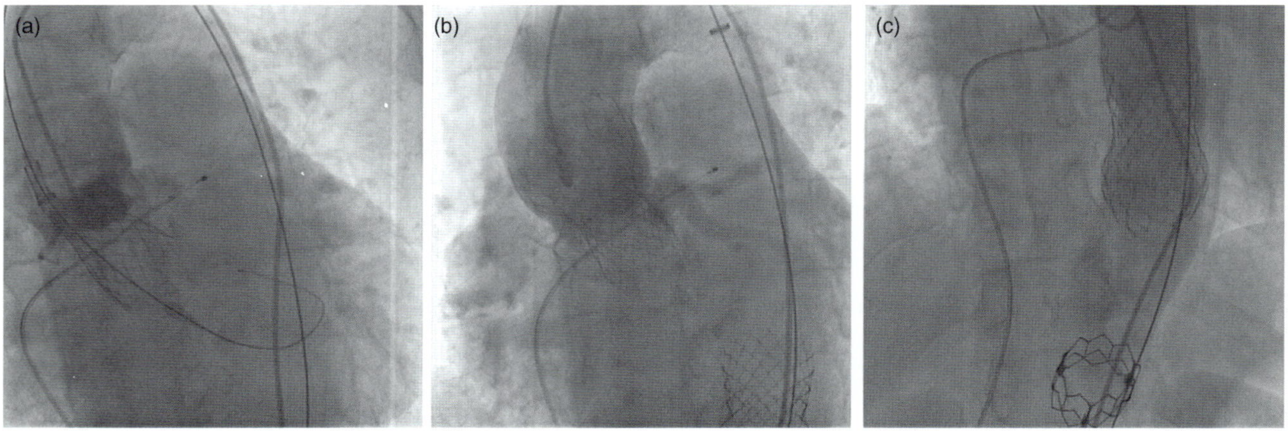

FIGURE 11.17
(a, b) A second 29-mm CoreValve prosthesis was deployed successfully. (c) Note the embolized Core Valve and Edwards Sapien valve as they are deployed in the descending thoracic aorta and abdominal aorta, respectively.

CASE ANALYSIS

This case illustrates the use of TAVI in a patient with severe aortic regurgitation, which is not an approved indication for this procedure, and several associated complications. Besides the fact that the Edwards Sapien valve is not approved for use in patients with aortic regurgitation, its use in this patient was erroneous for the following reasons: *(1)* successful implantation of this prosthesis require the presence of calcifications (which were absent in this case) to help anchor the prosthesis to the aortic annulus, and *(2)* the prosthesis was clearly undersized, given that the aortic annulus was 24 to 26 mm. It is not surprising, therefore, that the valve migrated to the left ventricle. The subsequent choice of the 29-mm CoreValve was correct, and its migration was a result of faulty deployment (retrieval of the deployment catheter before detachment of the prosthesis). This case illustrates that prosthesis migration to the aorta is well tolerated so long as the wire position in the left ventricle is maintained to prevent the valve from flipping over and obstructing antegrade blood flow.

On the other hand, management of prosthesis migration to the left ventricle is more challenging and is fraught with risk, as was illustrated in this case. The laudable, and eventually successful, attempts to retrieve the prosthesis from the left ventricle were complicated by ventricular perforation. Most likely, the perforation occurred during the failed attempts to snare the embolized valve with the 0.035-inch wire loop. Using a soft Simmons-shaped catheter to follow the wire through the valve and back from the LV into the aorta was essential for success and is clearly safer because it prevents contact between the body of the wire and the LV apex.

LESSONS

- The use of the CoreValve to treat patients with pure severe aortic regurgitation is feasible, but it remains experimental.
- Avoidance of prosthesis undersizing is critical to prevent prosthesis migration, particularly with the Edwards Sapien valve.
- In cases of prosthesis embolization to the aorta, maintaining wire position in the left ventricle is critical to successful stabilization.
- In cases of prosthesis embolization to the left ventricle, one should avoid using bare wire loops to extract the prosthesis. Instead, soft 5-Fr Simmons catheters can be valuable in this situation.

SUGGESTED READING

Erdoes G, Wenaweser P, Kadner A, et al. Ventricular prosthesis embolization during transapical aortic valve implantation: The role of transesophageal echocardiography in diagnosis and management. *J Am Soc. Echocardiogr.* e-pub July 2010.

Moss RR, Ivens E, Pasupati S, et al. Role of echocardiography in percutaneous aortic valve implantation. *J Am Coll Cardiol Img.* 2008;1:15–24.

Ng AC, Delgado V, van der Kley F, et al. Comparison of aortic root dimensions and geometries before and after transcatheter aortic valve implantation by 2- and 3-dimensional transesophageal echocardiography and multislice computed tomography. *Circ Cardiovasc Imaging.* 2010;3:94–102.

Tops LF, Wood DA, Delgado V, et al. Noninvasive evaluation of the aortic root with multislice computed tomography implications for transcatheter aortic valve replacement. *JACC Cardiovasc Imaging.* 2008;1(3):321–330.

Wood DA, Tops LF, Mayo JR, et al. Role of multislice computed tomography in transcatheter aortic valve replacement. *Am J Cardiol.* 2009;103(9):1295–1301.

CASE 11.3

Left Ventricular Rupture

CLINICAL HISTORY AND DIAGNOSTIC TESTING RESULTS

An 82-year-old woman with severe aortic stenosis (mean gradient, 52 mm Hg; valve area, 0.9 cm^2; left ventricle ejection fraction (LVEF), 62%) was referred to our institution for evaluation for Transcatheter aortic valve implantation (TAVI). She had several episodes of syncope over the past 6 months and was recommended for surgical valve replacement but declined, opting for the percutaneous procedure. Patient underwent coronary and aorto-iliac angiography that showed no evidence of coronary artery disease (CAD) and adequate iliac and femoral vessels without significant calcifications (Figure 11.18).

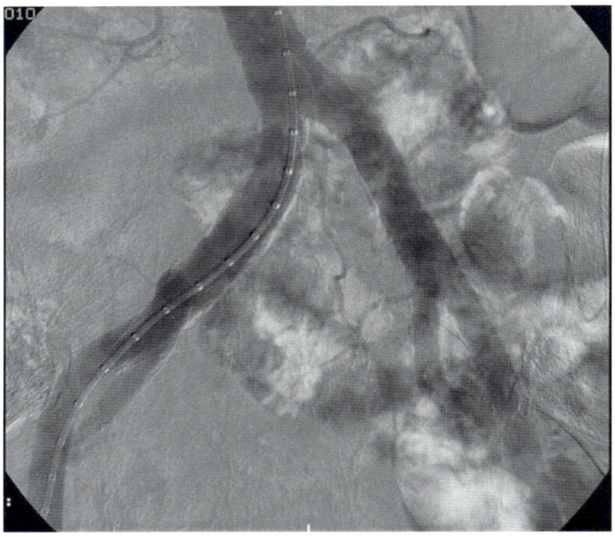

FIGURE 11.18
Diagnostic angiography of iliofemoral vessels showing adequate diameters, mild tortuosity, and absence of calcifications.

PLANNED PROCEDURE

TAVI with a 26-mm CoreValve.

PROCEDURE

The TAVI procedure was performed per standard technique, and the 26-mm CoreValve was deployed successfully (Figure 11.19).

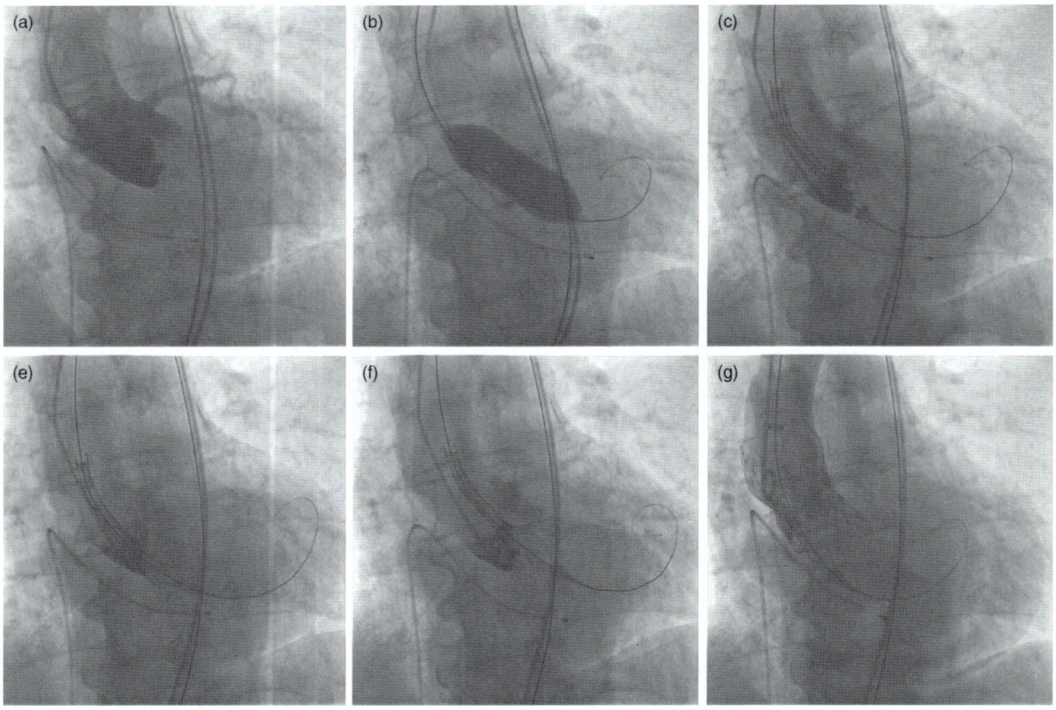

FIGURE 11.19
(a–f) These Figures demonstrate procedural steps from balloon valvuloplasty to CoreValve deployment.
(g) Aortic root angiography performed immediately after hemodynamic collapse showing proper prosthesis position and no paravalvular regurgitation.

COMPLICATION AND MANAGEMENT

Immediately after valve deployment, the patient became hypotensive and was found to have pulseless electrical activity (PEA) requiring cardiopulmonary resuscitation (CPR). The adequacy of valve implantation has already been assessed, with no evidence of paravalvular regurgitation or aortic rupture (Figure 11.19g). Transthoracic echocardiography showed massive pericardial effusion and cardiac tamponade. Left ventriculography showed left ventricle (LV) rupture (Figure 11.20). Pericardiocentesis was immediately performed and the drained blood was reinfused in the femoral venous access (approximately total 5 liters). Blood transfusions and vasopressors were also initiated, and the patient was transferred to the operating room. At surgical exploration, a large LV tear was found, but multiple attempts to suture and patch the defect failed, and the patient died 5 hours later.

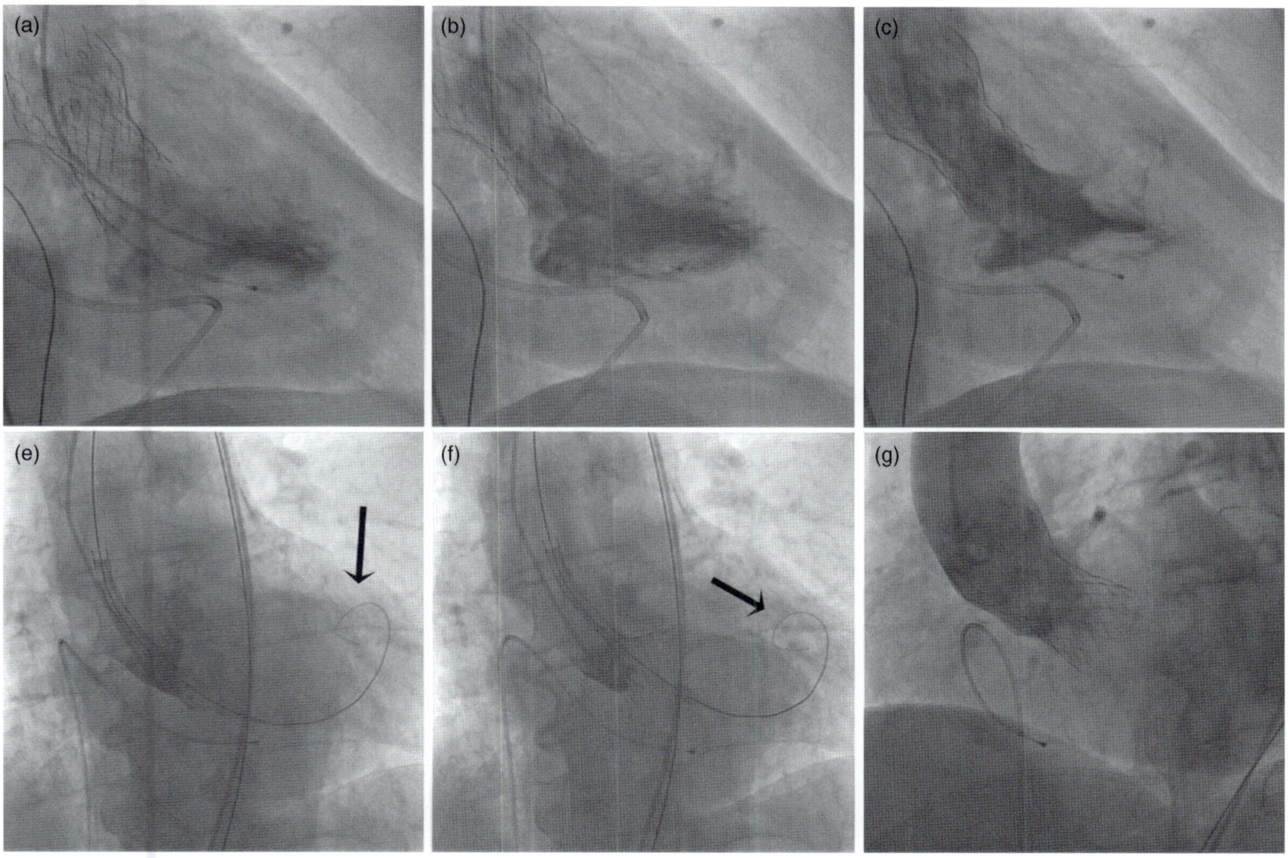

FIGURE 11.20
(a–c) Left ventriculography demonstrating LV free wall rupture (most likely due to aggressive manipulation of the superstiff Amplatz wire during prosthesis deployment [d–e]). (f) A pericardiocentesis catheter in place.

CASE ANALYSIS

Left ventricular rupture is a rare but catastrophic complication of TAVI procedures. This complication occurs either because of the mishandling of the 0.035-inch Amplatz Superstiff wire or the inadvertent advancement of the prosthesis deployment catheter without sufficient length of properly shaped wire tip. In this case, the Amplatz wire was initially placed beneath a mitral cord and subsequently freed and repositioned in the LV. Most likely, inadvertent wire movement is what led to ventricular rupture in this case. Proper shaping of the tip of the Amplatz wire and proper positioning of the tip are key elements to avoid ventricular rupture. Shaping the tip of the Amplatz wire as a large coil, with the heal of the coil at the LV apex, can be risky because it may lacerate the myocardium. Surgical repair is the only viable option when LV rupture involves the free wall; however, even with surgical intervention, the outcome remains poor.

LESSONS

- Left ventricular rupture is a catastrophic but avoidable complication of TAVI procedures.
- Proper shaping and positioning of the tip of the Amplatz wire and meticulous handling are key factors to prevent this complication.
- Early recognition of left ventricular rupture and immediate surgical intervention are key to improve patient outcomes.

SUGGESTED READING

Ussia GP, Scarabelli M, Mulè M, et al. Postprocedural management of patients after transcatheter aortic valve implantation procedure with self-expanding bioprosthesis. *Catheter Cardiovasc Interv.* 2010;76:767–768.

12

Paul Poommipanit, Zahid Amin, and Jonathan Tobis

Complications of Transcatheter Closure of Atrial Septal Defects and Patent Foramen Ovale

INTRODUCTION

Percutaneous closure of an atrial septal defect (ASD) or patent foramen ovale (PFO) has become a common procedure in the cardiac catheterization lab. There have been more than 200,000 Amplatzer septal occluder devices (AGA Medical, Plymouth, MN), more than 10,000 Helex septal occluder devices (Gore Medical, Flagstaff, AZ), and more than 32,000 CardioSEAL family of septal occluder devices (NMT Medical, Boston, MA) implanted since the mid-1990s (1–3). As the frequency of implants increases, it is conceivable that the number of complications will also increase. These risks range from device embolization to thrombus formation on the device, arrhythmias, and device-related cardiac perforation requiring emergent pericardiocentesis and surgery. The risk of pulmonary embolism, bleeding requiring blood transfusion, or death remains extremely low. In a meta-analysis of 1,355 patients, the combined risk of these major events was 1.5% (4,5). In this chapter, we will focus on device embolization, thrombus formation on the device, air embolization, and erosion.

DEVICE EMBOLIZATION

This is the most common complication following device placement (as reported to the medical device companies and FDA). The rate of this complication is dependent upon the type of defect for which the device is implanted. It is less than 1% among most devices implanted for PFO closure (6). The embolization of septal occluder devices for ASD closure is on the order of 0.55% to 4%, depending on the type of device implanted (7–9). Levi and Moore reported that the incidence of Amplatzer atrial septal occluder (ASO) device embolization was 0.55% (21 embolizations in 3,824 device placements) among company-designated proctors (7). The incidence of Helex septal occluder device embolization was 1.7% in the U.S. multicenter pivotal study of the Helex septal occluder for percutaneous closure of secundum ASDs (8). The incidence of embolization for the CardioSEAL and STARflex family of septal occluder devices was 4% when implanted for ASD closure (9). The majority of septal occluder devices that embolize are able to be retrieved percutaneously with use of snares and forceps. The clinical impact of device embolization is the possibility of palpitations, syncope, atrial or ventricular arrhythmias, chest pain, dyspnea, hemolysis, and other sequelae dependent on the location of the embolized device.

AIR EMBOLISM

A rare complication during device deployment is air embolization. Air may be inadvertently introduced through the delivery catheter during preparation and deployment of the device. Studies suggest that the incidence of air embolism is 0.5% or less for ASD closure (10) and 0.48% for PFO closure (11). ST segment elevation typically occurs in the inferior leads as the right coronary artery is in an anterior position while the patient is supine. Management of coronary air embolism is dependent on the patient's symptoms. Small volumes of air can typically be managed conservatively with high-flow oxygen and pain control. Large volumes of air may cause arrhythmias and hemodynamic compromise. Management includes aspiration, forceful saline injection, intraaortic balloon pump placement, defibrillation, and CPR. The long-term impact from these transient events is unknown.

THROMBUS FORMATION

Another potential complication of percutaneous device implantation is thrombus formation on the device. Complete endothelialization of an implanted device tends to occur by 6 months. In a study by Krumsdorf et al, the rates of thrombus formation were 0%, 7.1%, 5.7%, and 6.6% among Amplatzer PFO, CardioSEAL, StarFLEX, and PFO Star, respectively. The difference between the Amplatzer PFO device and the other devices was statistically significant. In that study, postprocedural atrial fibrillation and the presence of an atrial septal aneurysm were predictors for thrombus formation. Two of the patients required surgical removal of the device, and one had the thrombus evacuated (12). Another study with transesophageal echocardiography (TEE) found that the incidence of thrombus formation on the CardioSEAL device was as high as 23%. The risk of thrombus formation on the left atrial side of the device is the possibility of peripheral embolization producing myocardial infarction or stroke. The incidence of thrombus formation on the Helex septal occluder device is low compared with the Amplatzer family of devices.

A survey of 18 centers that implanted close to 14,000 devices revealed that surgical explantation of PFO devices occurred in 0.27% of implants. However, this risk was device dependent. For the CardioSEAL device, the explantation rate was 1/120 cases. For the Amplatzer device, it was 1/425 cases, and for the Helex device, it was 1/603 cases (13).

DEVICE EROSION

Device erosion is a rare complication of device implantation. The Amplatzer registry documented 28 cases of erosion from 1998 to 2004 with the ASO device. Device oversizing was the most common reason resulting in erosion (14). In a separate study, the incidence of erosion with the Amplatzer PFO device was found to be 0.018% (15). Erosion has been reported with the STARFlex and CardioSEAL family of devices (16). There have been no documented cases of erosion with the Helex device; however, mitral valve perforation secondary to wire fracture was described in a case report. Device-related erosion may lead to atrial wall injury (hemopericardium), formation of aorta to atrial fistula without hemodynamic compromise, or cardiac tamponade if atrial and aortic wall injury occurs (14). Fortunately, the incidence of erosion has decreased since the publication of these observations, presumably due to the use of more appropriately sized devices.

CASE 12.1

Embolization of a Helex Device Several Months After Suboptimal PFO Closure

CLINICAL HISTORY AND DIAGNOSTIC TESTING RESULTS

A 45-year-old man without prior medical history presented with right-sided hemiparesis 1 week after varicose vein stripping. Magnetic resonance imaging demonstrated left anterior cerebral artery occlusion. Transcranial Doppler showed a Spencer Grade-5 shunt, a lower extremity ultrasound demonstrated a greater saphenous vein occlusive thrombus, and transesopheageal echocardiography (TEE) showed a PFO.

PLANNED PROCEDURE

Intracardiac echo (ICE)-guided PFO closure.

PROCEDURE

The patient was premedicated with aspirin 325 mg and clopidogrel 600 mg. After ultrasound demonstrated the absence of thrombus, 8- and 11-Fr sheaths (Terumo Medical, Somerset, NJ) were placed in the right femoral vein. An 8-Fr Acuson AcuNav ICE probe (Siemens Medical, Malvern, PA) was used to guide placement of a Helex 25-mm septal occluder device (Figure 12.1a, b). Five minutes after release of the device, the right atrial disk slipped off the limbus of the septum secundum and was resting in the PFO tunnel (Figure 12.2a, b). Although the position of the device within the PFO tunnel was not ideal, we thought it was stable enough and that fibrous tissue would seal it to the tunnel. A trans-throacic echo (TTE) the following week and 1 month later showed that the device was in a stable position in the interatrial septum.

COMPLICATION AND MANAGEMENT

The patient returned for a follow-up TEE after 3 months (per our standard protocol). The TEE revealed a PFO, but the closure device was not visualized. The patient was asymptomatic. Fluoroscopy demonstrated that the Helex device had embolized to the descending abdominal aorta just below the renal arteries (Figure 12.3a). The patient was brought to the catheterization laboratory for percutaneous retrieval of the Helex device and for reattempting PFO closure.

Two 8-Fr sheaths were placed in the right femoral vein and a 6-Fr sheath (Terumo Medical) was placed in the left femoral artery. Intravenous heparin (3,000 units) was administered. The arterial site was preclosed using two Perclose Proglide closure devices (Abbott, Abbott Park, IL). A 10-Fr Flexor sheath (Cook Medical, Bloomington, IN) was inserted into the femoral artery and placed caudal to the Helex device. We obtained multiple views of the device in relation to the sheath in order to identify the position of the LA and RA islets. A 6-Fr pigtail catheter (Cordis Corp, Warren, NJ) was used to perform aortography (Figure 12.3b). A 6-Fr multipurpose diagnostic catheter (Cordis) with a 12- to 20-mm EnSnare (Angiotech Medical Device Technologies, Inc., Gainesville, FL) followed by a 6-Fr JR4 diagnostic catheter (Cordis) with a 35-mm Amplatz gooseneck snare (eV3 Inc., Plymouth, MN) was used to capture the left atrial eyelet. By pulling on the left atrial eyelet, the locking loop was successfully released and allowed the device to unravel. The unlocked Helex device was retracted into the Flexor sheath (Figure 12.4a). The right atrial eyelet was hooked on the distal tip of the sheath, which prevented the device from entering the catheter (Figure 12.4b). We did not remove the whole assembly because we were concerned that upon removal of the catheter, the device would hook on the femoral arteriotomy site and traumatize the artery. Attempts were made to retrieve the RA eyelet, but this resulted in partial migration of the device back into the aorta. The sheath was pulled back until the balloon and device were partially out of the body. Two large hemostat clamps were placed at 90° across the sheath, and the sheath and device were removed together (Figure 12.5). Hemostasis was achieved with the Perclose devices.

The patient's PFO was then closed successfully with a 30-mm Amplatzer cribriform device (AGA Medical) (Figure 12.6). The patient was discharged home the same day.

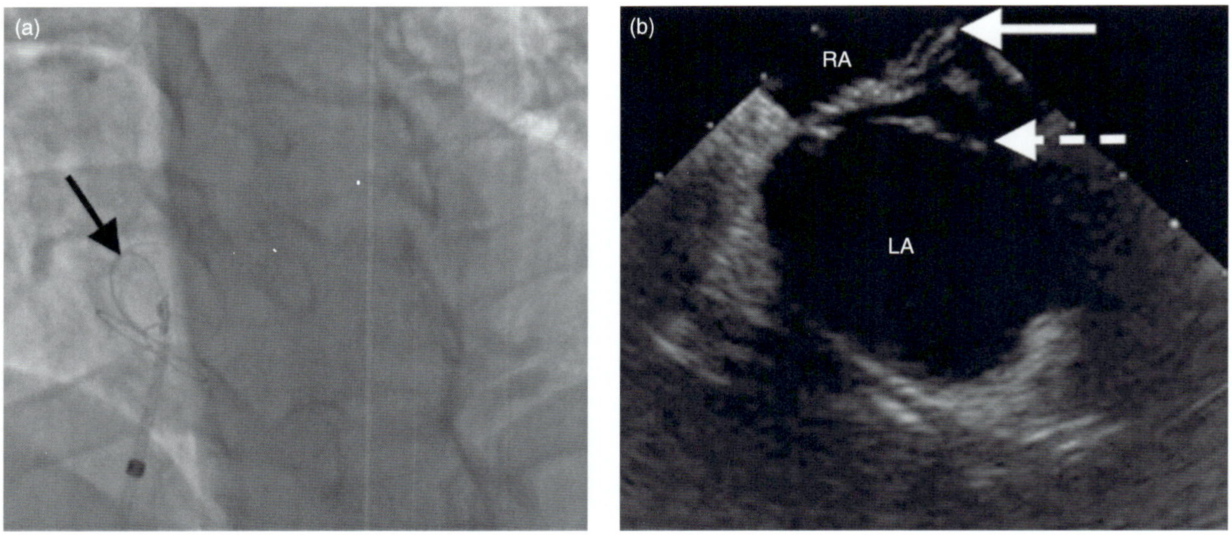

FIGURE 12.1

(a) Fluoroscopic image of the Helex device (black arrow) in place across the PFO with both atrial disks splayed across the septum secundum. (b) Typical intracardiac echo appearance of the Helex device with the right atrial disc (solid white arrow) and left atrial disc (dashed white arrow) straddling the septum secundum. The right atrium (RA) and left atrium (LA) are labeled.

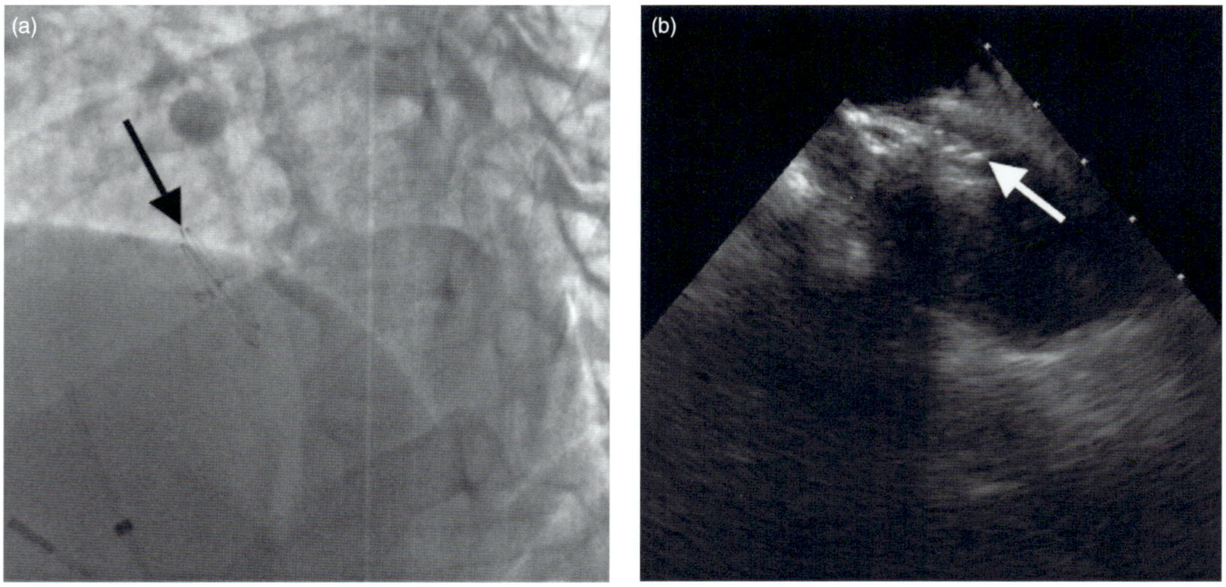

FIGURE 12.2

(a) Fluoroscopic image of the Helex device with the right atrial disc within the PFO tunnel (black arrow). (b) Intracardiac echo (ICE) image of the Helex device with the right atrial disc (white arrow) within the PFO tunnel. This was felt to be stable enough to allow for healing and fibrosis of the device within the tunnel.

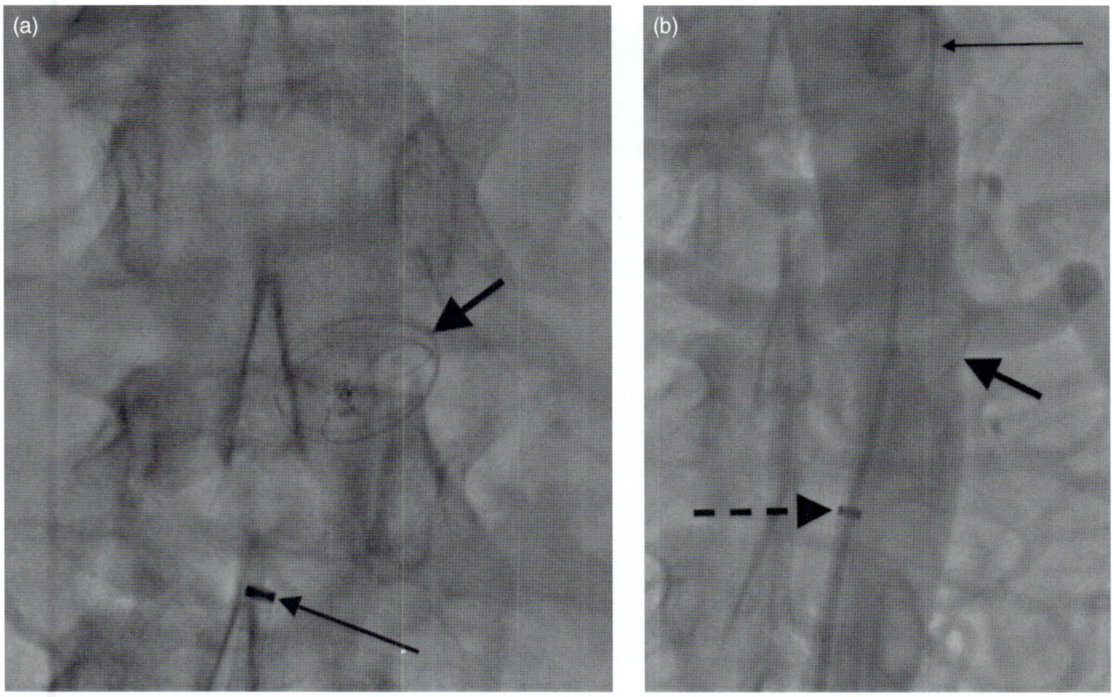

FIGURE 12.3

(a) Fluoroscopic image of the Helex device (short arrow) in relationship to the 10-Fr rescue sheath (long arrow). (b) Abdominal aortic angiography with a pigtail catheter (narrow black arrow) demonstrating the Helex device (wide black arrow) in relationship to the Flexor sheath (dashed arrow) and the renal arteries.

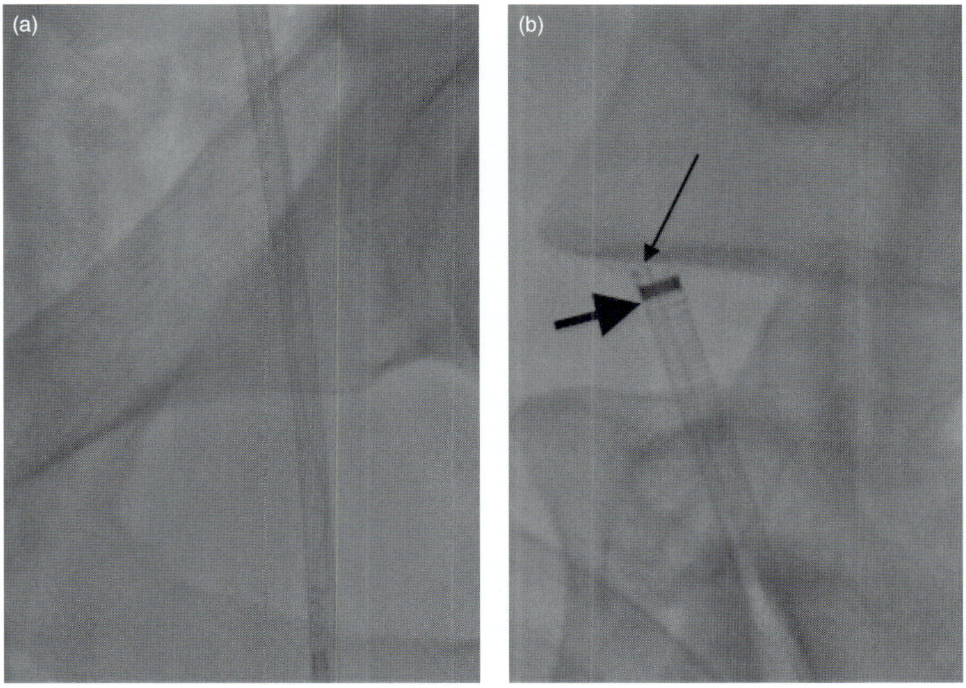

FIGURE 12.4

(a) Left atrial side of the Helex device retracted into the Flexor sheath. (b) Right atrial eyelet (narrow black arrow) caught on the end of the sheath (wide black arrow).

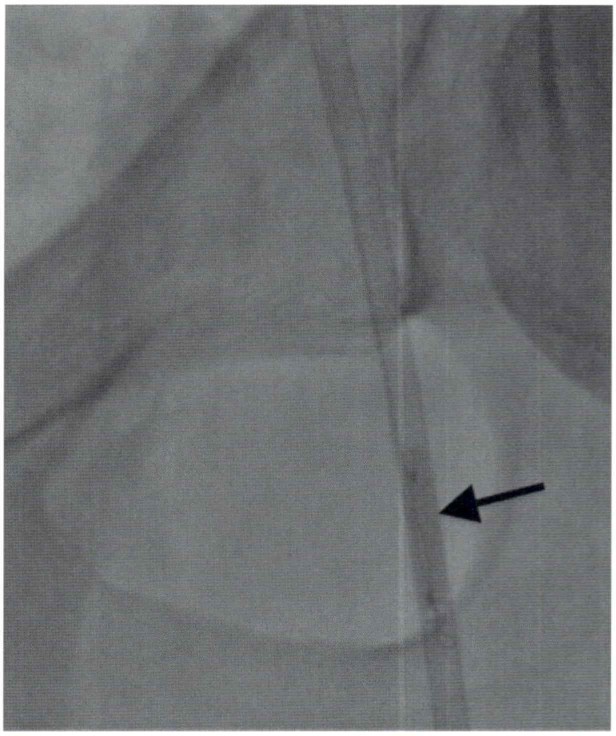

FIGURE 12.5

A Voyager 4- × 15-mm coronary balloon (Abbott) [black arrow] inflated within the sheath to trap the device.

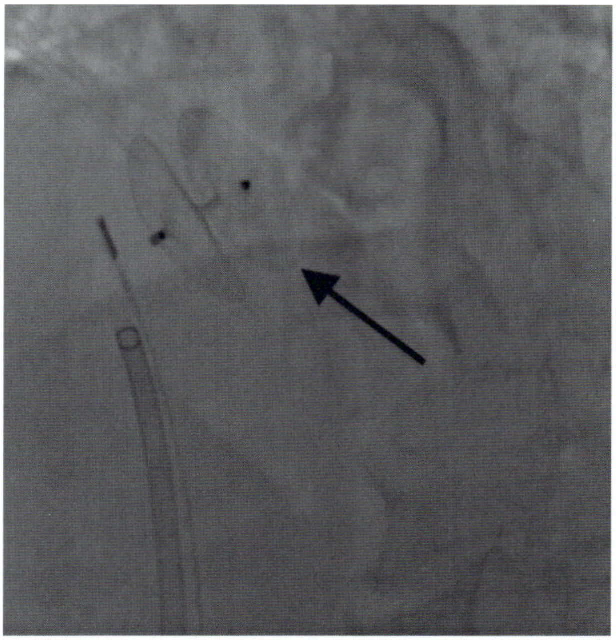

FIGURE 12.6

Amplatzer 30-mm cribriform device (arrow) within the PFO tunnel.

CASE ANALYSIS

Embolization of the Helex device 3 months after deployment was a result of suboptimal positioning due to device undersizing. In retrospect, the 25-mm device should have been retrieved and a larger device placed instead.

LESSONS

- During PFO closure, device undersizing predisposes to early and late device embolization.
- When using the Helex device for PFO closure, splaying of the right atrial disc over the septum secundum is essential for device stability.

SUGGESTED READING

Levi DS, Moore JW. Embolization and retrieval of the Amplatzer septal occluder. *Catheter Cardiovasc Interv.* 2004;61(4):543–547.

CASE 12.2

Air Embolism to the Right Coronary Artery During PFO Closure

CLINICAL HISTORY AND DIAGNOSTIC TESTING RESULTS

A 46-year-old woman with a history of breast cancer, status postmastectomy, radiation, and chemotherapy, which were complicated by radiation pneumonitis was being considered for lung transplantation. Patient's baseline oxygen saturation was 90%, and it dropped to 80% after minimal exercise, such as walking or bending down. Her oxygenation at rest with supplemental oxygen is 98%. It was felt that the degree of hypoxemia was out of proportion to the amount of pulmonary fibrosis. A TEE demonstrated a PFO confirming a diagnosis of orthodeoxia. Subsequently, the patient was referred for PFO closure hoping that this would improve her hypoxemia and avoid the need for lung transplantation.

PLANNED PROCEDURE

ICE-guided PFO closure.

PROCEDURE

The patient was premedicated with aspirin 325 mg and clopidogrel 600 mg. Two 8-Fr sheaths were placed in the right femoral vein. Intravenous heparin was given to maintain an activated coagulation time (ACT) over 300 seconds. A 6-Fr MPA-1 catheter was advanced over a 0.038-inch J-tipped guidewire into the right atrium. An 8-Fr Acuson AcuNav catheter (Siemens Medical) was advanced into the right atrium. Bubble studies were performed at rest and with forced expiration (up to 40 mmHg) into a manometer. The right-to-left shunt grade was recorded using both ICE and transcranial Doppler (TCD). A J-tipped guidewire was used to cross the PFO. The MPA catheter was advanced into the left superior pulmonary vein (LSPV), and the wire was removed. A 0.035-inch Amplatz extra stiff wire was advanced into the LSPV. The MPA catheter was removed. The 8-Fr sheath was exchanged for a 13-Fr sheath (St. Jude Medical, St. Paul, MN). The 9-Fr Helex delivery catheter could not pass across the interatrial septum.

An Amplatzer 24-mm sizing balloon was advanced into the interatrial septum. The balloon was inflated and demonstrated a PFO tunnel size of 6 mm (Figure 12.7). The Helex device was reinserted and crossed the interatrial septum. The device was deployed per standard technique (Figure 12.8).

COMPLICATION AND MANAGEMENT

During deployment of the left atrial disc, air bubbles were observed on fluoroscopy within the left atrium. The patient developed throat burning, and the ECG manifested ST-segment elevations in the inferior leads (baseline ECG in Figure 12.9; subsequent ECG in Figure 12.10). It was apparent that the patient had air embolization to the right coronary artery (RCA). The patient remained hemodynamically stable. The patient was given sublinguinal nitroglycerin and placed on high flow oxygen. Subsequently, the patient's symptoms resolved and the ST segment elevation normalized (Figure 12.11). TTE obtained 2 hours later showed normal wall motion, and troponin levels were normal. Patient was discharged home the second day in stable condition.

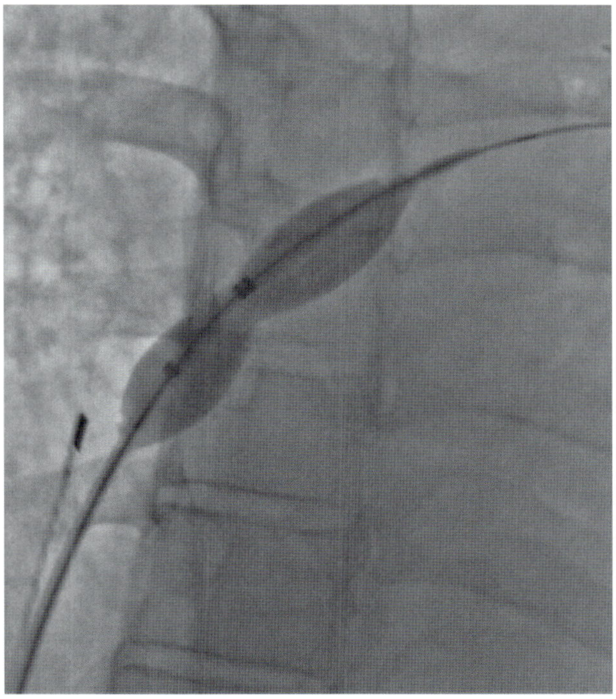

FIGURE 12.7
Flouroscopic image of an Amplatzer sizing balloon (24 mm) through the PFO.

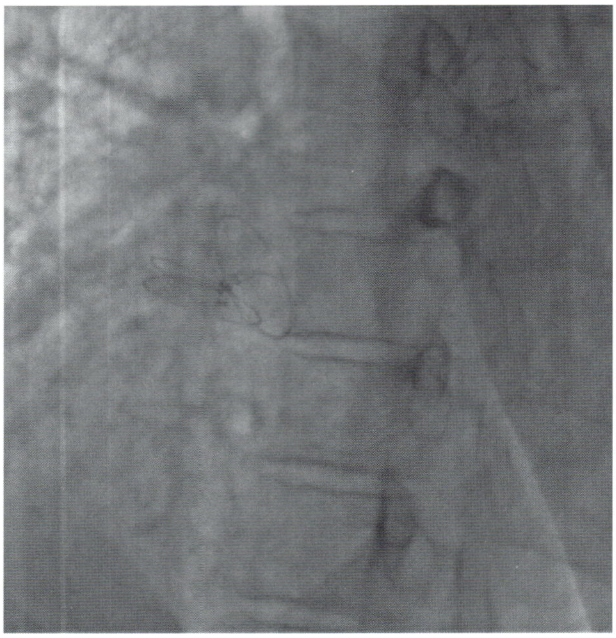

FIGURE 12.8
Flouroscopic image of a deployed 25-mm Helex device through the FFO.

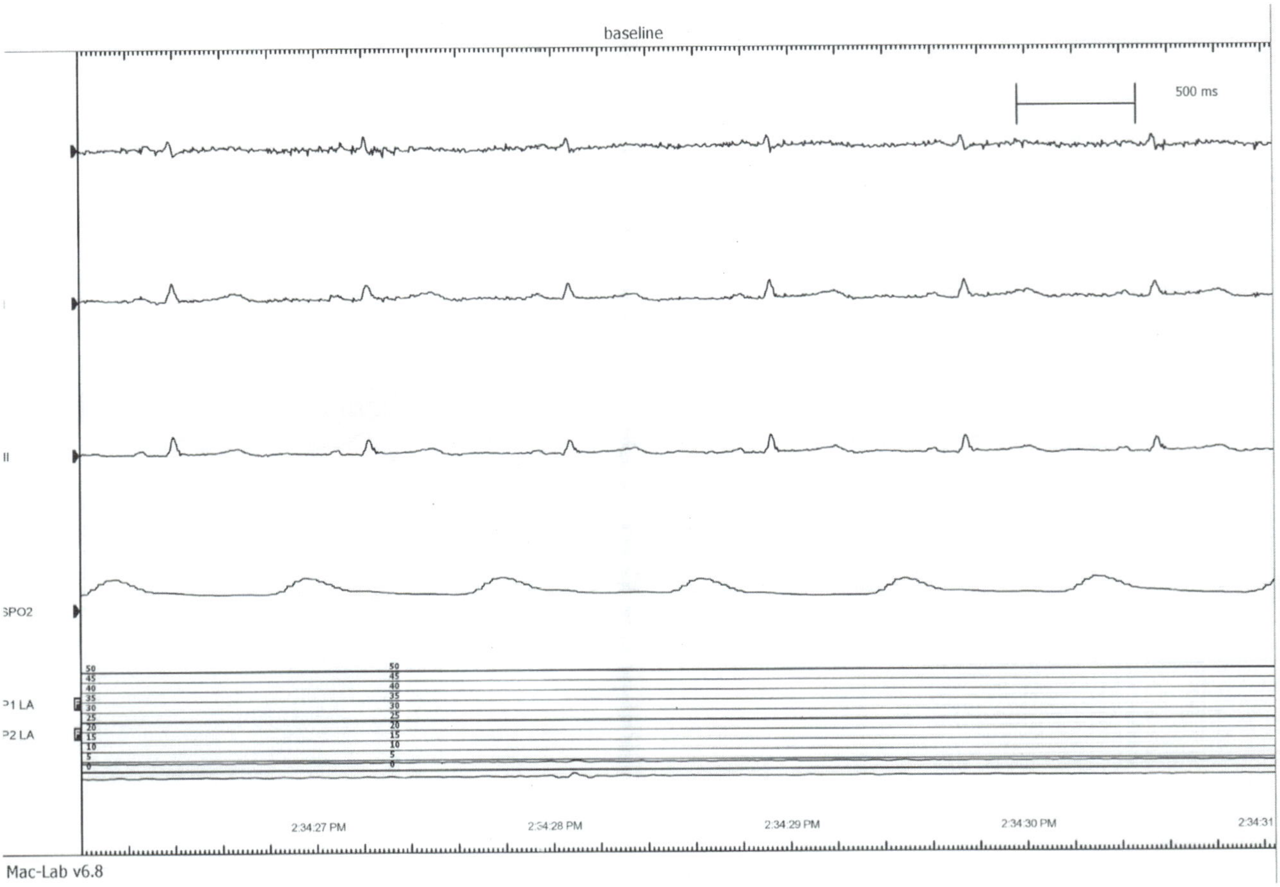

FIGURE 12.9
Baseline ECG.

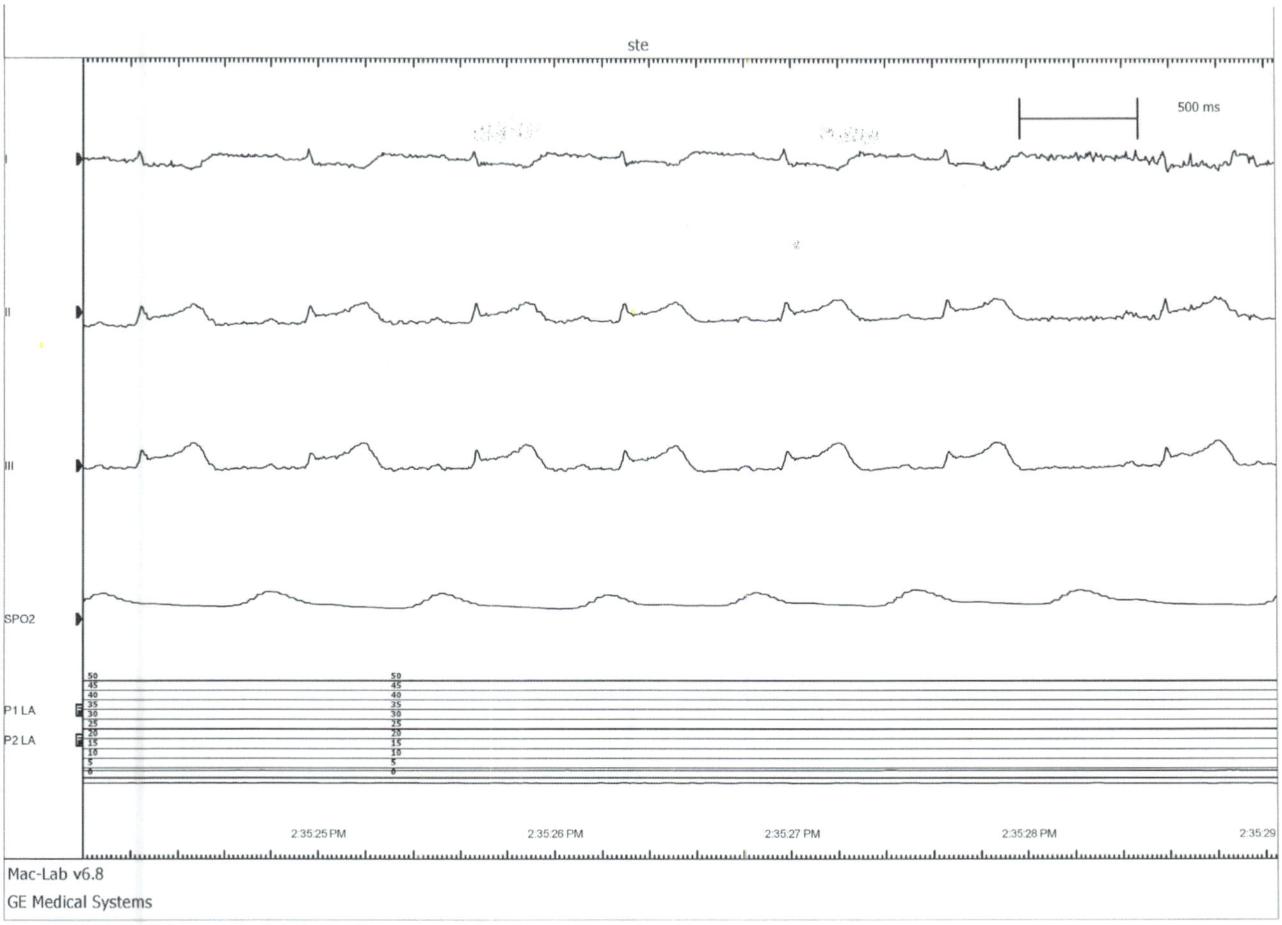

FIGURE 12.10
Intraprocedure ECG after air embolization demonstrating ST segment elevations in the inferior leads.

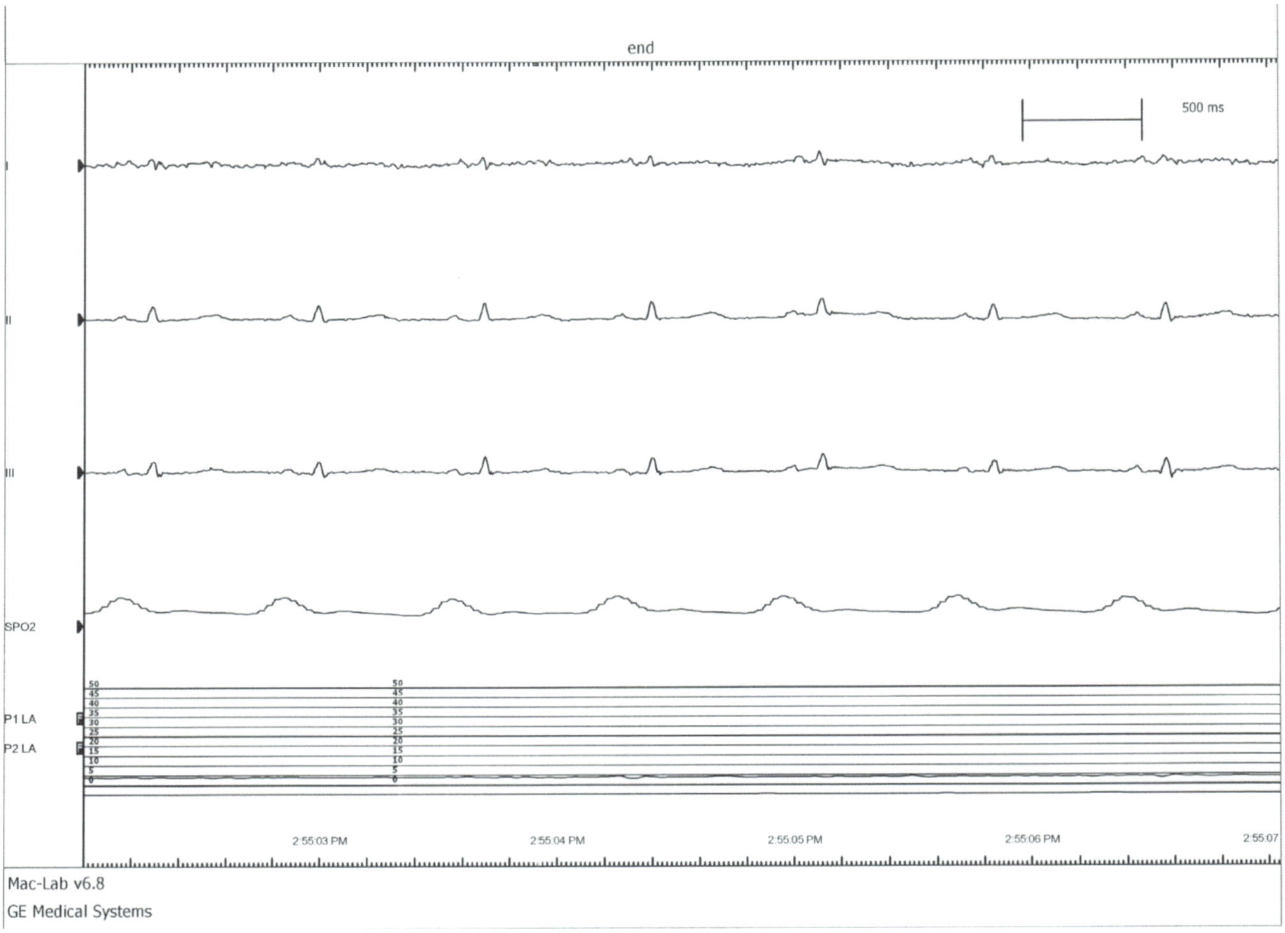

FIGURE 12.11
Postprocedure ECG demonstrating resolution of ST segment changes.

CASE ANALYSIS

The introduction of air from the delivery catheter was likely the cause of air embolization into the right coronary artery. This complication occurred because the device delivery catheter was removed and then reinserted, since it initially could not be manipulated through the PFO.

Meticulous flushing of all catheters is needed during all intravascular procedures. Even though this catheter was prepared with caution, saline probably leaked out of the delivery catheter after it was removed, and adequate flushing prior to catheter reinsertion was not performed.

LESSONS

- During PFO closure, the closure device delivery catheter should be flushed meticulously, and the backend of the catheter should be kept below the heart level.

SUGGESTED READING

Khan M, Schmidt DH, Bajwa T, Shalev Y. Coronary air embolism: Incidence, severity, and suggested approaches to treatment. *Cathet Cardiovasc Diagn*. 1995;36(4):313–318.

Wahl A, et al. Safety and feasibility of percutaneous closure of patent foramen ovale without intra-procedural echocardiography in 825 patients. *Swiss Med Wkly*. 2008;138(39–40):567–572.

CASE 12.3

Thrombosis of a CardioSEAL Device

CLINICAL HISTORY AND DIAGNOSTIC TESTING RESULTS

A 32-year-old man with a history of multiple transient ischemic attacks (TIAs) and a cerebellar stroke was found to have a PFO with right-to-left shunting on routine workup after his stroke. He had been on medical therapy since his stroke and was referred for PFO closure.

PLANNED PROCEDURE

TEE-guided PFO closure.

PROCEDURE

The patient was premedicated with aspirin and clopidogrel. An 8-Fr sheath was placed in the right femoral vein. TEE demonstrated a long PFO tunnel, approximately 18 to 20 mm. Bubble studies performed with agitated saline demonstrated a grade 3 shunt with coughing. Because the tunnel length was long, we were concerned that the CardioSEAL arms would not open up and lie flat against the septum. Therefore, a transseptal puncture was performed with an 8-Fr Mullins sheath and a Brockenbrough needle to place the CardioSEAL device (NMT Medical) in a central location within the interatrial septum. Intravenous heparin was given to produce an ACT above 250 seconds. An Amplatz 0.035-inch super stiff wire was placed into the left atrium and the sheath removed. Based on TEE measurements, a 30-mm CardioSEAL device was deployed in the usual manner without complications. The patient remained on aspirin and clopidogrel after the procedure.

COMPLICATION AND MANAGEMENT

Routine TEE at 4 weeks follow-up demonstrated a 1-cm thrombus on the left atrial side of the CardioSEAL device (Figure 12.12). The patient was asymptomatic. Since the patient was already on dual antiplatelet therapy, anticoagulation with warfarin was initiated. Repeat TEE 2 weeks later revealed progression of the thrombus with multiple pedunculated mobile echogenic structures on the left atrial disc (Figure 12.13). The patient was admitted to the hospital and placed on intravenous argatroban. Given the potential risk of embolization with continued medical therapy, the patient elected to undergo surgical explantation. Surgical views of the CardioSEAL device and thrombus are shown in Figures 12.14, 12.15, and 12.16. Continuous TEE monitoring during surgery documented that no thrombi were dislodged during the explantation procedure. The patient did well postoperatively and was discharged home. There were no subsequent neurologic events.

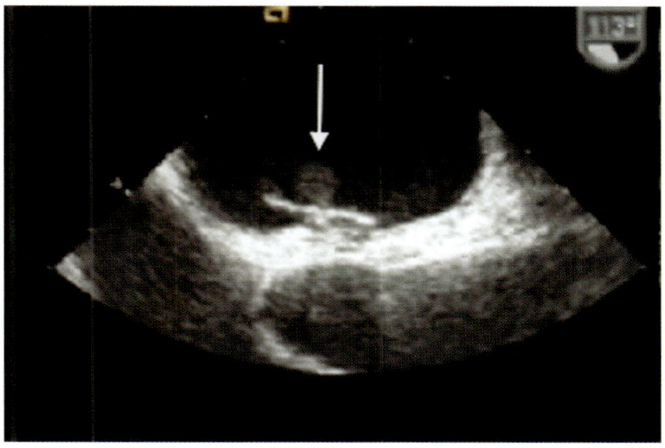

FIGURE 12.12

TEE of the CardioSEAL device at 4 weeks follow-up showing a thrombus on the left atrial disc.

CASE ANALYSIS

Thrombosis of the CardioSEAL device could not have been predicted in this case because implantation and postprocedure care was standard at that time. If it was not for the routine echo follow-up, the thrombus would not have been recognized, and the patient may have had a catastrophic event.

Although warfarin is considered the treatment of choice for left atrial thrombi, this case demonstrates that success cannot always be assumed and echo follow-up after warfarin initiation is essential to document thrombus resolution.

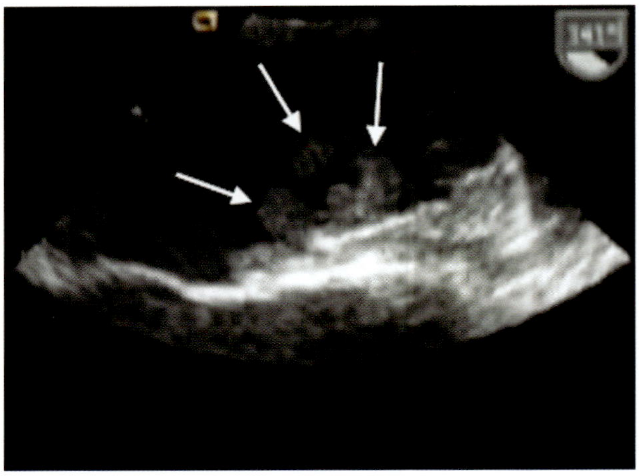

FIGURE 12.13
TEE of the CardioSEAL device at 6 weeks follow-up (2 weeks on warfarin) shows multiple thrombi on the left atrial disc.

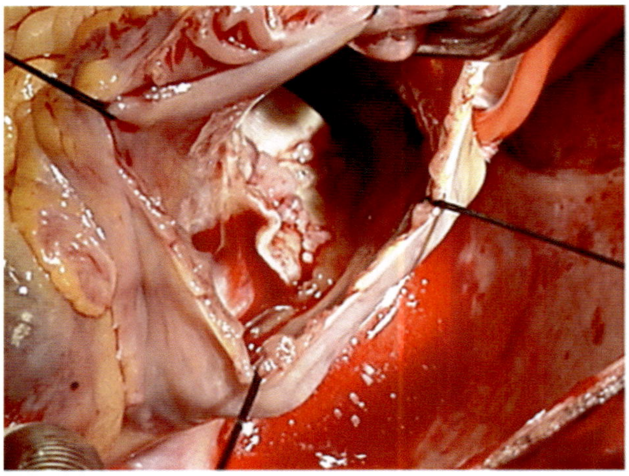

FIGURE 12.14
View of the CardioSEAL device at surgery.

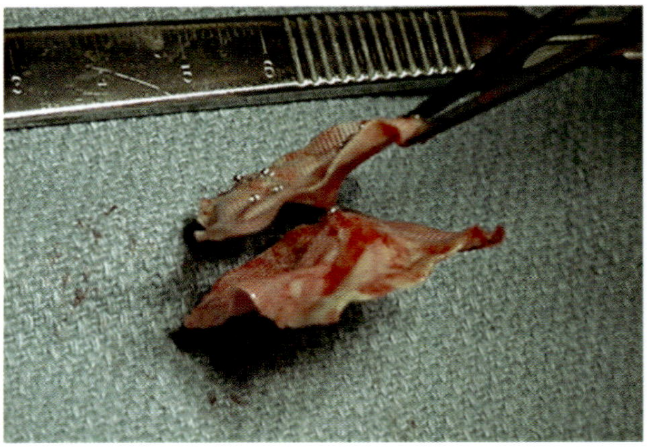

FIGURE 12.15
Explanted CardioSEAL device.

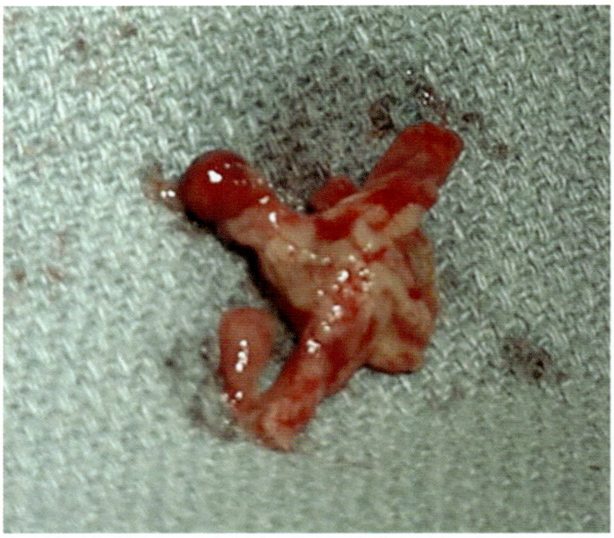

FIGURE 12.16
The extracted thrombus from the left atrial disc of the CardioSEAL device.

LESSONS

- Routine echo follow-up is essential after PFO/ASD closure.
- Although warfarin is the treatment of choice for left atrial thrombi, it is not successful in all cases.

SUGGESTED READING

Krumsdorf U, Ostemayer S, Billinger K, et al. Incidence and clinical course of thrombus formation on atrial septal defect and patient foramen ovale closure devices in 1,000 consecutive patients. *J Am Coll Cardiol.* 2004;43(2):302–309.

Zaidi AN, Cheatham JP, Galantowicz M, Astor T, Kovalchin JP. Late thrombus formation on the Helex septal occluder after double-lung transplant. *J Heart Lung Transplant.* 2010;29(7):814–816.

CASE 12.4

Aorto-Atrial Fistula After ASD Closure With an Oversized Amplatzer Device

CLINICAL HISTORY AND DIAGNOSTIC TESTING RESULTS

A 20-year-old man with secundum ASD and right atrial and ventricular enlargement by echocardiography was referred for transcatheter closure of the ASD. Preprocedure TEE revealed a large secundum ASD with deficient aortic rim in several views (Figure 12.17a–c).

PLANNED PROCEDURE

TEE-guided transcatheter ASD closure.

PROCEDURE

The cardiac catheterization procedure was performed per our standard protocol. TEE was utilized during the procedure. The defect was balloon-sized using the stop-flow technique and measured 22 mm in diameter. A 26-mm Amplatzer septal occluder device was placed without any incident. Thorough evaluation of the device after the placement (Figure 12.18) and next day revealed that the device was in good position.

COMPLICATION AND MANAGEMENT

The patient was seen after 1 month for routine follow up. Physical examination revealed a loud continuous murmur at the left upper and lower sternal border. Echocardiography showed a fistula between the aorta and the right atrium (Figure 12.19). There was no pericardial effusion. The patient was asymptomatic. The patient underwent cardiac surgery in which the Amplatzer device was removed, the fistula repaired, and the ASD closed with a patch. The surgical procedure went well and the patient was discharged home 3 days after surgery.

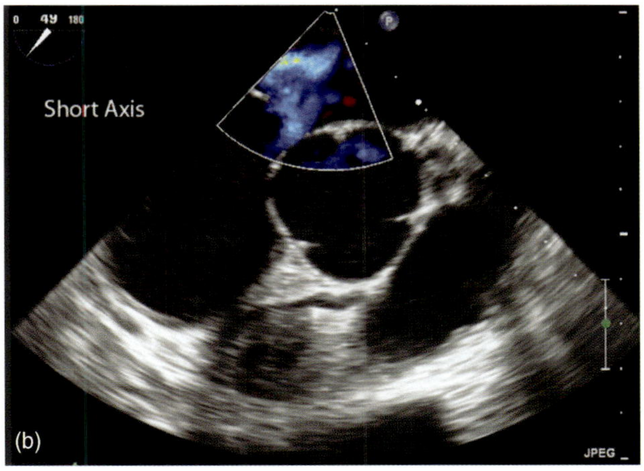

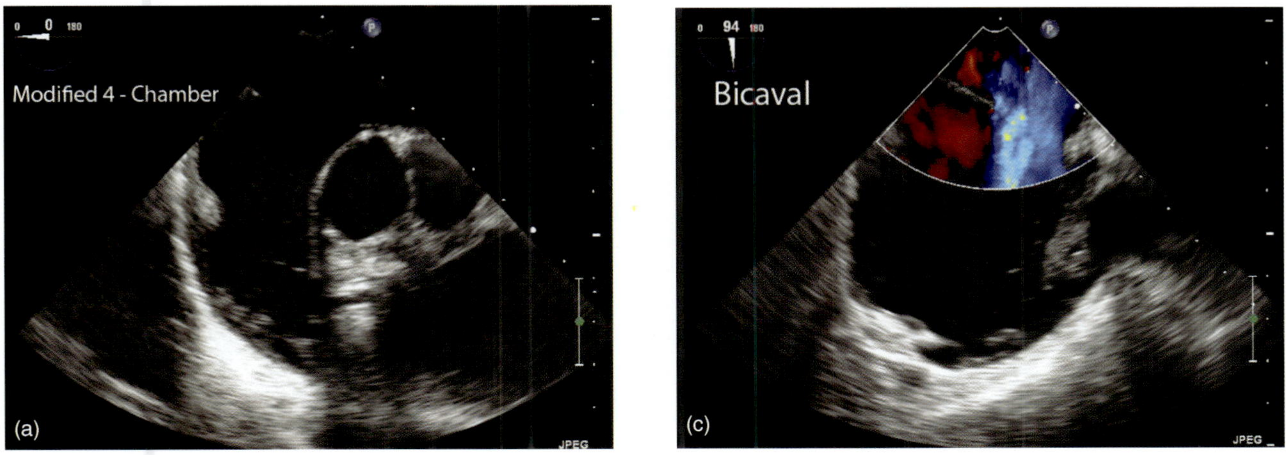

FIGURE 12.17

(a) Preprocedure TEE in modified four-chamber view: Aortic rim absence is seen. The posterior rim is thin but adequate in length. (b) Aortic short-axis view: aortic rim deficiency is noted. (c) Bicaval view: adequate SVC and IVC rims are seen.

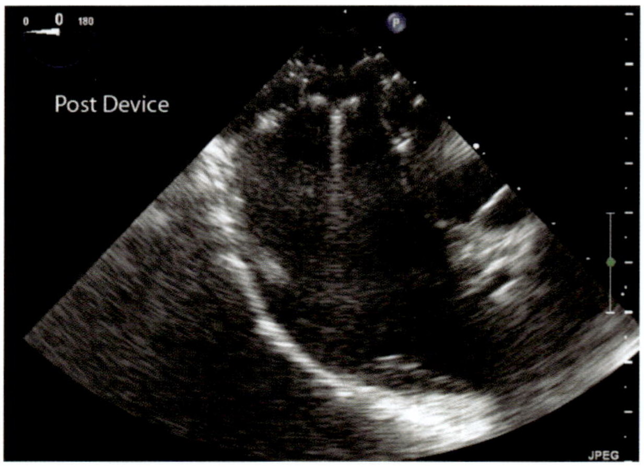

FIGURE 12.18
TEE short-axis aortic view after device implantation.

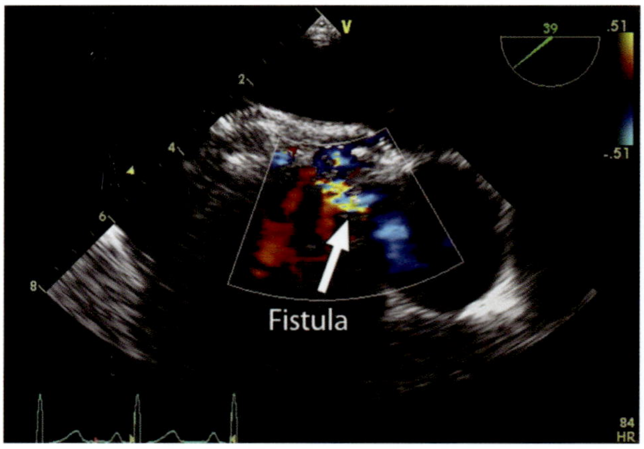

FIGURE 12.19
TEE short-axis view at 1 month follow-up. Note the fistula between the aorta and the right atrium (arrow points toward the fistula).

CASE ANALYSIS

In this case, we believe that oversizing of the Amplatzer device (26 mm) in the presence of aortic rim deficiency caused the aortic root perforation and the aorto-atrial fistula. In this case, a 22- or 24-mm device would have worked well. However, because of aortic rim deficiency, a larger device was chosen. Anatomically, the aortic root is wedged between the mitral and the tricuspid valves, and the ascending aorta is in close proximity to the ASD edge.

LESSONS

- Avoid oversizing the device beyond the stop-flow diameter of the ASD defect.
- Patients who have aortic rim deficiency in multiple views are at higher risk for developing cardiac trauma.

SUGGESTED READING

Amin Z. Transcatheter closure of secundum atrial septal defects. *Cathet Cardiovasc Interv.* 2006;68:778–787.

References

1. St. Jude Medical. http://www.amplatzer.com/products/.
2. www.goremedical.com/resources/dam/assets/AN1014EN1.HLX.NEWSLETTERFall09.FNL.MR.singles.pdf.
3. http://www.snl.com/irweblinkx/FinancialDocs.aspx?iid=4148066.
4. Khairy P, O'Donnell CP, Landzberg MJ. Transcatheter closure versus medical therapy of patent foramen ovale and presumed paradoxical thromboemboli: A systematic review. *Ann Intern Med.* 2003;139:753–760.
5. Chessa M, Carminati M, Butera G, et al. Early and late complications associated with transcatheter occlusion of secundum atrial septal defect. *J Am Coll Cardiol.* 2002;39:1061–1065.
6. Schwerzmann M, Salehian O. Hazards of percutaneous PFO closure. *Eur J Echocardiogr.* 2005;6(6):393–395.
7. Levi DS, Moore JW. Embolization and retrieval of the Amplatzer septal occluder. *Catheter Cardiovasc Interv.* 2004;61(4):543–547.
8. Jones TK, Latson LA, Zahn E, et al. Results of the U.S. multicenter pivotal study of the HELEX septal occluder for percutaneous closure of secundum atrial septal defects. *J Am Coll Cardiol.* 2007 Jun 5;49(22):2215–2221.
9. Carminati M, Giusti S, Hausdorf G, et al. A European multicentric experience using the CardioSEAL and Starflex double umbrella devices to close interatrial communications holes within the oval fossa. *Cardiol Young.* 2000;10(5):519–526.
10. Fischer G, Stieh J, Uebing A, Hoffmann U, Morf G, Kramer HH. Experience with transcatheter closure of secundum atrial septal defects using the Amplatzer septal occluder: A single centre study in 236 consecutive patients. *Heart.* 2003;89(2):199–204.
11. Wahl A, Praz F, Stinimann J, Windecker S, et al. Safety and feasibility of percutaneous closure of patent foramen ovale without intra-procedural echocardiography in 825 patients. *Swiss Med Wkly.* 2008;138(39–40):567–572.
12. Krumsdorf U, Ostermayer S, Billinger K, et al. Incidence and clinical course of thrombus formation on atrial septal defect and patient foramen ovale closure devices in 1,000 consecutive patients. *J Am Coll Cardiol.* 2004;43(2):302–309.
13. Verma and Tobis. Surgical explantation of PFO devices. Unpublished data.
14. Amin Z, Hijazi ZM, Bass JL, Cheatham JP, Hellenbrand WE, Kleinman CS.. Erosion of Amplatzer septal occluder device after closure of secundum atrial septal defects: Review of registry of complications and recommendations to minimize future risk. *Catheter Cardiovasc Interv.* 2004;63(4):496–502.
15. Amin Z, Hijazi ZM, Bass JL, Cheatham JP, Hellenbrand W, Kleinman CS. PFO closure complications from the AGA registry. *Catheter Cardiovasc Interv.* 2008;72(1):74–79.
16. Motreff P, Dauphin C, Souteyrand G. Cardiac perforation and tamponade 3 months after transcatheter PFO closure by STARFlex device: A case report. *Catheter Cardiovasc Interv.* 2008;71(3):412–416.

13 *Damien Kenny, Thomas J. Forbes, and Zahid Amin*

Complications of Ventricular Septal Defect Closure

INTRODUCTION

Transcatheter ventricular septal defect (VSD) closure was first described in 1987 (1), and since then, thousands of defects have been closed worldwide using different devices (2–6). Initial reports described closure of muscular VSDs, and the majority of the experience is based upon muscular VSD closure. About 80% of defects are present in the perimembranous region of the intraventricular septum. The juxtaposed nature of the perimembranous VSD to the aortic, mitral, and tricuspid valves precluded placement of muscular devices in this location. Thus, new devices were developed to assist closure with consideration to the surrounding anatomic structures, the aortic valve in particular (7,8). Complete heart block, however, has plagued this approach (9,10). As the hemodynamic impact of clinically significant VSDs may affect both pulmonary vascular resistance and the size and function of the left ventricle, closure of these defects is advised in childhood, and therefore most reports include this age group. There have been a number of reports of transcatheter closure of VSDs in the adult population, with indications that include symptoms with progressive left ventricular dilatation, residual postoperative and iatrogenic VSDs, and previous endocarditis (11,12). Reported experience with transcatheter VSD closure in adults has also occurred in the setting of postinfarct VSDs with mixed results (13,14). The general approach to VSD closure is independent of age and etiology and involves creation of an arteriovenous wire loop (wire from femoral artery through the VSD and femoral vein) to guide device delivery, venovenous (wire femoral vein through the atrial septum, mitral valve, and VSD) wire loop, or direct left ventricular approach (closure from the left ventricle side). Reported complications relate predominantly to device malposition or embolization and impingement of the device on surrounding structures, including the conduction tissue as described above and the aortic valve in the setting of perimembranous VSDs (15). Variable significant complication rates have been reported, ranging from 6.5% in a large European registry (3) to 10.7% in the US registry, including device embolization, cardiac perforation, stroke, and two deaths (8).

This chapter deals with the potential procedural complications of

- Device embolization
- Complete heart block

The cases will highlight each of the above complications. Other arrhythmic complications although seen with this procedure are not specific to it, and therefore not discussed. Hemolysis has been reported with residual leak, although this is uncommon.

DEVICE EMBOLIZATION

Although a number of devices have been reported in transcatheter closure of VSDs, the Amplatzer (St. Jude Medical, Plymouth, MN) family of devices is by far the most commonly used. The incidence of device embolization may be related to the operator's experience, but overall the rates are low (1.2% in the large European registry) (3). This may also be related to a tendency toward device oversizing to reduce the likelihood of embolization. This strategy may not be an issue with muscular defects, but this approach has been implicated in the incidence of complete heart block following transcatheter closure of perimembranous defects and thus should be avoided. Recommendations exist for proper sizing of devices (16) and when possible should be followed to minimize either under sizing or oversizing. Intraprocedural echocardiographic imaging is vital in this process. Devices may embolize to either the venous or arterial circulation, and location of the device may guide whether retrieval should be attempted by transcatheter or surgical routes. In general if the device in entangled within the chordae of either atrioventricular valve, surgical removal may be preferable (17). If transcatheter retrieval is attempted, it is vital to ensure that the catheterization laboratory is stocked with appropriate large diameter sheaths and snares before embarking on the procedure.

Embolization may be seen more commonly with postinfarct VSDs (up to 14%) (14) when the defect is often lacunar in shape and therefore difficult to size accurately. This may be compounded by the presence of seminecrotic tissue surrounding the defect that may not provide adequate support for the rims of the device.

COMPLETE HEART BLOCK

The reported incidence of complete heart block with transcatheter closure of perimembranous VSDs using the Amplatzer (St. Jude Medical, Plymouth, MN) membranous device has been quite variable. Larger series describe rates of complete heart block of 5%; (3,18) however, some centers have reported rates of up to 22% citing higher occluder-to-VSD size ratios as a particular risk factor (19). Sizing of defects is a particular problem, as a great heterogeneity exists with regard to defect morphology and variation in measurements between color Doppler, and 2D imaging during transesophageal echocardiography (TEE) may lead to choice of the largest recorded measurement. To counteract this, a larger range of membranous occluder sizes in 1-mm increments and new sizing recommendations have been introduced. Recovery of atrioventricular block has been reported with early treatment with steroid (20) or early surgical removal of the membranous occluder (21); Comparable rates of complete heart block following surgical closure have been reported at less than 1% (22). Unlike postsurgical patients, the timing of presentation of heart block with transcatheter closure is difficult to predict, and such uncontrolled presentation leading to syncope and potential death may be a concern for both patient and physician. Alternative approaches have been reported. The Amplatzer muscular VSD occluder has been used for perimembranous VSDs when distance of the defect to the aortic valve was >4 mm or in those with associated aneurysmal tissue surrounding the defect (16,23). This approach in theory may either reduce the continued mechanical motion of the asymmetric nitinol occluder exerting pressure on the conducting system or indeed avoid it altogether when positioned within the aneurysm away from both the conduction tissue and the aortic valve. Newer devices are being tested to avoid these issues. Phase II trials of transcatheter perimembranous VSD closure with the Amplatzer membranous occluder are on hold in the United States.

CASE 13.1

Device Embolization

CLINICAL HISTORY AND DIAGNOSTIC TESTING RESULTS

A 73-year-old man presented with chest pain and an EKG finding consistent with ST-elevated myocardial infarction (STEMI). He had significant initial hemodynamic compromise and required continuous inotrope infusion and intra-aortic balloon pump to support ventricular function. There was some improvement in his clinical condition after 72 hours; however, he deteriorated again the following day, and clinical examination was consistent with that of VSD. Transesophageal echocardiogram confirmed the presence of inferior ventricular septal rupture with significant left-to-right shunting. Surgery was not a consideration due to the degree of ventricular dysfunction, and hence the patient was managed conservatively for a few days. He was subsequently discussed with the interventional cardiologists for consideration of transcatheter postinfarct VSD closure.

PLANNED PROCEDURE

Postinfarct VSD closure.

PROCEDURE

The procedure was performed in a dedicated biplane cardiac catheterization laboratory. The right internal jugular vein and femoral artery were accessed with 7-Fr and 5-Fr short sheaths, respectively. Following diagnostic catheterization, left ventriculogram confirmed the presence of a large inferior VSD. VSD was confirmed on TEE, and it measured 20 mm on largest color flow Doppler image. The VSD was crossed from the left ventricle using a diagnostic right Judkins catheter and Glidewire (Terumo, Japan), which was advanced into the superior vena cava. The wire was snared using an Amplatzer Gooseneck snare (Microvena Corporation, White Bear Lake, MN) and exteriorized out of the right internal jugular vein, establishing an arterial-venous circuit. A 10-Fr delivery sheath was advanced through the jugular vein into the left ventricle. The 24-mm Amplatzer postinfarct VSD device was prepped and advanced through the delivery sheath across the septal rupture into the left ventricle. The device was pushed partially out of its catheter sheath until release of the first disc. The delivery catheter was drawn back into the right ventricle until the left-sided disc was positioned against the left ventricular septum. Finally, the right-sided disc was released, covering the VSD from the right side. Angiography following release demonstrated some residual shunting (Figure 13.1). The patient remained hemodynamically stable and was extubated following the procedure.

COMPLICATION AND MANAGEMENT

The following day, the patient became hypotensive, and chest x-ray (CXR) revealed the device had embolized to the right pulmonary artery. The patient was taken back to the catheterization laboratory, and the position of the device in the right pulmonary artery was confirmed (Figure 13.2). The right femoral vein was accessed and the VSD device was snared with a 25-mm Amplatzer Gooseneck snare (Figure 13.3) and pulled into the main pulmonary artery, where it was retracted into a 14-Fr Mullins sheath and exteriorized through the femoral vein. The patient recovered from this procedure. Two days later, he underwent a second attempt at VSD closure with a similar approach to that described above. He made significant progress over the following 72 hours but became acutely ill and died two days later of presumed sepsis with the device still in place.

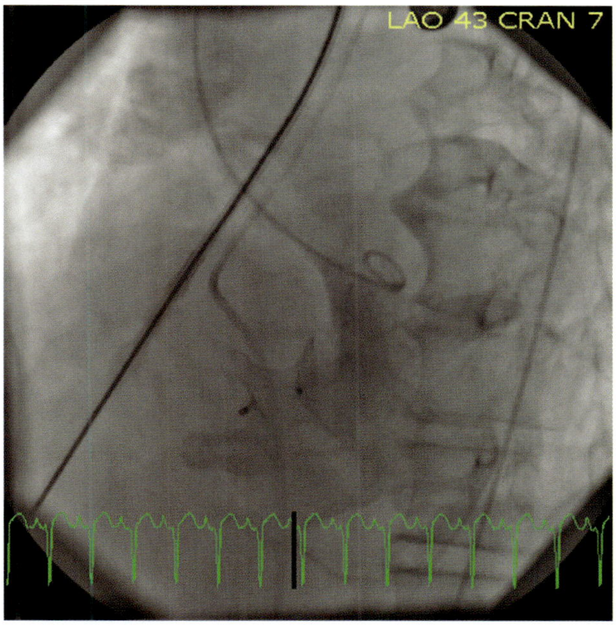

FIGURE 13.1
Left ventricular angiogram following initial device release.

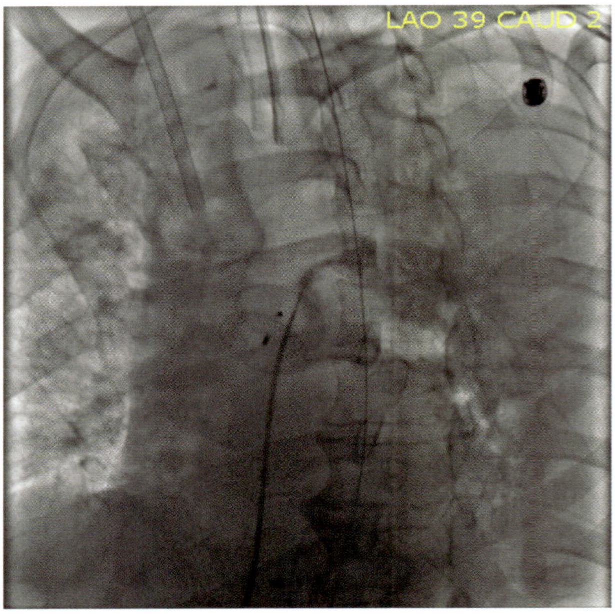

FIGURE 13.2
Device embolization to the right pulmonary artery.

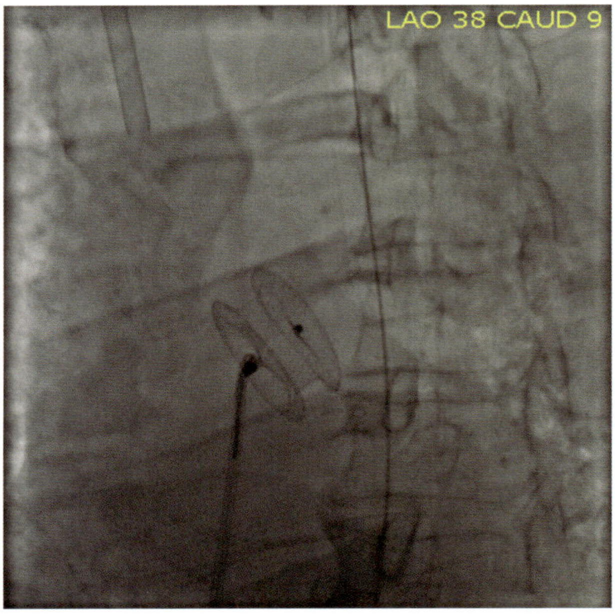

FIGURE 13.3
Snaring of embolized device in the right pulmonary artery.

CASE ANALYSIS

Ventricular septal rupture in the setting of myocardial infarction is uncommon; however death is the usual outcome without intervention (24). Until recently, surgical closure has been the mainstay of treatment. Mortality remains high at over 50% in some series. Technical success with transcatheter closure of congenital VSDs allowed adaptation of the technique for postinfarct VSDs with a device designed specifically for this indication, although other devices, including Amplatzer atrial septal occluders, have been used with success. Complication rates are high and include left ventricular rupture and device embolization rates up to 20%. (14). Device embolization and significant residual shunts are a reflection of the difficulty in defining the morphology and margins of these VSDs surrounded by partially necrotic myocardium. The necrotic tissue secedes for up to 3 weeks after the infarction, and hence it is difficult to predict the actual size of the defect when closing these defects in the first week. Some centers have used more advanced forms of imaging, such as MRI (or CT if intra-aortic balloon pump is in place) to assess the size, shape, and the viability of the surrounding tissues of these defects prior to attempted transcatheter closure. These forms of imaging suggest that postinfarction ventricular septal defects (PIVSDs) are often crescent in shape, and thus TEE imaging may underestimate the true defect size.

LESSONS

- A larger device (Amplatzer Atrial Septal Occluder) may have been more appropriate in this case; however, device stability was achieved with a 24-mm PIVSD device 2 days following the embolization.
- Case selection and significant device oversizing are of paramount importance in these cases to avoid multiple interventions. Advanced preprocedural imaging may be useful in achieving this and assessing the dimensions of the future size of the defect.
- When retrieving devices, it is essential to have the appropriate equipment available, including snare catheters and a variety of long sheaths. In general for device retrieval, it is prudent to choose a sheath size at least 2-Fr to 4-Fr larger than the recommended delivery size for the device.

SUGGESTED READING

Amin Z, Cao QL, Hijazi ZM. Closure of muscular ventricular septal defects: Transcatheter and hybrid techniques. *Catheter Cardiovasc Interv.* 2008;72:102–111.

Kim MS, Klein AJ, Carroll JD. Transcatheter closure of intracardiac defects in adults. *J Interv Cardiol.* 2007;20:524–545.

Thiele H, Kaulfersch C, Daehnert I et al. Immediate primary transcatheter closure of postinfarction ventricular septal defects. *Eur Heart J.* 2009;30:81–88.

CASE 13.2

Complete Heart Block

CLINICAL HISTORY AND DIAGNOSTIC TESTING RESULTS

An adolescent male with trisomy 21 was under ongoing follow-up for a restrictive perimembranous VSD. Although asymptomatic, serial transthoracic echocardiograms demonstrated increasing indexed left-ventricular end-diastolic dimensions suggestive of a significant left-to-right shunt, and hence a decision was made to attempt transcatheter closure of the defect. Preprocedural electrocardiogram demonstrated sinus rhythm with normal PR interval (Figure 13.4), and preprocedural transthoracic echocardiogram (TTE) suggested there was a 3-mm subaortic rim to the defect.

PLANNED PROCEDURE

Closure of perimembranous VSD.

PROCEDURE

The procedure was performed in a biplane catheterization laboratory under general anesthesia with TEE guidance. The defect measured 5 mm on short axis view with color Doppler. Initial diagnostic catheterization revealed a pulmonary-to-systemic shunt of 1.9:1, with mildly elevated mean pulmonary arterial pressures. Left ventricular angiography demonstrated a perimembranous defect with mild left ventricular dilatation (Figure 13.5a). Creation of an arteriovenous loop with a guidewire was achieved as described above. The wire was exteriorized on the venous side through the right femoral vein. An 8-mm Amplatzer membranous occluder was advanced through a 7-Fr delivery sheath, and the left disc was deployed on the left ventricular aspect of the defect. Proper alignment of the device was confirmed, and the left disc was pulled to approximate the ventricular septum. The right disc was then deployed (Figure 13.5b). The device was released (Figure 13.5c), and repeat left ventricular angiogram demonstrated complete occlusion of the defect (Figure 13.5d). The patient recovered well from the procedure, and EKG the following day demonstrated sinus rhythm (Figure 13.6) with the device maintaining a good position on TTE.

COMPLICATION AND MANAGEMENT

Four days following the procedure, the patient presented with an episode of syncope and Holter monitoring demonstrated episodes of complete heart block with little or no escape rhythm (Figure 13.7).

The patient was started on high dose oral steroids due to evidence that this approach may reduce the inflammatory effect of the device on the conduction tissue (10). However with no escape rhythm, this was only seen as a temporary measure until the patient was discussed with the surgeons and taken to the operating room for removal of the device and surgical closure of the defect. External pacing wires were fitted as the patient was in sinus rhythm at the end of cardiopulmonary bypass and removed on day 5 postoperatively as there were no further episodes of complete heart block. Transvenous pacemaker was not considered following the initial presentation due to the long-term complications of chronic pacing in patients of this age.

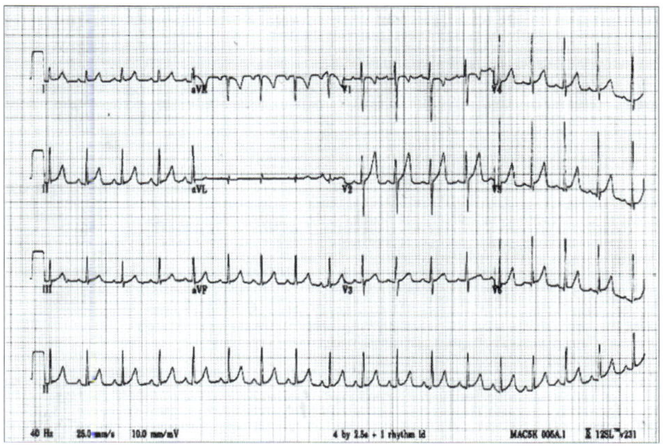

FIGURE 13.4
Electrocardiogram prior to perimembranous VSD closure.

CASE ANALYSIS

Device oversizing may be implicated in the development of postprocedural complete heart block in this patient. At the time of the procedure, devices were only available in 2-mm size increments, and there were concerns regarding device embolization with the use of a 6-mm device in a defect measuring 5 mm; hence an 8-mm device was used. The radial force exerted by this device on the conduction tissue may have lead to mechanical trauma and swelling of the conduction system, which recovered with surgical removal of the device as previously reported. The patient had trisomy 21, and defects in this setting are more prone to develop complete heart block because the course of conduction tissue may be different.

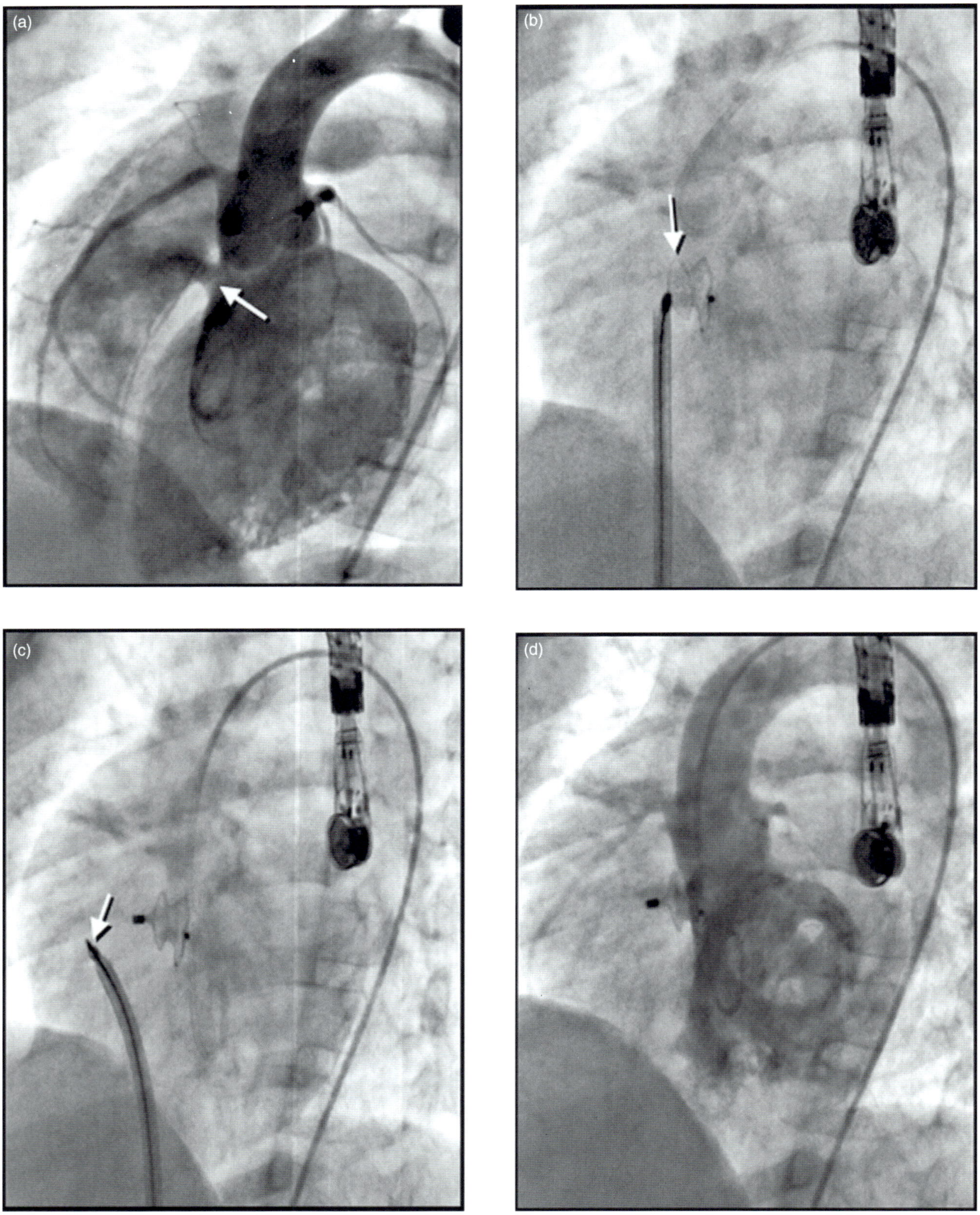

FIGURE 13.5
(a–d) Series of images demonstrating the stages of VSD closure with the membranous occluder.

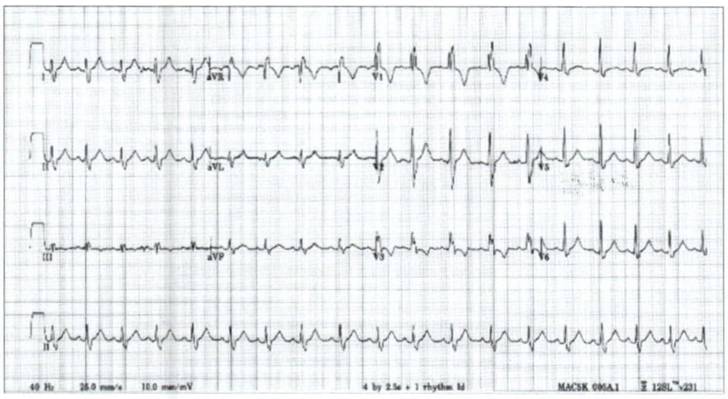

FIGURE 13.6
Electrocardiogram following the procedure, demonstrating interventricular conduction delay but no evidence of complete heart block.

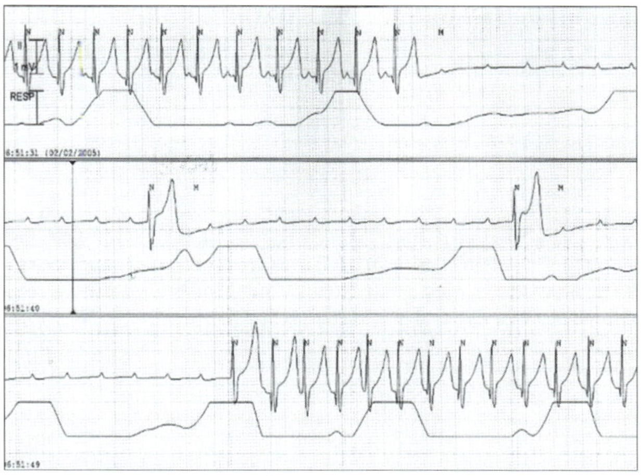

FIGURE 13.7
Holter monitor recording demonstrating periods of complete heart block with, for the most part, no ventricular escape rhythm.

Proper AMPLATZER Membranous VSD Device Size Selection
During end diastole, Orthogonal measurements of the ventricular septal defect should be obtained on the left and right ventricular aspects of the defect, and the major and minor axes of the elliptical defect recorded.

- The smaller of the two elliptical areas (LV vs. RV aspect) should be chosen.
- Use the formula below and the smaller of the two elliptical areas (LV vs. RV aspect) to determine the size of the device.

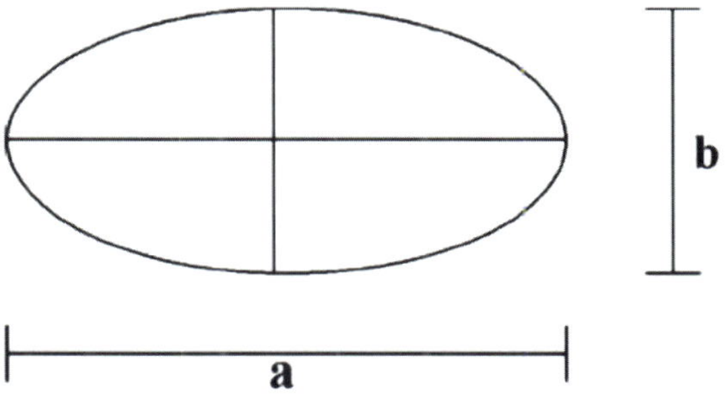

D (Diameter of Device) = $\sqrt{a \times b}$
(D = diameter of device; a = major axis of VSD ellipse; b= minor axis of VSD ellipse)

For example, if a = 8 and b = 4, device size should equal $\sqrt{32}$ = 5.7. Therefore a 6 mm device would be selected (rounded up to nearest millimeter size).

FIGURE 13.8
New sizing recommendations from Amplatzer using the membranous occluder.

LESSONS

- Device oversizing is a significant risk factor for complete heart block when using the Amplatzer membranous occluder for transcatheter perimembranous VSD closure.
- This approach is no longer approved in the United States with currently available devices; however, new sizing recommendations exist from Amplatzer (Figure 13.8) and using these recommendations a 6-mm device would have been more appropriate.

SUGGESTED READING

Kenny D, Morgan G, Bajwa A, et al. Evolution of transcatheter closure of perimembranous ventricular septal defects in a single centre. *Catheter Cardiovasc Interv.* 2009;73:568–575.

Yip WC, Zimmerman F, Hijazi ZM. Heart block and empirical therapy after transcatheter closure of perimembranous ventricular septal defect. *Catheter Cardiovasc Interv.* 2005;66:436–441.

References

1. Lock JE, Block PC, McKay RG, et al. Transcatheter closure of ventricular septal defects. *Circulation.* 1988;78:361–368.
2. Bridges ND, Perry SB, Keane JF, et al. Preoperative transcatheter closure of congenital muscular ventricular septal defects. *N Engl J Med.* 1991;324:1312–1317.
3. Carminati M, Butera G, Chessa M, et al; Investigators of the European VSD Registry. Transcatheter closure of congenital ventricular septal defects: Results of the European Registry. *Eur Heart J.* 2007;28:2361–2368.
4. Rigby ML, Redington AN. Primary transcatheter umbrella closure of perimembranous ventricular septal defect. *Br Heart J.* 1994;72:368–371.
5. Sideris EB, Walsh KP, Haddad JL, et al. Occlusion of congenital ventricular septal defects by the buttoned device. "Buttoned device" Clinical Trials International Register. *Heart.* 1997;77:276–279.
6. Lim DS, Forbes TJ, Rothman A, Lock JE, Landzberg MJ Transcatheter closure of high-risk muscular ventricular septal defects with the CardioSEAL occluder: Initial report from the CardioSEAL VSD registry. *Catheter Cardiovasc Interv.* 2007;70:740–744.
7. Hijazi ZM, Hakim F, Haweleh AA, et al. Catheter closure of perimembranous ventricular septal defects using the new Amplatzer membranous VSD occluder: Initial clinical experience. *Catheter Cardiovasc Interv.* 2002;56:508–515.
8. Fu YC, Bass J, Amin Z, et al. Transcatheter closure of perimembranous ventricular septal defects using the new Amplatzer membranous VSD occluder: Results of the U.S. phase I trial. *J Am Coll Cardiol.* 2006;47:319–325.
9. Yip WC, Zimmerman F, Hijazi ZM. Heart block and empirical therapy after transcatheter closure of perimembranous ventricular septal defect. *Catheter Cardiovasc Interv.* 2005;66:436–441.
10. Walsh MA, Bialkowski J, Szkutnik M, et al. Atrioventricular block after transcatheter closure of perimembranous ventricular septal defects. *Heart.* 2006;92:1295–1297.
11. Chessa M, Butera G, Negura D, et al. Transcatheter closure of congenital ventricular septal defects in adult: Mid-term results and complications. *Int J Cardiol.* 2009;133:70–73.
12. Al-Kashkari W, Balan P, Kavinsky CJ, et al. Percutaneous device closure of congenital and iatrogenic ventricular septal defects in adult patients [published online ahead of print September 17,2010]. *Catheter Cardiovasc Interv.*
13. Holzer R, Balzer D, Amin Z, et al. Transcatheter closure of postinfarction ventricular septal defects using the new Amplatzer muscular VSD occluder: Results of a U.S. Registry. *Catheter Cardiovasc Interv.* 2004;61:196–201.
14. Thiele H, Kaulfersch C, Daehnert I, et al. Immediate primary transcatheter closure of postinfarction ventricular septal defects. *Eur Heart J.* 2009;30:81–88.
15. Kenny D, Tometzki A, Martin R. Significant aortic regurgitation associated with transcatheter closure of perimembranous ventricular septal defects with a deficient aortic rim. *Catheter Cardiovasc Interv.* 2007;70:445–449.
16. Kenny D, Morgan G, Bajwa A, et al. Evolution of transcatheter closure of perimembranous ventricular septal defects in a single centre. *Catheter Cardiovasc Interv.* 2009;73:568–575.
17. Amin Z, Cao QL, Hijazi ZM. Closure of muscular ventricular septal defects: Transcatheter and hybrid techniques. *Catheter Cardiovasc Interv.* 2008;72:102–111.
18. Butera G, Carminati M, Chessa M, et al. Transcatheter closure of perimembranous ventricular septal defects: Early and long-term results. *J Am Coll Cardiol.* 2007;50:1189–1195.
19. Predescu D, Chaturvedi RR, Benson LN, et al. Occluder closure of hemodynamically significant perimembranous ventricular septal defects. *Catheter Cardiovasc Interv.* 2007;70:S6-S7.
20. Walsh MA, Bialkowski J, Szkutnik M, et al. Atrioventricular block after transcatheter closure of perimembranous ventricular septal defects. *Heart.* 2006;92:1295–1297.
21. Ovaert C, Dragulescu A, Sluysmans T, et al. Early surgical removal of membranous ventricular septal occluder might allow recovery of atrioventricular block. *Pediatr Cardiol.* 2008;29:971–975.
22. Tucker EM, Pyles LA, Bass JL, Moller JH. Permanent pacemaker for atrioventricular conduction block after operative repair of perimembranous ventricular septal defect. *J Am Coll Cardiol.* 2007;50:1196–2000.
23. Szkutnik M, Qureshi SA, Kusa J, et al. Use of the Amplatzer muscular ventricular septal defect occluder for closure of perimembranous ventricular septal defects. *Heart.* 2007;93:355–358.
24. Menon V, Webb JG, Hills LD, et al. Outcome and profile of ventricular septal rupture with cardiogenic shock after myocardial infarction: A report from the SHOCK Trial Registry. Should we emergently revascularize occluded coronaries in cardiogenic shock? *J Am Coll Cardiol.* 2000;36:1110–1116.

14

Damien Kenny and Zahid Amin

Complications of Patent Arterial Duct Closure

INTRODUCTION

Transcatheter occlusion of a patent arterial duct (PDA) was first described by Porstmann in 1967 (1). Since then, a variety of devices have been designed for PDA closure, with mixed results (2–13). The majority of these reports have focused on closure within the pediatric population; closure experience specific to the adult population is on the rise (14–18). The complication rate following PDA closure remains very low. There are some reports that indicate closure-related issues specific to the adult population, including larger defects (15), calcification of the arterial duct (16), and pulmonary hypertension (18). Change in the orientation of the arterial duct with age may lead to a more horizontal entry into the pulmonary artery, and this may have implications for transcatheter approach and closure. Despite these issues, closure rates are high, with low procedure-related morbidity even in adult population. The most widely reported device for PDA closure is the Amplatzer ductal occluder (St. Jude Medical, Plymouth, MN). Amplatzer muscular and atrial septal occluders have been used in larger defects, particularly those with pulmonary artery hypertension, as the symmetrical disc design may limit the risk of embolization to the aorta (18,19). Other reported complications in the adult population include hemolysis, but luckily the incidence of this complication in adults is very low. Hemolysis was encountered more commonly with older devices, such as the Rashkind occluder (15,16), or with the use of coils (14) and is not seen as frequently with newer device design. If hemolysis does occur, it is usually possible to deploy another device to abolish the residual shunt and hence the mechanical effect of the device on red blood cell breakup, although in some cases, surgery has been required. Some issues relating to closure in the pediatric population, particularly left pulmonary artery stenosis and pseudocoarctation of the aorta due to device protrusion into the aorta, are usually not relevant to the adult population.

In this chapter, we will highlight device embolization. Other procedural complications as mentioned above will not be discussed further.

DEVICE EMBOLIZATION

With such a variety of devices reported in the literature, detailed review of risk of embolization with each device is beyond the scope of this chapter. The only currently approved device in the United States for transcatheter closure of PDA is the Amplatzer ductal occluder. Coils and other devices, such as the Amplatzer vascular plug, are also currently used. Coil occlusion in adult patients, although reported (14), is not common, and residual shunting with risk of hemolysis is an issue. Ductal closure with the Amplatzer occluder was evaluated in a large multicentre U.S. trial, which included adult patients (20). There were two device embolizations reported from a total of 439 cases. One of these devices embolized to the pulmonary artery was retrieved surgically with ductal ligation. This approach was chosen due to the large size of the ductus in a small patient and the possibility of further embolization with further transcatheter device deployment. The second device embolized to the descending aorta was retrieved with a snare catheter without complication. Sizing recommendations for this device state that the pulmonary end of the device used should be 2 mm larger than the minimum measured diameter of the PDA. Care must be taken in evaluating PDA size, as ductal spasm may occur with angiography and an erroneously small ductal measurement may increase the risk of embolization. Significant pulmonary hypertension may increase the risk of embolization to the aorta with this device, and other more symmetrical devices may be more appropriate in this setting. Balloon occlusion may be warranted in this setting to temporarily assess the effect of closure on the pulmonary artery resistance. The Amplatzer Ductal Occluder II is currently under Food and Drug Administration–approved trials in the United States but is available outside of the United States for ductal closure and has a more symmetrical design. It is a much softer device and may not be appropriate for patients with pulmonary hypertension. It does offer the potential for retrograde closure from the arterial side, making it an attractive option for smaller babies. Arterial deployment of the device is not recommended with the currently regular Amplatzer ductal occluder device. Embolization rates with this device are difficult to estimate as most studies to date have reported only small numbers.

CASE 14.1

Device Embolization and Ductal Spasm

CLINICAL HISTORY AND DIAGNOSTIC TESTING RESULTS

A child was referred for assessment of recurrent respiratory infections and heart murmur. Clinical examination revealed full peripheral pulse volume with a continuous murmur in the left infraclavicular region. Transthoracic echocardiogram (TTE) confirmed the presence of a moderate to large arterial duct with left heart dilatation and hyperdynamic left ventricular performance.

PLANNED PROCEDURE

Transcatheter PDA closure.

PROCEDURE

The procedure was performed in a biplane cardiac catheterization laboratory under general anesthesia. The right femoral artery and right femoral vein were accessed with 4-Fr and 5-Fr short sheaths, respectively. Diagnostic right heart catheterization was performed to delineate the size and morphology of the arterial duct so as not to precipitate potential ductal spasm with a catheter in the pulmonary arteries. The aortogram demonstrated a very small PDA (Figure 14.1a), which was inconsistent with the previous clinical and echocardiographic findings. Based on the cardiac catheterization measurements, a 5/4-mm Amplatzer ductal occluder was prepared and advanced via an anterograde approach from the right femoral vein through a 6-Fr-long delivery sheath, which was advanced into the descending aorta over a standard 0.035-inch wire. The device was deployed in a good position, and follow-up angiogram demonstrated minimal residual shunting through the device, and hence the device was released. The patient recovered well and had an uneventful postprocedural course.

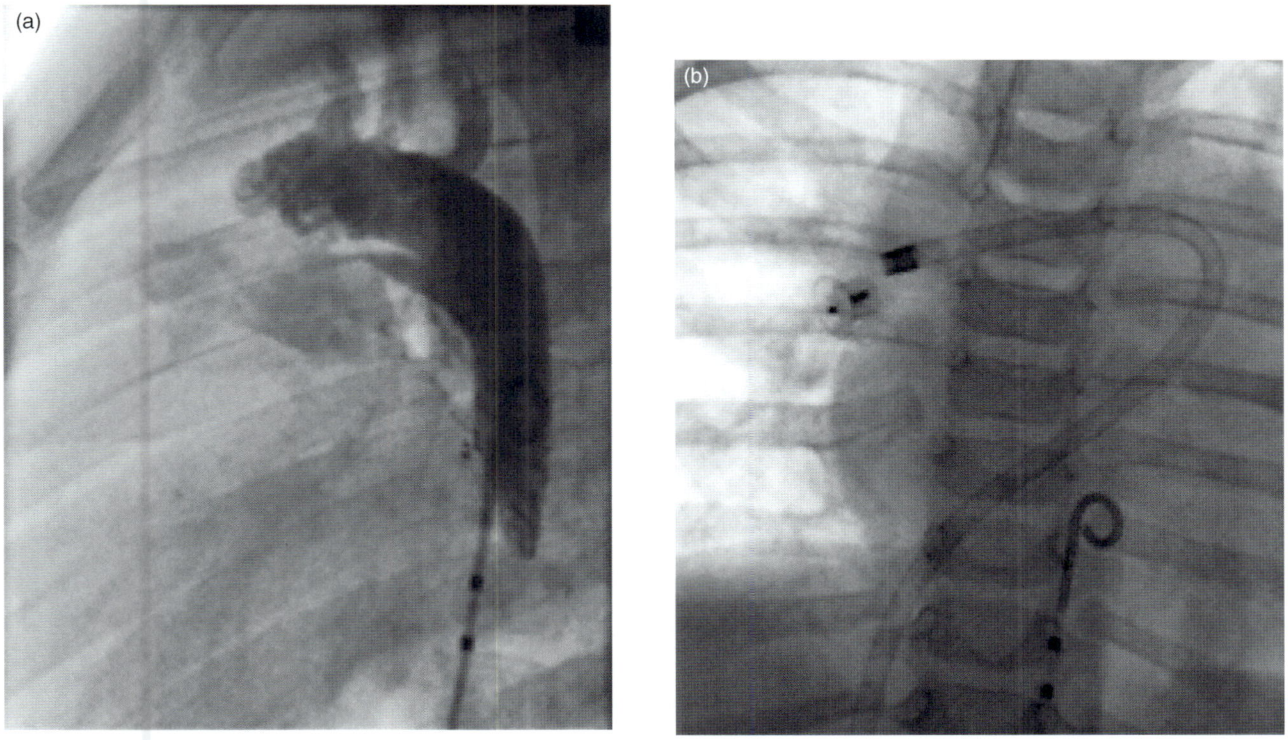

FIGURE 14.1 a–b

(a) Initial descending aortic angiogram in the lateral plane demonstrating small arterial duct with significant restriction at the pulmonary end. (b) Fluororscopic image of the embolized Amplatzer ductal occluder and the long retrieval sheath in the right pulmonary artery.

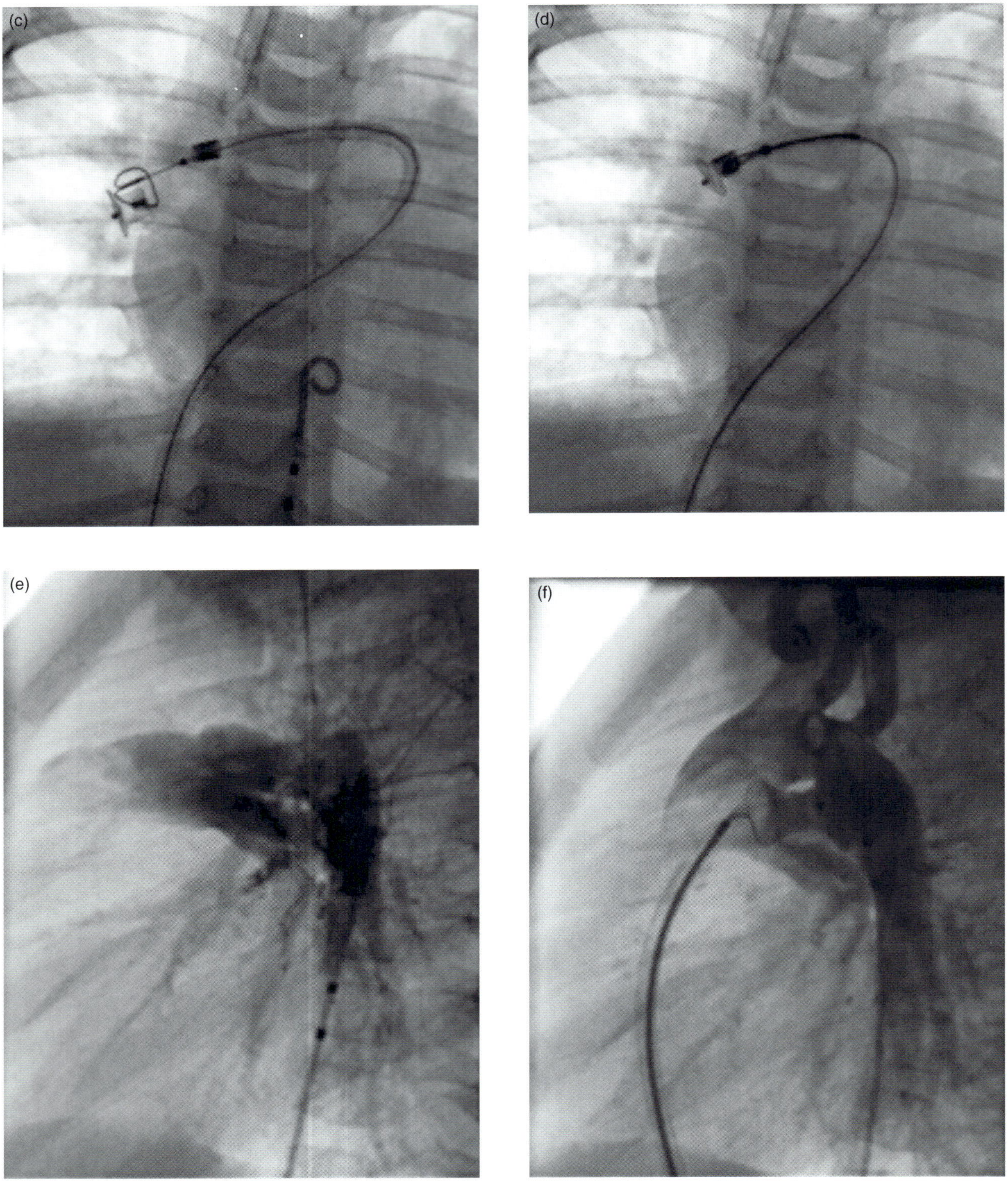

FIGURE 14.1 c–f

(c) Advancement of the snare catheter through the long sheath to grasp the embolized device. (d) Retrieval of the device into the long sheath within the right pulmonary artery. (e) Subsequent descending aortic angiogram demonstrating large tubular arterial duct. (f) Aortogram following closure of the PDA with a larger Amplatzer ductal occluder.

COMPLICATION AND MANAGEMENT

The following morning, clinical examination revealed a loud continuous murmur, and TTE revealed the presence of a large PDA. Chest x-ray confirmed the embolization of the device to the right pulmonary artery.

The patient was brought back to the catheter laboratory for retrieval of the device. An 8-Fr sheath was placed in the right femoral vein. A balloon wedge catheter was advanced into the pulmonary artery. This catheter was removed over an exchange length wire. The short sheath was removed, and an 8-Fr-long sheath was advanced from the left femoral vein into the right pulmonary artery (Figure 14.1b). The device was snared with a 10-mm gooseneck snare and pulled into the large delivery sheath (Figures 14.1c and 14.1d). The device was removed through the sheath without difficulty. Subsequent descending aortogram with a 4-Fr pigtail catheter in the left femoral artery demonstrated a large tubular PDA measuring 6 mm at its narrowest point (Figure 14.1e). Thus a 10/8 Amplatzer ductal occluder was prepared and again advanced through the long sheath in place from the venous side across the arterial duct. The device maintained a stable position following deployment, and aortogram demonstrated negligible residual shunt through the defect prior to release (Figure 14.1f). The device was released following assessment of the pressure gradient across the aortic arch to ensure the device was not causing a pseudocoarctation of the aorta. The patient recovered well, and TTE the following day demonstrated the device in a good position with no residual shunt and no significant obstruction of the left pulmonary artery.

CASE ANALYSIS

Despite attempts to minimize the potential for ductal spasm, the discrepancy in the size of the PDA between the original and follow-up angiograms indicate that ductal spasm had occurred following the first angiogram, and this led to placement of an undersized device with subsequent embolization. Although the initial clinical examination and echocardiogram was more consistent with a larger defect, it is possible for the arterial duct to spasm significantly during the cardiac catheterization procedure. Device retrieval was relatively straightforward with appropriate equipment, and a long sheath, at least 2-Fr larger than the original delivery sheath, is advised. It is always worth assessing the impact of larger devices on both the descending aorta and the left pulmonary artery to ensure relative narrowing of these vessels is not present secondary to device protrusion.

LESSONS

- Beware of ductal spasm, particularly when there is a discrepancy in the angiographic and preprocedural clinical and imaging data. If concerns exist, it may be more prudent to repeat angiography after at least 15 to 20 minutes.
- While advancing pigtail catheter in the descending aorta over the wire, care should be taken to avoid wire advancement into the PDA.
- Right heart catheterization should be delayed until after aortic angiography has been performed.
- Postprocedural review and imaging is essential in these patients to evaluate device position prior to discharge.
- Device retrieval is achievable via the transcatheter route in majority of cases; however, a full range of equipment is necessary to facilitate this.

SUGGESTED READING

Jang GY, Son CS, Lee JW, et al. Complications after transcatheter closure of patent ductus arteriosus. *J Korean Med Sci.* 2007;22:484–490.

Pass RH, Hijazi Z, Hsu DT, et al. Multicenter USA Amplatzer patent ductus arteriosus occlusion device trial: Initial and one-year results. *J Am Coll Cardiol.* 2004;44:513–519.

Yan C, Zhao S, Jiang S, et al. Transcatheter closure of patent ductus arteriosus with severe pulmonary arterial hypertension in adults. *Heart.* 2007;93:514–518.

References

1. Porstmann W, Wierny L, Warneke H. Closure of the persistent ductus arteriosus without thoracotomy. *Ger Med Mon.* 1967;12:259–261.
2. Rashkind WJ, Mullins CE, Helenbrand WE, et al. Nonsurgical closure of patent ductus arteriosus: Clinical application of the Rashkind PDA occluder system. *Circulation.* 1987;75:583–592.
3. Rao PS, Sideris EB, Haddad J, et al. Transcatheter occlusion of patent ductus arteriosus with adjustable buttoned device: Initial clinical experience. *Circulation.* 1993;88:1119–1126.
4. Verin VE, Saveliev VS, Kolody SM, et al. Results of transcatheter closure of the patent ductus arteriosus with the Botalloocluder. *J Am Coll Cardiol.* 1993;22:1509–1514.
5. Moore JW, George L, Kirkpatrick SE, et al. Percutaneous closure of the small patent ductus arteriosus using occluding spring coils. *J Am Coll Cardiol.* 1994;23:759–765.
6. Hijazi ZM, Geggel RL. Results of anterograde transcatheter closure of patent ductus arteriosus using single or multiple Gianturco coils. *J Am Coll Cardiol.* 1994;74:925–929.
7. Tometzki AJ, Arnold R, Peart I, et al. Transcatheter occlusion of the patent ductus arteriosus with Cook detachable coils. *Heart.* 1996;76:531–535.
8. Uzun O, Hancock S, Parsons JM, et al. Transcatheter occlusion of the arterial duct with Cook detachable coil: Early experience. *Heart.* 1996;76:269–273.
9. Podnar T, Masura J. Percutaneous closure of patent ductus arteriosus using special screwing detachable coil. *Cath Cardiovasc Diagn.* 1997;41:386–391.
10. Masura J, Kevin P, Thanopoulos B, et al. Catheter closure of moderate- to large-sized patent ductus arteriosus using the new Amplatzer duct occluder: Immediate and short-term results. *J Am Coll Cardiol.* 1998;31:878–882.
11. Masura J, Gavora P, Podnar T. Transcatheter occlusion of patent ductus arteriosus using a new angled Amplatzer duct occluder: Initial clinical experience. *Catheter Cardiovasc Interv.* 2003; 58:261–267.
12. Tometzki A, Chan K, De Giovanni J, et al. Total UK multicenter experience with a novel arterial occlusion device (DuctOcclud pfm). *Heart.* 1996;76:520–524.
13. Forsey J, Kenny D, Morgan G, et al. Early clinical experience with the new Amplatzer Ductal Occluder II for closure of the persistent arterial duct. *Catheter Cardiovasc Interv.* 2009;74(4):615–623.
14. Oishi Y, Okamoto M, Sueda T, et al. Transcatheter coil embolization of large-size patent ductus arteriosus in adult patients: Usefulness and problems. *Jpn Circ J.* 1999;63:994–998.
15. Bonhoeffer P, Borghi A, Onorato E, et al. Transfemoral closure of patent ductus arteriosus in adult patients. *Int J Cardiol.* 1993;39:181–186.
16. Schenck MH, O'Laughlin MP, Rokey R, et al. Transcatheter occlusion of patent ductus arteriosus in adults. *Am J Cardiol.* 1993;72:591–595.
17. Lee CH, Leung YL, Kwong NP, et al. Transcatheter closure of patent ductus arteriosus in Chinese adults: Immediate and long-term results. *J Invasive Cardiol.* 2003;15:26–30.
18. Yan C, Zhao S, Jiang S, et al. Transcatheter closure of patent ductus arteriosus with severe pulmonary arterial hypertension in adults. *Heart.* 2007;93:514–518.
19. Eicken A, Balling G, Gildein HP, et al. Transcatheter closure of a non-restrictive patent ductus arteriosus with an Amplatzer muscular ventricular septal defect occluder. *Int J Cardiol.* 2007;117:e40-e42.
20. Pass RH, Hijazi Z, Hsu DT, et al. Multicenter USA Amplatzer patent ductus arteriosus occlusion device trial: Initial and one-year results. *J Am Coll Cardiol.* 2004;44:513–519.

15 Damien Kenny, Robin Martin, and Zahid Amin

Complications of Transcatheter Treatment of Aortic Coarctation

INTRODUCTION

Coarctation of the aorta (CoA) accounts for 5% of congenital heart disease, making it the fourth most common abnormality requiring surgical or catheter-based intervention (1). Surgery remains the standard treatment in infancy, but in older children and adults, catheter-based interventions are being undertaken with increasing frequency.

Balloon angioplasty for coarctation was first reported in 1982, with widespread use during the past 2 decades (2). Medium-term outcome studies of balloon angioplasty showed good initial relief of stenosis but high rates of recoarctation and aneurysm formation (3–6). Hence, stent implantation is now the preferred intervention for coarctation, with persistent relief of stenosis and lower incidence of aneurysm formation compared to balloon angioplasty alone (7,8). Stent technology has evolved rapidly and includes primarily balloon expanding and occasionally self-expanding stents, in addition to expanded polytetrafluoroethylene-covered stents. Covered stents have also been used to treat increasingly complex aortic arch obstructions and aneurysm formation (9,10). Covered stents offer the advantage of excluding any stretch-induced wall trauma from the endoluminal aspect of the aorta particularly in the catastrophic event of aortic rupture, which has been reported (11).

Short-term efficacy of stent implantation is well recognized, but accurate long-term follow-up assessment is sparse. Recent reports have demonstrated potential physiological benefits following stenting, including mid-term left ventricular mass regression and long-axis function improvement, and amelioration in central aortic function with associated reduction of daytime ambulatory systolic blood pressure (12,13). Long-term evaluation of both stent and aortic wall integrity is essential to monitor potentially life-threatening complications. Follow-up with computed tomography (CT) examination suggest that overall aneurysm rate is low (14); however, other reports have variable results (15,16). In this chapter, we will highlight the following potential procedural complications:

- Aneurysm formation
- Stent migration
- Aortic rupture

Other complications, such as stent fracture, which is a direct function of the recalcitrant nature of the coarctation segment and occurs weeks to months after the procedure, will not be dealt with. In addition, some stents are more prone to fracture. Complications such as pacing-induced arrhythmias, paraplegia secondary to occlusion of spinal cord vessels, or left arm claudication secondary to occlusion of the subclavian artery though reported are rare and therefore will not be discussed further.

ANEURYSM FORMATION

Any form of intervention aimed at relieving stenosis at the site of coarctation can lead to trauma to the aortic wall. Differentiating therapeutic tears and pathological tears is important (17). Defining the preprocedural characteristics and exact procedural mechanisms that lead to pathological tears has so far eluded interventionalists. Definition of what constitutes an aneurysm had previously been derived from adult surgical literature. However, more relevant angiographic definitions have since been published (17). Although some still advocate the use of balloon angioplasty in older patients (18), it is generally accepted that the aneurysm rate of 30% is very high (4,6). Rates of aneurysm formation with stenting were lower than that with balloon angioplasty in early reports and ranged from 6% to 15% (7,17,19,20). More recent data with complete poststenting imaging follow-up suggest that rates are as low as 1% (14, 21), and large follow-up studies suggest that overall complication rates have decreased in later years, suggesting that as technical competence and understanding have increased, complication rates have reduced (22). Certain approaches, such as aggressive prestenting balloon angioplasty, may precipitate aneurysm formation and are best avoided (22). Some reports advocate aggressive prestent balloon angioplasty; we believe that prestent balloon angioplasty may precipitate aneurysm formation and should be avoided (22). Some authors advocate the use of aortic wall balloon compliance testing before stent implantation. There is, however, no evidence that this maneuver helps in screening patients for potential aneurysm formation. In the large follow-up study previously mentioned, higher balloon–coarctation ratios were not associated with immediate aortic wall complications of any type (22). In a recent study, however, ratio of over 4 was associated with aortic wall complications at intermediate follow-up (15). Older age was associated with increased risk of aortic wall tears. Covered stents may be a more appropriate choice in this setting. Covered stents may offer a sealant effect between the lumen of the aorta and any stretch-induced damage caused to the aortic wall. Apposition of the edges of the covered stent is important, and hourglass appearance of the stent in the coarctation segment may result in suboptimal apposition and allow flow into the site of aneurysm formation.

The incidence of aneurysm formation in surgically repaired CoA varies according to the type of operative repair (23), with most aneurysms seen with Dacron patch aortoplasty, and consequently this approach has largely been abandoned. Conservative management of these aneurysms is unacceptable however, with 100% rupture rates reported at 15 years follow-up (24), and surgical treatment is associated with not-insignificant rates of morbidity and mortality (24, 25).

STENT MIGRATION

In the largest follow-up series to date evaluating acute complications in 565 stenting procedures for CoA, stent migration was the most frequently encountered technical complication, occurring in 5% of cases (22). The major cause for stent migration was delivery of the stent on a balloon, catheter that was larger than the aorta proximal to the coarctation site (>2 mm). The second most common cause of stent migration was related to deployment of the stent on an undersized balloon, where the coarctation site was not a true stenosis, but more of a fold in the aortic arch. Stent migration occurred with larger balloon sizes, with 64% of stents migrating when the delivery balloon diameter was greater than or equal to 15 mm. Of the 28 migrated stents, 13 were successfully repositioned and did not require any further intervention. Eight stents were placed in a suboptimal location, requiring a second stent for successful outcome. Methods employed to reduce the incidence of stent migration during deployment include the use of the balloon-in-balloon (BIB) catheter (NuMED Inc, Hopkinton, NY), with initial inflation of the inner balloon and subsequent angiography to confirm optimum stent position prior to inflation of the outer balloon. Reduction in arterial pressure with either adenosine or more commonly rapid right ventricular pacing may also help reduce the potential for distal migration during balloon inflation. Generally, stent migration tends to occur in mild forms of CoA. The use of covered stents increases the risk associated with migration, as occlusion of the spinal arteries or mesenteric vessel can occur.

AORTIC DISSECTION/RUPTURE

Terminology has often been confusing in differentiating between aortic dissection and rupture. According to one study (17), aortic dissection is "a tear in the intima and media that extends beyond the coarcted segment in the axial dimension, permitting extraluminal contrast to track proximally or distally from the dilated segment." An aortic rupture on the other hand occurs when there is "a frank disruption of the aortic wall, which angiographically appears as extravasation of contrast beyond the confines of the aorta into the mediastinum or pleural space." Thus, a dissection is contained within the aortic wall and a rupture is not. Most cases of aortic rupture have been confined to case reports (11,26), and it is noteworthy that rupture may also occur with covered stents although it may buffer the blood loss, leading to delayed recognition (26). In another large cohort follow-up study (22), aortic dissection or rupture occurred in 1.5% of the cases. Three patients were sent to surgery and two of these patients did not survive. Three patients had covered stent implanted and three were managed medically. Risk factors for acute significant aortic wall injury included older age, with postulated mechanism secondary to progressive loss of aortic wall compliance (11, 22). Recent reports have measured aortic compliance in patients with coarctation using MRI and this may provide risk analysis in the future (27).

CASE 15.1

Stent Migration

CLINICAL HISTORY AND DIAGNOSTIC TESTING RESULTS

A 28-year-old, status post aortic valvotomy for aortic stenosis, was noted on routine follow-up to have progressive increases in descending aortic Doppler velocities on transthoracic echocardiography associated with systolic hypertension. He underwent MRI assessment of his aorta, which demonstrated severe discrete CoA distal to the left subclavian artery with numerous collateral arteries. The lesion was deemed suitable for stenting.

PLANNED PROCEDURE

Bare-metal stenting of a discrete native CoA.

PROCEDURE

The procedure was performed under general anesthesia. Following insertion of a 6-Fr sheath to the right femoral artery and vein, a femoral angiogram was taken in the right anterior oblique view to evaluate both the puncture site and size of the right femoral artery. The patient was given an initial intravenous bolus of heparin and intravenous antibiotics. The CoA site was crossed with a 5-Fr Judkins right catheter and advanced into the right subclavian artery. A 0.035-inch stiff wire was then inserted into the right subclavian artery, and the Judkins catheter was exchanged for a 5-Fr multitrack catheter through an 8-Fr short sheath. The pullback gradient was 51 mmHg with angiography demonstrating a tight distal discrete CoA (Figure 15.1a). A Palmaz 4014 stent (Cordis Corporation, Warren, NJ) was crimped onto a 15-mm Cristal balloon (Balt Extrusion, Montmorency, France) and advanced across the coarctation through a 12-Fr long sheath with multiple angiograms to ensure good positioning (Figure 15.1b).

COMPLICATION AND MANAGEMENT

On inflation of the balloon, the stent slipped proximally and was no longer fully across the coarctation site (Figure 15.1c). As this was a bare-metal stent, stent deployment across the left subclavian artery was unlikely to occlude the vessel, and thus the stent was deployed in this position.

Although the stent migrated, it was now secure and a second P4014 stent was prepared and mounted on a 15-mm balloon and positioned across the coarctation just distal to the embolized stent. Gentle traction on the balloon during inflation ensured a more stable position during inflation, and the balloon was inflated maintaining a good position (Figure 15.1d). Final angiography demonstrated good resolution of the coarctation with stable position of both stents (Figure 15.1e). There was no gradient across the stent on pullback following deployment of the second stent.

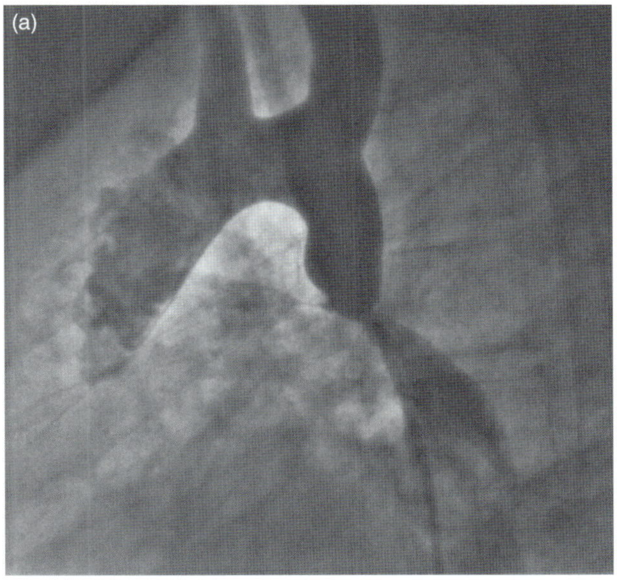

FIGURE 15.1 a

(a) Initial angiogram demonstrating severe distal coarctation. (*Continues on next page*)

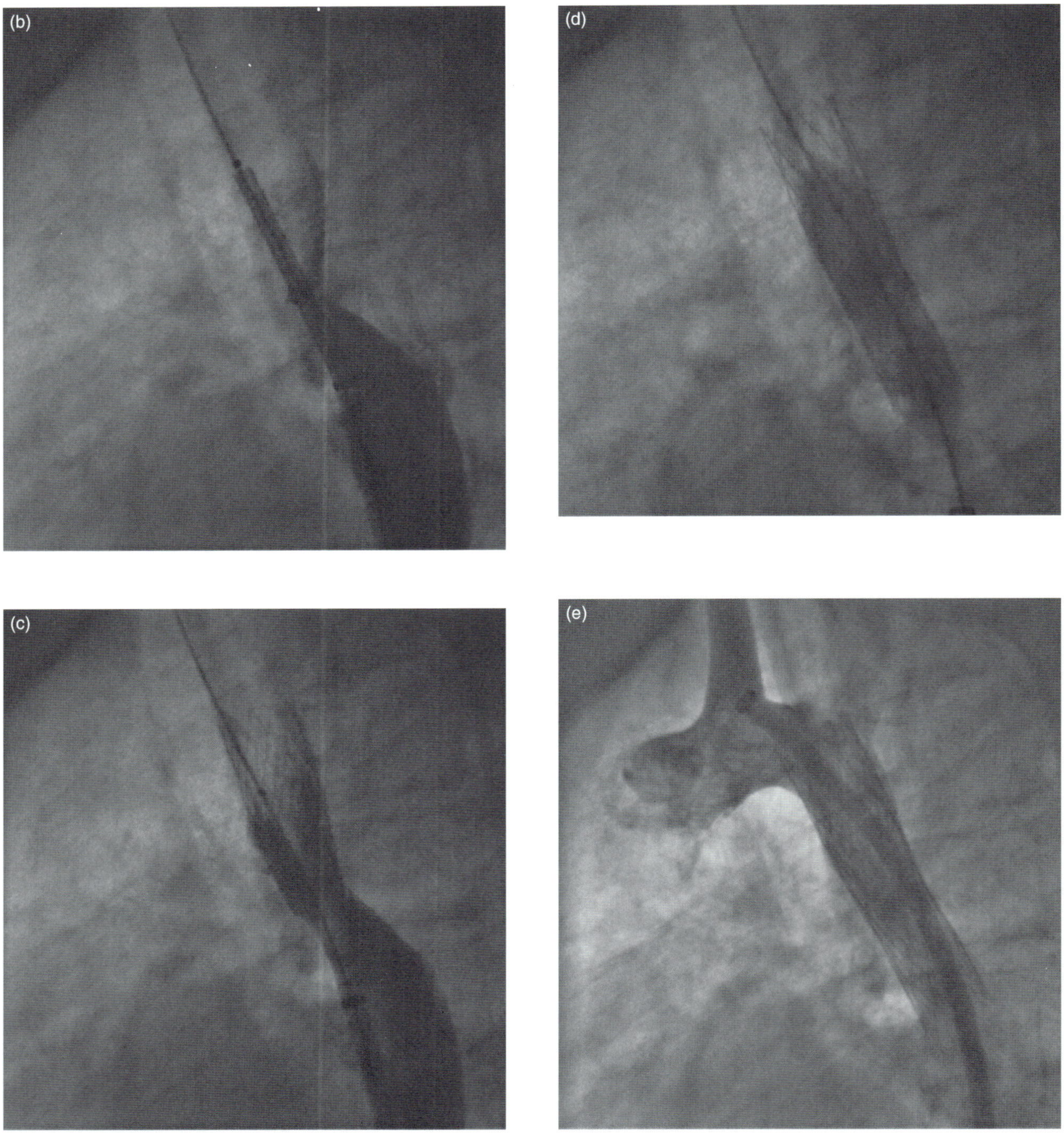

FIGURE 15.1 b–e

(b) Initial stent positioning angiogram. (c) Proximal migration of the stent balloon following balloon dilatation. (d) Inflation of the second stent across the coarctation. (e) Final angiogram showing the two stents in place with resolution of the coarctation and no evidence of aneurysm formation.

CASE ANALYSIS

As discussed above, one of the main risk factors for stent migration identified from the large follow-up study was either under- or oversizing of the balloon in relation to the size of the proximal aorta (15). The diameter of the proximal aorta prior to initial stent deployment was 14 mm and hence the rationale for choosing the 15-mm balloon. It may be prudent however to measure this in two planes, as the aorta in this region may not always be completely circular. Use of a single balloon with stent deployment is another risk factor for migration, and it is now more common practice to use a BIB catheter (NuMed, Hopkington, NJ) with inflation of the inner balloon, offering potential for stent repositioning should migration occur prior to full inflation of the outer balloon. Lastly, due to the tight morphology of the coarctation in this patient, rapid right ventricular pacing was not employed. It is possible that this may have improved stent stability during deployment, although some authors feel it is only necessary with less severe coarctation or when other factors likely to affect stent stability, such as concomitant aortic regurgitation, are present (14).

LESSONS

- Prevention of stent migration is becoming increasingly important because of the increased use of covered stents.
- Measures to reduce the likelihood of stent migration are optimal profiling of the coarctation segment, accurate sizing of the proximal and distal aorta in two planes, use of the BIB catheter for deployment, and rapid right ventricular pacing in appropriate cases.

SUGGESTED READING

Forbes TJ, Garekar S, Amin Z, et al. Procedural results and acute complications in stenting native and recurrent coarctation of the aorta in patients over 4 years of age: A multi-institutional study. *Catheter Cardiovasc Interv.* 2007;70:276–285.

CASE 15.2

Contained Aortic Rupture

CLINICAL HISTORY AND DIAGNOSTIC TESTING RESULTS

A 23-year-old woman's status postprevious arterial switch operation for d-transposition of the great arteries and subclavian flap repair for a discrete juxtaductal CoA was noted on routine follow-up MRI to have developed a large saccular aortic aneurysm at the site of previous coarctation repair (Figure 15.2a). The aneurysm measured approximately 2 × 2 cm. There was no associated recoarctation.

PLANNED PROCEDURE

Implant a covered stent to occlude the aneurysm. As the aneurysm was large, we requested a custom-made 65-mm-long covered Cheatham Platinum (CP) stent (NuMED Inc, Hopkinton, NY) premounted on a 24-mm BIB catheter. The balloon diameter requested was larger than the diameter of the aorta at either end of the aneurysm; however, the intention was not to maximally inflate the outer balloon, the rationale being that it was better to have a slightly larger balloon rather than a slightly smaller balloon in this setting.

PROCEDURE

The initial procedural details are similar to those described above. Two Perclose devices (Abbott Vascular Laboratories, Abbott Park, IL) were preplaced in femoral artery. As there was no recoarctation, initial angiography was performed using a 5-Fr pigtail catheter in the frontal and lateral planes, which confirmed the presence, and dimensions of the aneurysm detected by preprocedural MRI. A 0.035-inch stiff wire was then placed in the right subclavian artery and a 14-Fr-long delivery sheath advanced proximal to the site of the aneurysm. The stent was advanced over the wire through the delivery sheath and deployed using rapid right ventricular pacing. Repeat angiography demonstrated good stent position with no residual flow into the aneurysm (Figure 15.2b). The patient remained hemodyanically stable.

COMPLICATION AND MANAGEMENT

Twenty minutes after the procedure, the patient became hemodynamically unstable with tachycardia and hypotension. A follow-up angiogram demonstrated leakage from the proximal aspect of the stent, with dense opacities seen within the left lung field (Figure 15.2c). Hemothorax was confirmed by emergency chest CT (Figure 15.2d).

The patient was stabilized with fluid and blood replacement. Implantation of a second covered stent was considered; however, owing to the gothic morphology of the aortic arch, the patient was taken to the operating room and had an 18-mm Gore-Tex interposition tube graft inserted. The operative note specifically mentioned that the aortic wall tissue was thin and friable at the site of aneurysm formation. Follow-up MRI demonstrated a satisfactory surgical repair (Figure 15.2e).

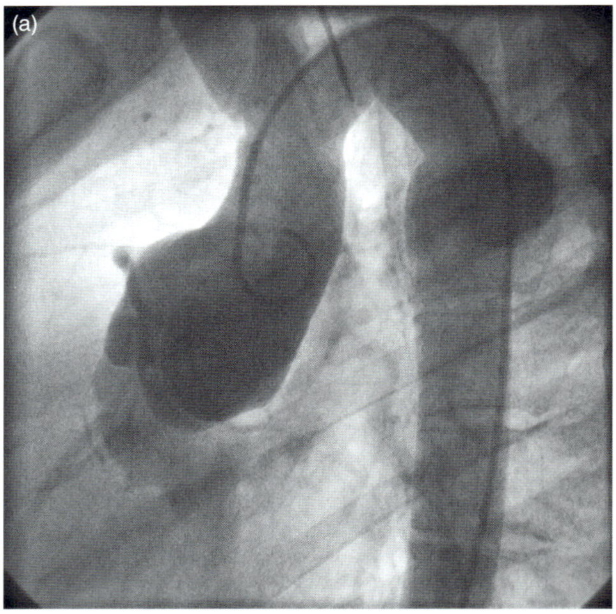

FIGURE 15.2 a

Continues on next page

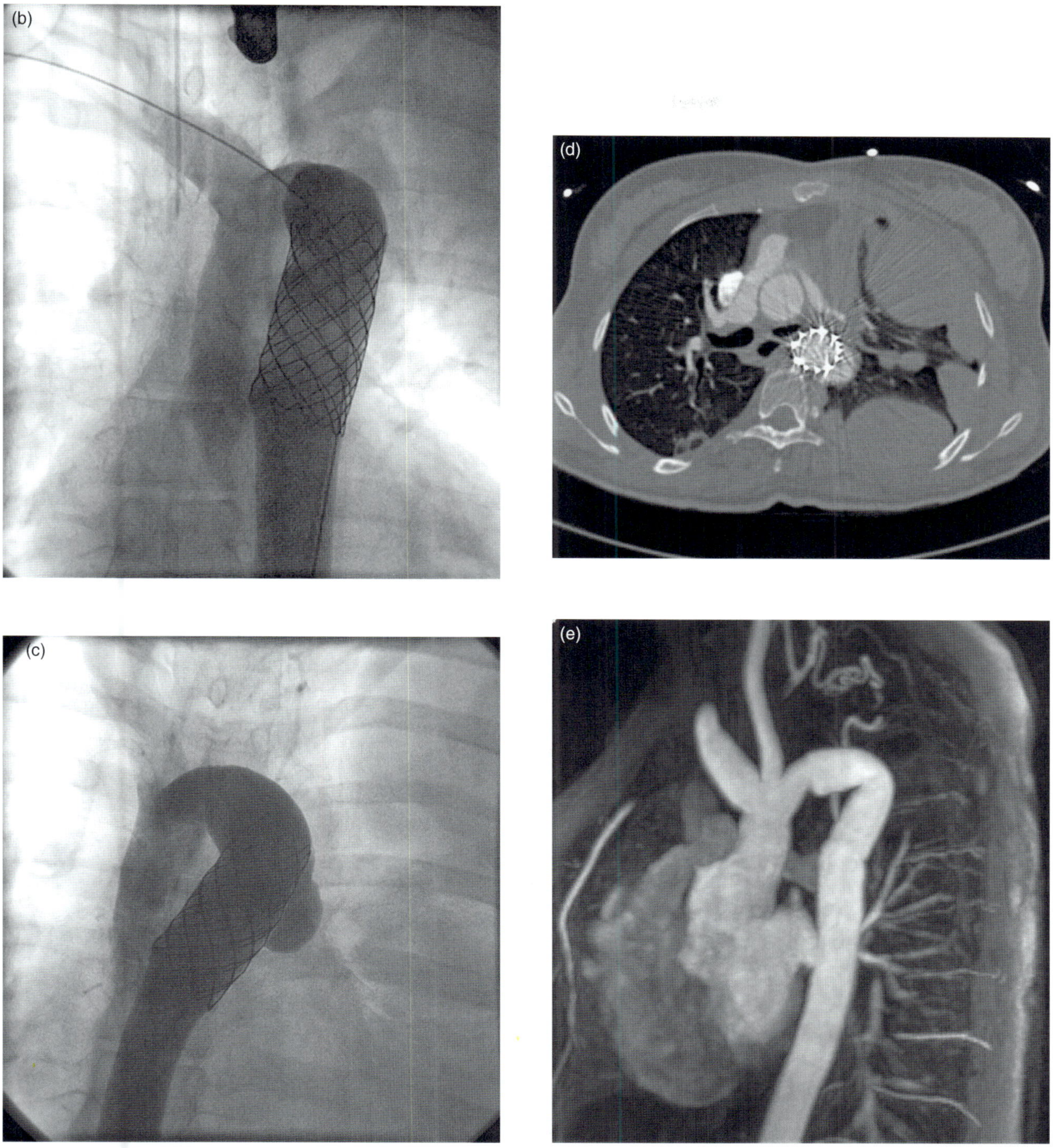

FIGURE 15.2 b–e

(a) Angiogram demonstrating large saccular aneurysm with no associated recoarctation. (b) Following stent deployment, with no residual flow seen within the aneurysm. (c) Angiogram demonstrating leak from the proximal aspect of the stent, with dense opacities seen within the left lung field. (d) Axial CT image of the chest demonstrating large collection of fluid in the left pleural space and periaortic hematoma. (e) Parasagittal MRI image of the aorta following repair with interposition grafting.

CASE ANALYSIS

The complication in this case was related to balloon oversizing. The custom-made stent was premounted on a 24-mm balloon. The aorta at either end of the aneurysm was 20 mm, and attempts were made at deployment not to fully inflate the balloon; in reality, this is difficult to achieve. Most published reports recommend choosing a balloon size no more than 1 to 2 mm larger than the proximal aorta when stenting for CoA. The stent was also longer than necessary, and protrusion of the proximal end toward the aneurysm was difficult to avoid with the given arch morphology and shape.

LESSONS

- Aggressive overdilation of the aorta when stenting for aneurysm formation may increase the likelihood of aortic rupture.
- This case also highlights the benefit of cardiac radiology and congenital surgical support when performing these complex interventions, and therefore, these should only be performed in centers where such support is available.

SUGGESTED READING

Kenny D, Margey R, Turner MS, Tometzki AJ, Walsh KP, Martin RP. Self-expanding and balloon expandable covered stents in the treatment of aortic coarctation with or without aneurysm formation. *Catheter Cardiovasc Interv.* 2008;72:65–71.

Varma C, Benson LN, Butany J, McLaughlin PR. Aortic dissection after stent dilatation for coarctation of the aorta: A case report and literature review. *Catheter Cardiovasc Interv.* 2005;64:495–506.

References

1. Fyler DC, Buckley LP, Hellenbrand WE, et al. Report of the New England regional infant cardiac program. *Pediatrics.* 1980;65:432–436.
2. Singer MI, Rowen M, Dorsey TJ. Transluminal aortic balloon angioplasty for coarctation of the aorta in the newborn. *Am Heart J.* 1982;103:131–132.
3. Fletcher SE, Nihill MR, Grifka RG, et al. Balloon angioplasty of native coarctation of the aorta: Midterm follow-up and prognostic factors. *J Am Coll Cardiol.* 1995;25:730–734.
4. Fawzy ME, Awad M, Hassan W, Al Kadhi Y, Shoukri M, Fadley F. Long-term outcome (up to 15 years) of balloon angioplasty of discrete native coarctation of the aorta in adolescents and adults. *J Am Coll Cardiol.* 2004;43:1062–1067.
5. Rao PS, Galal O, Smith PA, Wilson AD. Five- to nine-year follow-up results of balloon angioplasty of native aortic coarctation in infants and children. *J Am Coll Cardiol.* 1996;27:462–470.
6. Cowley CG, Orsmond GS, Feola P, McQuillan L, Shaddy RE. Long-term, randomized comparison of balloon angioplasty and surgery for native coarctation of the aorta in childhood. *Circulation.* 2005;111:3453–3456.
7. Chessa M, Carrozza M, Butera G, et al. Results and mid-long-term follow-up of stent implantation for native and recurrent coarctation of the aorta. *Eur Heart J.* 2005;26:2728–2732.
8. Zabal C, Attie F, Rosas M, Buendía-Hernández A, García-Montes JA. The adult patient with native coarctation of the aorta: Balloon angioplasty or primary stenting? *Heart.* 2003;89:77–83.
9. Kenny D, Margey R, Turner MS, Tometzki AJ, Walsh KP, Martin RP. Self-expanding and balloon expandable covered stents in the treatment of aortic coarctation with or without aneurysm formation. *Catheter Cardiovasc Interv.* 2008;72:65–71.
10. Holzer RJ, Chisolm JL, Hill SL, Cheatham JP. Stenting complex aortic arch obstructions. *Catheter Cardiovasc Interv.* 2008;71:375–382.
11. Varma C, Benson LN, Butany J, McLaughlin PR. Aortic dissection after stent dilatation for coarctation of the aorta: A case report and literature review. *Catheter Cardiovasc Interv.* 2005;64:495–506.
12. Lam YY, Kaya MG, Li W. Effect of endovascular stenting of aortic coarctation on biventricular function in adults. *Heart.* 2007;93:1441–1447.
13. Chen SS, Donald AE, Storry C, Halcox JP, Bonhoeffer P, Deanfield JE. Impact of aortic stenting on peripheral vascular function and daytime systolic blood pressure in adult coarctation. *Heart.* 2008;94:919–924.
14. Chakrabarti S, Kenny D, Morgan G, et al. Balloon expandable stent implantation for native and recurrent coarctation of the aorta–prospective computed tomography assessment of stent integrity, aneurysm formation and stenosis relief. *Heart.* 2010;96:1212–1216.
15. Forbes TJ, Moore P, Pedra CA, et al. Intermediate follow-up following intravascular stenting for treatment of coarctation of the aorta. *Catheter Cardiovasc Interv.* 2007; 70:569–577.
16. Hamdan MA, Maheshwari S, Fahey JT, Hellenbrand WE. Endovascular stents for coarctation of the aorta: Initial results and intermediate term follow-up. *J Am Coll Cardiol.* 2001;38:1518–1523.
17. Qureshi AM, McElhinney DB, Lock JE, Landzberg MJ, Lang P, Marshall AC. Acute and intermediate outcomes, and evaluation of injury to the aortic wall, as based on 15 years experience of implanting stents to treat aortic coarctation. *Cardiol Young.* 2007;17:307–318.
18. Walhout RJ, Suttorp MJ, Mackaij GJ, Ernst JM, Plokker HW. Long-term outcome after balloon angioplasty of coarctation of the aorta in adolescents and adults: Is aneurysm formation an issue? *Catheter Cardiovasc Interv.* 2009;73:549–556.
19. Harrison DA, McLaughlin PR, Lazzam C, Connelly M, Benson LN. Endovascular stents in the management of coarctation of the aorta in the adolescent and adult: One year follow up. *Heart.* 2001;85:561–566.
20. Hamdan MA, Maheshwari S, Fahey JT, Hellenbrand WE. Endovascular stents for coarctation of the aorta: Initial results and intermediate-term follow-up. *J Am Coll Cardiol.* 2001;38:1518–1523.
21. Thanopoulos BV, Eleftherakis N, Tzanos K, Skoularigis I, Triposkiadis F. Stent implantation for adult aortic coarctation. *J Am Coll Cardiol.* 2008;52:1815–1816.
22. Forbes TJ, Garekar S, Amin Z, et al. Procedural results and acute complications in stenting native and recurrent coarctation of the aorta in patients over 4 years of age: A multi-institutional study. *Catheter Cardiovasc Interv.* 2007;70:276–285.
23. von Kodolitsch Y, Aydin MA, Koschyk DH, et al. Predictors of aneurysmal formation after surgical correction of aortic coarctation. *J Am Coll Cardiol.* 2002;39:617–624.
24. Knyshov GV, Sitar LL, Glagola MD, Atamanyuk MY. Aortic aneurysms at the site of the repair of coarctation of the aorta: A review of 48 patients. *Ann Thorac Surg.* 1996;61:935–939.
25. Ala-Kulju K, Heikkinen L. Aneurysms after patch graft aortoplasty for coarctation of the aorta: Long-term results of surgical management. *Ann Thorac Surg.* 1989;47:853–856.
26. Collins N, Mahadevan V, Horlick E. Aortic rupture following a covered stent for coarctation: Delayed recognition. *Catheter Cardiovasc Interv.* 2006;68:653–655.
27. Ou P, Celermajer DS, Raisky O, et al. Angular (Gothic) aortic arch leads to enhanced systolic wave reflection, central aortic stiffness, and increased left ventricular mass late after aortic coarctation repair: Evaluation with magnetic resonance flow mapping. *J Thorac Cardiovasc Surg.* 2008;135:62–68.

16

Jeffrey D. Booker and Charanjit S. Rihal

Complications of Paravalvular Leak Closure Interventions

INTRODUCTION

Device closure of paravalvular regurgitant defects is a technically challenging procedure. Patients referred for device closure of these defects commonly have undergone multiple cardiac surgical procedures and have significant medical comorbidities. Percutaneous treatment has been advocated as a less-invasive option, but anatomic, patient, and lesion factors and lack of purpose-designed devices increase the risk of procedural complications (1–3).

The basic technique for device closure of a paravalvular defect involves positioning a catheter near the defect, crossing with a guidewire, advancing a catheter across the defect, and positioning an occlusion device. Various approaches can be used, including antegrade, retrograde, and transapical—each carrying its own risks and benefits. Crossing irregular and serpiginous defects with delivery catheters can often be difficult, occasionally necessitating creation of an arteriovenous rail by snaring a wire and exteriorizing it to provide added support, or attempting an alternate approach to the defect.

Selection of an appropriate closure device is influenced by the geometry of the defect and the proximity to the prosthetic valve leaflets and surrounding cardiac structures. Currently available "round" closure devices may not provide adequate closure of crescentic or oblong defects. The devices with larger waists and retention disks are favored, but the added stability and greater effective closure comes with a risk of device interference with prosthetic valve function (4).

Potential procedural complications include access-site bleeding—those related to the transseptal puncture (perforation, tamponade), air or thrombo-embolism, device embolization, prosthetic valve disruption, device interference with prosthetic leaflet function, late erosion, and worsening or new-onset hemolysis. High radiation doses may be observed in particularly long and challenging cases (5).

The technical challenges and potential serious complications associated with this new procedure necessitate a high degree of technical skill, expertise, and ability to manage complications. These are often best achieved with a team approach consisting of an adult interventional cardiologist, a pediatric congenital interventionalist, and an interventional imaging specialist.

CASE 16.1

Embolized Amplatzer Vascular Plug After Deployment in a Mitral Paravalvular Leak

CLINICAL HISTORY AND DIAGNOSTIC TESTING RESULTS

A 69-year-old man with two prior sternotomies presented with class IV heart failure due to severe paravalvular mitral regurgitation. He had had two-vessel coronary bypass and bioprosthetic mitral valve replacement for mitral regurgitation, followed by a second bioprosthetic aortic valve replacement for aortic stenosis 5 months prior to presentation. There was no clinical or laboratory evidence of hemolysis or endocarditis. Ejection fraction was 45% to 50%, and severe paravalvular mitral regurgitation was seen through a defect in the intervalvular fibrosa (Figure 16.1). The aortic valve bioprosthesis was functioning normally. Comorbidities included chronic renal insufficiency, diabetes mellitus, and hypothyroidism.

PLANNED PROCEDURE

Device closure of paravalvular mitral defect.

PROCEDURE

The planned approach was antegrade from the left atrium to the left ventricle via a transseptal puncture. Fluoroscopic visualization of the sewing rings of both the bioprosthetic aortic and mitral valves was challenging (Figure 16.2), and obtaining useable orthogonal planes was difficult.

A transseptal puncture was performed and the interatrial septum dilated with a 14-Fr Inoue dilator (Toray Medical Co. Ltd, Tokyo, Japan). An 11-Fr deflectable sheath was placed in the left atrium (Agilis, St. Jude Medical Inc., St. Paul, Minnesota). A telescoping catheter system of a 6-Fr 125-cm multipurpose diagnostic catheter through an 8-Fr 100-cm multipurpose guiding catheter was placed through the Agilis sheath and the sewing ring of the mitral valve probed using a 260-cm stiff angled Glidewire (Terumo Medical Corporation, Somerset, NJ). The defect was successfully crossed with the wire and followed by the 6-Fr and 8-Fr catheters.

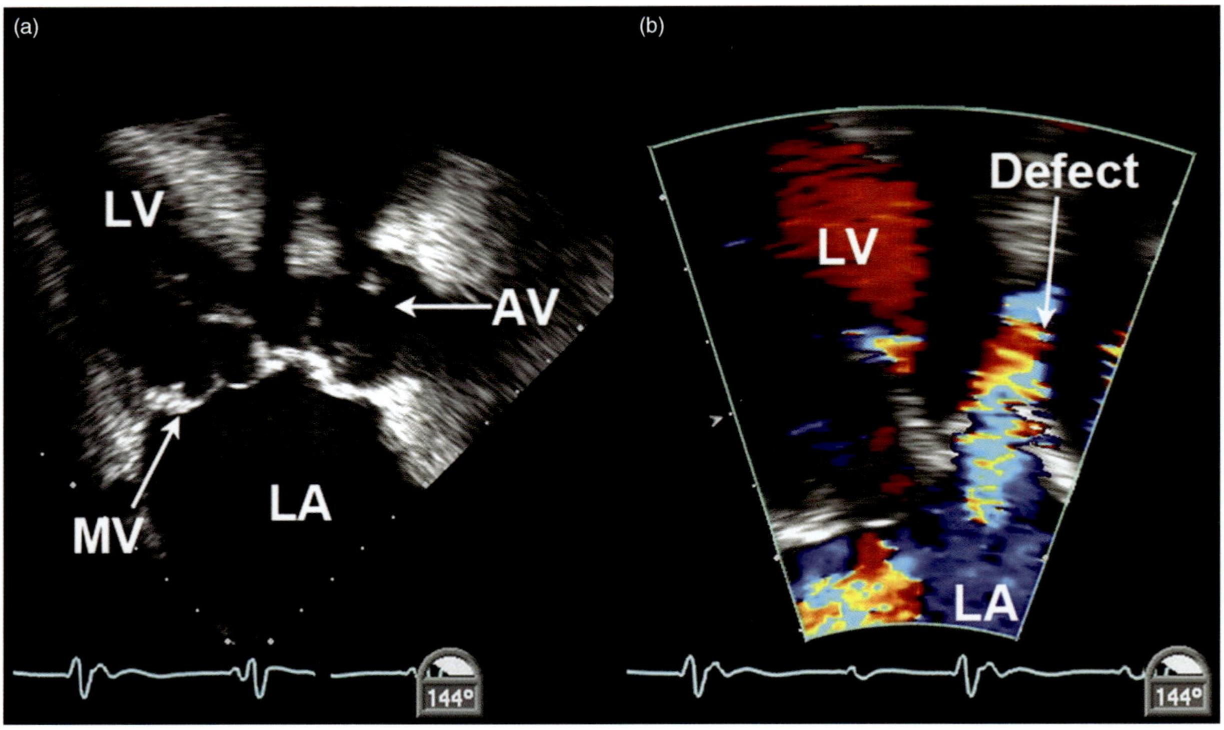

FIGURE 16.1

Transesophageal echocardiographic images demonstrating the anterior position of the paravalvular defect in the intervalvular fibrosa. LA=left atrium, LV=left ventricle, AV=aortic valve, MV=mitral valve. (LOOPS 16.1a, b)

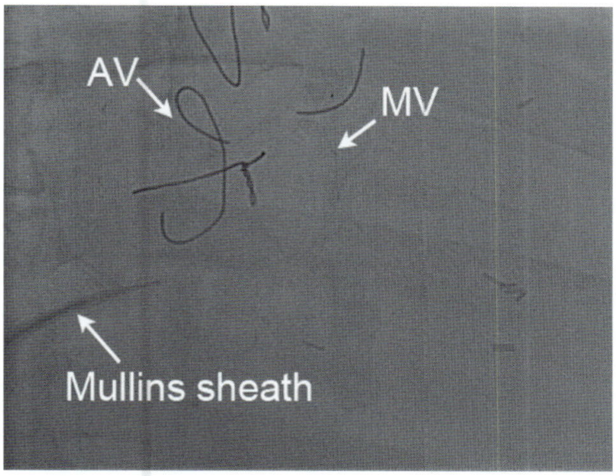

FIGURE 16.2

Fluoroscopic image demonstrating the difficult visualization of the aortic and mitral valve sewing rings. AV=aortic valve, MV=mitral valve. (LOOP 16.2)

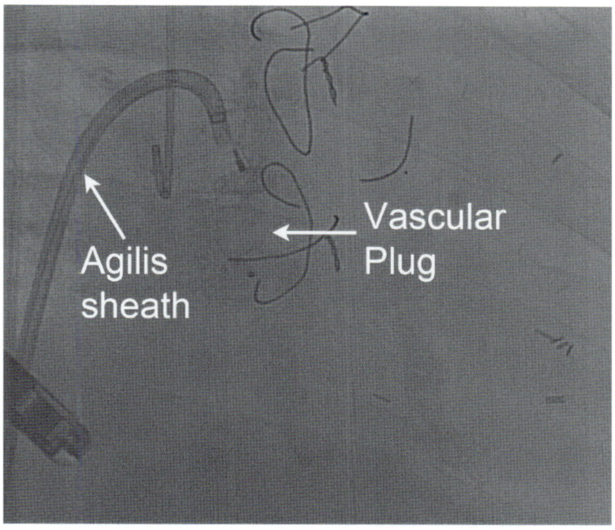

FIGURE 16.3

Fluoroscopic image of the initial deployment of the Amplatzer Vascular Plug (AVP-II). (LOOP 16.3)

COMPLICATION AND MANAGEMENT

A 14-mm Amplatzer Vascular Plug (AVP-II, AGA Medical Inc., Plymouth, MN) was placed; however, difficult visualization of the valve resulted in the device becoming stuck in the struts of the bioprosthetic valve, and it was deployed in the left ventricular outflow tract (Figure 16.3). Unfortunately, echocardiographic visualization at that point was also suboptimal and could not confirm the position of the device. Following release, the device was held in position by the struts of the prosthetic mitral valve but began to prolapse in the left ventricular outflow tract (LVOT), moving back and forth across the aortic valve (Figure 16.4). The patient remained stable. The right femoral arterial sheath was upsized to an 8-Fr sheath, an 8-Fr multipurpose catheter was brought into the ascending aorta, and a 15-mm gooseneck snare (ev3 Inc., Plymouth, MN) was used to snare the retention disk of the device, allowing it to be withdrawn from the LVOT (Figure 16.5). The patient did develop a single episode of ventricular fibrillation requiring defibrillation. The device, was pulled down to the level of the right external iliac. Due to the angulation of the device and the snare, it could not be removed through the right femoral arterial sheath. Left femoral arterial access was obtained with a 14-Fr sheath. The device was snared from both ends, stretched, and removed successfully. To provide sufficient force to remove the device, a bioptome was used to grasp the device and extract it through the 14-Fr sheath (Figure 16.6). Further attempts to place a device were not made.

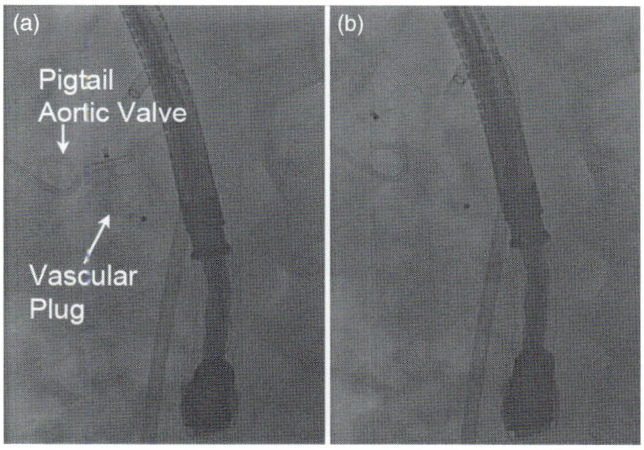

FIGURE 16.4

Fluoroscopic images demonstrating the motion of the device prolapsing from the left ventricular outflow tract out the aortic valve. (LOOP 16.4)

The patient subsequently had surgical mitral valve replacement and insertion of a 31-mm St. Jude Biocor valve. Unfortunately, postoperative infectious complications led to a prolonged hospitalization, and the patient died 4 months after surgery.

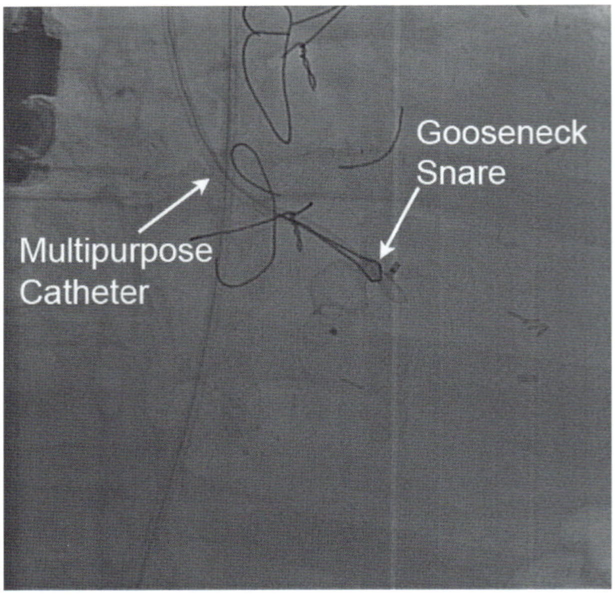

FIGURE 16.5

Fluoroscopic image illustrating snaring the device through the aortic valve. (LOOP 16.5)

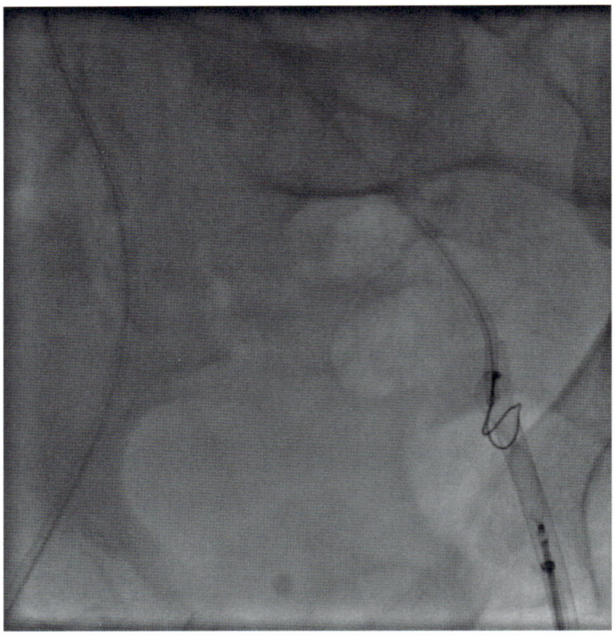

FIGURE 16.6

Fluoroscopic image of the device removal using a bioptome through a 14-Fr left femoral arterial sheath. (LOOP 16.6)

CASE ANALYSIS

A combination of factors led to malpositioning of the device during deployment. The fluoroscopic imaging challenges as described led to the device deployment in a view that was not orthogonal to the plane of the valve orifice. Difficulties in obtaining adequate echocardiographic images at that point in time led to reliance on the fluoroscopic appearance of the device. The struts of the bioprosthetic valve held the distal retention disk firmly and falsely provided tactile feedback to the operator that the device was securely in the defect. The malpositioned device was ultimately retrieved without major immediate complication, apart from an episode of ventricular fibrillation. The most significant complication was an ultimately unsuccessful percutaneous procedure followed by an unfortunate postsurgical outcome.

LESSONS

- Imaging with both fluoroscopy and echocardiography is essential for successful percutaneous closure of paravalvular leaks.
- Various techniques for device retrieval may be necessary to bail out an operator with a malpositioned or embolized device.

CASE 16.2

Amplatzer Muscular VSD Ocluder Impingement on a Mechanical Mitral Valve After Deployment in a Paravalvular Leak

CLINICAL HISTORY AND DIAGNOSTIC TESTING RESULTS

A 59-year-old woman with five prior cardiac surgeries over 12 years presented with severe paravalvular leak and New York Heart Association (NYHA) class III heart failure symptoms. There was a history of prior prosthetic valve infective endocarditis and subsequently a recurrent paravalvular leak. The prosthetic mitral valve was a 27-mm ATS mechanical bileaflet valve. Transesophageal echocardiographic images demonstrated the perimitral anterior crescentic defect lateral to the intervalvular fibrosa with severe regurgitation (Figure 16 7) and normal ejection fraction. Comorbidities included severe pulmonary hypertension (pulmonary artery systolic pressure, 75 mmHg), moderately severe tricuspid regurgitation, right ventricular enlargement with reduced systolic function, paroxysmal atrial tachycardia, and a permanent pacemaker for sinus node dysfunction.

PLANNED PROCEDURE

Device closure of paravalvular mitral defect.

PROCEDURE

An antegrade approach to the perimitral defect was selected. A transseptal puncture was performed with great difficulty due to scarring and patching of the septum. The paravalvular defect was quickly crossed, and an Inoue wire was placed in the left ventricular cavity. Over this wire, an 8-Fr Flexor shuttle sheath (Cook Medical, Bloomington, IN) was advanced across the defect.

Initial deployment of a 20-mm AVP-II revealed persistent significant regurgitation, and thus this device was removed. An 18-mm Amplatzer muscular ventricular septal defect (VSD) device (AGA Medical Inc., Plymouth, MN) was deployed. There was significant improvement in the regurgitation, but the left atrial retention disk could not be expanded; the device was not felt to be stable and it was thus removed. A retrograde approach to the defect was taken next. The defect was crossed retrograde through the aortic valve with a stiff-angled glide wire guided with an internal mammary artery (IMA) catheter (Figure 16.8), and an 8-Fr Flexor shuttle sheath placed over a stiff wire.

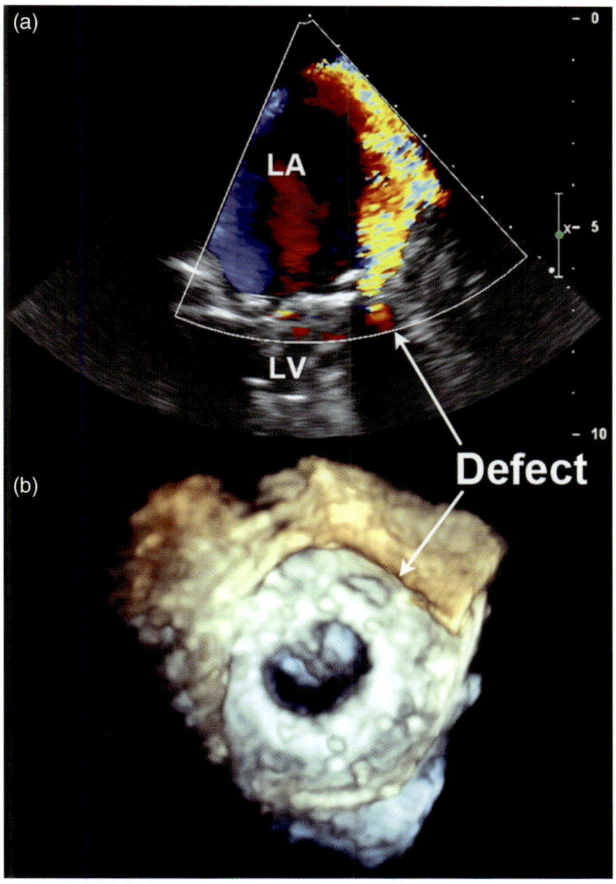

FIGURE 16.7

(a) Transesophageal echocardiographic image of color doppler flow through the regurgitant perimitral defect. LA=left atrium, LV=left ventricle. (b) Three-dimensional echocardiographic images of an en face view of the prosthetic mitral valve with the defect visualized. **(LOOP 16.7a, b)**

COMPLICATION AND MANAGEMENT

An 18-mm Amplatzer muscular VSD occluder was placed, with marked reduction in regurgitation. While tethered to the delivery cable and sheath, the device position appeared favorable, and the mechanical valve leaflet occluders were functioning normally (Figure 16.9). Once released, the ventricular portion of the device shifted toward the adjacent valve leaflet

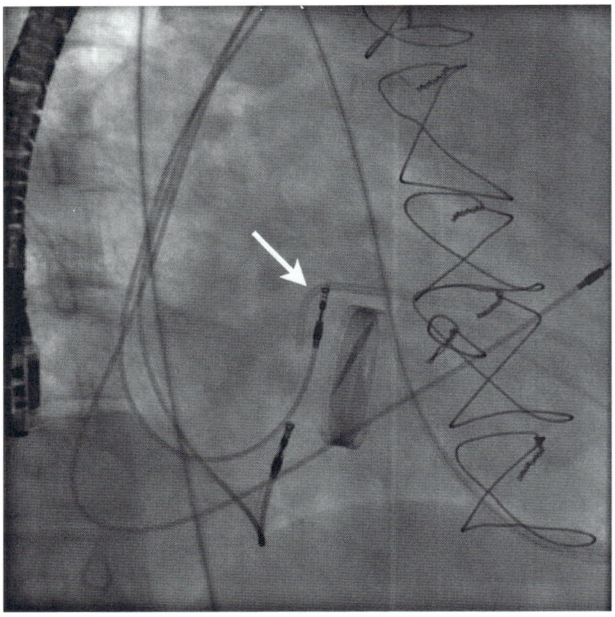

FIGURE 16.8

Fluoroscopic image of the internal mammary catheter (arrow) advanced retrogradely across the paravalvular defect. (LOOP 16.8)

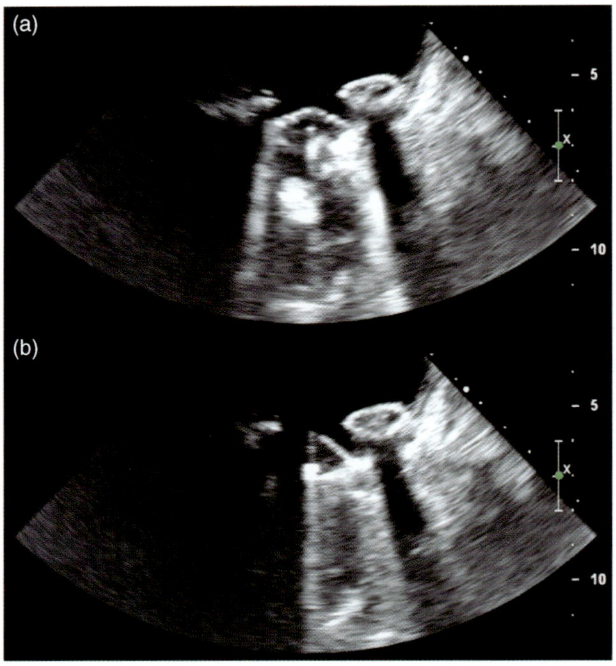

FIGURE 16.10

(a and b) Echocardiographic images demonstrating the motion of the prosthetic mitral valve leaflet being restricted by the deployed muscular VSD occluder device. (LOOP 16.10)

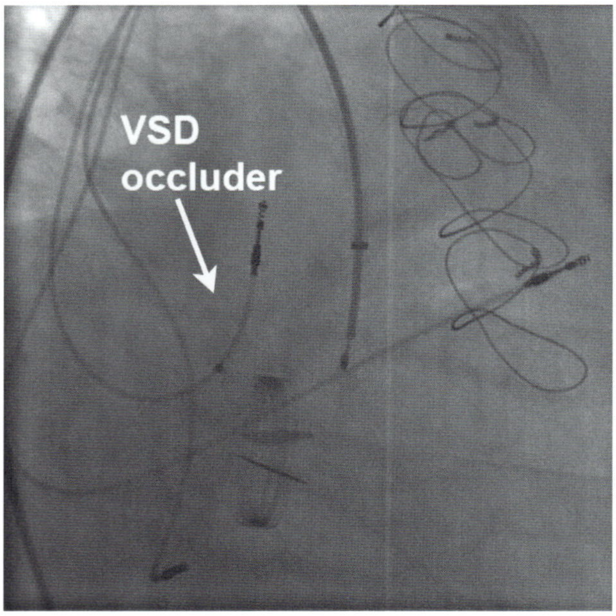

FIGURE 16.9

Fluoroscopic image of the muscular VSD occluder device deployed in the paravalvular defect. (LOOP 16.9)

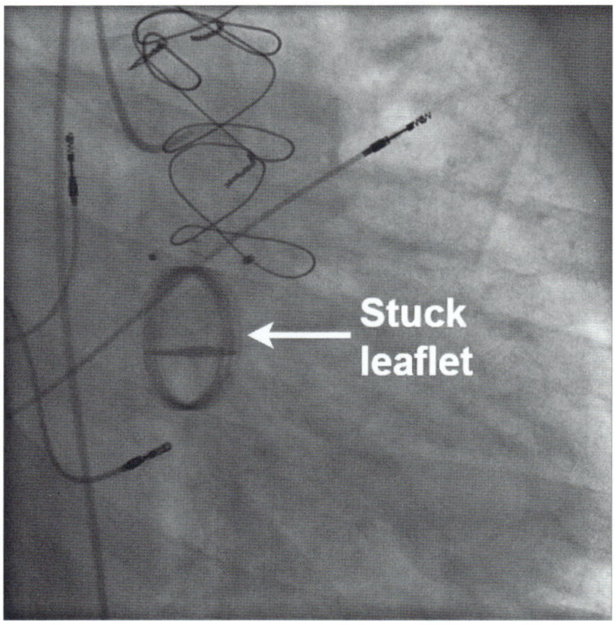

FIGURE 16.11

Fluoroscopic image of the obstructed mechanical leaflet occluder during preoperative angiography of the left coronary circulation. (LOOP 16.11) occluder and obstructed its motion. The leaflet became stuck in a partially closed position (Figures 16.10 and 16.11). The patient remained hemodynamically stable. Attempts to snare the device were unsuccessful, and the valve remained obstructed. The mitral inflow gradient was severely elevated and a surgical consultation obtained. Emergent surgery was performed with removal of the occluder device, suture closure of the paravalvular defect, and a tricuspid valve annuloplasty. The patient made an uneventful recovery from her surgery, and at 6-month follow-up, she was asymptomatic with a normal functional capacity. There was trivial mitral and tricuspid regurgitation, and her pulmonary pressures had fallen to 39 mmHg.

CASE ANALYSIS

Device impingement on prosthetic valve leaflets is a complication more commonly seen with mechanical valve prostheses. The distance of the defect from the leaflets and the location on the sewing ring relative to the leaflet hinges may predict occurrence of this complication. Leaflet obstruction is typically apparent immediately upon device deployment. When an antegrade approach is used, the distal retention disk can be pulled back slowly while visualizing the prosthetic leaflet motion. If leaflet impingement is seen, the device can be repositioned and "tucked in" to the defect or retrieved, and an alternate device can be used. The retrograde approach requires a careful assessment of the proximal retention disk once deployed. In this case, a large device was chosen due to the large defect size. The angulation of the delivery catheter and cable prevented accurate assessment of the final device position, despite attempting to test potential for valve interference by moving the device with the delivery cable and catheter. Once released, snaring the device proved exceedingly difficult—primarily due to the large size of the proximal occluder disc. Anterolateral perimitral defects frequently have a vertical orientation, and devices may be more apt to tilt across the mechanical leaflets.

The frequency of valve leaflet impingement can be reduced by choosing multiple smaller devices with a lower profile rather than one larger device to close large crescentic or oblong defects. Multiple devices can be deployed simultaneously via multiple delivery catheters (a feasible option for venous access and antegrade approaches to perimitral defects) or sequentially using a single delivery catheter and leaving a retained wire through the defect. These techniques also allow the devices to self-position and anchor within irregularly shaped defects providing more-effective closure.

LESSONS

- Prosthetic valve leaflet obstruction is not uncommon when deploying large devices in paravalvular defects, particularly with mechanical valves.
- Careful assessment of the movement of the valve leaflet occluders is essential prior to the release of a newly deployed device.
- Consider multiple smaller devices when attempting closure of large defects.
- Surgical backup is essential in complex structural heart disease interventions.

CASE 16.3

Hemolysis Acceleration After Partial Closure of a Mitral Paravalvular Leak

CLINICAL HISTORY AND DIAGNOSTIC TESTING RESULTS

A 63-year-old man with two prior sternotomies for radiation-induced valvular heart disease and coronary artery disease presented with class II heart failure and hemolysis secondary to severe paravalvular mitral regurgitation. The current state of his valves included aortic and mitral bioprosthetic valve replacements (Medtronic Hancock, 22 and 29 mm [Medtronic, Minneapolis, MN]). Echocardiography revealed two paravalvular mitral defects, a moderate- medial and large posterolateral, with severe regurgitation (Figure 16.12a, b). The aortic valve prosthesis was normal, and comorbidities included a left ventricular ejection fraction of 45%, sick sinus syndrome, dual chamber pacemaker implantation, hypertension, dyslipidemia, and Hodgkin's lymphoma with mantle radiation 30 years prior.

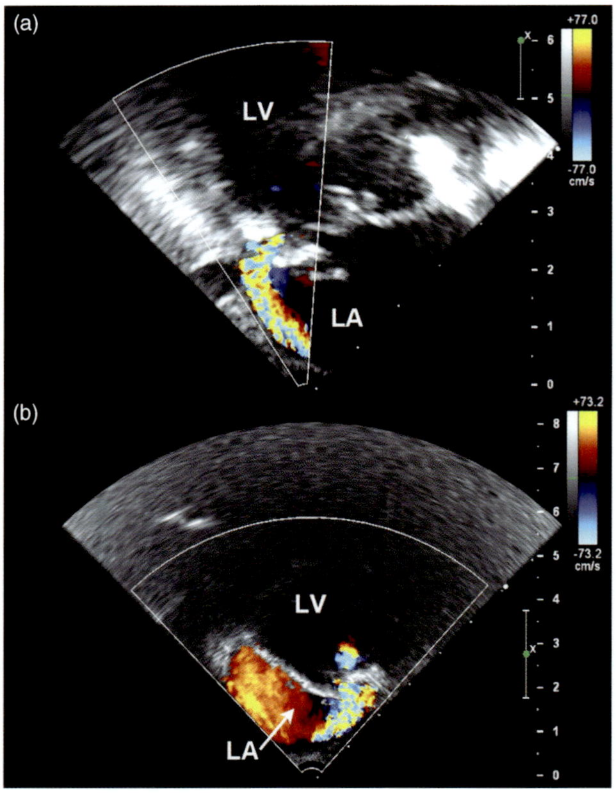

FIGURE 16.12

Transesophageal echo images demonstrating color Doppler flow through the medial (a) and posterolateral (b) perimitral defects. LA=left atrium, LV=left ventricle. **(LOOP 16.12a, b)**

PLANNED PROCEDURE

Device closure of paravalvular mitral defect.

PROCEDURE

The planned approach was antegrade via a transseptal puncture. A telescoping catheter system consisting of a 5-Fr 125-cm multipurpose diagnostic catheter is passed through a 6-Fr 100-cm multipurpose guiding catheter in turn through an 8.5-F Agilis deflectable left atrial catheter. A 260-cm stiff-angled guidewire was used to cross the defect, was looped in the left ventricular cavity, and advanced out the aortic valve into the ascending aorta. Over this wire, the catheters were advanced across the defect into the left ventricle (Figure 16.13), and a 12-mm AVP-II device was placed, but echocardiography revealed significant residual medial regurgitation. The device was retrieved and the guidewire readvanced into the left ventricle. A 7-Fr Flexor shuttle sheath was placed across the defect over

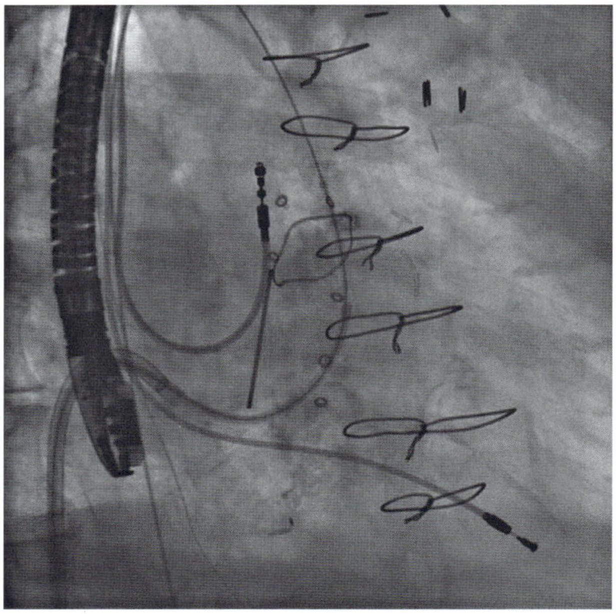

FIGURE 16.13

Fluoroscopic image of telescoping catheters advanced across the paravalvular defect in an antegrade fashion over a stiff glide wire. **(LOOP 16.13)**

an arteriovenous (A-V) rail created by snaring of the guidewire in the ascending aorta and exteriorization through the femoral arterial sheath. A 16-mm AVP-II was deployed in the defect (Figure 16.14) with obliteration of the medial regurgitation. The function of the mitral bioprosthesis was intact and the device was released.

A 12/10 Amplatzer patent arterial duct (PDA) occluder (AGA Medical Inc., Plymouth, MN) was advanced and deployed in the posterolateral defect using similar techniques (Figure 16.15a, b). This was well seated, but there remained moderate residual regurgitation adjacent to the deployed device (Figure 16.16). Given the length and difficulty of the procedure and a significant reduction in the severity of the regurgitation, the procedure was concluded.

COMPLICATION AND MANAGEMENT

The patient made an uneventful early recovery following the procedure. Unfortunately, acceleration of hemolysis developed and required weekly blood transfusions. He ultimately proceeded to a second device closure procedure as described in Case 4 (below).

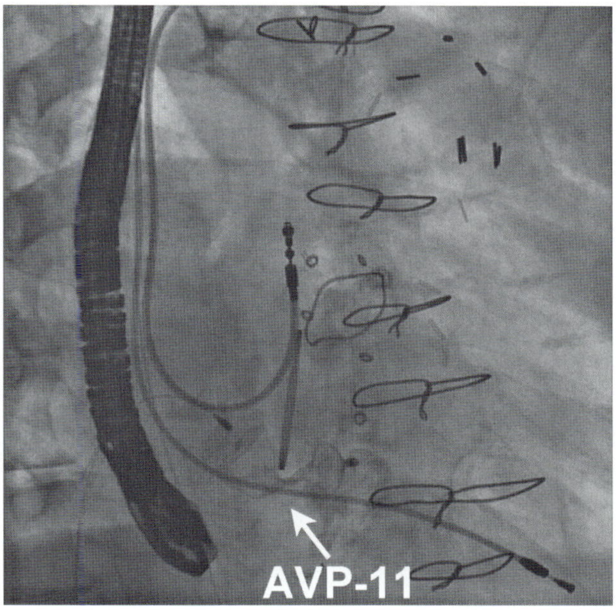

FIGURE 16.14

Fluoroscopic image of the Amplatzer Vascular Plug II (AVP-II) deployed in the medial paravalvular defect. **(LOOP 16.14)**

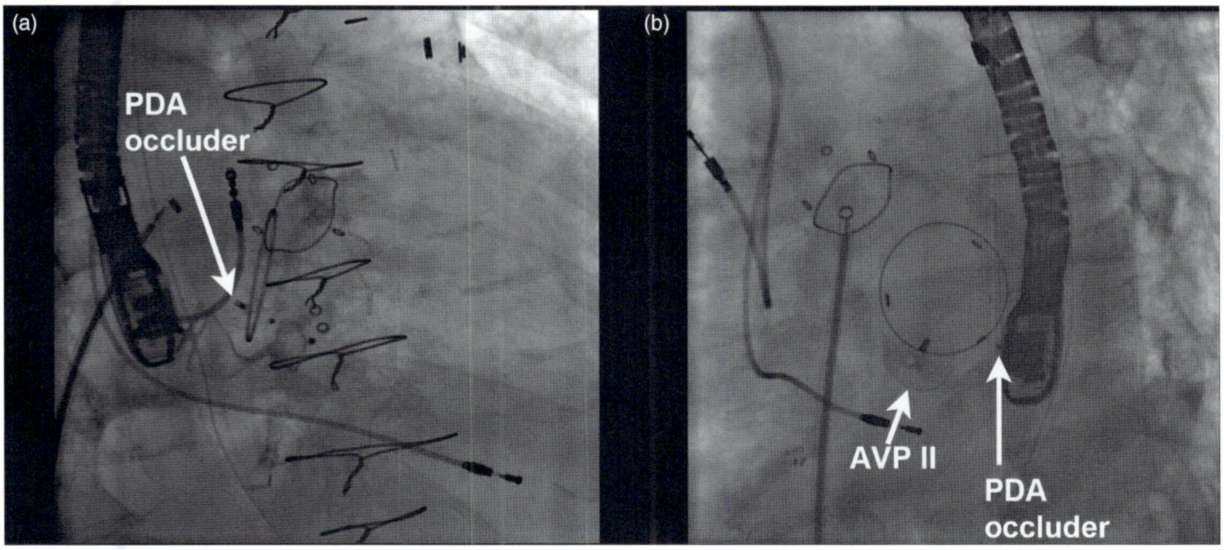

FIGURE 16.15

Fluoroscopic images of the Amplatzer PDA occluder device deployed in the posterolateral defect. (a) Right anterior oblique projection. (b) Left anterior oblique with caudal angulation. **(LOOP 16.15)**

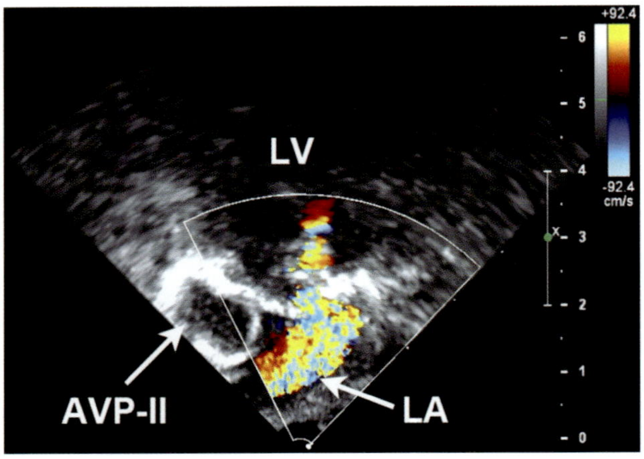

FIGURE 16.16

Echocardiographic image demonstrating residual paravalvular regurgitation following deployment of both occluder devices. LA=left atrium, LV=left ventricle, AVP-II=Amplatzer Vascular Plug II. **(LOOP 16.16)**

CASE ANALYSIS

The indications for device closure of paravalvular leaks include congestive heart failure and hemolysis. Reduction in the regurgitant volume can result in substantial improvements in heart failure symptoms, even with incomplete closure of the paravalvular defect. The response of hemolysis due to a paravalvular leak following device closure is more variable. It can improve (2) or worsen due to increased flow velocity and shear stress through a residual defect. Clearly, the goal of closure should be as little residual regurgitation as possible when treating patients for hemolysis.

LESSONS

- Device closure of paravalvular leaks may provide effective treatment of hemolysis.
- Residual regurgitation may result in acceleration of hemolysis and there should be less tolerance for residual regurgitation as compared to the treatment of heart failure due to paravalvular leaks.

CASE 16.4

Embolization of an Amplatzer PDA Occluder From a Paravalular Leak Site While Attempting to Deploy a Second Adjacent Occluder

CLINICAL HISTORY AND DIAGNOSTIC TESTING RESULTS

The patient described in Case 3 returned 6 weeks later with acceleration in his hemolysis for a second attempt at device closure. In addition, he had also developed worsening heart failure symptoms. Persistent moderate paravalvular regurgitation adjacent to the patent arterial duct (PDA) occluder device AGA Medical Inc., Plymouth, MN) in the posterior region was present (Figure 16.17), and only trace regurgitation in the medial defect was observed. A surgical consultation was obtained, and the patient elected to proceed with a second percutaneous device closure procedure.

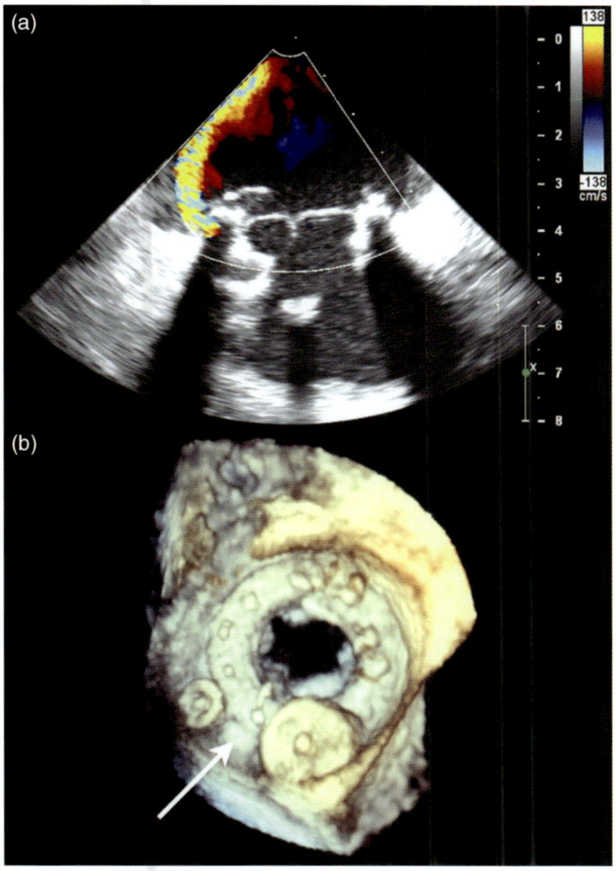

FIGURE 16.17

(a) Transesophageal echocardiographic image with color Doppler flow illustrating the residual posterior paravalvular defect. (b) Three-dimensional transesophageal echocardiographic images outlining the position of the two previously deployed closure devices and the residual defect (arrow). **(LOOP 16.17a, b)**

PLANNED PROCEDURE

Device closure of the residual paravalvular mitral defect.

PROCEDURE

A telescoping catheter system as previously described was placed transseptally in the left atrium, and an exchange-length stiff angled glide wire was used to cross the defect. In attempting to advance the catheters across the residual defect, the adjacent PDA occluder device was dislodged (Figure 16.18a, b) and embolized to the right common iliac artery. Next, device closure of the paravalvular defect was performed, with two devices using a simultaneous deployment technique. The defect was crossed with a 6-Fr multipurpose guiding catheter, through which two 260-cm and 0.032-inch Amplatz extra-stiff exchange wires with broad curves were placed in the left ventricular cavity. The delivery catheters were removed and two separate telescoping catheter delivery systems were advanced over the wires, across the defect, and into the left ventricular cavity. This allowed two 12-mm AVP-II devices to be advanced and simultaneously deployed in the defect (Figures 16.19 and 16.20). An excellent result with very mild residual regurgitation and no interference with the prosthetic valve function was achieved. The devices were released and attention was then given to the embolized device.

COMPLICATION AND MANAGEMENT

An 8-Fr 45-cm sheath was placed in the right femoral artery. This was advanced to the embolized device in the right common iliac, and a bioptome was brought into the sheath. The bioptome did not have sufficient strength to pull the device into the 8-Fr sheath (Figure 16.21), although it was pulled further distally into the right external iliac artery. The femoral sheath was replaced with a 10-Fr sheath and the device grasped using the bioptome and withdrawn through the sheath (Figure 16.22). Final angiography demonstrated no arterial injury. The patient experienced marked clinical benefit and at 2-month follow-up had required no further blood transfusions. There were no vascular sequelae.

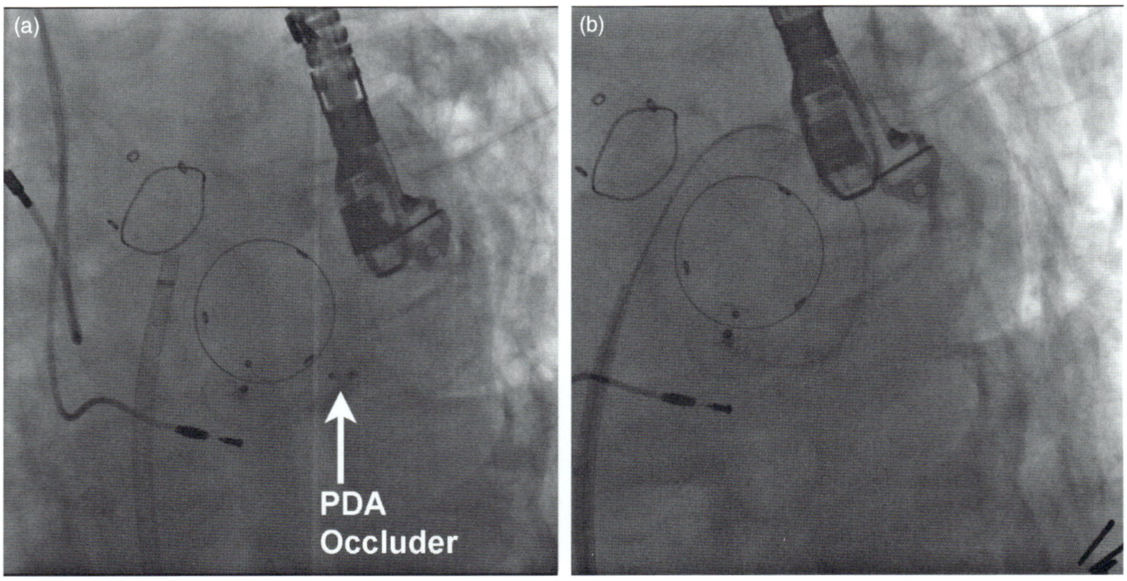

FIGURE 16.18

(a) Fluoroscopic images showing the two previously placed occluder devices and an Agilis sheath in the left atrial cavity. (b) The previously seen Amplatzer PDA occluder device is no longer visualized adjacent to the prosthetic valve. **(LOOP 16.18a, b)**

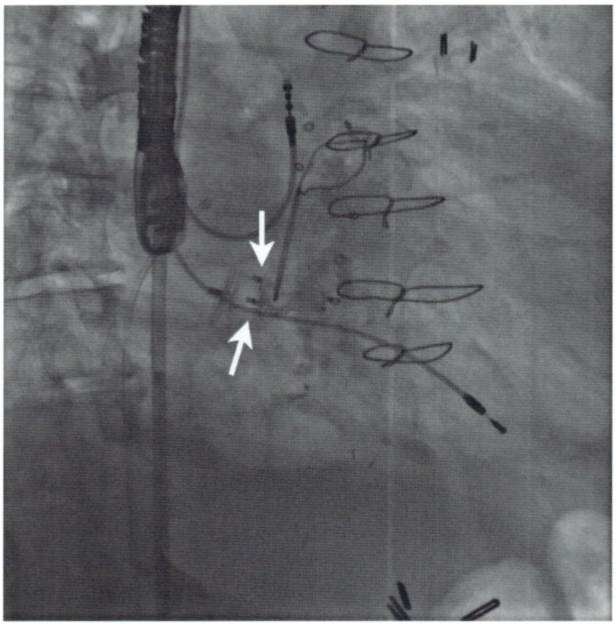

FIGURE 16.19

Fluoroscopic image of two new Amplatzer Vascular Plugs (AVP-IIs, arrows) deployed in the residual paravalvular defect adjacent to the prior device. **(LOOP 16.19)**

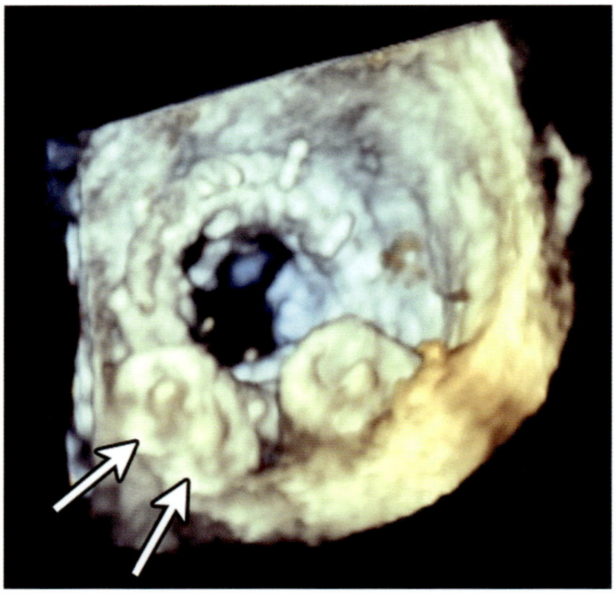

FIGURE 16.20

Three-dimensional transesophageal echocardiographic image of two new AVP-II devices (arrows) now deployed in the paravalvular defect. **(LOOP 16.20)**

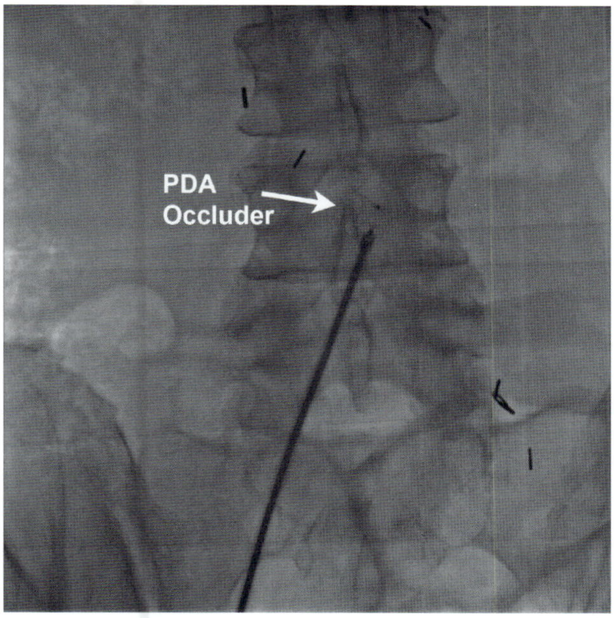

FIGURE 16.21

Fluoroscopic image of the embolized PDA occluder at the origin of the right common iliac artery. It is grasped with a bioptome through an 8-Fr sheath. **(LOOP 16.21)**

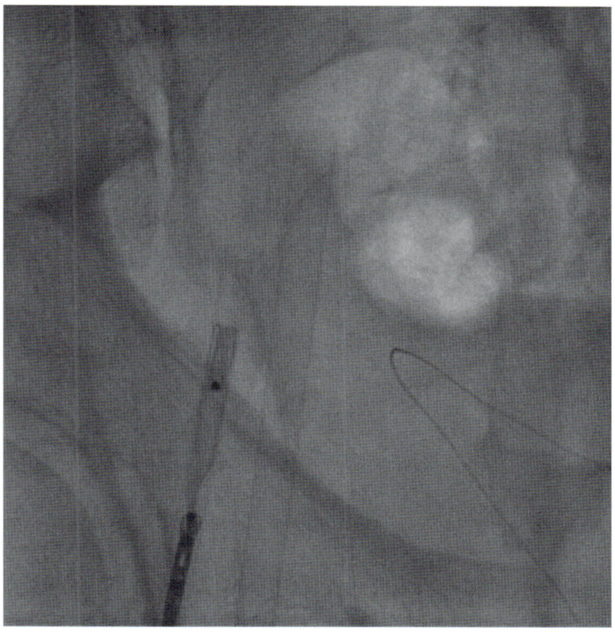

FIGURE 16.22

Fluoroscopic image of the embolized device being withdrawn through a 10-Fr femoral sheath using a bioptome. **(LOOP 16.22)**

CASE ANALYSIS

Attempting to cross a defect adjacent to a previously deployed device in a paravalvular defect can be difficult. The device may obstruct passage of the catheter and necessitate significant force to advance the catheter. The Amplatzer PDA occluder has only a distal retention disk and this, coupled with minimal healing and endothelialization, likely caused dislodgment of the occluder and embolization. A device with a proximal retention disk may be less likely to embolize in this circumstance. Solutions to defects that are large or irregularly shaped and likely to require multiple devices include advancement of multiple delivery catheters, as described in this case, or sequential device deployment techniques. In the sequential strategy, an anchor wire is exteriorized and used to retain access to the left ventricle. This allows repetitive crossing of the defect with a delivery system and sequential multiple device deployment. This technique reduces the risk of embolization as the deployed device is not yet released. Device obstruction to passage of the catheter remains a challenge.

LESSONS

- Care must be taken when crossing defects adjacent to recently deployed devices.
- The use of multiple smaller closure devices, either simultaneously or sequentially deployed, can result in more-effective closure of large irregularly shaped defects.

References

1. Cortes M, Garcia E, Garcia-Fernandez MA, Gomez JJ, Perez-David E, Fernandez-Aviles F. Usefulness of transesophageal echocardiography in percutaneous transcatheter repairs of paravalvular mitral regurgitation. *Am J Cardiol.* 2008:101:382–386.
2. Sorajja P, Cabalka AK, Hagler DJ, Reeder GS, Chandrasekaran K, Cetta F, Rihal CS. Successful percutaneous repair of perivalvular prosthetic regurgitation. *Catheter Cardiovasc Interv.* 2007;70:815–823.
3. Pate GE, Al Zubaidi A, Chandavimol M, Thompson CR, Munt BI, Webb JG. Techniques for percutaneous closure of prosthetic paravalvular leaks. *Catheter Cardiovasc Interv.* 2006;67:158–166.
4. Nietlispach F, Johnson M, Moss RR, et al. Transcatheter closure of paravalvular defects using a purpose-specific occluder. *JACC Cardiovasc Interv.* 2010;3(7):759–765.
5. Kim MS, Casserly IP, Garcia JA, Klein AJ, Salcedo EE, Carroll JD. Percutaneous transcatheter closure of prosthetic mitral paravalvular leaks: Are we there yet? *JACC Cardiovasc Interv.* 2009;2(2):81–90.

III

COMPLICATIONS OF PERIPHERAL VASCULAR INTERVENTIONS

17

Andrea Pacchioni, Luca Favero, Dimitrios Nikas, Salvatore Saccà, Giampaolo Pasquetto, Carlo Cernetti, Carlo Penzo, and Bernhard Reimers

Complications of Carotid Artery Stenting

INTRODUCTION

Carotid artery stenting (CAS) has emerged as an effective therapy for extracranial carotid artery stenosis in both symptomatic and asymptomatic patients if periprocedural complications are low. Therefore, efforts to reduce periprocedural complications are pivotal to improve the short- and long-term outcome of patients undergoing CAS.

Prevention of complications after CAS begins before the procedure by way of proper patient selection and initiation of antiplatelet therapy; continues during the procedure through appropriate diagnostic and interventional device selection, procedure execution, and adequate intraprocedural pharmacological treatment; and extends postprocedure through blood pressure control and neurological monitoring. The experience of the operator and the support staff is critical for complications prevention and management through all these phases.

CASE 17.1

Intrastent Plaque Prolapse

CLINICAL HISTORY AND DIAGNOSTIC TESTING RESULTS

A 71-year-old woman with history of type II diabetes mellitus and hypertension presented with crescendo TIAs and right internal carotid artery (RICA) stenosis, which were demonstrated by duplex ultrasound. Medical therapy was initiated with dual antiplatelet therapy (aspirin and clopidogrel) and a high-dose statin. Carotid angiography demonstrated high-grade ulcerated RICA stenosis (Figure 17.1a–c).

PLANNED PROCEDURE

CAS of the RICA with proximal protection with the MoMa device.

PROCEDURE

After administration of intravenous unfractionated heparin, the innominate artery was engaged with a 5-Fr AR mod catheter. A 0.035-inch hydrophilic J-wire (Terumo Glidewire®, Tokyo, Japan) was advanced to the external carotid artery using a road map. The 5-Fr AR mod catheter was advanced over the Terumo wire into the external carotid artery, and this wire was exchanged for a Hi-Torque Supracore® wire (Abbott Vascular, Abbott Park, IL). Once the Supracore wire was stable in the external carotid artery, the diagnostic catheter was retrieved and the 9-Fr MoMa proximal protection device (MoMa® Ultra Proximal Cerebral Protection Device, Medtronic Invatec, Roncadelle, Italy) advanced to the common carotid artery. CAS with flow blockage was then successfully performed per standard technique. A flexible open-cell self-expandable nitinol stent (Cordis Precise® 7 × 30 mm, Bridgewater, NJ) was chosen due to the severe angulation at the lesion site. Postdilation was performed with a semicompliant Sterling® balloon, 5 × 20 mm. (Boston Scientific, Natick, MA).

COMPLICATION AND MANAGEMENT

After postdilation, active blood aspiration, and deflation of the MoMa device, carotid angiography showed an intraluminal filling defect prolapsing through the stent (Figure 17.2a). The elastomeric balloons of the MoMa device were inflated again, and gentle intrastent balloon inflation was performed. Repeat carotid angiography showed persistence of the plaque prolapse (Figure 17.2b), therefore, a second overlapping stent was deployed (Cordis Precise, 7 × 30 mm) and

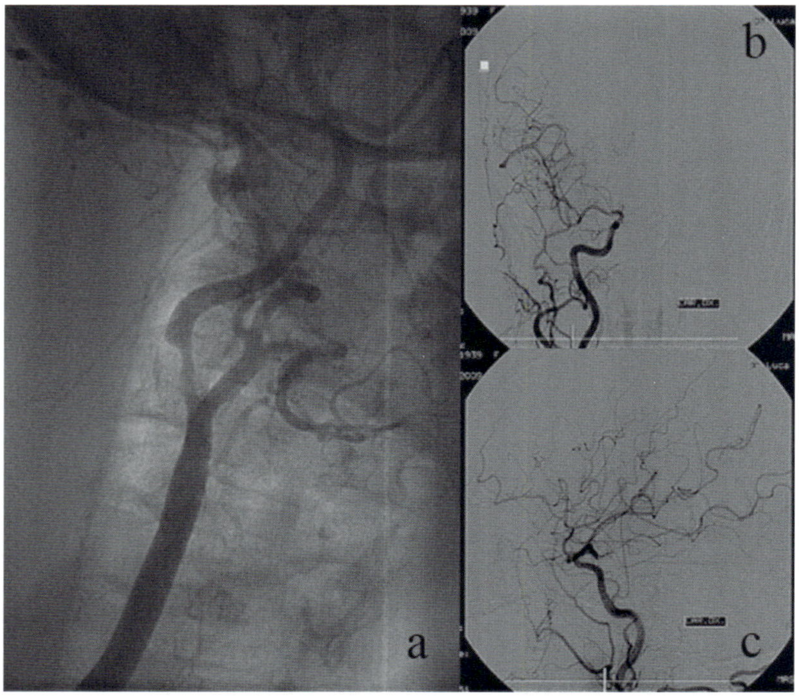

FIGURE 17.1

(a) Baseline angiography of right internal carotid artery showing high-grade ulcerated soft plaque. (b, c) Preprocedure cerebral angiography showing patent intracerebral vessels.

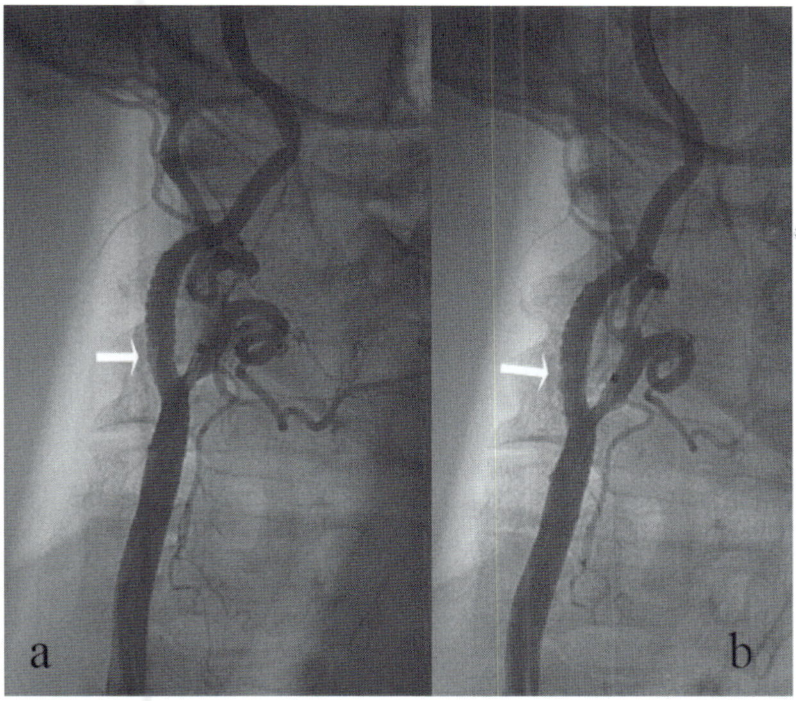

FIGURE 17.2
(a) An intraluminal filling defect through the stent cells (plaque prolapse) is present after stenting and post-dilation (arrow). (b) Plaque prolapse is still present after prolonged low-pressure balloon inflation (arrow).

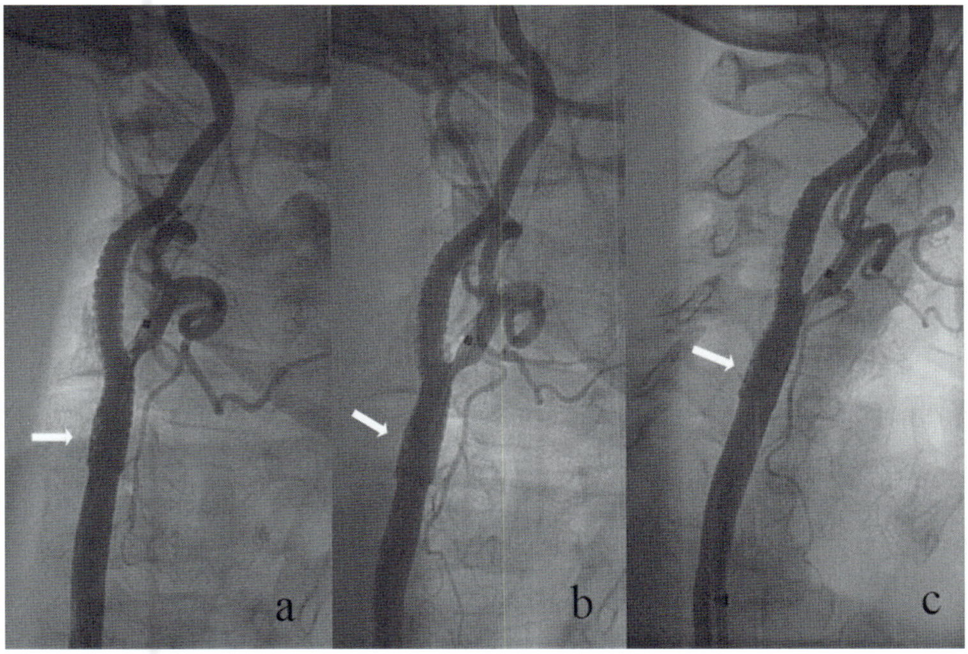

FIGURE 17.3
(a) The second stent led to resolution of the original plaque prolapsed, but a new more proximal plaque prolapse appeared (arrow). (b, c) The new plaque prolapse persisted after two more balloon dilations.

postdilated under protection of the MoMa device. Repeat carotid angiography showed improvement of the original plaque prolapse, but a new plaque prolapse appeared proximally in the common carotid artery (Figure 17.3a). This prolapse persisted despite two more balloon postdilations (Figure 17.3b, c). A third stent (Cordis Precise 9 × 20 mm) was implanted at the site of the new plaque prolapse under proximal protection, obtaining complete plaque sealing without prolapse (Figure 17.4a–d).

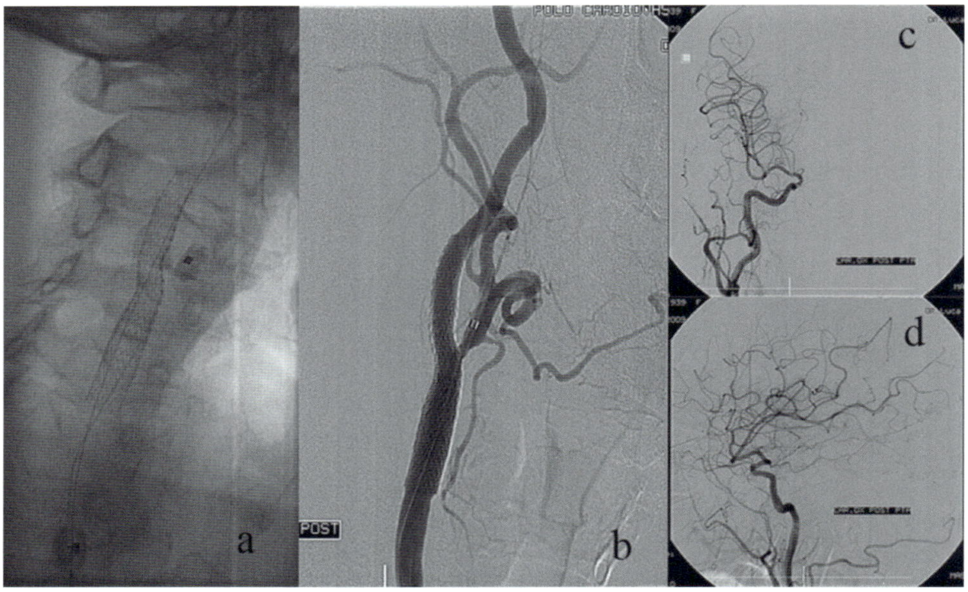

FIGURE 17.4

(a, b) A third stent was implanted with proximal protection, leading to resolution of the proximal plaque prolapse. (c, d) Postprocedure cerebral angiography showed no change from baseline.

CASE ANALYSIS

In this case, plaque prolapse through the stent occurred because an open-cell design stent was implanted in a soft lesion with large plaque burden. Ideally, this lesion should have been treated with a closed-cell design stent (mesh braided wire Carotid Wallstent®, Boston Scientific, Natick, MA; or nitinol Xact®, Abbott Vascular, Abbott Park, IL) to reduce the likelihood of plaque protrusion and fragments dislodgement. However, this design reduces flexibility of the stent, limiting its application in highly tortuous carotid arteries. Plaque prolapse may predispose to stent thrombosis, or it may lead to material embolization with subsequent ischemic neurological events. The best treatment for intrastent plaque prolapse remains uncertain. Minor plaque prolapse with limited lumen encroachment can be treated with dual antiplatelet therapy and early (1 month postprocedure) ultrasound evaluation. Large protruding plaques that encroach on the lumen should be eliminated with repeat balloon inflations or restenting if necessary. In these cases, postdilation must be performed with adequately sized balloon to minimise the risk of stent thrombosis, which appears to be higher with this technique.

LESSONS

- When CAS is planned in symptomatic patients with large plaque burden, closed-cell design stents reduce the chances of plaque prolapse.
- When intrastent plaque prolapse occur, its treatment depends on the degree it encroaches on the lumen.
- If balloon dilation does not adequately reduce the prolapsed plaque restenting should be considered.

SUGGESTED READING

Cremonesi A, Setacci C, Manetti R, et al. Carotid angioplasty and stenting: Lesion related treatment strategies. *EuroIntervention.* 2005;13:289–295.

Bosiers M, de Donato G, Deloose K, et al. Does free cell area influence the outcome in carotid artery stenting? *Eur J vasc Endovasc Surg.* 2007;33:135–141.

Hart JP, Peeters P, Verbist J, et al. Do device characteristics impact outcome in carotid artery stenting? *J Vasc Surg.* 2006;44:725–730.

CASE 17.2

Common Carotid Artery Dissection

CLINICAL HISTORY AND DIAGNOSTIC TESTING RESULTS

A 74-year-old man with history of type II diabetes, hypertension, dyslipidemia, and ischemic cardiomyopathy with recent symptoms of transient ischemic attacks (TIAs) (1 month ago). The patient was started on aspirin 100 mg/day and clopidogrel 75 mg/day and referred for carotid duplex ultrasound that showed subtotal occlusion of the left internal carotid artery (LICA). Carotid and cerebral angiography confirmed the presence of critical LICA stenosis and patent intracerebral vessels (Figure 17.5a–e).

PLANNED PROCEDURE

CAS of the LICA with proximal protection (MoMa device).

PROCEDURE

After administration of intravenous unfractionated heparin, the left common carotid artery was engaged with a 5-Fr JR4 catheter. A 0.035-inch hydrophilic J-wire (Terumo Glidewire®, Tokyo, Japan) was advanced to the external carotid artery using a road map. The 5-Fr JR4 catheter was advanced over the Terumo wire into the external carotid artery, and this wire was exchanged for a Hi-Torque Supracore® wire (Abbott Vascular, Abbott Park, IL). Once the Supracore wire was stable in the external carotid artery, the diagnostic catheter was retrieved, and the 9-Fr MoMa proximal protection device (Mo.Ma® Ultra Proximal Cerebral Protection Device, Medtronic Invatec) was advanced to the common carotid artery. CAS with flow blockage was then successfully performed over a 0.014-inch balanced middle weight (BMW) wire using a 6- to 8- × 40-mm Xact stent (Abbott Vascular, Abbott Park, IL) that was postdilated with a 5.5- × 20-mm Sterling semicompliant balloon (Boston Scientific, Natick, MA) (Figure 17.6a).

COMPLICATION AND MANAGEMENT

Carotid angiography after stent postdilation showed a flow-limiting dissection in the left common carotid artery proximal to the stent (Figure 17.6b, c). The patient was asymptomatic. A multipurpose 4-Fr catheter was advanced through the MoMa device over the BMW wire (that was used for CAS) into the LICA (Figure 17.7a). The 0.014-inch wire was then exchanged for a Supracore wire (Figure 17.7b). On further

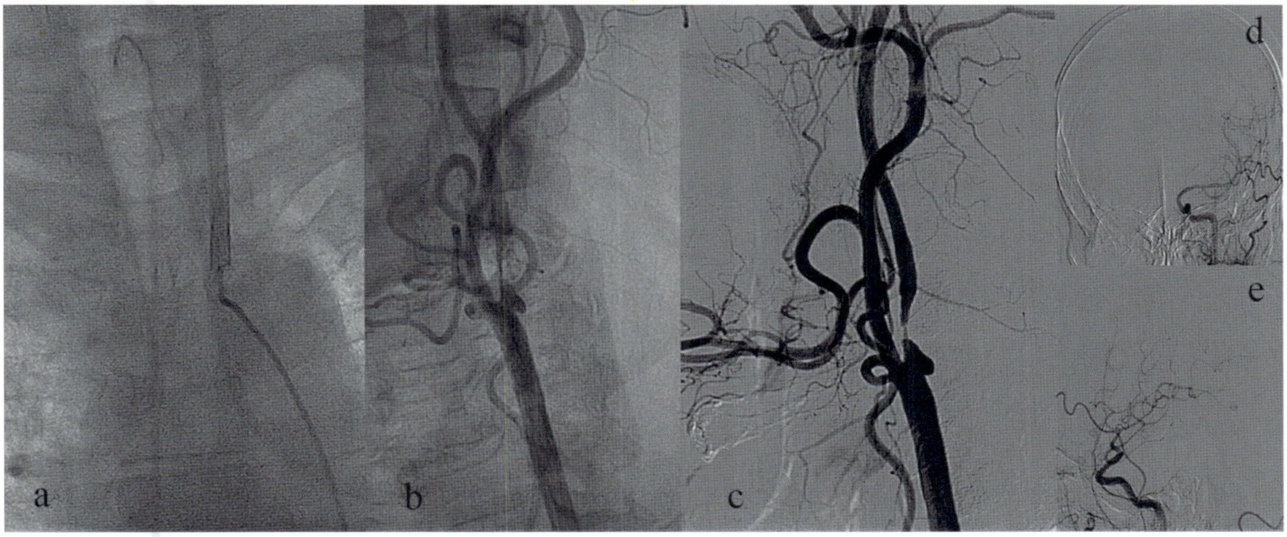

FIGURE 17.5

(a) Engagement of the left common carotid artery with a 6-Fr JR4 catheter. (b, c) Note the critical stenosis of the LICA. (d, e) Preserved intracerebral blood flow.

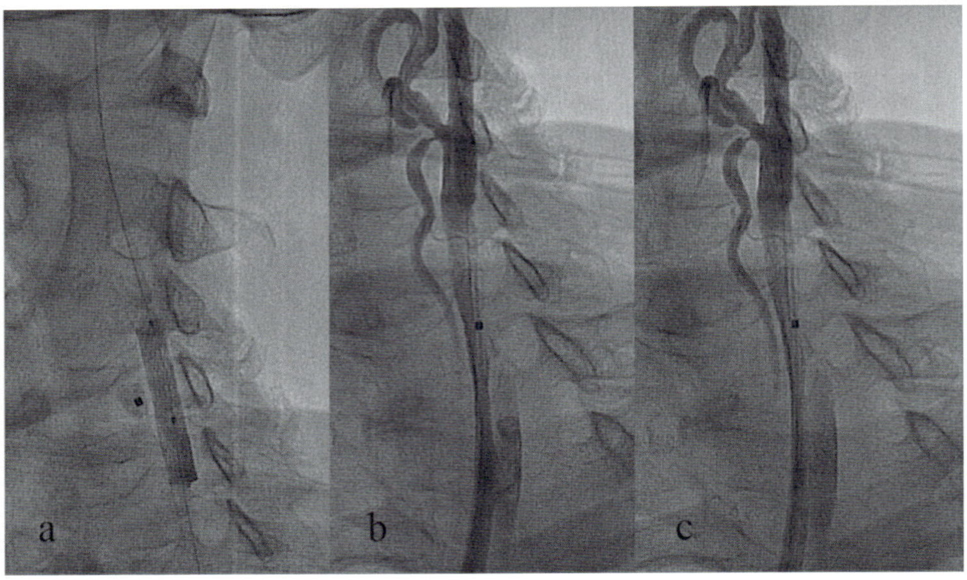

FIGURE 17.6
(a) CAS with proximal flow blockage. (b, c) Note the extensive flow-limiting dissection of the left common carotid artery (CCA).

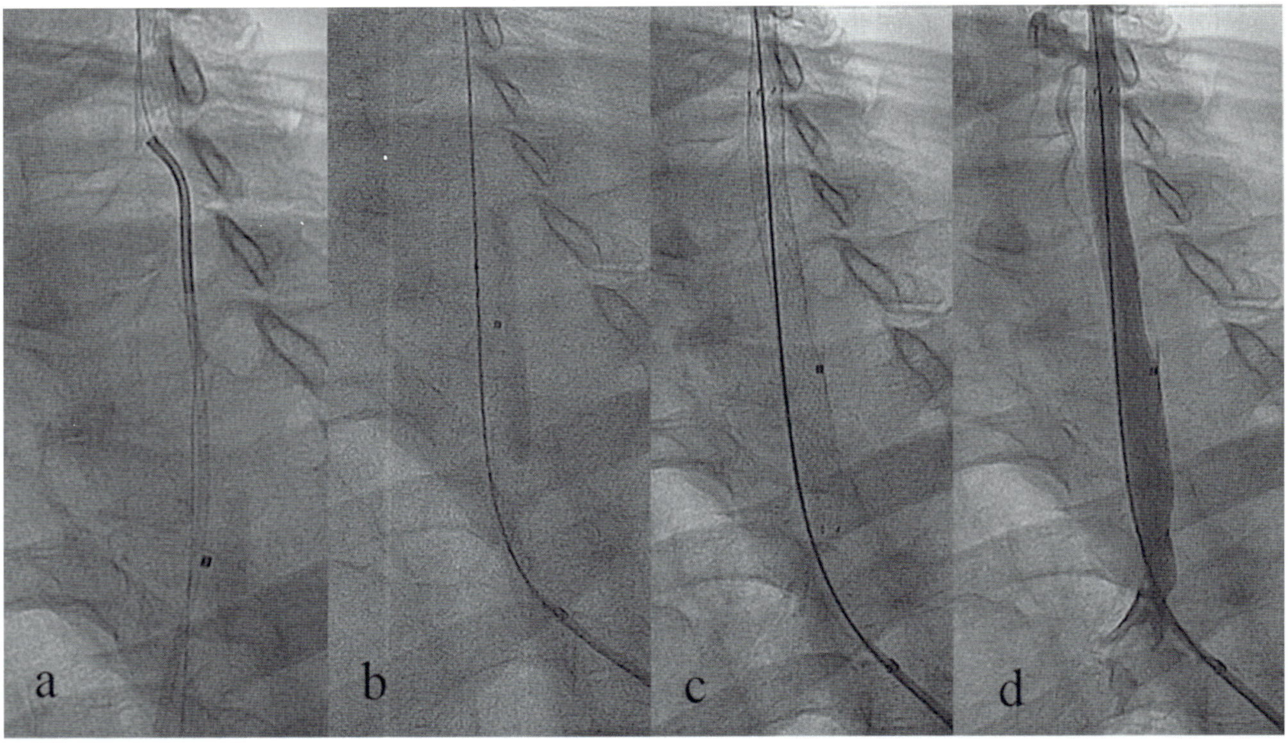

FIGURE 17.7
(a) A multipurpose diagnostic catheter was gently advanced into the implanted stent over the 0.014-inch BMW wire. (b) Exchange of the 0.014-inch BMW wire for a 0.035-inch Supracore wire. (c, d) Self-expandable stent implantation in the proximal and mid CCA.

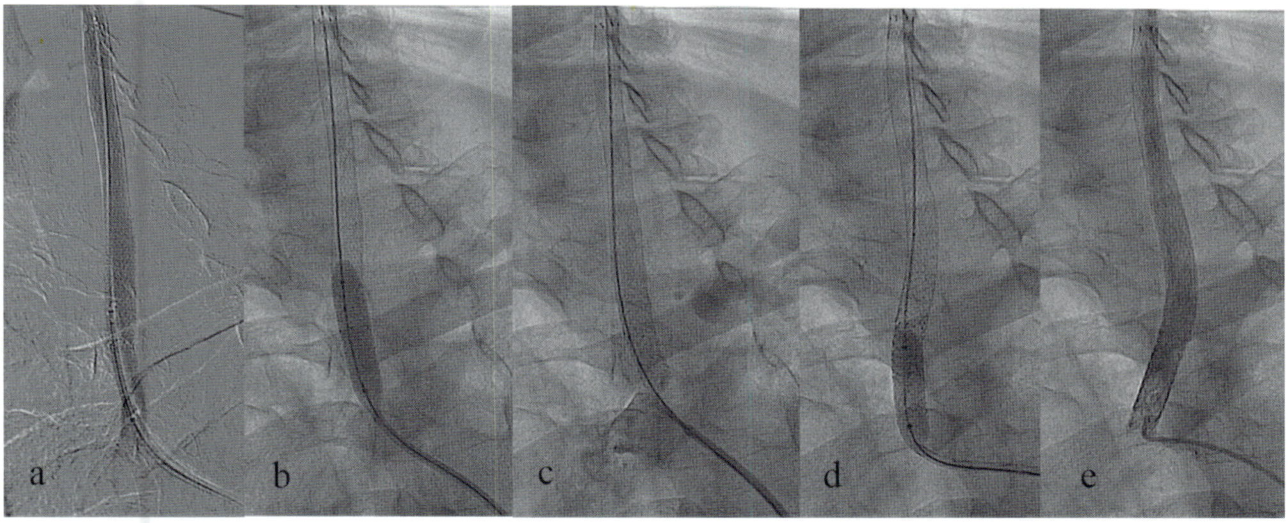

FIGURE 17.8
(a–e) Balloon-expandable stent implantation at the dissection origin in the left CCA ostium.

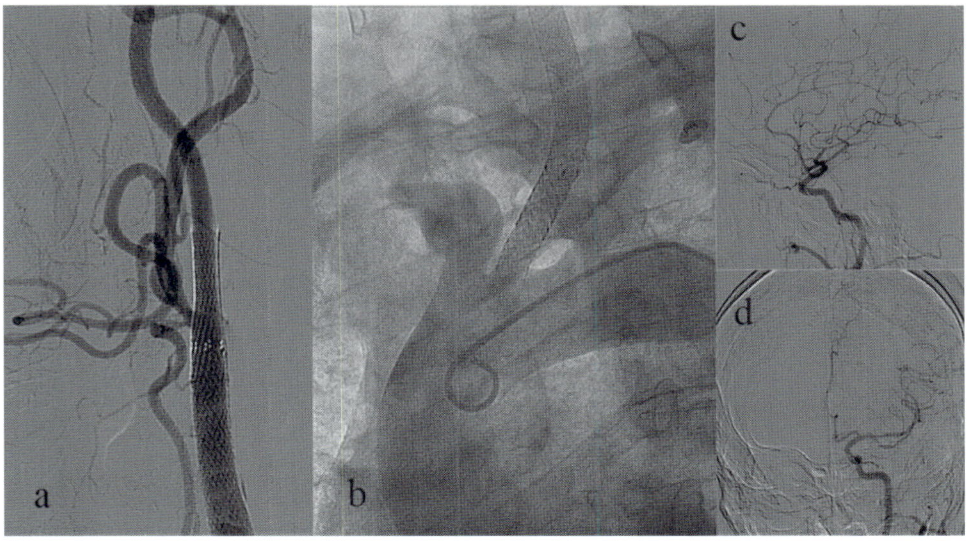

FIGURE 17.9
(a) Final carotid angiography; (b) aortic arch angiography; and (c, d) intracerebral angiography.

examination, the left common carotid artery dissection appeared to extend from the ostium of the common carotid artery upward, necessitating stenting the whole length of the left common carotid artery. An 8- × 80-mm Smart Control® stent (Cordis, Bridgewater, NJ) was deployed proximal to the LICA stent (Figure 17.7c, d) and two Omnilink® (Abbott Vascular, Abbott Park, IL) balloon-expandable stents (9 × 29 mm and 9 × 19 mm) were positioned more proximally, extending to the ostium of the common carotid artery. All stents were then postdilated with adequately sized balloons (Figure 17.8a–e). Final carotid, cerebral, and aortic angiography is shown in Figure 17.9.

CASE ANALYSIS

Although the cause of the left common carotid artery dissection in this case cannot be determined for certain, it is probably related to initial wiring with the Terumo wire. The operator did feel resistance to wire progression; nonetheless, he persisted with wire advancement through the common carotid artery. Most likely, the Terumo wire went subintimal through the proximal segment of the common carotid artery and then reentered the true lumen more distally. Advancement of the MoMa device through the dissection plane and subsequent inflation of the common carotid balloon extended the dissection to its full length. Although not all common carotid artery dissections need to be stented, the dissection in this case certainly needed to be treated because of its extent and encroachment on the lumen. Such dissections can cause thrombotic arterial occlusion or embolization, leading to major ischemic cerebral events. The successful management of this complication depended on its recognition before removing the 0.014-inch wire from the LICA.

LESSONS

- The operator should always be sensitive to any resistance to wire advancement into the carotid arteries. "Road mapping" during wire advancement is a valuable tool to avoid complications.
- After CAS, always perform carotid angiography prior to removal of the wire/filter from the internal carotid artery to ensure the presence of dissections.
- Extensive common carotid artery dissections should be stented.

SUGGESTED READING

Kremer C, Mosso M, Georgiadis D, et al. Carotid dissection with permanent and transient occlusion or severe stenosis: Long-term outcome. *Neurology.* 2003;60:271–275.

Nicosia A, Nikas D, Castriota F, et al. Classification for carotid artery stenting complications: Manifestation, management and prevention. *J Endovasc Ther.* 2010;17:275–294.

CASE 17.3

Common Carotid Artery Rupture

CLINICAL HISTORY AND DIAGNOSTIC TESTING RESULTS

An 82-year-old man with history of hypertension and prior right carotid endarterectomy (CEA) was found to have RICA restenosis and 90% de novo stenosis of the LICA (mixed hypoechogenic and calcified plaque) on routine duplex ultrasound evaluation. Brain MRI did not show any cerebral defects. Patient was referred for diagnostic carotid angiography, which showed severe and calcified LICA stenosis (Figure 17.10).

PLANNED PROCEDURE

CAS of the LICA with distal protection.

PROCEDURE

After administration of intravenous unfractionated heparin, the left common carotid artery was engaged with an Amplatz right modified catheter. A 0.035-inch hydrophilic J-wire (Terumo Glidewire®, Tokyo, Japan) was advanced to the external carotid artery using a road map. The diagnostic catheter was advanced over the Terumo wire into the external carotid artery, and this wire was exchanged for a Hi-Torque Supracore® wire (Abbott Vascular, Abbott Park, IL). Once the Supracore wire was stable in the external carotid artery, the diagnostic catheter was retrieved and a 6-Fr × 90-cm-long introducer sheath (Pinnacle Destination®, Terumo, Tokyo, Japan) was advanced and positioned in the left common carotid artery. A 5.5-mm Accunet filter (Abbott Vascular, Abbott Park, IL) was advanced through the lesion and positioned in the distal LICA. The lesion was predilated with a Maverick® 4- × 20-mm semicompliant balloon (Boston Scientific, Natick, MA) at 10 atm. CAS was then performed using a 7- × 40-mm Precise stent (Cordis, Bridgewater, NJ). The stent was postdilated with a 6- × 20-mm Sterling balloon at 10 atm (Figure 17.11a–d).

COMPLICATION AND MANAGEMENT

Carotid angiography after postdilatation showed extravasation at the site of the calcified plaque, which is consistent with that of vessel wall rupture (Figure 17.12a). Immediate flow blockage was instated, heparin was partially reversed with protamine sulphate, and prolonged low-pressure balloon inflation was performed. These measures resulted in almost complete sealing of the extravasation (Figure 17.12b–d). The patient remained hemodynamically stable without any neurologic events. Follow-up carotid duplex ultrasound prior to discharge showed complete vessel healing (Figure 17.13).

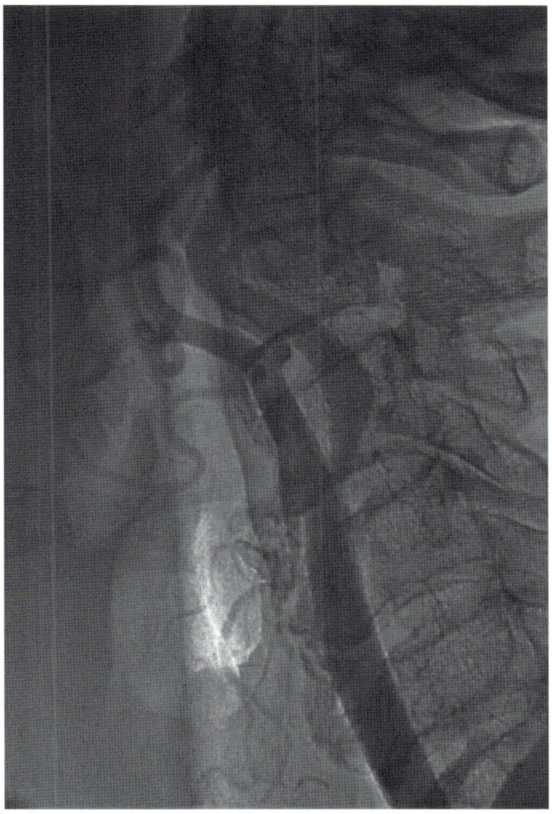

FIGURE 17.10
Heavily calcified stenosis of the LICA.

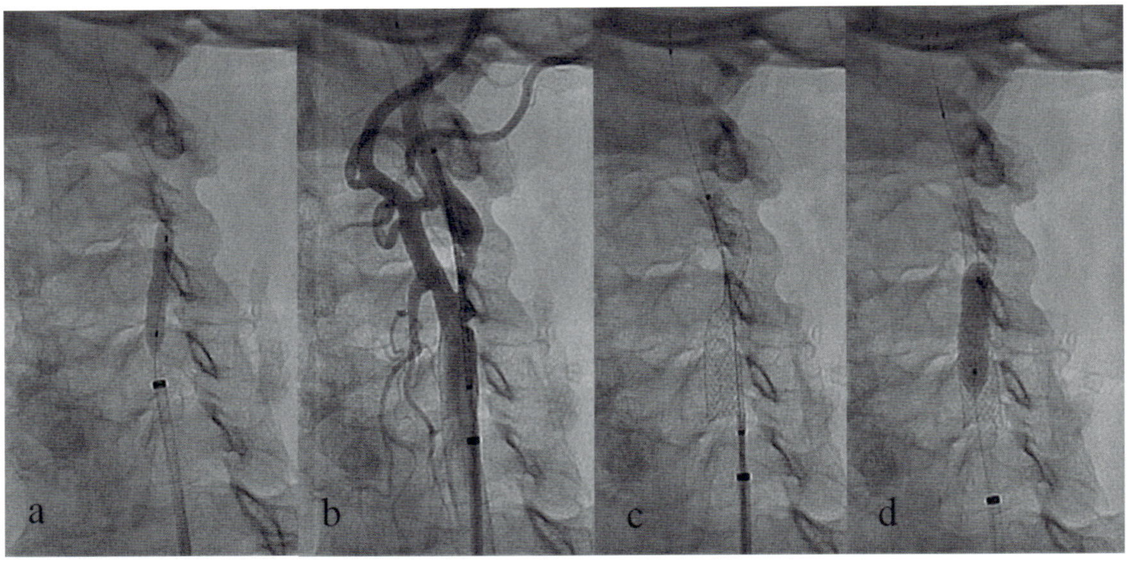

FIGURE 17.11
(a) Predilatation with a 4-mm semicompliant balloon at 10 atm, (b) stent positioning, and (c, d) postdilatation with a semicompliant 6-mm balloon at 10 atm.

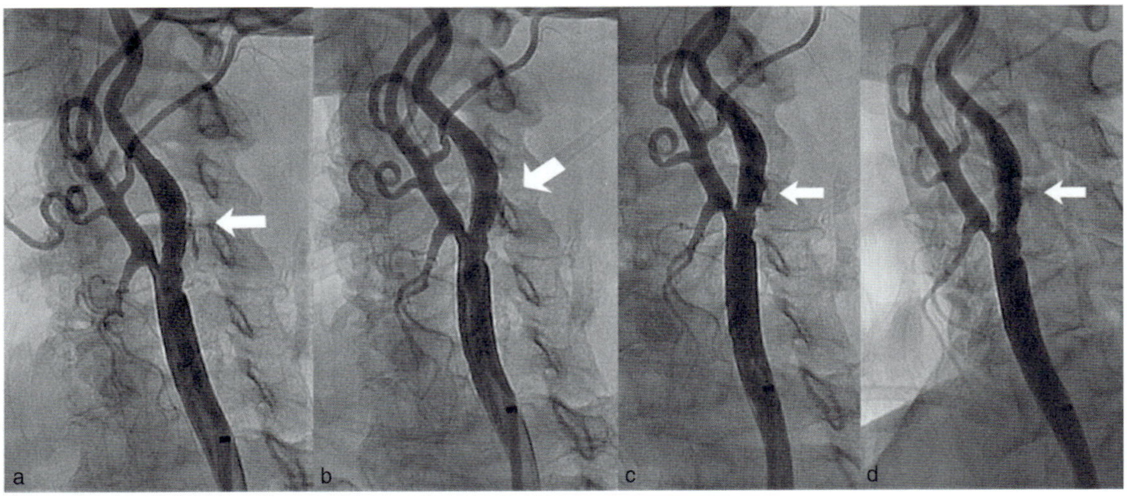

FIGURE 17.12
(a–d) Extravasation (arrows) was significantly reduced after heparin reversal and prolonged low-pressure balloon inflation.

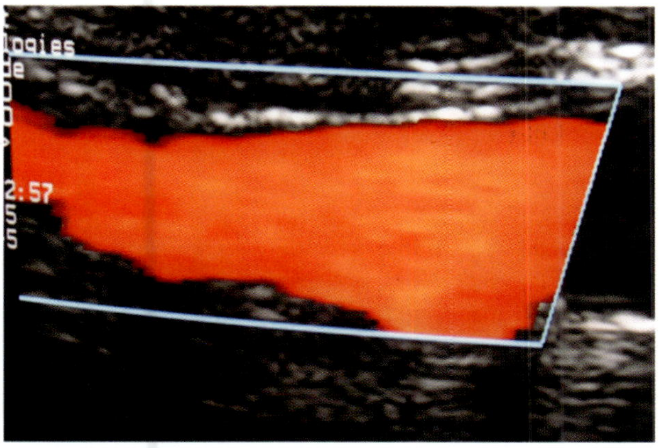

FIGURE 17.13

Follow-up duplex ultrasound prior to discharge showed complete vessel wall healing without pseudo-aneurysm or dissection.

CASE ANALYSIS

In this case, carotid vessel rupture occurred because of the use of an oversized balloon (6 mm) for postdilatation to overcome the resistance of a calcified lesion. In most likelihood, this complication would have been avoided if we used a 5.5-mm balloon for postdilatation. Although the use of an undersized balloon may have resulted in a suboptimal result in terms of residual percent diameter stenosis (DS), this is often inconsequential except for the possibility of higher restenosis rate.

Management of vessel wall rupture begins with immediate reversal of anticoagulation and prolonged low-pressure balloon inflation at the site of rupture as long as it is tolerated by the patient. If extravasation persists, referral to immediate surgical exploration is needed. If this option is not available, implantation of a covered stent should be considered. It is also crucial to continuously inspect the neck for any signs of hematoma or compromise in respiratory status. There should be a very low threshold for intubation to preserve the airway.

LESSONS

- Balloon oversizing should be avoided when postdilating carotid stents during CAS. In the majority of patients, a 5- to 5.5-mm noncompliant balloon would be sufficient. Rarely, there is a need for a 6-mm balloon.
- When faced with a nondilatable carotid stenosis, the operator should opt for a noncompliant undersized balloon inflated at high pressure rather than an oversized balloon. In these cases, one may accept a suboptimal results (i.e., residual %DS of 30%–50%).
- Carotid vessel wall rupture is an emergency that should be taken seriously. Immediate reversal of anticoagulation, low-pressure balloon inflation, maintaining the airways, and alerting surgical colleagues are keys for successful management.

SUGGESTED READING

Wada H, Piotin M, Boissonnet H, et al. Carotid rupture during stent-assisted aneurysm treatment. *AJNR Am J Neuroradiol.* 2004;25(5):827–829.

Rigatelli G, Sacco LL, Sacco A, et al. Iliac stent graft for common carotid artery rupture. *Cardiovasc Revasc Med.* 2007;8(3):226–227.

CASE 17.4

Filter Occlusion

CLINICAL HISTORY AND DIAGNOSTIC TESTING RESULTS

An 84-year-old man with multiple cardiovascular risk factors and previous myocardial infarction was found to have a carotid bruit during routine examination. Carotid duplex ultrasound showed occlusion of the RICA and critical stenosis of the LICA (echolucent plaque). Carotid angiography confirmed the diagnosis of LICA stenosis (Figure 17.14a–d).

PLANNED PROCEDURE

CAS of the LICA with distal protection.

PROCEDURE

Patient was pretreated with dual antiplatelet therapy (aspirin 100 mg and clopidogrel 75 mg). After systemic heparinization, an 8-Fr Guider softip™ XF (Boston Scientific, Natick, MA) was used to engage the ostium of the left common carotid artery. A 6.5-mm Accunet® filter (Abbott Vascular, Abbott Park, IL) was advanced through the lesion and positioned in a straight landing zone in the distal LICA. An 8.0- × 30-mm Vascuflex® nitinol open-cell self-expandable stent (Braun, Betlehem, PA) was deployed, and postdilatation was performed using a 5- × 20-mm Sterling semicompliant balloon.

COMPLICATION AND MANAGEMENT

Carotid angiography after postdilatation demonstrated slow flow, but the patient remained asymptomatic (Figure 17.15a–c). The slow flow resolved after filter removal without angiographic or neurological consequences (Figure 17.16).

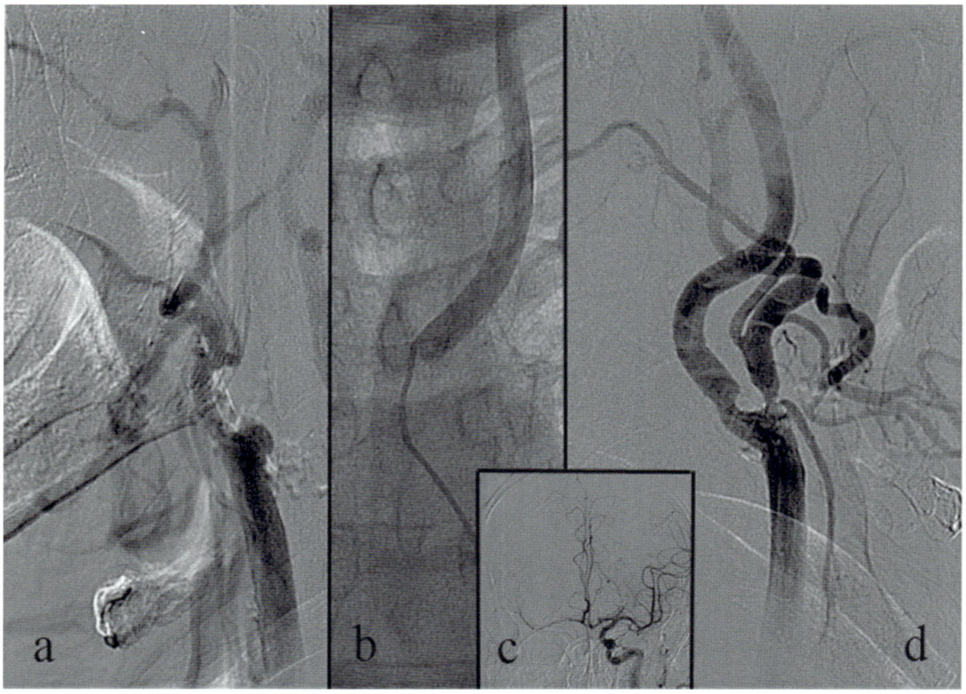

FIGURE 17.14

(a) RICA occlusion. (b) Engagement of the left CCA. (c) Intracerebral blood flow is almost exclusively provided by the LICA. (d) LICA stenosis.

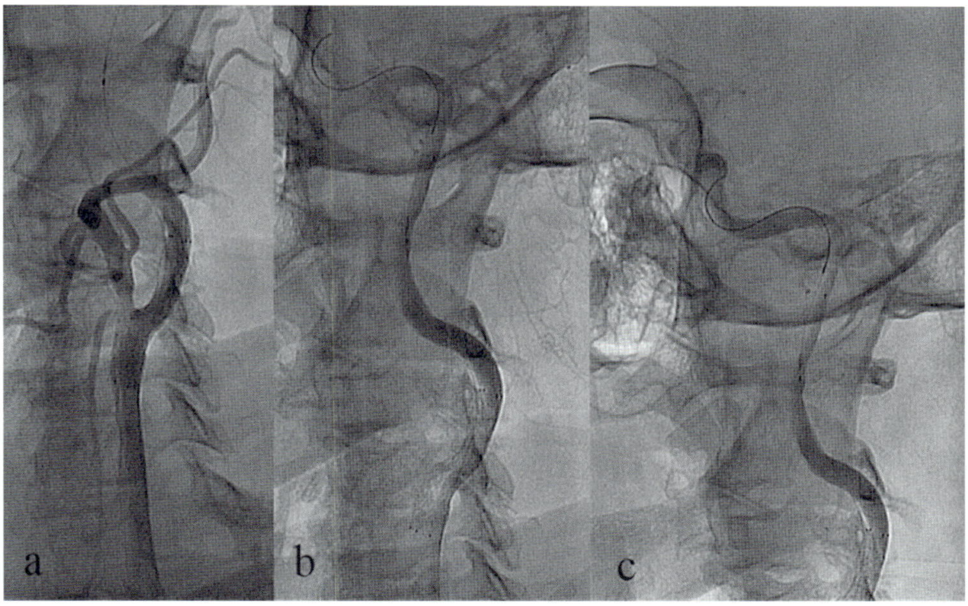

FIGURE 17.15

(a–c) Carotid slow flow after balloon postdilatation. Note the complete blockage of flow at the filter site. (LOOP 17.15)

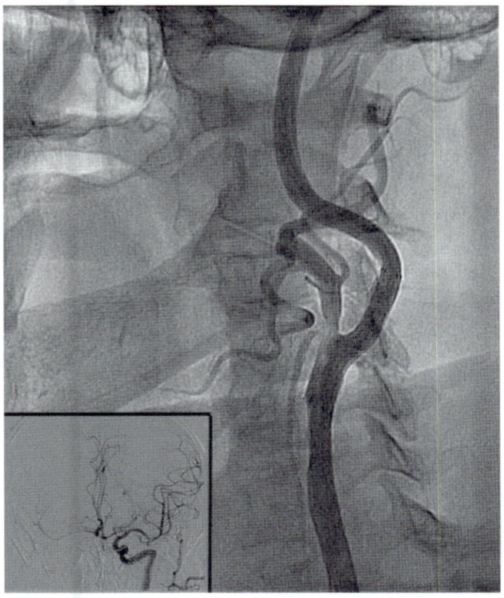

FIGURE 17.16

Normalized carotid flow after filter removal. (LOOP 17.16)

CASE ANALYSIS

The slow flow in this case occurred because the filter occluded with embolized material. In this situation, filter removal generally restores blood flow immediately in almost all cases, as was demonstrated in this case. However, catheter-based aspiration of debris from inside the filter should be attempted before retrieval to reduce the amount of material in the basket. In addition, the filter should never be fully withdrawn into the retrieval sheath because the retained embolic material may be squeezed out through the filter pores. It has been demonstrated that symptomatic patients, vulnerable carotid plaques (as defined by MR plaque imaging), and larger stent sizes are risk factors for filter occlusion during CAS. The differential diagnosis of slow flow after CAS should include intracranial shower of microemboli, carotid spasm, and common carotid artery dissection.

LESSONS

- Distal filter device occlusion during CAS occurs more often in symptomatic patients, in asymptomatic patients with "vulnerable plaques," and in association with large stent sizes.
- Distal filter device occlusion should be suspected in any case with slow flow after CAS.
- If distal filter device occlusion is suspected, filter aspiration should be attempted to reduce the burden of the embolized material before filter retrieval.

SUGGESTED READING

Casserly IP, Abou-Chebl A, Fathi RB, et al. Slow-flow phenomenon during carotid artery intervention with embolic protection devices: predictors and clinical outcome. *J Am Coll Cardiol.* 2005;46(8):1466–1472.

Sakamoto M, Taoka T, Nakagawa H, et al. Magnetic resonance plaque imaging to predict the occurrence of the slow-flow phenomenon in carotid artery stenting procedures. *Neuroradiology.* 2010;52(4):275–283.

CASE 17.5

Filter Device Embolization and Intracerebral Vessel Rupture

CLINICAL HISTORY AND DIAGNOSTIC TESTING RESULTS

A 77-year-old man with history of type II diabetes, hypertension, dyslipidemia, and previous myocardial infarction was referred to us after a routine carotid duplex ultrasound showed a heavily calcified stenosis of the LICA. The patient was asymptomatic. Carotid angiography confirmed the diagnosis (Figure 17.17a–c).

PLANNED PROCEDURE

CAS of the LICA with distal protection.

PROCEDURE

After administration of intravenous unfractionated heparin, the left common carotid artery was engaged with an Amplatz right modified catheter. A 0.035-inch hydrophilic J-wire (Terumo Glidewire®, Tokyo, Japan) was advanced to the external carotid artery using a road map. The diagnostic catheter was advanced over the Terumo wire into the external carotid artery, and this wire was exchanged for a Hi-Torque Supracore® wire (Abbott Vascular, Abbott Park, IL). Once the Supracore wire was stable in the external carotid artery, the diagnostic catheter was retrieved and a 6-Fr × 90-cm-long introducer sheath (Pinnacle Destination®, Terumo, Tokyo, Japan) was advanced and positioned in the left common carotid artery. A 7-mm Angioguard filter was advanced through the lesion and positioned in the distal LICA. The lesion was predilated with a 4- × 20-mm cutting balloon (Boston Scientific, Natick, MA). CAS was then performed using a 7- × 30-mm Precise stent (Cordis, Bridgewater, NJ). The stent was postdilated with a 6- × 20-mm Sterling balloon (Figure 17.18a–c).

COMPLICATION AND MANAGEMENT

During retrieval of the filter, the very distal part of the filter wire detached and embolized to the middle cerebral artery (Figure 17.19a–c). Several attempts were made to capture the filter with a gooseneck snare and with a maverick 1.5- × 8-mm balloon, which was moved up and down to mobilize the embolized wire (Figure 17.20a–f). During these attempts, the embolized wire penetrated the vessel wall, causing small intracerebral haemorrhage (Figure 17.21a–c). Anticoagulation was immediately reversed with protamine sulphate, and the procedure was aborted. The patient was transferred to the stroke unit, where he was closely monitored and conservatively managed with intravenous mannitol. The intracerebral haemorrhage stopped without clinical consequences. The patient was discharged home after 1 week on dual antiplatelet therapy. At 1 year follow-up, the patient was alive and free of events.

CASE ANALYSIS

In this case, filter fracture and embolization were not predicted because we did not encounter technical difficulties during filter retrieval. On the other hand, the intracerebral haemorrhage occurred because of the aggressive attempts to retrieve the embolized filter fragment.

Typically, filter disruption occurs during technically challenging retrieval either because of the operator inability to manipulate the retrieval catheter through a tortuous internal carotid artery (ICA) or because of filter entrapment in the stent struts during removal. The latter occurs when the filter is pulled back with the mouth partially open. Filter entrapment carries the risk of filter disruption and potential embolization of debris. There are several technical tips to deal with this complication and avoid deleterious consequences. First, ask the patient to rotate the neck or to swallow. If this fails, three techniques can be attempted: advance the introducer sheath or guiding catheter into the stent to provide adequate support to capture the filter with the retrieval catheter, or advance a "buddy-wire" to the ICA or external carotid artery (ECA) to modify the course of the vessel and facilitate filter retrieval, or advance a 5-Fr diagnostic catheter with a Judkins right or vertebral curve to retrieve the filter instead of the dedicated retrieval catheter. Pulling the filter aggressively downward should never be attempted because it may result in filter disruption or even basket entrapment into the stent struts. On the contrary, the operator should try to advance the filter carefully to reduce the surface contact between the filter and the stent, allowing advancement of the retrieval sheath. Surgical removal of the entrapped filter should be considered when all maneuvers have failed.

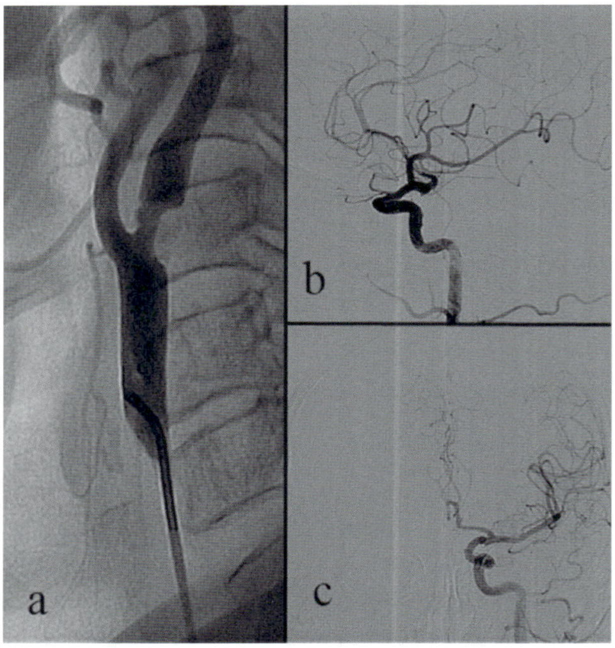

FIGURE 17.17
(a–c) Baseline LICA angiography demonstrating calcified stenosis and preserved cerebral circulation.

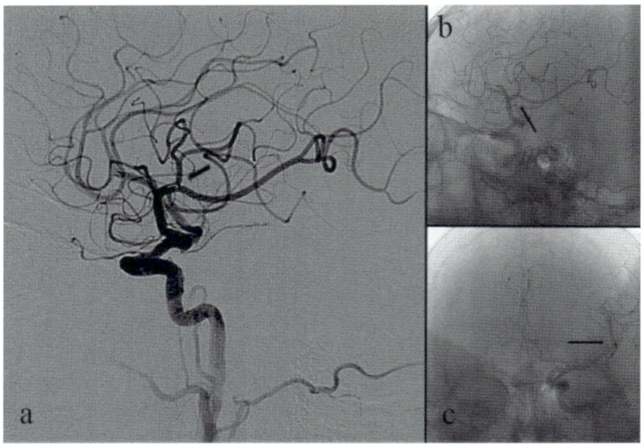

FIGURE 17.19
(a–c) Intracerebral angiography demonstrating embolization of the distal tip of the filter wire to the middle cerebral artery (arrows). Note that filter retrieval was performed without noticeable difficulties.

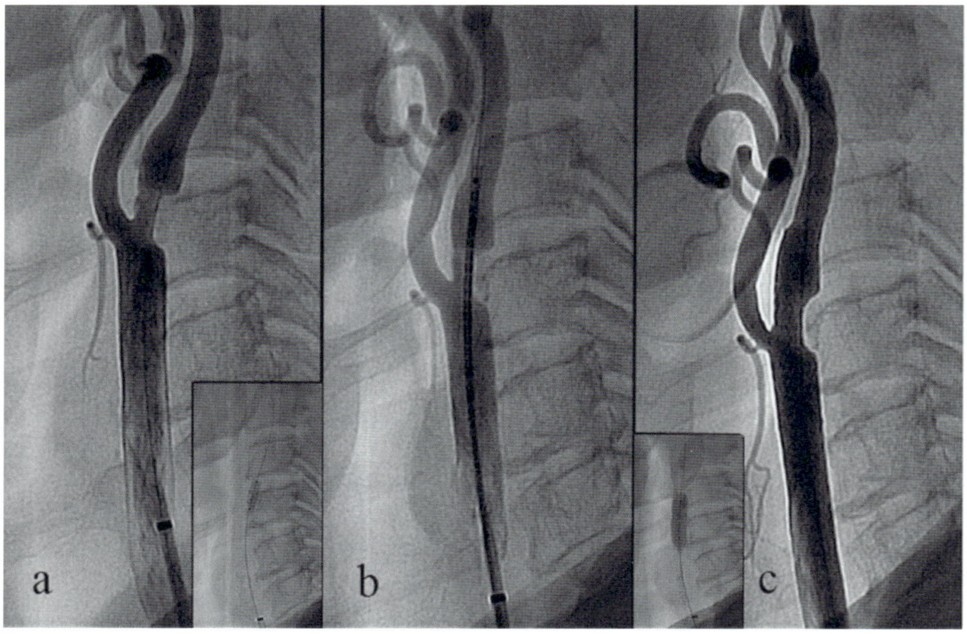

FIGURE 17.18
(a–c) CAS with distal protection was performed as planned.

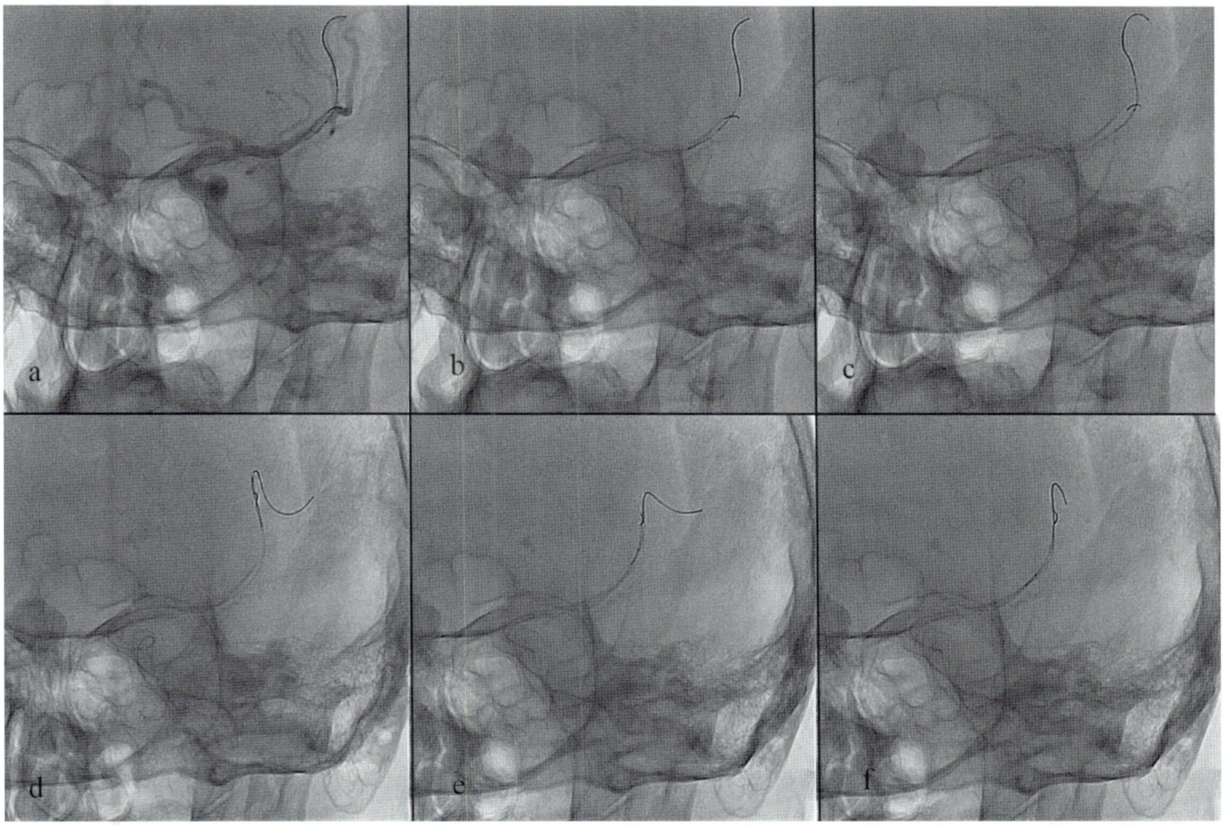

FIGURE 17.20
(a–f) Multiple attempts to remove the fractured wire with a gooseneck catheter and a low profile balloon failed.

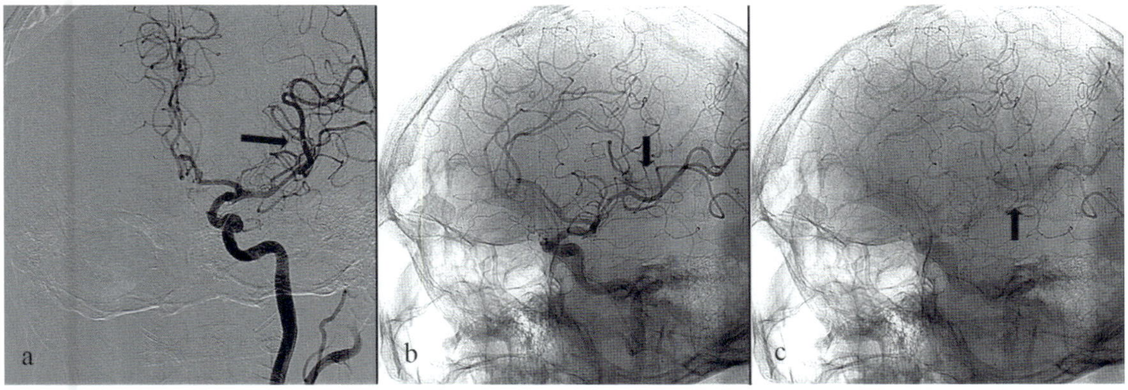

FIGURE 17.21
(a–c) Note the extravasation due to vessel wall rupture by the tip of the wire (arrows).

LESSONS

- When resistance is encountered during advancement of the filter retrieval sheath, the operator should make sure that the filter does not get pulled down toward the stent struts. All the manuevers described above to facilitate retrieval sheath advancement should be attempted.
- If the filter device is inadvertently pulled down and entrapped with the distal stent struts, several techniques can facilitate its disengagement. Never forcefully pull the filter down. The easiest manuever is to ask the patient to rotate the neck and swallow. If this does not work, then other techniques (described above) can be attempted.
- If filter fragments embolize to the intracranial cerebral vessels retrieval attempts should be very judicious and conservative because aggressive attempts at retrieval can easily cause vessel rupture.

SUGGESTED READING

Ganim RP, Muench A, Giesler GM, et al. Difficult retrieval of the EPI filterwire with a 5 French JR4 coronary catheter following carotid stenting. *Catheter Cardiovasc Interv.* 2006;67:309–311.

Schilling K, Uretsky BF, Hunter GC. Entrapment of a cerebral embolic protection device—A case report. *Vasc Endovascular Surg.* 2006;40:229–233.

18

Giovanni B. Torsello and Giovanni F. Torsello

Complications of Endovascular Repair of Abdominal Aortic Aneurysms

CASE 18.1

Inadverent Occlusion of the Renal Arteries During EVAR

CLINICAL HISTORY AND DIAGNOSTIC TESTING RESULTS

A 72-year-old man with history of hypertension, renal insufficiency, and coronary artery disease (CAD) was recently diagnosed with asymptomatic infrarenal abdominal aortic aneurysm (AAA) by duplex ultrasound. Preprocedure CT angiography confirmed the presence of AAA and dilatation of the common iliac arteries.

PLANNED PROCEDURE

Implantation of a Fortron (Cordis Bridgewater, NJ) aortoiliac endograft.

PROCEDURE

Implantation of the Forton endograft proceeded as per standard technique. The main body of the graft was introduced from the right femoral access. At the last stage of the main body deployment, the graft "jumped" proximally and the patient reported abdominal pain.

COMPLICATION AND MANAGEMENT

Abdominal aortogram after graft upward motion revealed occlusion of both renal arteries (Figure 18.1). As the main body of the graft was already deployed, a double curved catheter was inserted from the right side, and a glide wire was used to canulate the left iliac artery (crossover approach) (Figure 18.2). After snaring the wire through the contralateral access, the stent graft was pulled down by carefully retracting both ends of the crossover wire. Subsequently, the patency of the renal arteries and the integrity of the aorta was verified by aortic angiography (Figure 18.3). and follow-up CT scan.

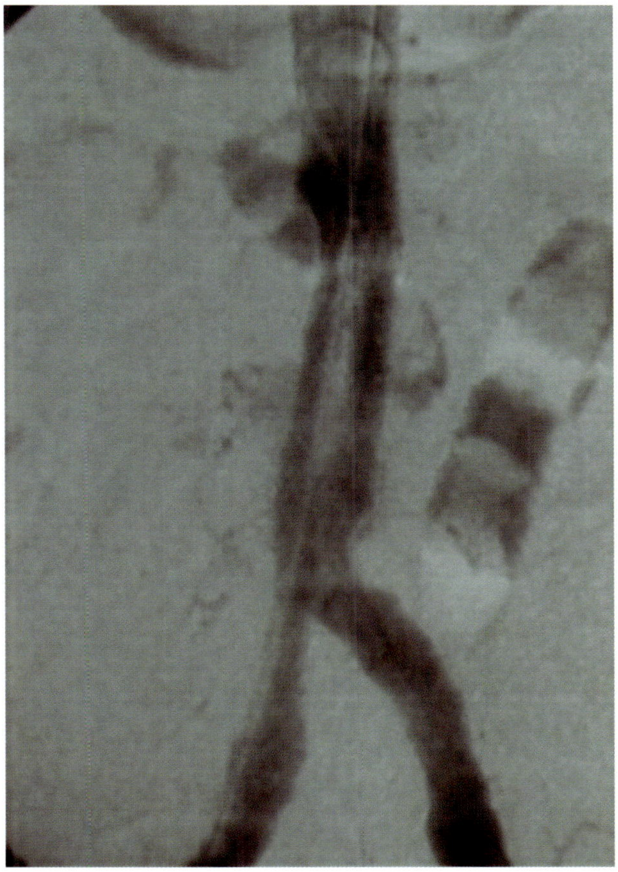

FIGURE 18.1
Occlusion of the renal arteries after deployment of the main body of the stent graft.

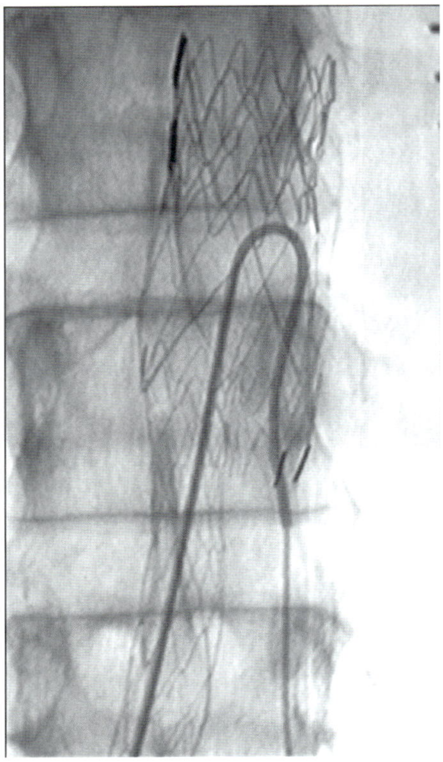

FIGURE 18.2
Crossover approach. After snaring the wire through the contralateral access, the stent graft was pulled down.

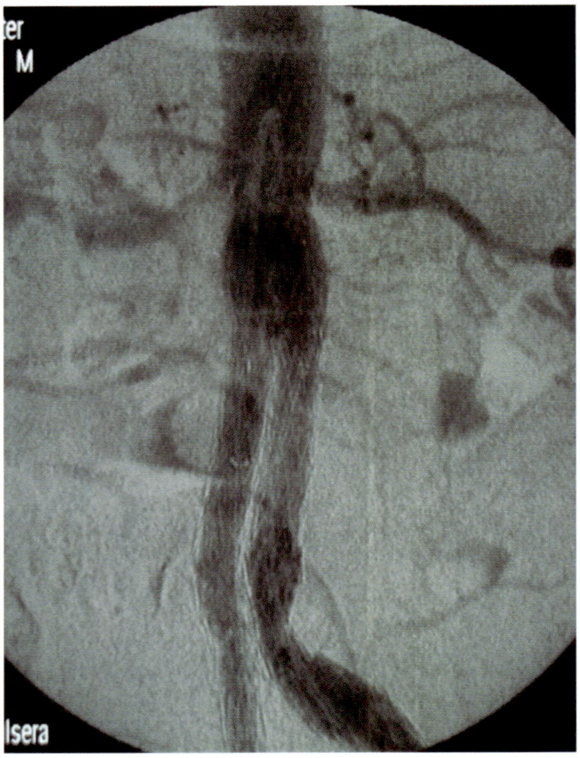

FIGURE 18.3
After pulling down the stent graft, completion angiography demonstrated patency of the renal arteries and integrity of the aorta.

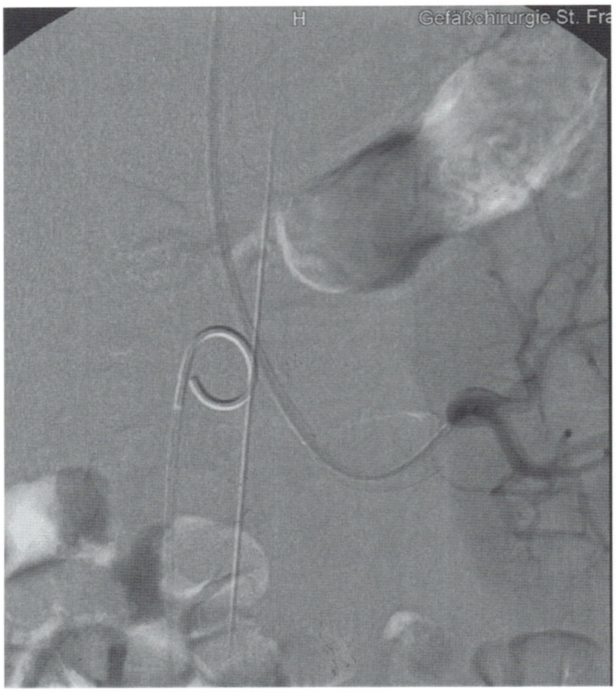

FIGURE 18.4
Cannulation of the lower renal artery using a 6-Fr-long sheath allows exact deployment of the stent graft in patients with extremely short aneurysm necks.

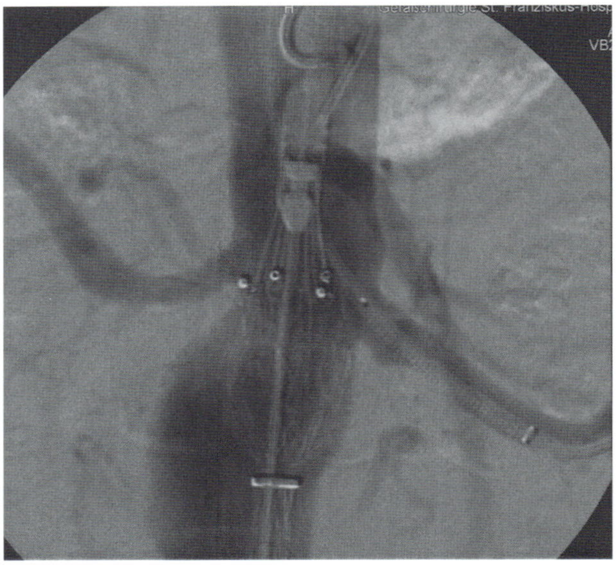

FIGURE 18.5
Implantation of a bare or covered stent at the renal artery ostium in bailout situations.

CASE ANALYSIS

This complication occurred because of inadverent upward motion of the stent graft. The inadvertent coverage of one or both renal arteries is a rare complication of endovascular aneurysm repair (EVAR). Inadvertent coverage of the renal artery is related to the morphology and length of the AAA infrarenal neck. Short, conical, and angulated necks and aneurysms with perirenal thrombus are important risk factors. Poor angiographic imaging during EVAR can also lead to misinterpretation of the anatomical structures. Other causes include the use of too long or too large grafts, especially in inverted conical necks.

In patients with AAA and unfavorable aortic neck, it is essential to use maximum magnification of the perirenal aorta during graft deployment to avoid paralaxis. In extremely short necks, cannulation of the lower renal artery using a 6-Fr-long sheath (Figure 18.4). allows exact deployment of the stent graft and the implantation of a bare or covered stent in the renal artery in bailout situations (Figure 18.5).

In this case, we were able to uncover the renal arteries by carefully pulling down the stent graft using a crossover approach. However, this maneuver may lead to aortic wall disruption if the stent graft is equipped with pins at its proximal end.

LESSONS

- In patients undergoing EVAR, optimum visualization is critical to avoid inadvertent coverage of the renal arteries.
- Patients with AAA and short and angulated neck are at risk for this complication.
- Once the renal artery, or arteries, is covered with the stent graft, management depends on whether the ipsilateral graft leg is still constrained inside the delivery system or is fully deployed. In the former, inflating a 12-mm percutaneous transluminal angioplasty (PTA) balloon in the contralateral short leg and pulling the graft down can be attempted. Alternatively, if the main body is fully deployed, the crossover approach can be utilized. Either way, graft retrieval can cause aortic wall disruption in the presence of graft barbs.
- Conversion to open surgery is technically demanding but can be performed as a last resort.

SUGGESTED READING

Malina M, Brunkwall J, Ivancev K, et al. Renal arteries covered by aortic stents: clinical experience from endovascular grafting of aortic aneurysms. *Eur J Vasc Surg.* 1997;14:109–113.

Walker SR, Yusuf SW, Wenham PW, Hopkinson BR. Renal complications following endovascular repair of abdominal aortic aneurysms. *J Endovasc Surg.* 1998;5:318–322.

CASE 18.2

Consequences of Coverage of a Solitary Hypogastric Artery During EVAR

CLINICAL HISTORY AND DIAGNOSTIC TESTING RESULTS

A 78-year-old man with history of hypertension and CAD was diagnosed with an abdominal aortic aneurysm (AAA) on screening duplex ultrasound. Preprocedure CT angiography confirmed the presence of AAA (Figure 18.6). with aneurysmal dilatation of both common iliac arteries and occlusion of the left hypogastric artery. Aortic angiography confirmed these findings (Figure 18.7).

PLANNED PROCEDURE

Implantation of a Zenith aortoiliac endograft (Cook Medical, Bloomington, IN) with coverage of both hypogastric arteries.

PROCEDURE

The Zenith endograft was implanted as per standard technique without postoperative complications.

COMPLICATION AND MANAGEMENT

The patient returned 2 months after EVAR with severe buttock claudication that was treated conservatively. Symptoms persisted, and 3 months later, the patient underwent right external-to-internal iliac artery bypass after ligation of the hypogastric artery (Figure 18.8). After 2 years, the patient developed left leg claudication, with a rest ankle-brachial index (ABI) of 0.6 (ABI on the right side, 1.0). Peripheral angiography showed occlusion of the left iliac limb of the stent graft (Figure 18.9). The cause of the occlusion was kinking of the left limb of the endograft (Figure 18.10). An attempt to recanalize the occlusion percutaneously failed, but surgical intervention was not necessary because of preserved pelvic collateralization through the right hypogastric artery (Figure 18.11).

At follow-up 2 years later, the patient has no claudication, and the CT-scan demonstrated aneurysm shrinkage, with persistent occlusion of the left iliac limb of the endograft (ABI 0.8 on the left and 1.0 on the right side).

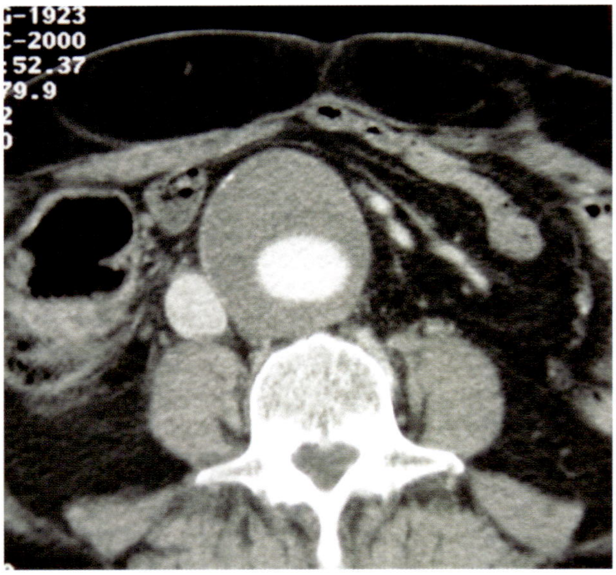

FIGURE 18.6

CT angiography demonstrating AAA involving both common iliac arteries with occlusion of the left hypogastric artery.

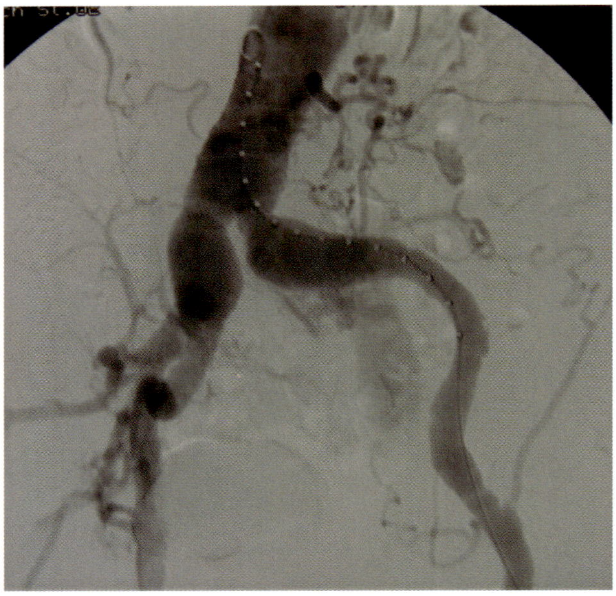

FIGURE 18.7

Abdominal angiography with a calibrated catheter demonstrating AAA involving both common iliac arteries with occlusion of the left hypogastric artery.

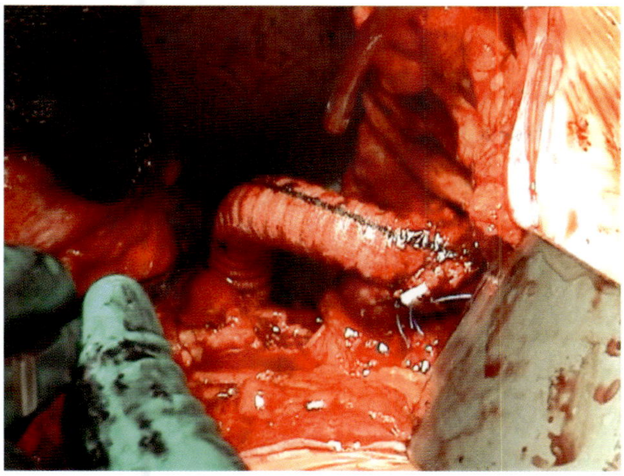

FIGURE 18.8
Implantation of an alloplastic bypass graft from the right external-to-internal iliac artery through a retroperitoneal approach.

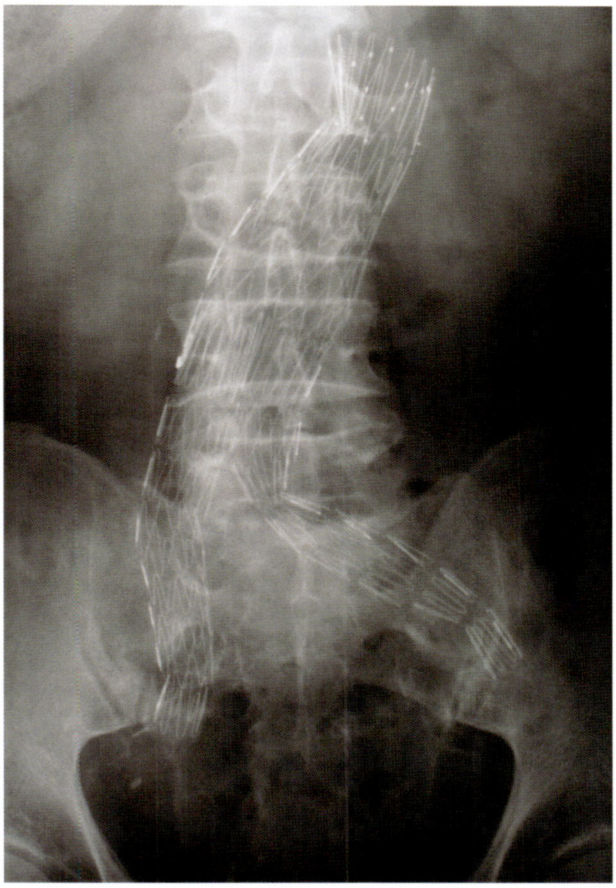

FIGURE 18.10
An abdominal x-ray demonstrating narrowing and kinking of the left limb of the endograft.

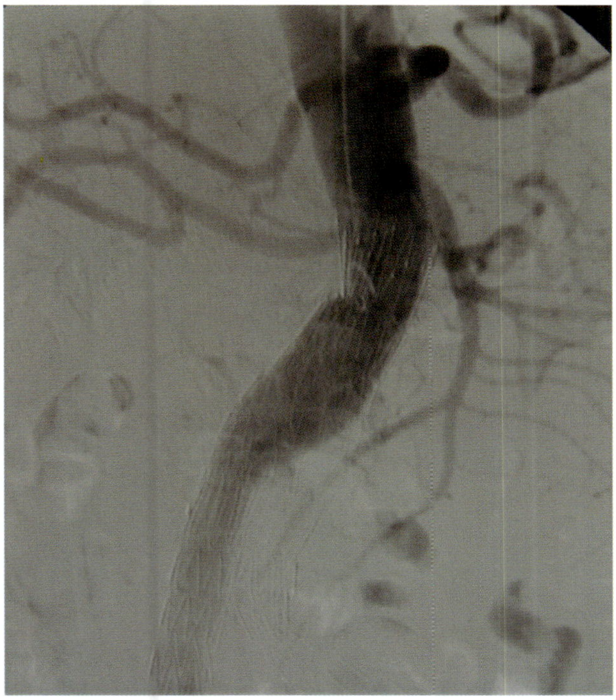

FIGURE 18.9
Follow-up aortoiliac angiography shows occlusion of the left iliac limb of the stent graft.

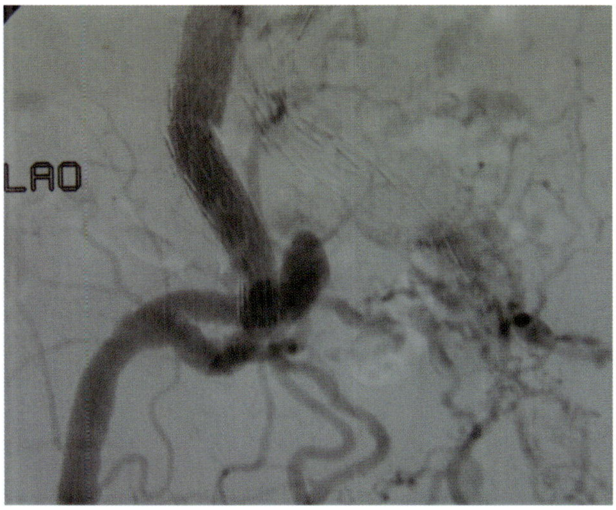

FIGURE 18.11
Iliac angiography demonstrating good pelvic collateralization through the revascularized right hypogastric artery.

CASE ANALYSIS

In this case, coverage of the right hypogastric artery was intended because of aneurysmal involvement of the right common iliac artery. Typically, occlusion of a single hypogastric artery is well tolerated, but when the contralateral hypogastric artery is already occluded, symptoms of buttock claudication may ensue. Occlusion of the main trunk is not as dangerous as peripheral embolization because of the preservation of pelvic collaterals. Bilateral embolization of the hypogastric arteries results in buttock claudication and erectile dysfunction in 40% of patients. Although pelvic and colonic ischemia are rarely observed even in bilateral occlusions, they can be devastating when they occur. In our experience, unilateral hypogastric occlusion occurred in 38 patients and bilateral occlusion in 8 patients out of 1000 consecutive EVAR procedures. Among these patients, 70% developed buttock claudication, but only one patient underwent surgical intervention for colonic ischemia.

In patients with only one patent hypogastric artery, occlusion during EVAR can be avoided using iliac side-branched stent grafts, if available. If this technology is not available, prophylactic external–internal iliac bypass should be considered.

LESSONS

- During EVAR, coverage of the hypogastric artery with the stent graft should be avoided, particularly in patients with contralateral occlusion.
- If coverage of a unilateral hypogastric artery is deemed unavoidable due to aneurysmal dilatation of the common iliac artery, use of iliac side-branch endografts should be considered. If this is unavailable, then prophylactic external to internal iliac artery bypass should be considered.

SUGGESTED READING

Engelke C, Elford J, Morgan RA, Belli AM. Internal iliac artery embolization with bilateral occlusion before endovascular aortoiliac aneurysm repair—Clinical outcome of simultaneous and sequential intervention. *J Vasc Interven Radiol.* 2002;13(7):667–676.

Rayt HS, Bown MJ, Lambert KV, Fishwick NG, et al. Buttock claudication and erectile dysfunction after internal iliac artery embolization in patients prior to endovascular aortic aneurysm repair. *Cardiovasc Intervent Radiol.* 2008;31: 728–734.

Unno N, Inuzuka K, Yamamoto N, et al. Preservation of pelvic circulation with hypogastric artery bypass in endovascular repair of abdominal aortic aneurysm with bilateral iliac artery aneurysms. *J Vasc Surg.* 2008;44(6):1170–1175.

Yano OJ, Morrissey N, Eisen L, et al. Intentional internal iliac artery occlusion to facilitate endovascular repair of aortoiliac aneurysms. *J Vasc Surg.* 2001;34(2):204–211.

CASE 18.3

Type I Endoleak

CLINICAL HISTORY AND DIAGNOSTIC TESTING RESULTS

A 68-year-old man with history of hypertension, peripheral arterial disease, and CAD was diagnosed with an asymptomatic AAA on screening duplex ultrasound. Preprocedure CT angiography confirmed the presence of AAA.

PLANNED PROCEDURE

Implantation of a Vanguard stent graft (Boston Scientific, Natick, MA).

PROCEDURE

The Vanguard endograft was implanted as per standard technique without evidence of endoleak on completion angiography (Figure 18.12). and without postoperative complications. Routine follow-up CT angiography at first month did not reveal any endoleak (Figure 18.13).

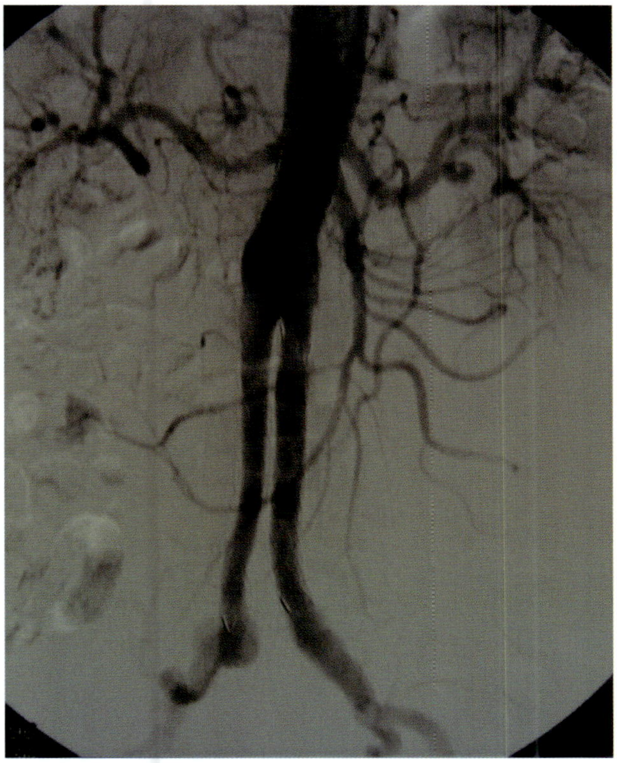

FIGURE 18.12
Postprocedure abdominal aortic angiography showing no endoleak.

COMPLICATION AND MANAGEMENT

Routine follow-up Duplex ultrasound after 3.4 years showed type I endoleak with a 5-cm AAA. The patient was asymptomatic. CT angiography confirmed the endoleak and showed dislodgement of the iliac limbs

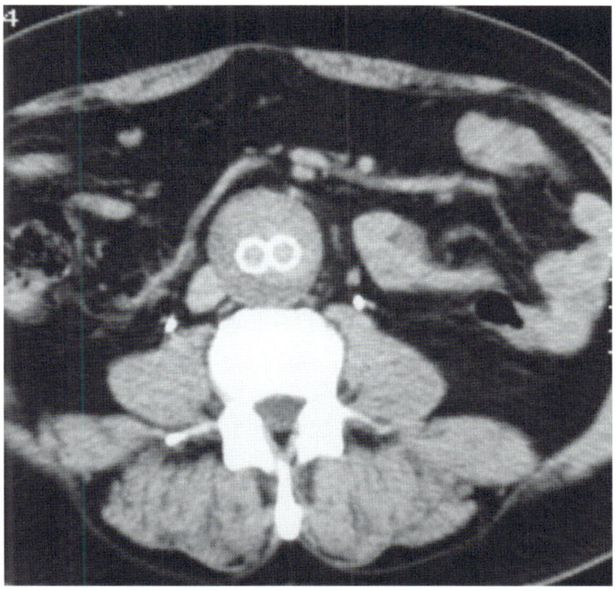

FIGURE 18.13
Follow-up CTA at 1-month without evidence of endoleak.

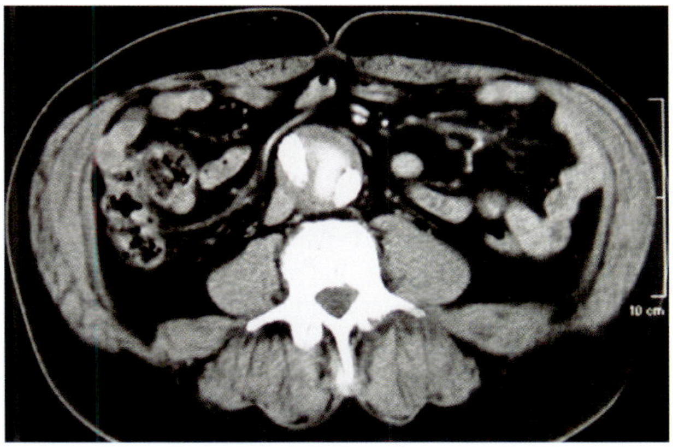

FIGURE 18.14
Follow-up CTA after 3.4 years showed type I endoleak and dislodgement of the left iliac limb.

(Figure 18.14). Aortoiliac angiography demonstrated kinking and retraction of the left limb into the aneurysm sack causing a distal type I endoleak (Figure 18.15). This endoleak was treated with implantation of a Talent graft extension (Medtronic, Santa Rosa, CA) (Figures 18.16 and 18.17).

A follow-up CT angiography 3.6 years later showed recurrence of the type I endoleak (Figure 18.18), and the patient was scheduled for endovascular repair. However, the patient had aneurysm rupture prior to repair, which was successfully treated by open surgery at a different institution.

CASE ANALYSIS

Migration of first-generation flexible endografts due to remodelling of the aorta, as in this patient, can cause distal and proximal type I endoleak. Type I endoleak is associated with significant pressure elevation in the aneurysm sac and can be considered equivalent to aneurysm recurrence. Routine follow-up using plain radiography of the graft and duplex scan is essential to recognize the problem. The implantation of a stiff leg extension can correct the kinking and the endoleak for a while. Only implantation of a new second-generation stent graft would stabilize the prosthesis and avoid future rupture. Rupture after endovascular repair is usually contained; hemodynamic shock is not frequent, allowing survival after open or endovascular repair.

In general, an important cause of late migration is aneurysmal degeneration of the proximal aneurysm neck with successive proximal detachment. As a large proximal neck negatively influences the radial force, endograft oversizing (by ~ 20%) and suprarenal fixation are recommended to reduce the rate of proximal type I endoleak. On the other hand, excessive graft oversizing of a stiff stent graft can lead to infolding of the graft and thus causing endoleak. In such cases, proximal type I endoleaks can be corrected by ballooning. Large balloon-expandable or self-expandable bare metal stents are good options for achieving seal if aortic graft extensions are not feasible.

LESSONS

- The incidence of type I endoleak after implantation of first-generation flexible endografts is not insignificant.
- Routine imaging at follow-up is critical for early detection of this complication.
- Type I endoleaks should be promptly treated as soon as they are identified to prevent aneurysm rupture.
- Type I endoleak is usually corrected by iliac or aortic extensions at the sealing zones (**CASE 18.3 LOOPS**). If the endoleak is caused by device failure, it is necessary either to implant a second stent-graft into the lumen of the initial one in order to achieve sealing or alternatively to convert to open surgery.

SUGGESTED READING

Buth J, Laheij R. Early complications and endoleaks after endovascular abdominal aortic aneurysm repair: Report of a multicenter study. *J Vasc Surg.* 2000;31:134–146.

Cao P, De Rango, Verzini F, Parlani G. Endoleak after endovascular aortic repair: Classification, diagnosis and management following endovascular thoracic and abdominal repair. *J Cardiovasc Surg.* 2010;51:53–69.

Donas K, Torsello G, Austermann M. The use of abdominal chimney grafts is feasible and safe: Short term results. *J Endovasc Ther.* 2010;17:589–593.

Torsello G, Klenk E, Kasprzak B, Umscheid Th. Rupture of abdominal aortic aneurysm previously treated by endovascular stentgraft. *J Vasc Surg.* 1998;28:184–187.

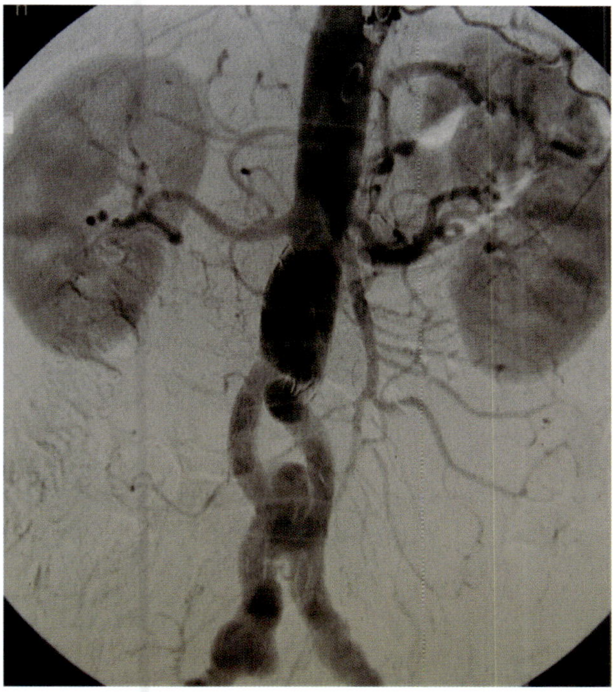

FIGURE 18.15
Follow-up aortic angiography after 3.4 years showed kinking and retraction of the left limb into the aneurysm sack causing a distal type I endoleak.

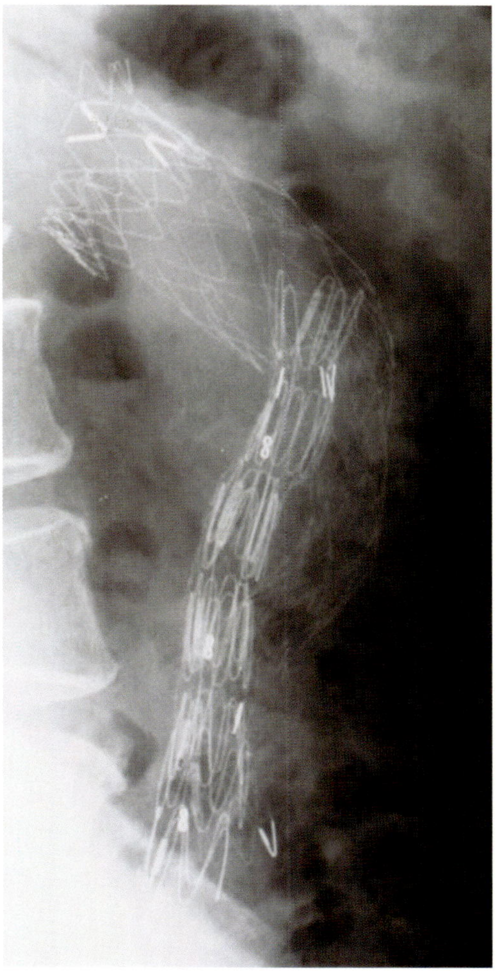

FIGURE 18.17
An x-ray demonstrating implantation of a Talent leg and repairing the kink.

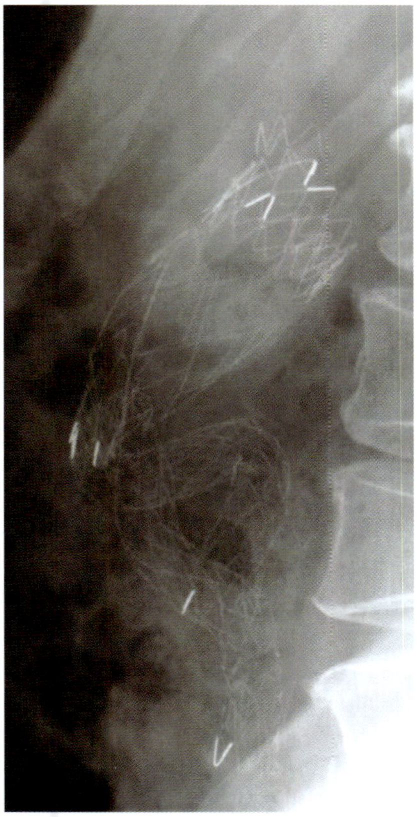

FIGURE 18.16
An x-ray demonstrating straightening of the left graft limb after introducing a Lunderqvist wire (Cook Medical, Bloomington, IN).

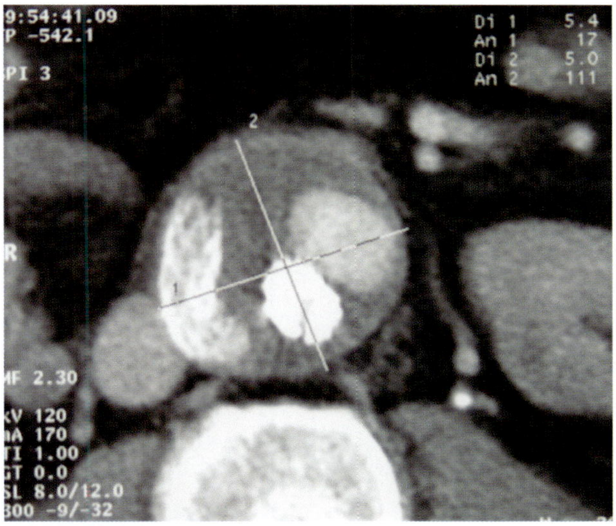

FIGURE 18.18
Follow-up CTA on 18/10/2004 showed recurrence of the type I endoleak.

CASE 18.4

Type II Endoleak

CLINICAL HISTORY AND DIAGNOSTIC TESTING RESULTS

A 74-year-old man with history of hypertension, atrial fibrillation (on coumadine), and COPD was diagnosed with an AAA on screening duplex ultrasound. Preprocedure CT angiography confirmed the presence of a 5.6-cm AAA with dilatation of both common iliac arteries. Aortoiliac angiography confirmed these findings and demonstrated severe bilateral iliac tortousity. Also, antegrade perfusion of the inferior mesenteric artery and four lumbar arteries was demonstrated (Figure 18.19).

PLANNED PROCEDURE

Implantation of a Zenith bifurcated stent graft (Cook Medical, Bloomington, IN).

PROCEDURE

The Zenith bifurcated stent graft was implanted as per standard technique. Completion angiography demonstrated type II endoleak.

COMPLICATION AND MANAGEMENT

The decision was made to manage the type II endoleak conservatively. Follow-up CT angiography at 6 months showed an aneurysm diameter of 5.7 cm with retrograde filling of the aneurysm sack. At 1 year, CT angiography showed similar findings with no change of aneurysm size. Duplex ultrasound follow-up after 1.5 years showed minimal growth of the aneurysm to 5.8 cm, with aneurysm filling through the inferior mesenteric artery. At that point, coumadine was replaced with aspirin. At 2 years follow-up, CTA showed significant aneurysm growth (6.3 cm), but the patient remained asymptomatic. The patient underwent aortic

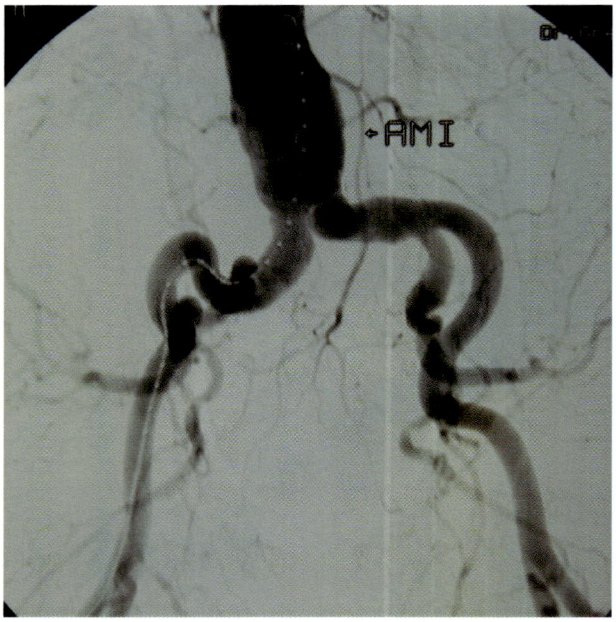

FIGURE 18.19
Aortic angiography shows retrograde filling of the aneurysm sack by the inferior mesenteric artery.

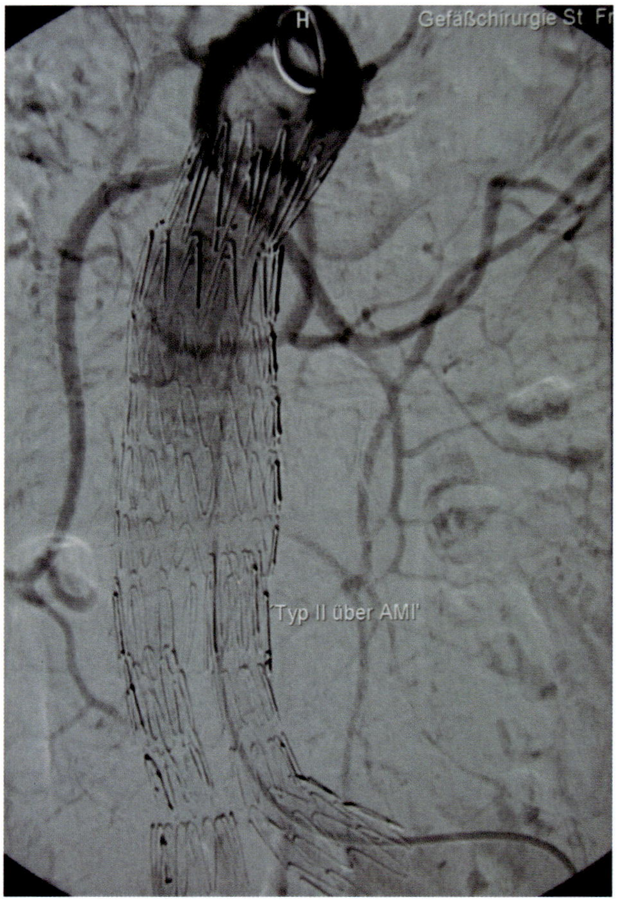

FIGURE 18.20
Superselective catheterization of the Riolan anastomosis of the inferior mesenteric artery with a microcatheter.

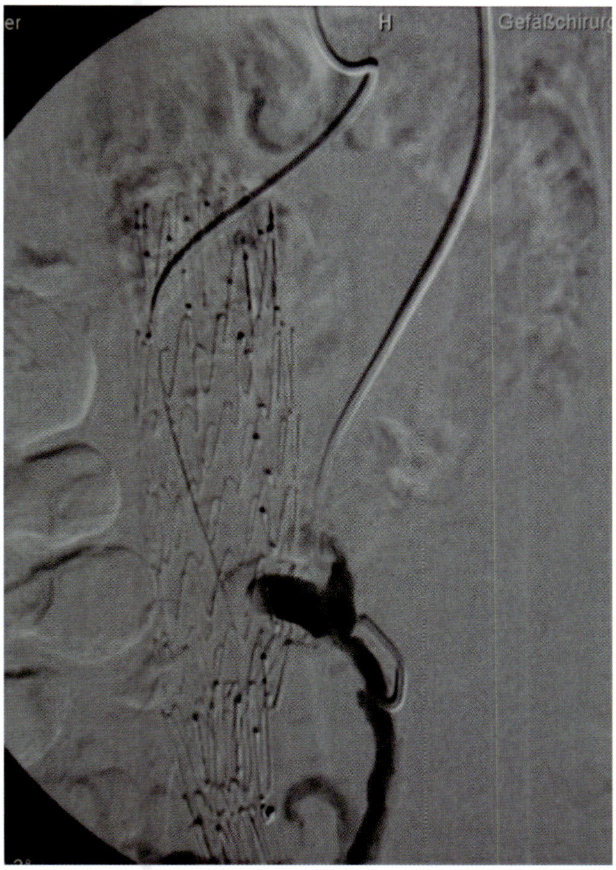

FIGURE 18.21
Embolization of the inferior mesenteric artery at its junction with the aneurysm using coils.

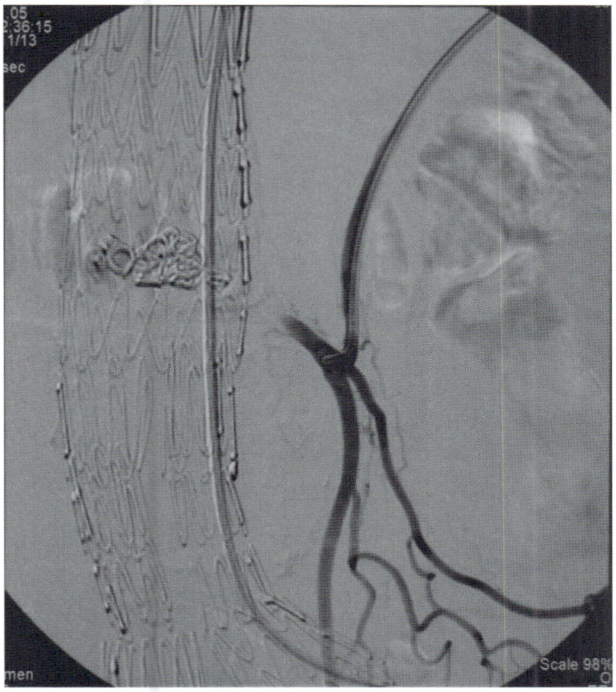

FIGURE 18.22
Completion angiography shows obliteration of perfusion of the aneurysm sack.

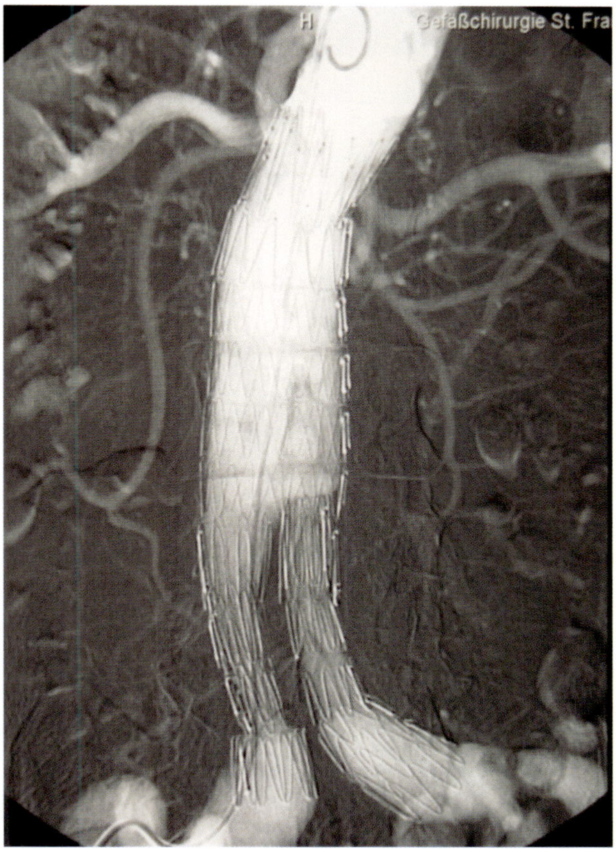

FIGURE 18.23
Preprocedure CT angiography showing an aneurysm of the infrarenal aorta with a narrow distal aortic neck and severe circular calcification of both the iliac arteries and the aortic bifurcation.

angiography that demonstrated persistence of retrograde filling of the aneurysm from the inferior mesenteric artery (Figure 18.20). The superior mesenteric artery was engaged with a 6-Fr sheath, and an over-the-wire microcatheter was advanced to the Riolan anastomosis of the inferior mesenteric artery (Figure 18.21). The inferior mesenteric artery was embolized at its junction with the aneurysm using coils (Figure 18.22). Completion angiography confirmed absence of perfusion of the aneurysm sack (Figure 18.23). Follow-up CT angiography 6 months later demonstrated absence of endoleak and an aneurysm diameter of 5.8 cm.

CASE ANALYSIS

Type II endoleak is defined as continuous blood flow to the aneurysm sack from collateral vessels, such as the lumbar arteries and the inferior mesenteric artery, as was the case in this patient. It is the most common form of endoleak and is usually detected at the time of endovascular aneurism repair (EVAR). During the first year, many type II endoleaks resolve spontaneously, but in about 8% of patients, type II endoleaks persist long term. In these cases, as in this patient, an intervention is required to obliterate the source of blood flow to arrest aneurysm growth.

While technology continues to evolve and newer endografts are associated with a lower incidence of complications, the incidence of type II endoleaks remains unchanged. Predictors of type II endoleaks include the extent of parietal thrombus in the aneurysm sac and prior use of oral anticoagulants. Spontaneous remission is frequent particularly if the retrograde filling originates from the lumbar arteries.

LESSONS

- Type II endoleak is a common complication after EVAR.
- Type II endoleak seldom lead to aneurysm rupture.
- Type II endoleaks should be initially managed by regular follow-up noninvasive imaging. Persistent type II endoleaks leading to aneurysm growth should be treated.
- The treatment of choice for type II endoleaks is transcatheter occlusion of the culprit vessel (s) at their junction with the aneurysm sack using coils or other embolic agents, such as Onyx (ev3 Plymouth, MN).
- Open surgery is recommended if the endoleak does not resolve with endovascular technique, and the AAA continues to expand.

SUGGESTED READING

Jones J, Atkins M, Brewster D, et al. Persistent type 2 endoleak after endovascular repair of abdominal aortic aneurysm is associated with adverse late outcomes. *J Vasc Surg.* 2007;46:1–8.

Steinmetz E, Rubin B, Sanchez L, et al. Type II endoleak after endovascular abdominal aneurysm repair: A conservative approach with selective intervention is safe and cost-effective. *J Vasc Surg.* 2004;39:306–313.

Tolia A, Landis R, Lamparello P, et al. Type II endoleaks after endovascular repair of abdominal aortic aneurysms: Natural history. *Radiology.* 2005;235(2):683–686.

CASE 18.5

Aorto-Iliac Rupture

CLINICAL HISTORY AND DIAGNOSTIC TESTING RESULTS

An 83-year-old woman with history of hypertension and CAD was diagnosed with symptomatic AAA by duplex ultrasound. Preprocedure CT angiography showed a 6.2-cm infrarenal AAA with a 20–mm-long proximal neck and 14–mm-long distal aortic neck (diameter 12 mm). Also, the CT showed severe circular calcification of both iliac arteries and the aortic bifurcation (Figure 18.24).

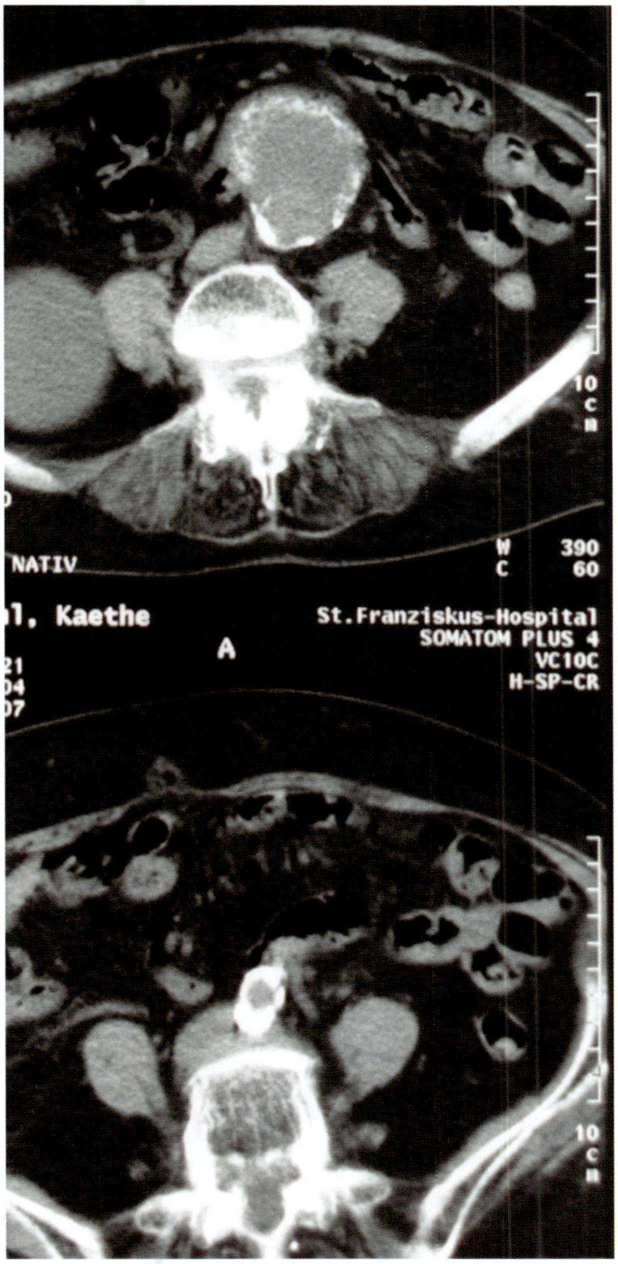

FIGURE 18.24

Aortoiliac angiography demonstrating tortuosity and dilatation of both the iliac arteries and antegrade perfusion of the inferior mesenteric artery and four lumbar arteries.

PLANNED PROCEDURE

EVAR of the AAA using an aorto-uniliac or straight endograft due to the narrow distal aortic neck.

PROCEDURE

An attempt to introduce the aorto-uniliac stent graft through the iliac artery failed due to tortousity and cacifications. Subsequently, a decision was made to use a "double tube" approach, which requires the use of two short straight grafts (two iliac legs or one leg in combination with an aortic extension, which usually has a smaller profile). The left iliac leg graft was successfully deployed. Advancement of the right iliac leg graft encountered resistance. Flouroscopy demonstrated that the tip of the introducer was held at the aortic bifurcation, and the body of the introducer showed a 90° bend in the right iliac artery (Figure 18.25). As the graft could not be advanced into the aorta, the introducer was removed.

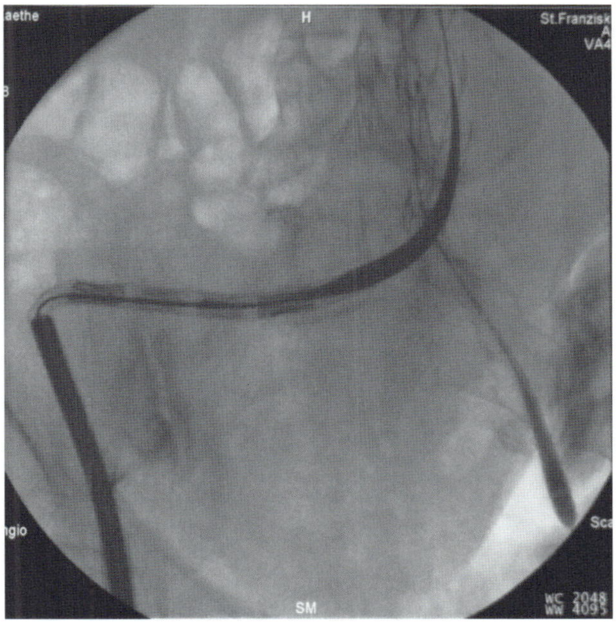

FIGURE 18.25

After successful deployment of the first iliac leg, the introducer of the second graft shows a 90° bending.

COMPLICATION AND MANAGEMENT

After sheath removal, the patient became suddenly hypotensive, and immediate angiography showed perforation at the external common iliacartery junction (Figure 18.26). Immediately, an aortic occlusion balloon was introduced from the left arterial access. An attempt to deliver a covered stent from the right arterial access failed. A longer Talent graft leg was implanted with successful sealing of the perforation (Figure 18.27). However, the patient died 2 days later due to multiorgan failure.

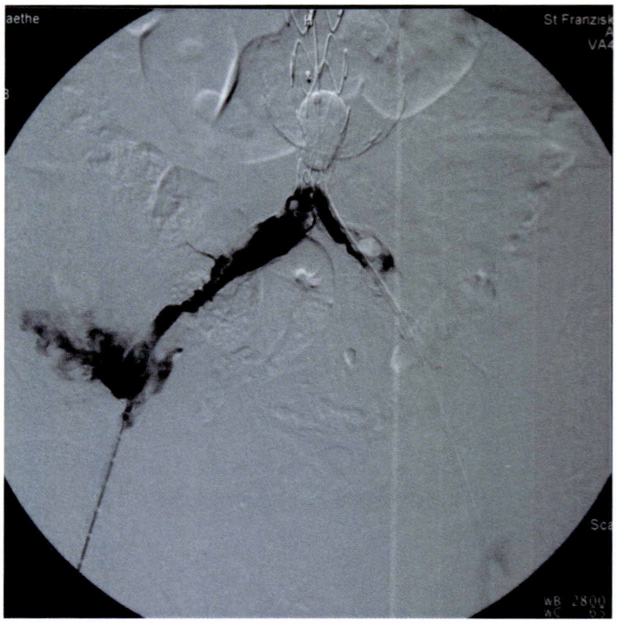

FIGURE 18.26
Contrast medium extravasation at level of external-common iliac junction.

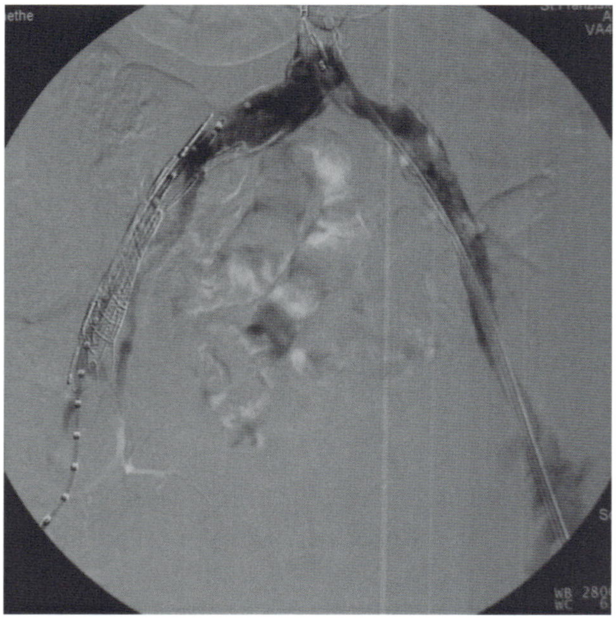

FIGURE 18.27
Implantation of a Talent leg for controlling the bleeding.

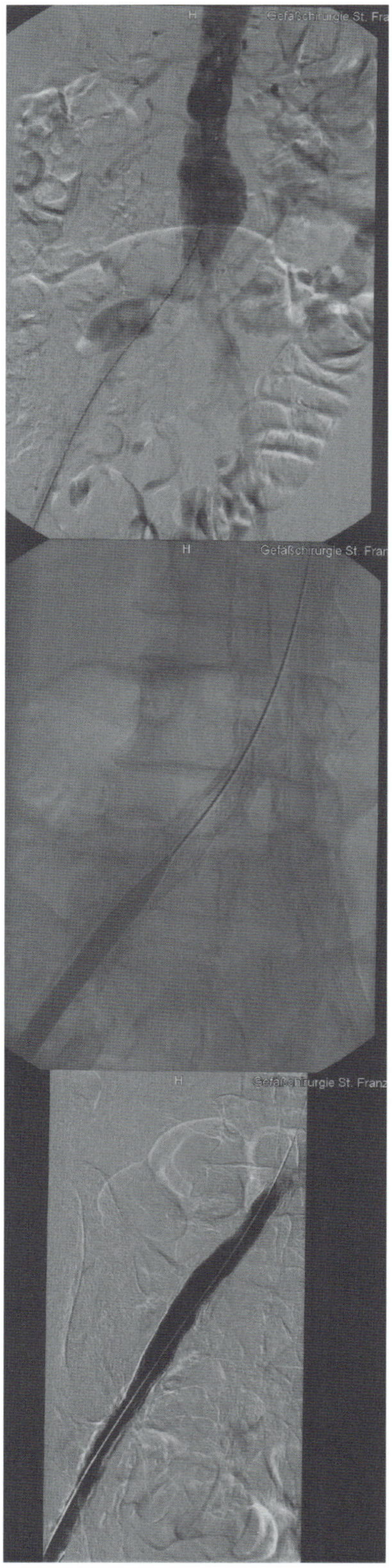

FIGURE 18.28
Use of an endoconduit implanting a long low-profile balloon expandable covered stent "cracking and paving" the calcified iliac artery.

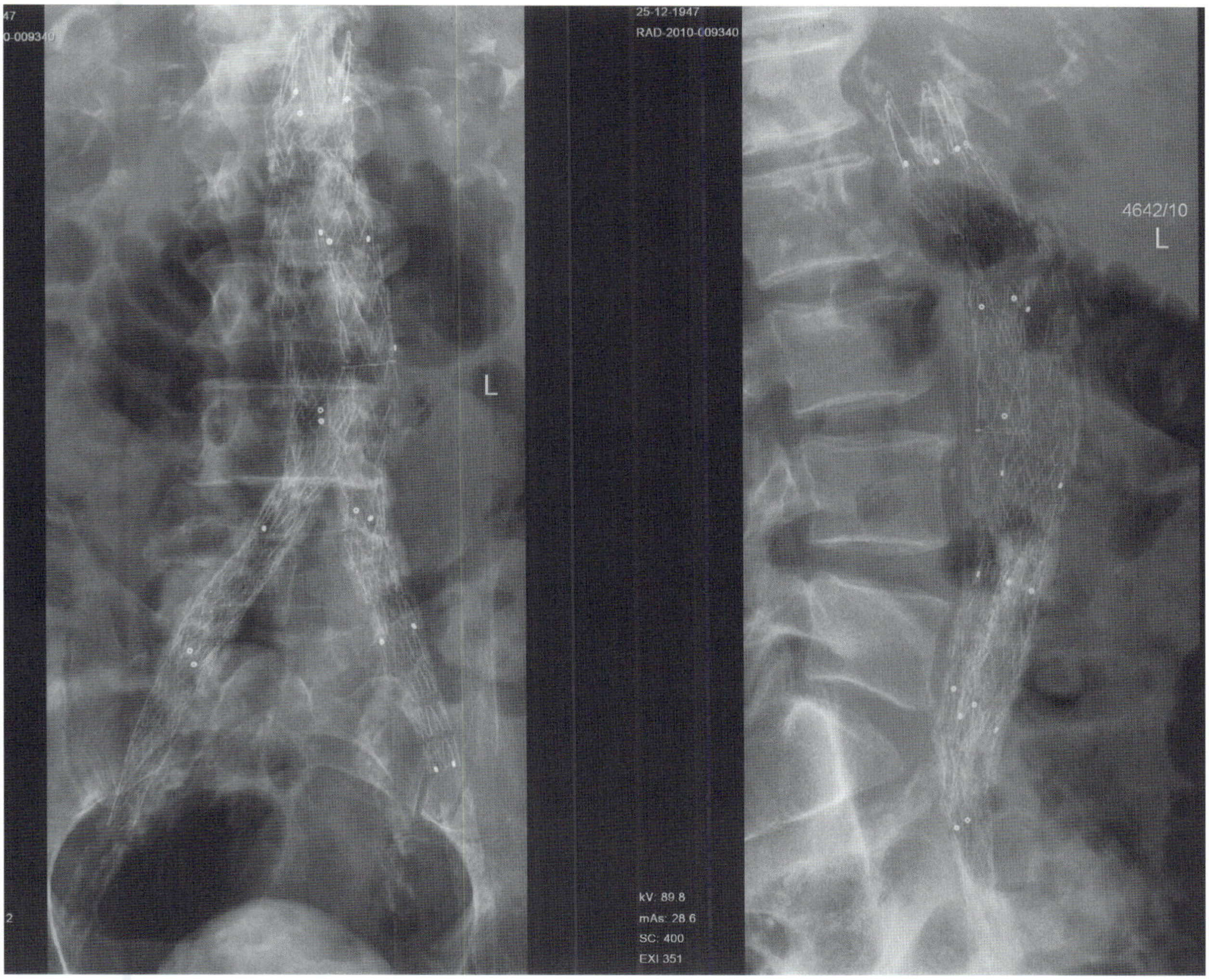

FIGURE 18.29
Completion angiography after endografting using an endoconduit.

CASE ANALYSIS

In this case, the iliac perforation occurred as a consequence of forceful advancement of the graft introducer due to severely calcified and tortuous iliac vessel and lower abdominal aorta. This complication could have been avoided if the operator ceased to advance the introducer at the first sign of resistance. There are several other techniques that can be utilized to facilitate introducer advancement in these cases, such as lubrication of the delivery system with silicone, predilation of the iliac artery with a balloon or sequential dilators, and transbrachial through-and-through stiff wire technique. Recently, we successfully used an endoconduit by implanting a long balloon expandable covered stent (Advanta, Atrium Co, Hudson, NH) in similar cases (Figure 18.28 and 18.29). This technique is safe, particularly in patients with occluded internal iliac artery. Using these methods reduced the need for surgical conduit through a retroperitoneal or transperitoneal approach to <1% during the past 5 years.

Technological advances in introducer sheaths and endografts are likely to reduce further the incidence of these dreadful complications. Recently, the SoloPath TransFemoral sheath (Onset Medical Corporation, Irvine, CA) has been introduced into the market in Europe. This is a balloon expandable sheath with a folded distal section of 13-Fr outer diameter that can reach >21-Fr after deployment. In the last few years, an increasing number of low-profile endografts has been introduced in order to reduce access complications and expand indications for EVAR. For instance, the Endurant stent graft (Medtronic, Santa Rosa, CA) can be loaded into a low-profile delivery system, with an outer diameter of 18-Fr to 20-Fr for the main body and 14-Fr. to 16-Fr for the iliac legs. Its hydrophilic surface has reduced the drag force by 75%. Other devices are under investigation and will be introduced in the near future.

LESSONS

- The presence of moderate-to-severe calcification and tortousity in the iliac artery increases the risk of iliac perforation when using large profile catheters.
- Forceful advancement of large profile catheters/introducers should always be avoided.
- Flouroscopic guidance of introducer/catheter advancement can help detect early signs of potential arterial disruption.
- In the event of iliac rupture, hemodynamic compromise does not occur until sheath removal because the sheath prevents blood extravasation.
- When iliac rupture is recognized, internal aortic clamping using a large balloon from the contralateral side should be performed immediately.
- Covered stents or endografts can be used to cover the perforation site. If perforation persists, aortic blockage should be deployed and the patient should go to surgery.

SUGGESTED READING

Fernandez J, Craig J, Garrett H. Endovascular management of iliac rupture during endovascular aneurysm repair: A single-center experience. *J Vasc Surg.* 2009;50:1293–1299.

Gabrielli L, Baudo A, Molinari A, Domanin M. Early complications in endovascular treatment of abdominal aortic aneurysm. *Acta Cir Belg.* 2004;104:519–526.

Millon A, Delchand A, Feugier P, et al. Conversion to open repair after endovascular aneurysm repair: Causes and results. *Eur J Vasc Endovasc Surg.* 2009;38:429–434.

Torsello G, Troisi N, Tessarek J, et al. Endovascular aortic aneurysm repair with the Endurant stent-graft: Early and 1-year results from a European multicenter experience. *J Vasc Interv Radiol.* 2010;21:73–80.

19

Konstantinos P. Donas and Giovanni B. Torsello

Complications of Endovascular Thoracic Aortic Aneurysm Repair

CASE 19.1

External Iliac Rupture and Spinal Cord Ischemia During TEVAR

CLINICAL HISTORY AND DIAGNOSTIC TESTING RESULTS

An 84-year-old man with history of hypertension, renal insufficiency, and coronary artery disease (CAD) presented with ruptured thoracic aortic aneurysm (TAA) of 7.5 cm diameter, which was confirmed by thoracic computer tomography angiography (CTA) (Figure 19.1).

PLANNED PROCEDURE

Thoracic aorta endovascular aneurysm repair (TEVAR) with Valiant stent grafts (Medtronic Vascular, Santa Rosa, CA).

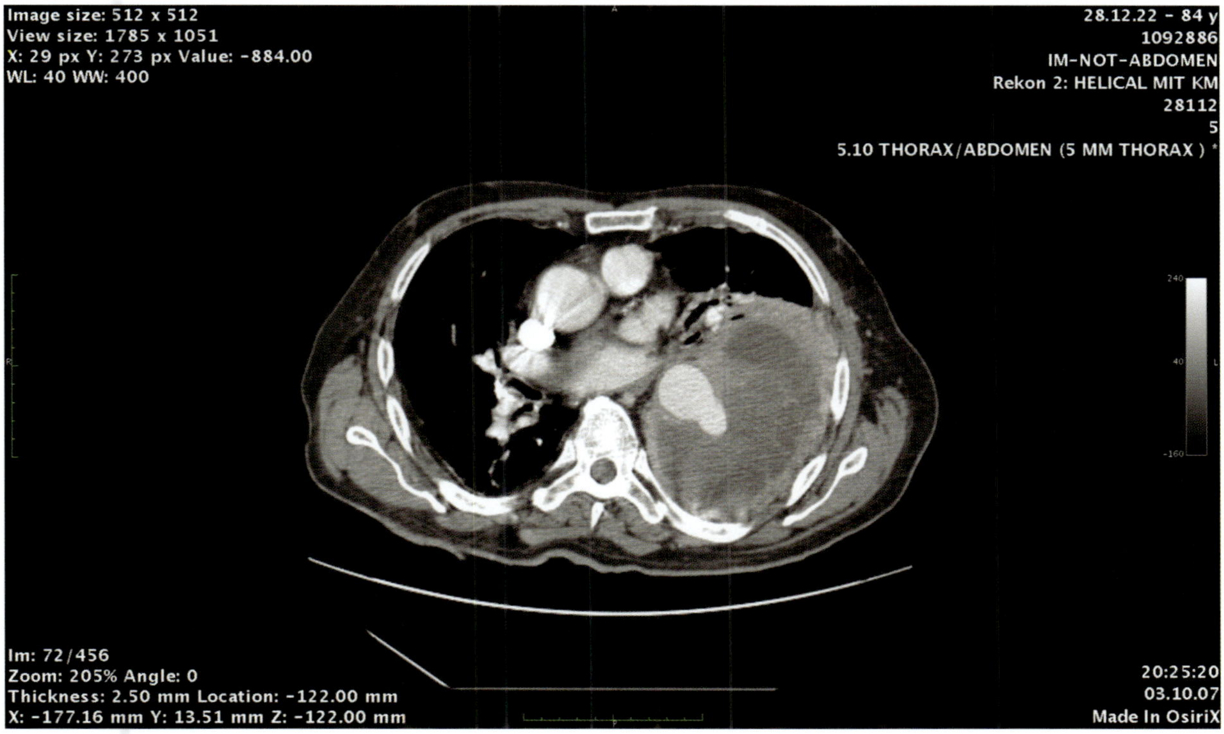

FIGURE 19.1
Thoracic CTA demonstrating rupture of the TAA.

PROCEDURE

Baseline intraoperative thoraco-abdominal angiography is shown in Figure 19.2. TEVAR was performed per standard technique. The diameter of the stent-graft was calculated from the largest diameter of the proximal landing zone and oversized by 20%. The side of insertion of primary introducer sheath was based on the size of the access vessels and distal extension of the aneurysm. We used three Valiant stent grafts (total length of 260 mm) (Figure 19.3). After removal of the delivery system of the third Valiant stent graft, sudden hypotension was noted.

COMPLICATION AND MANAGEMENT

Immediate iliac angiography showed right external iliac artery rupture (Figure 19.4). An additional stent-graft (Talent limb, Medtronic, Minneapolis, MN) was deployed at the site of the vessel rupture. As the bleeding could not be controlled at the level of the distal external iliac artery, surgical cut down had to be performed. The injury was repaired by interposition of dacron graft (8 mm). Subsequently, it was noted that the patient had suffered paraparesis due to spinal cord ischemia (SCI).

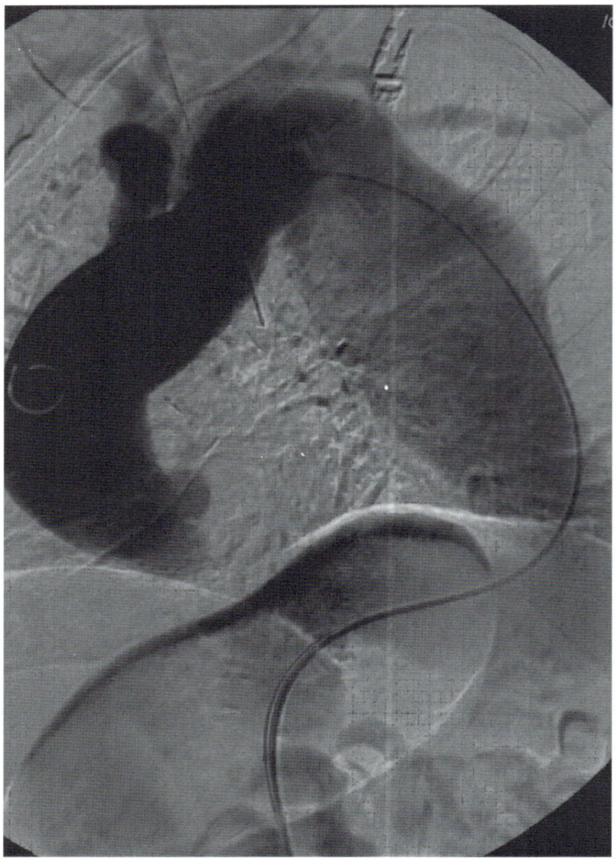

FIGURE 19.2
Baseline intraoperative thoracoabdominal angiography demonstrates the TAA.

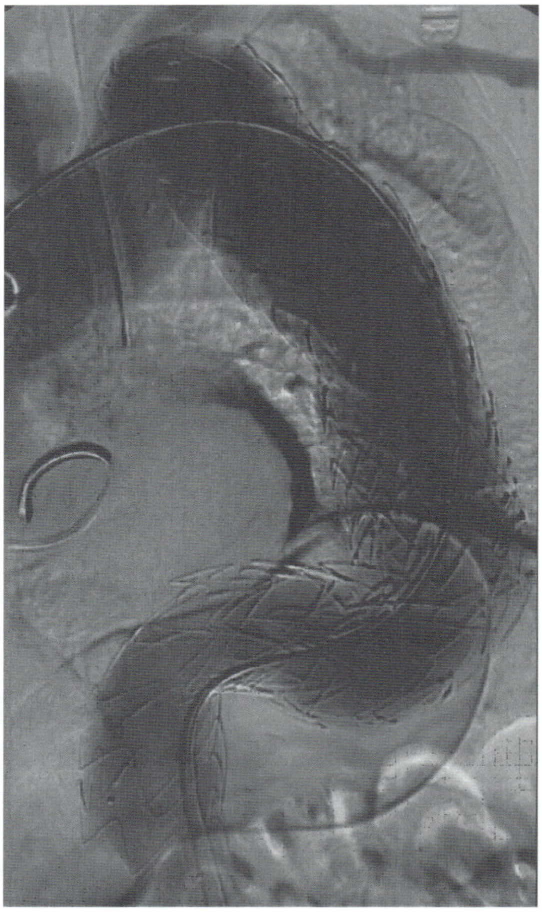

FIGURE 19.3
Thoracoabdominal angiography after implantation of the Valiant endografts to exclude the TAA.

CASE ANALYSIS

This patient suffered from two complications as a result of TEVAR. First, rupture of the external iliac artery, which occurred as a result of severe kinking and calcification of the vessel. This complication could have been avoided if the device was advanced carefully with fluoroscopic guidance. Despite proper management of the iliac rupture, the prolonged hypotension contributed to the occurrence of SCI.

SCI after TEVAR occur as a result of coverage of the entire descending aorta down to the visceral vessels, thereby occluding the intercostal arteries. Of course, concomitant hypotension would further reduce spinal perfusion as well as make spinal drainage more difficult. SCI after TEVAR can be immediate or of delayed onset. The immediate occurrence of SCI symptoms may be the result of occlusion of a critical feeding vessel of the anterior spinal artery. The delayed onset may be secondary to episodes of hypotension or due to loss of previously patent collateral vessels.

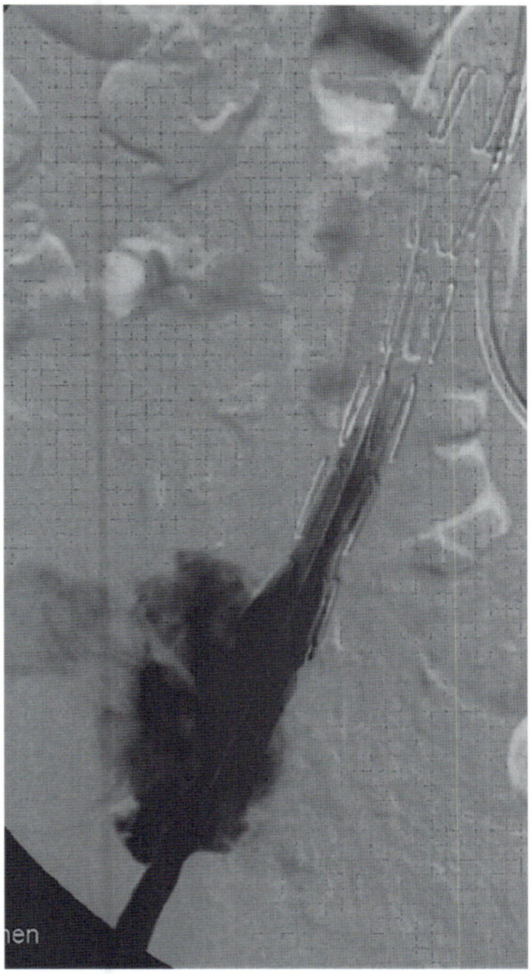

FIGURE 19.4
Rupture of the right external iliac artery.

LESSONS

- Kinked and severely calcified iliac arteries increase the risk of arterial rupture during advancement of large caliber stent grafts. In these cases, arterial pressure should be closely monitored during sheath withdrawal.
- Immediate placement of a covered stent can often restore vessel integrity.
- The risk of SCI after TEVAR increases with the increasing length of the covered thoracic aorta as well as concomitant hypotension.

SUGGESTED READING

Gravereaux EC, Faries PL, Burks JA, et al. Risk of spinal cord ischemia after endograft repair of thoracic aortic aneurysms. *J Vasc Surg.* 2001;34:997–1003.

CASE 19.2

Distal Type I Endoleak After TEVAR

CLINICAL HISTORY AND DIAGNOSTIC TESTING RESULTS

An 82-year-old woman with history of hypertension and CAD presented with symptomatic thoracoabdominal aneurysm as confirmed with CTA (Figure 19.5). The maximum aneurysm diameter was 69 mm. The aorta diameter at the left subclavian artery origin was 33 mm. A left subclavian-carotid transposition was previously performed to create a landing zone in the distal aortic arch.

PLANNED PROCEDURE

TEVAR with Valiant stent grafts (Medtronic Vascular, Santa Rosa, CA).

PROCEDURE

Under spinal anasthesia, baseline thoraco abdominal angiography was performed (Figure 19.6). TEVAR was performed per standard technique using three Talent stent grafts (Figure 19.7). The diameter of the stent graft was calculated from the largest diameter of the proximal landing zone and oversized by 20%. The side of insertion of the primary introducer sheath was based on the size of the access vessels and distal extension of the aneurysm.

COMPLICATION AND MANAGEMENT

Follow-up CTA at 6 months demonstrated type Ib endoleak (distal type). Thoraco abdominal angiography confirmed the presence of distal type I endoleak (Figure 19.8). The patient was managed with endovascular implantation of additional stent graft placement overlapping the existing endograft down to the celiac artery (Figure 19.9).

CASE ANALYSIS

The cause of delayed type Ib endoleak in this case is aneurysmal degeneration of the aortic segment just above the origin of the visceral vessels. This complication occurs more often in patients with Marfan syndrome.

LESSONS

- Sufficient stent graft overlapping and aortic coverage into normal segments beyond the aneurysm is critical to avoid type I endoleaks.
- Coverage of critical aortic branches (carotid artery and visceral arteries) can be avoided by selective angiography and utilization of the chimney technique or fenestrated grafts.
- Routine follow-up CTA is necessary to detect delayed endoleaks in a timely fashion.

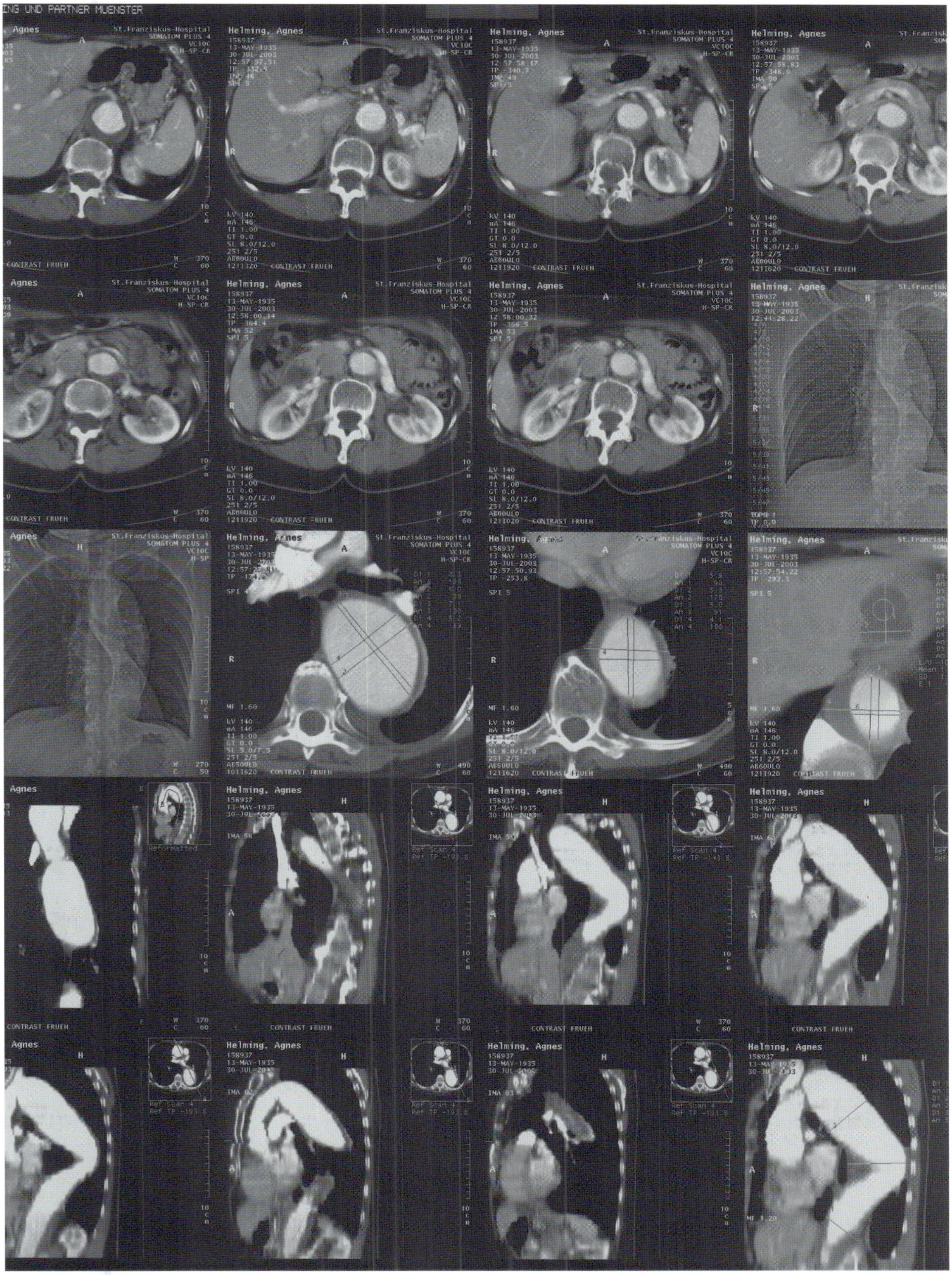

FIGURE 19.5
Baseline thoracic CTA demonstrating a thoracoabdominal aneurysm.

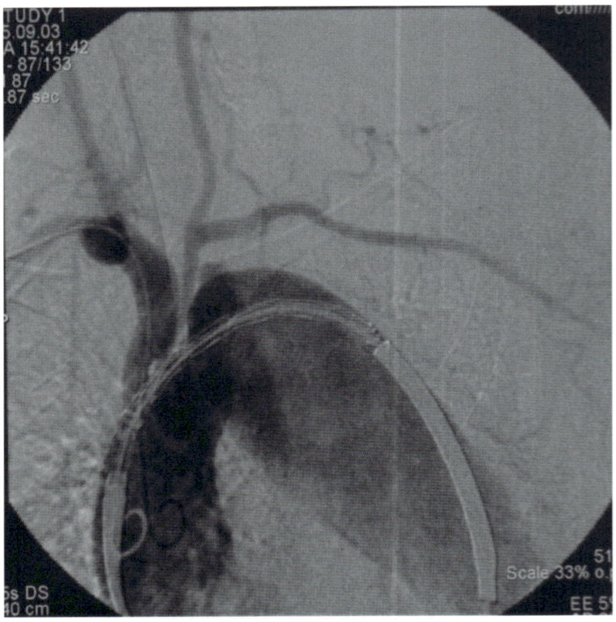

FIGURE 19.6
Baseline thoracoabdominal angiography demonstrating subclavian-carotid transposition.

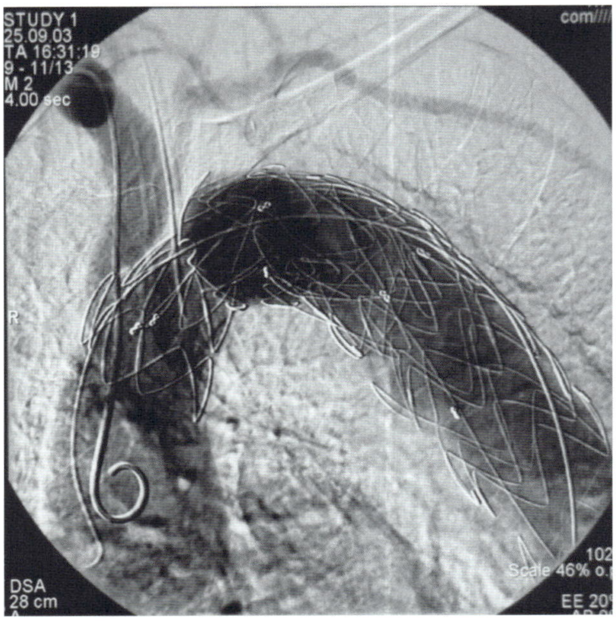

FIGURE 19.7
Aortic angiography after implantation of three Talent stent grafts.

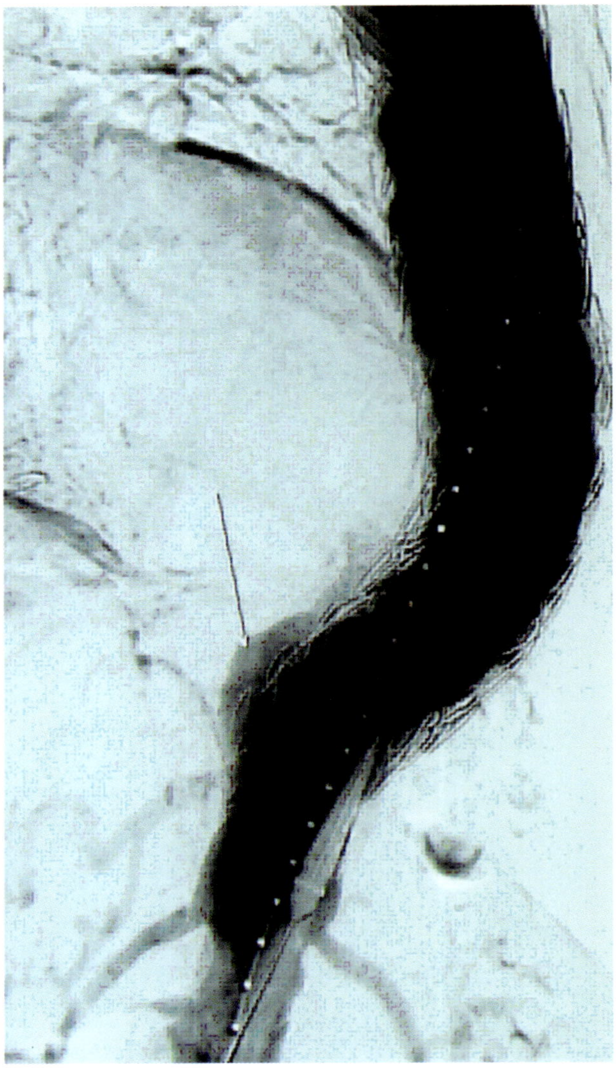

FIGURE 19.8
Follow-up aortic angiography demonstrating type Ib endoleak.

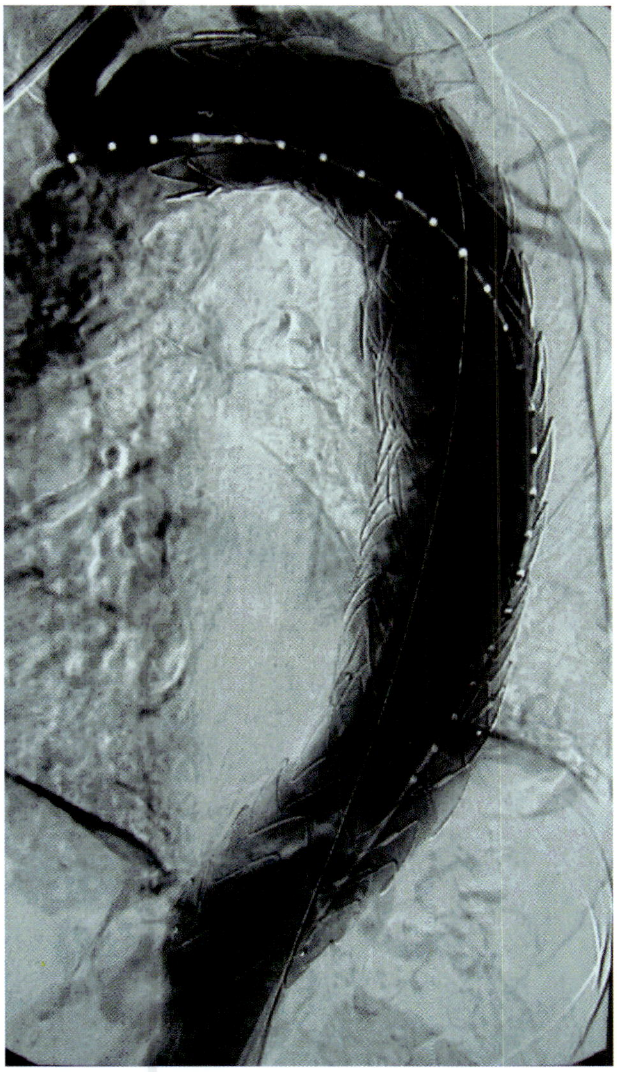

FIGURE 19.9
Successful treatment of the endoleak by additional stent graft placement.

CASE 19.3

Iliac Occlusion During TEVAR

CLINICAL HISTORY AND DIAGNOSTIC TESTING RESULTS

A 75-year-old man with hypertension and hyperlipidaemia presented with asymptomatic thoracoabdominal aneurysm with a maximum diameter of 67 mm. The aneurysm was detected on a CT scan that was performed for workup of a lumbar spinal syndrome.

PLANNED PROCEDURE

TEVAR with Valiant stent grafts (Medtronic Vascular, Santa Rosa, CA).

PROCEDURE

Baseline thoracoabdominal angiography showed TAA (Figure 19.10). TEVAR was performed per standard technique using Valiant stent-grafts (total length of 200 mm), which resulted in successful exclusion of the aneurysm (Figure 19.11). The diameter of the stent graft was calculated from the largest diameter of the proximal landing zone and oversized by 10% to 20%.

COMPLICATION AND MANAGEMENT

After endograft deployment and delivery catheter removal, right iliac angiography showed occlusion of the right common iliac artery (Figure 19.12). The patient was treated surgically with endarterectomy of the external iliac artery (Figure 19.13) and additional stent graft placement of the common iliac artery (Figure 19.14).

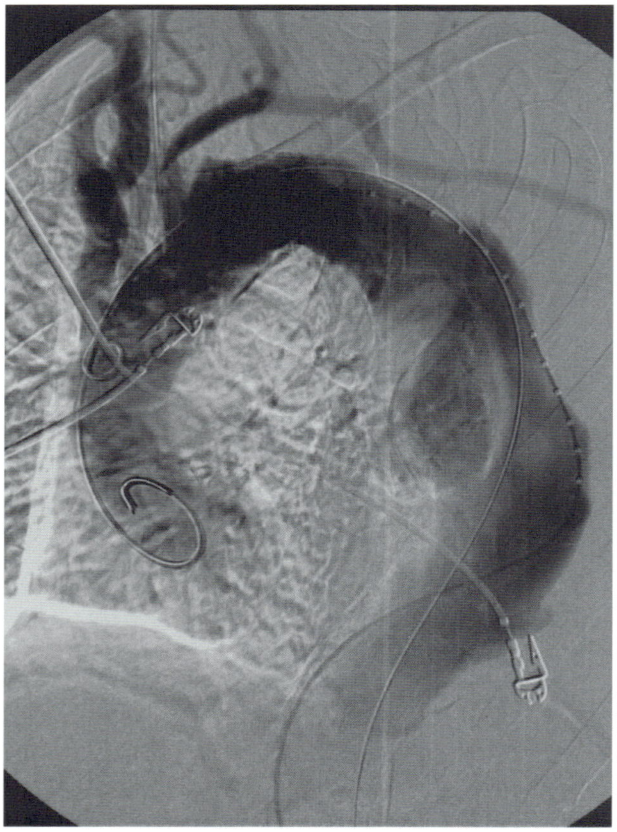

FIGURE 19.10
Baseline aortic angiography demonstrating a TAA.

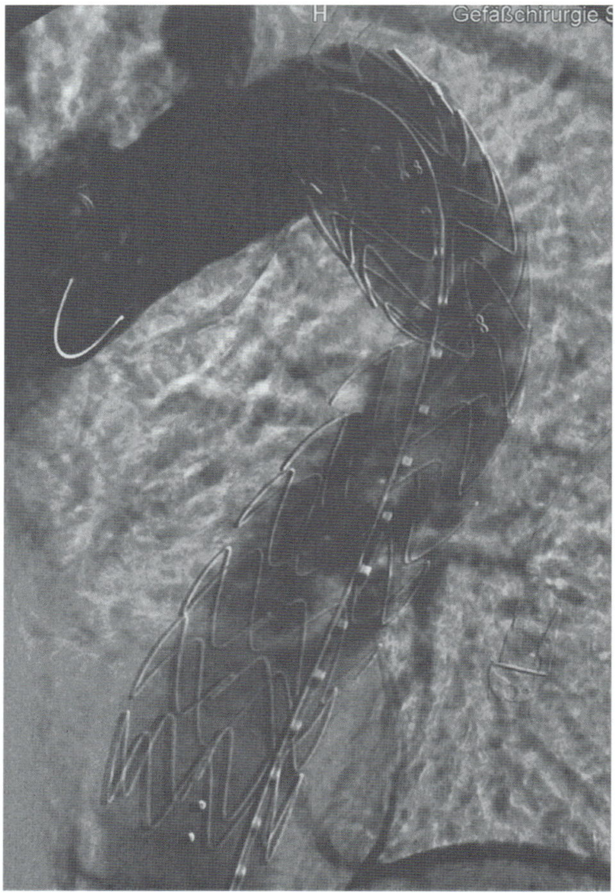

FIGURE 19.11
Intraoperative aortic angiography after endografting.

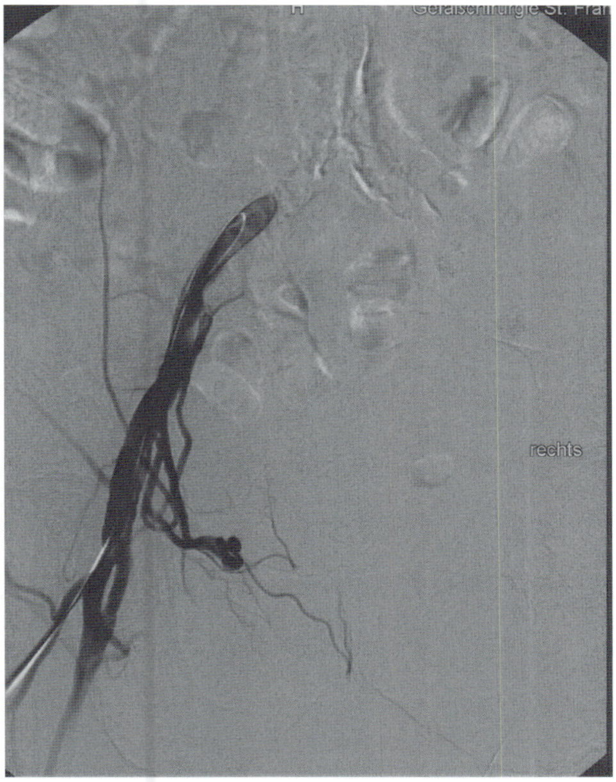

FIGURE 19.12
Acute intraoperative occlusion of the right common iliac artery.

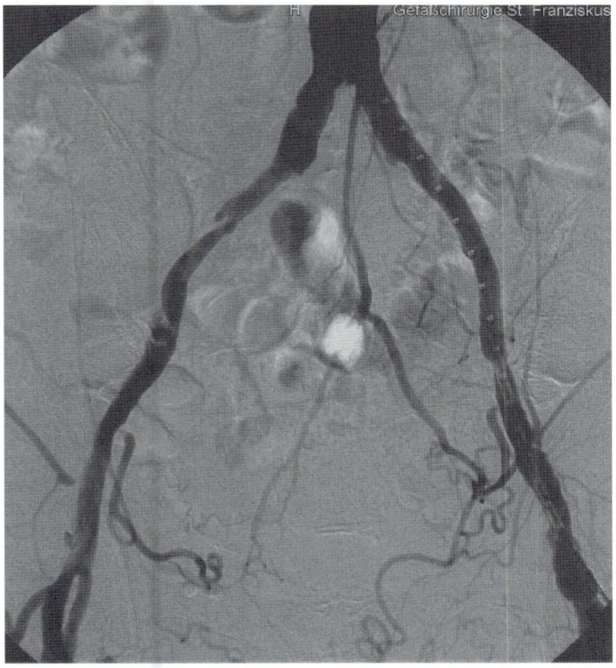

FIGURE 19.13
Ring endarterectomy of the right external iliac artery with restoration of perfusion of the right iliac axis. Significant residual stenosis of distal common iliac artery.

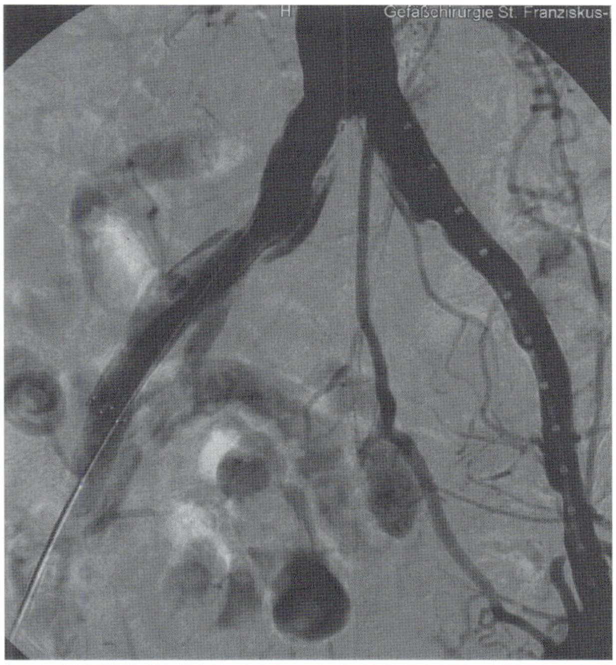

FIGURE 19.14
Additional stent graft placement of the common iliac artery to treat the stenosis of the distal common iliac artery.

CASE ANALYSIS

This complication occurred because of lack of adequate anticoagulation. Hybrid repair with surgical endarterectomy and additional stent placement allowed optimal management of this complication. Stand-alone stenting was not sufficient because the lesion involved the common femoral artery.

LESSONS

- Confirmation of adequate anticoagulation based on activated coagulation time (ACT) measurement during TEVAR is essential.
- Hybrid surgical and endovascular repair allows optimal management of post-TEVAR iatrogenic acute arterial occlusion.

SUGGESTED READING

Donas KP, Torsello G. Complications and reintervertions after EVAR: Are they decreasing in incidence? *J Cardiovasc Surg.* 2011 Apr;52(2):189–192.

CASE 19.4

Endograft Malposition during TEVAR

CLINICAL HISTORY AND DIAGNOSTIC TESTING RESULTS

A 77-year-old man with hypertension and diabetes mellitus presented with acute complicated aortic type B dissection confirmed with thoracic computer tomography angiography (CTA) (Figure 19.15).

PLANNED PROCEDURE

TEVAR with Valiant stent grafts (Medtronic Vascular, Santa Rosa, CA).

PROCEDURE

Baseline thoracoabdominal aortic angiography is shown in Figure 19.16. After deployment of the first two springs, the "wind sock" effect of the blood pressure on the flexible stent graft caused a "droop effect" with malposition of the endograft (Figure 19.17).

COMPLICATION AND MANAGEMENT

After completion of the deployment of the thoracic endograft, severe bending of the proximal portion of the stent graft was observed (Figure 19.18). This was addressed by retracting the graft distally and implanting an additional endograft proximally to achieve coverage of the dissection at the entry site (Figure 19.19).

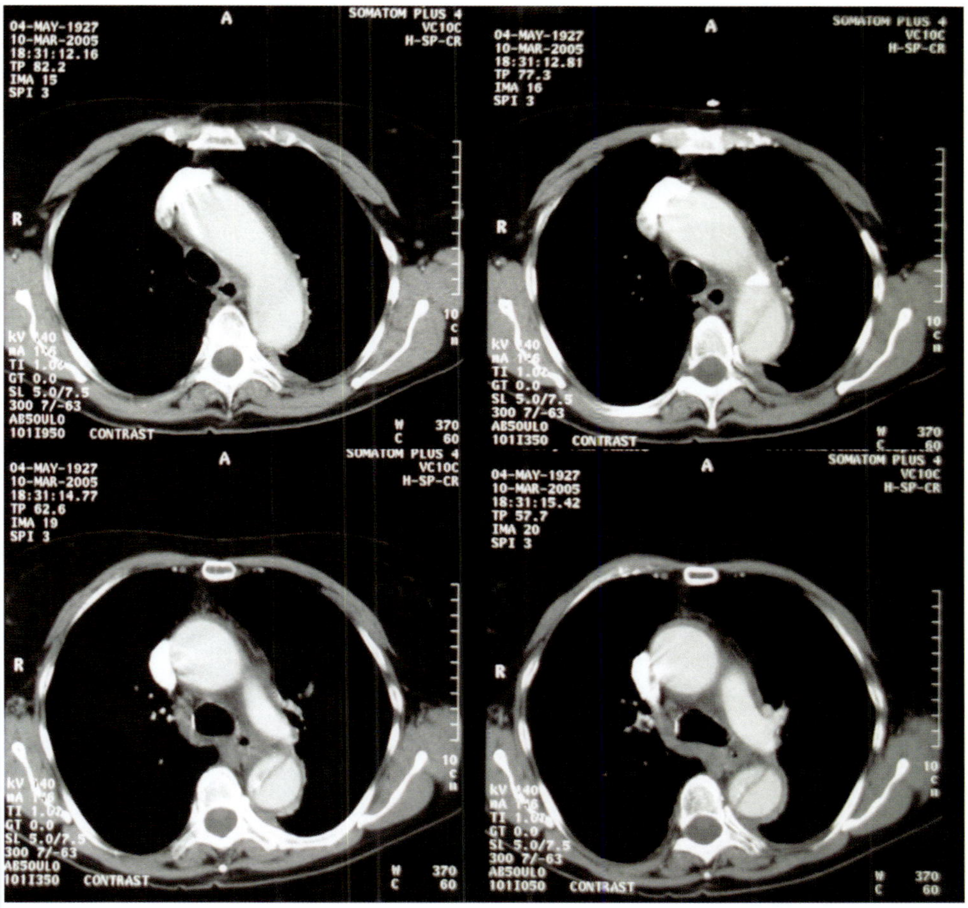

FIGURE 19.15

Baseline thoracic CTA demonstrating a type B dissection.

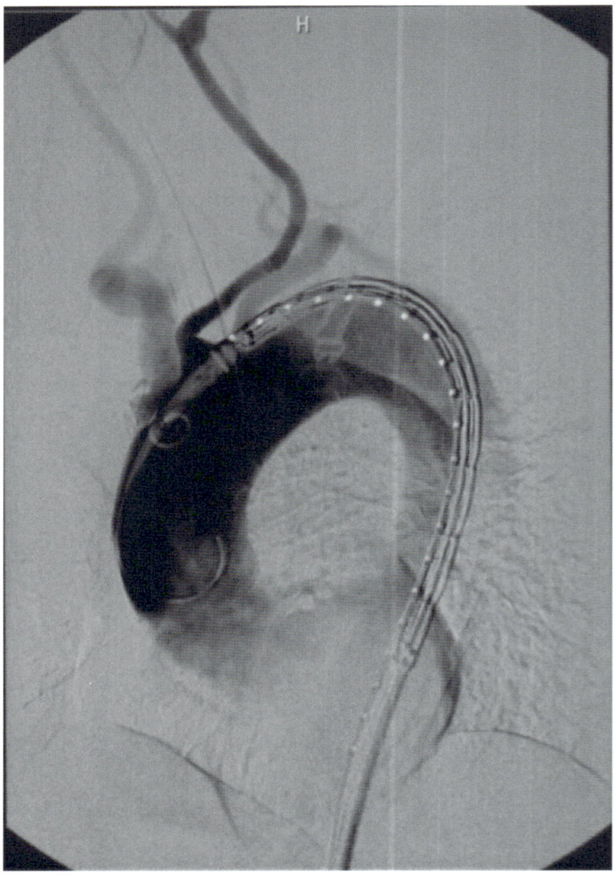

FIGURE 19.16
Baseline thoracoabdominal aortic angiography.

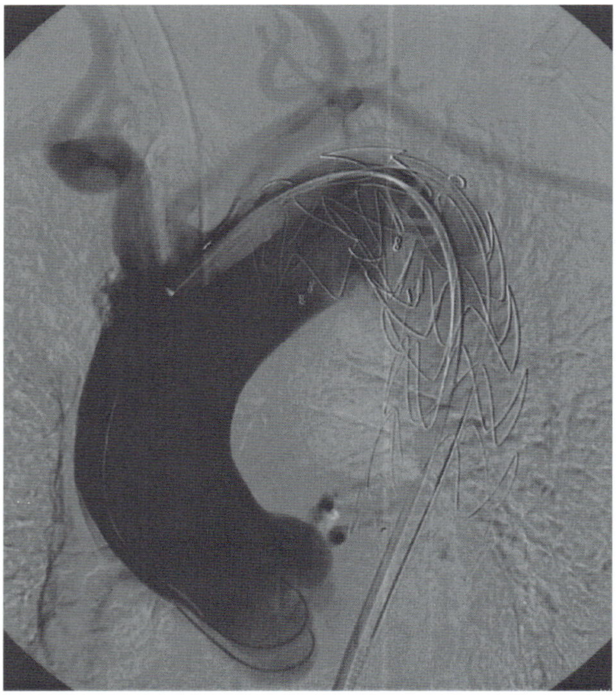

FIGURE 19.17
Malposition of the endograft.

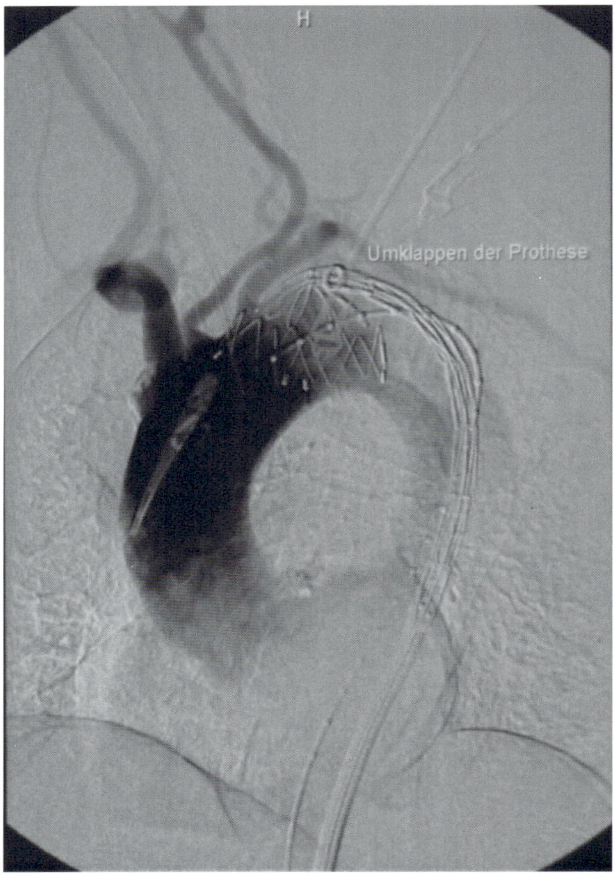

FIGURE 19.18
Note the severe bending of the proximal portion of the stent graft.

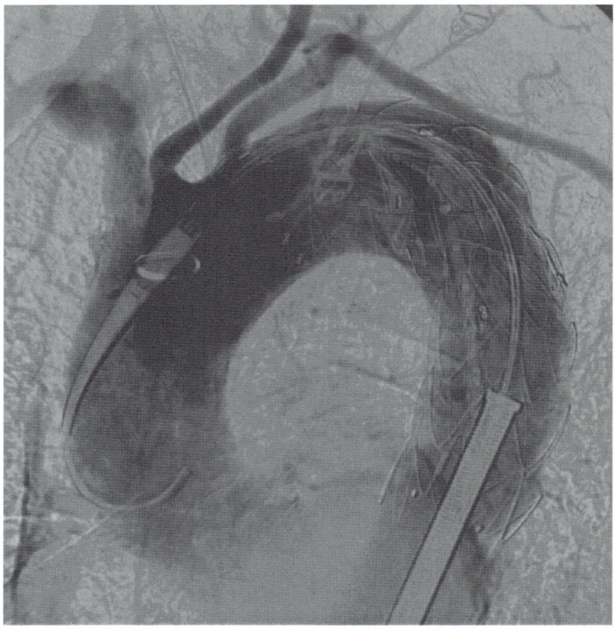

FIGURE 19.19
Deployment of a second endograft to correct the malposition.

CASE ANALYSIS

This complication occurred because the Valiant endograft lacks the longitudinal supporting bar that is present in the Talent device. This design allows greater flexibility and conformability in tortuous anatomy as well as better wall apposition, thus reducing the frequency of type I endoleak. However, this design predisposes to graft kinking in the distal arch and descending thoracic aorta.

Alternative devices with more longitudinal support, such as the Zenith endograft (Cook Medical, Bloomington, IN) may be indicated in this anatomy. Currently, the Valiant Captivia (Medtronic Vascular, Santa Rosa, CA) provides more accurate deployment in the aortic arch.

LESSONS

- Stent grafts without a longitudinal bar are more likely to be associated with kinking in the distal aortic arch.
- The probability of stent graft kinking can be reduced by better blood pressure control, faster graft release, and use of stent-grafts with tip control release mechanisms.

SUGGESTED READING

Donas KP, Torsello G. Performance of thoracic stent grafts. *Panminerva Med.* 2011 Mar;53(1):31–36.

CASE 19.5

Inadverent Occlusion of the Left Subclavian Artery During TEVAR

CLINICAL HISTORY AND DIAGNOSTIC TESTING RESULTS

A 77-year-old man with history of smoking, chronic obstructive pulmonary disease, and diabetes mellitus presented with acute complicated type B dissection confirmed with thoracic CTA (Figure 19.20).

PLANNED PROCEDURE

TEVAR with one stent graft using the chimney technique.

PROCEDURE

Baseline thoracoabdominal aortic angiography is shown in Figure 19.21a and 19.21b. The diameter of the stent-graft was calculated from the largest diameter of the proximal landing zone and oversized by 10% to 20%. TEVAR was performed per standard technique using Valiant stent graft.

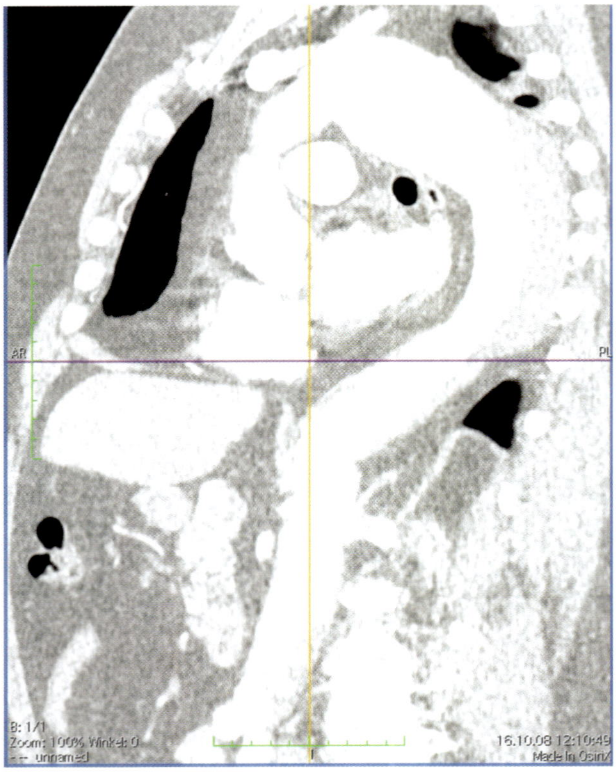

FIGURE 19.20
Baseline thoracoabdominal CTA demonstrating a type B dissection.

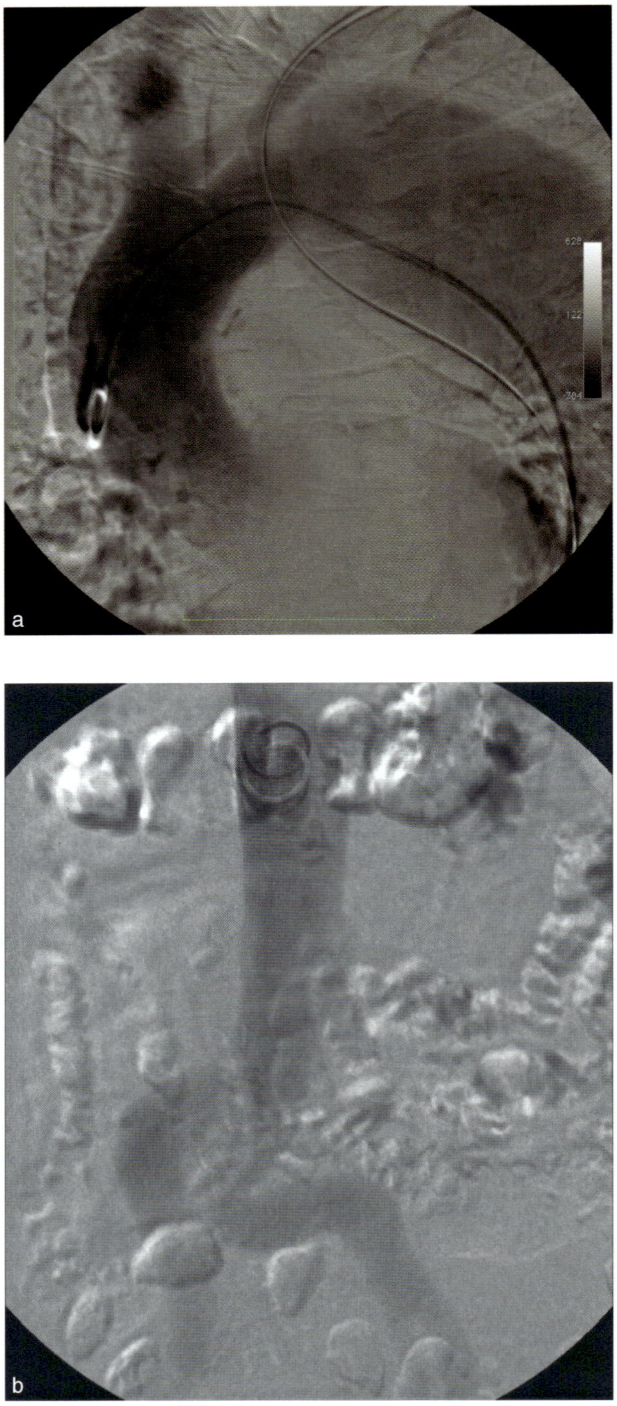

FIGURE 19.21 a, b
Baseline thoracoabdominal aortic angiography.

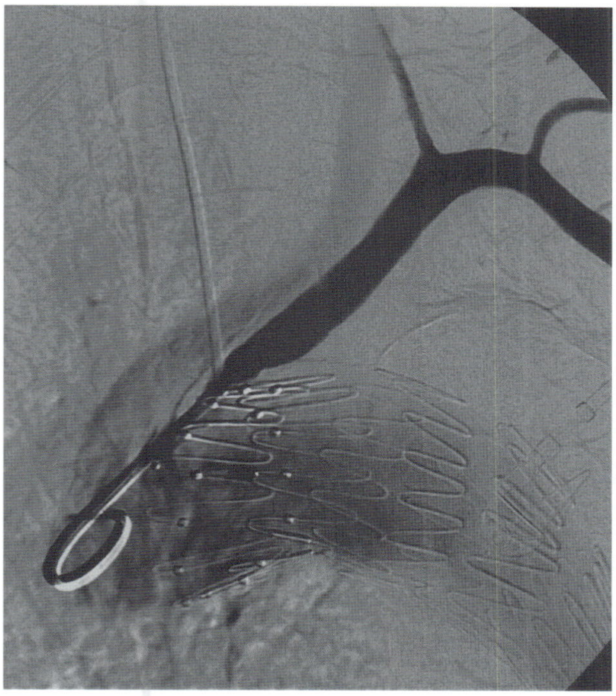

FIGURE 19.22
Aortic arch angiography after stent graft deployment demonstrating compromise of the left subclavian artery.

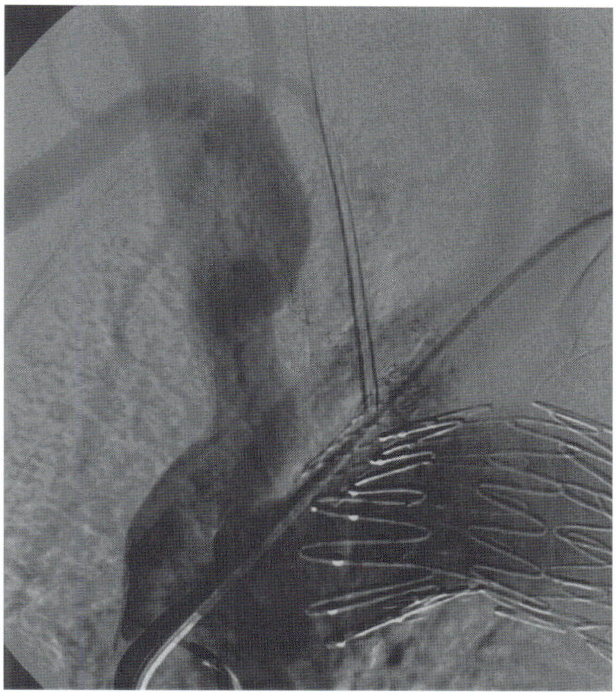

FIGURE 19.23
Successful placement of chimney graft and restoration of left subclavian artery perfusion.

COMPLICATION AND MANAGEMENT

Aortic arch angiography after stent graft deployment showed compromise of the left subclavian artery (Figure 19.22). This complication was managed with implantation of a 8-mm × 39-mm Advanta balloon expandable stent graft (Atrium, Hudon, NH) in the left subclavian artery with mild protrusion into the aortic arch beneath the aortic graft (a chimney graft) (Figure 19.23).

CASE ANALYSIS

Inadverent occlusion of the left subclavian artery during TEVAR occur as a result of insufficient neck and/or inaccurate graft placement due to motion. The use of chimney grafts is very useful in these cases.

LESSONS

- Inadverent left subclavian artery occlusion during TEVAR can be avoided by careful patient selection and procedure execution using optimal fluoroscopic visibility.
- If inadvertent left subclavian artery occlusion occurs, the use of the chimney technique can restore vessel perfusion.
- In these cases, balloon expandable stent-grafts are preferred due to its high radial force and visibility.

SUGGESTED READING

Dumfarth J, Michel M, Schmidli J, et al. Mechanisms of failure and outcome of secondary surgical interventions after thoracic endovascular aortic repair (TEVAR). *Ann Thorac Surg*. 2011 Apr;91(4):1141–1146.

20

John H. Rundback and Kevin "Chaim" Herman

Complications of Renal Artery Interventions

INTRODUCTION

Complications of percutaneous renal artery intervention (PRAI)—including selective renal artery catheterization, percutaneous transluminal renal artery angioplasty (PTRA), and renal artery stenting—are uncommon and can be described as major, minor, technical, or procedural. Major complications are generally considered as resulting in admission to a hospital for therapy (for outpatient procedures), an unplanned increase in the level of care, prolonged hospitalization, permanent adverse conditions, or death. This would include complications such as renal loss, dialysis, unplanned surgery, and transfusion. Minor complications include a wide range of events that result in no sequelae but may require a minimal amount of additional therapy or brief hospitalization, and include events ranging from groin hematoma to transient renal insufficiency or minor organ injury. Technical-procedural complications are events that occur during catheterization, PTRA, or stent deployment that have no clinical consequences but lead to an increase in procedural time and/or cost (1).

Thresholds for the occurrence of both minor and major events have been reported (Table 20.1) (1). Several older series have evaluated complication rates related to renal angioplasty varying from a high of 36% to a low of 12% (2–5); the weighted mean rate of all adverse events was 14%, excluding complications classified as radiological-technical. A more recent comparative effectiveness review described procedure related dissection in 0.3% to 13%, renal arterial thrombosis in 0.3% to 0.8%, transient renal failure in 1.5% to 13%, and peripheral emboli in 1.4% to 10% (6). Embolization results in segmental renal infarction in approximately 1% of cases (4).

Thirty-day mortality is approximately 1%, usually related to renal artery perforation, cholesterol embolization, acute renal failure, and retroperitoneal hemorrhage due to inadvertently high arterial puncture. Surgical rescue for emergent revascularization, hemorrhage, or secondary nephrectomy is below 1% in meta-analysis (6). Groin hematoma and puncture site trauma are the most commonly reported complications (7,8).

In the most contemporary and largest prospective study to date, the Angioplasty and Stenting for Renal Artery Lesions trial described procedure-related complications in 31 of 359 patients randomized to renal intervention, a composite rate of 9% (9). There was a 4.5% "serious" complication rate, including five occurrences of renal embolization, four renal artery

TABLE 20.1

Specific Major Complications From Percutaneous Renal Revascularization.

	REPORTED RATE	THRESHOLD
30-day mortality	1%	1%
Secondary nephrectomy	<1%	1%
Surgical salvage operation	1%	2%
Symptomatic embolization	3%	3%
Main renal artery occlusion	2%	2%
Branch renal artery occlusion	2%	2%
Access site hematoma requiring surgery, transfusion, or prolonging hospital stay	5%	5%
Acute renal failure	2%	2%
Worsening of chronic renal failure requiring an increase in the level of care	2%	5%

Source: Used with permission from Martin et al (1).

occlusions, four perforations of the renal artery, and three peripheral cholesterol embolizations resulting in amputations. In addition, there was one additional renal artery occlusion during 30-day follow-up; five patients with acute kidney injury not described in detail and four patients with groin hematomas required repeat hospital admission. Thirty-day mortality was 0.7% (9). These data are comparable to prior series and the global experience with renal interventions.

Transient contrast related declines in renal function may be seen in up to 13% of patients undergoing renal interventions (1). The risk factors for renal failure following administration of iodinated contrast material are well known and include preexisting renal insufficiency, dehydration, diabetic nephropathy, hyperuricemia, and multiple myeloma (10). Fortunately in patients with normal renal function, the risk of permanent renal impairment is small. CO_2 angiography may be routinely used in patients with marginal renal reserve (11). In addition, premedication with mucomyst or fenoldopam may decrease the renal toxicity of iodinated contrast material (12,13).

Arguably, the more routine use of modern low-profile systems and flexible stents has reduced the procedural hazard. In contemporary series utilizing modern technique, serious adverse events occur in 5% or less of treated patients (14–16). Distal embolic protection devices (DPDs) may mitigate embolic risk in selected cases (16). As with all invasive therapies, optimal outcomes of renal artery stenting are likely to be achieved by a combination of careful case selection, individualized interventional strategies, and familiarity and comfort with a wide range of available devices and techniques. Interventional suites must be equipped with both basic as well as less commonly used but potentially critical therapeutic systems, including specialized guidewires, selective catheters, guides, balloon, and stents of varying sizes and configurations. Finally, prompt recognition and management of complications are paramount to avoiding organ loss or potential mortality. The following case examples exemplify the management of some of the more fatal potential technological problems occurring with renal artery stenting.

CASE 20.1

Renal Artery Rupture During Renal Artery Angioplasty

CLINICAL HISTORY AND DIAGNOSTIC TESTING RESULTS

A 74-year-old Hispanic female with a 14-year history of hypertension, type 2 diabetes, obesity, and asymptomatic 70% right internal carotid artery stenosis, initially referred for evaluation for carotid artery stenting. Current medications are glipizide, clopidogrel, olmesartan, hydrochlorothiazide, metformin, nateglinide, and eszopiclone. On examination, blood pressure in the right arm was 174/65 mmHg, left arm 178/72 mmHg, and heart rate was 83 beats per minute. A renal duplex ultrasound demonstrated symmetrical kidney size with elevated peak systolic velocities (PSV) in the proximal and middle portion of both renal arteries (right PSV 240 cm/s, left PSV 215 cm/s).

PLANNED PROCEDURE

Bilateral renal angioplasty

PROCEDURE

An initial aortogram (not shown) demonstrated bilateral severe renal artery stenosis. After successful stent placement of the left renal artery, selective catheterization of the right renal artery was performed with a Sos 3 catheter (Angiodynamics, Queensbury, NY). Angiogarphy demonstrated diffuse fibromuscular dysplasia extending from the renal ostium into the right upper pole renal artery (Figure 20.1). Through a 7-Fr Renal Double Curve guide (Cordis Inc, Bridgewater, NJ), the lesion was crossed with a 0.014-inch Spartacore wire (Abbott Vascular, Abbott Park, IL) and 0.014-inch RADI wire (St. Jude Medical, St. Paul, MN) wire revealing a 20 mmHg systolic gradient. Initial angioplasty was performed with a 6-mm Sterling balloon (Boston Scientific, Nadick, MA), with angiography demonstrating residual weblike stenosis and a 15 mmHg residual gradient. Therefore, repeat angioplasty was performed over both wires with a 7-mm Ultrathin (Boston Scientific) balloon (Figure 20.2).

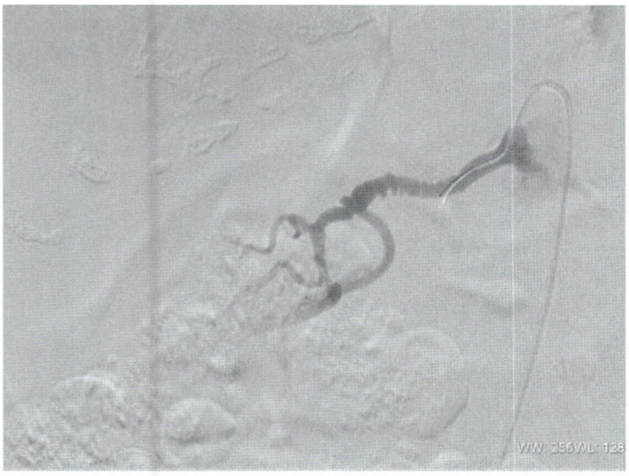

FIGURE 20.1

Selective right renal arteriography demonstrating a "string-of-beads" pattern typical of medial fibroplasias.

COMPLICATION AND MANAGEMENT

After balloon deflation, repeat angiography demonstrated a renal artery rupture with extensive retroperitoneal contrast extravasation (Figure 20.3). The patient experienced right flank pain and had sudden hypotension with a systemic blood pressure of 80/40 mmHg. A balloon was quickly advanced into the renal artery and inflated for hemostasis. Exchange was made for an 8-Fr vascular sheath (Cordis brite tip) over the two 0.014-inch wires. This was used to engage the ostium of the right renal artery, and a 7- × 38-mm long iCAST polytetrafluoroethylene covered stent graft (Atrium

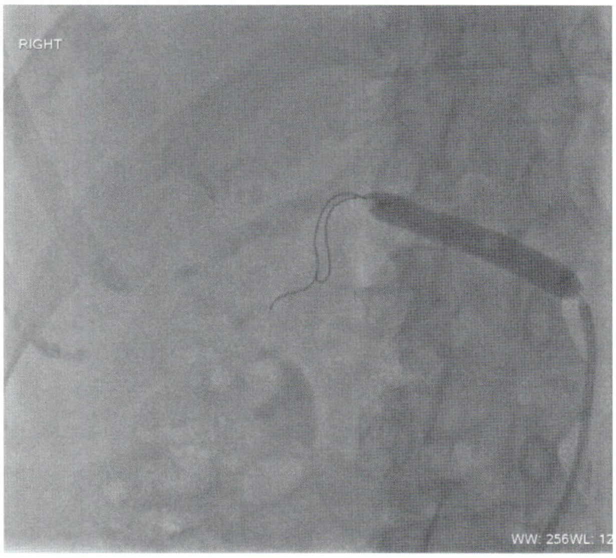

FIGURE 20.2

Repeat angioplasty of the right renal artery using a 7- × 40-mm Ultrathin balloon (Boston Scientific) advanced over two 0.014 inch wires, as described in the text. Prior angioplasty using a 6-mm diameter balloon resulted in inadequate dilation and a residual gradient, requiring more aggressive dilation.

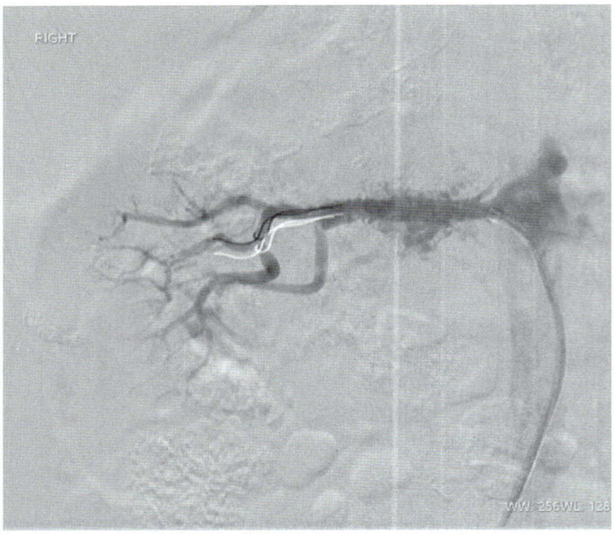

FIGURE 20.3
Angiography after 7-mm angioplasty demonstrated rupture along the length of the main renal artery with extensive perivascular extravasation (arrows).

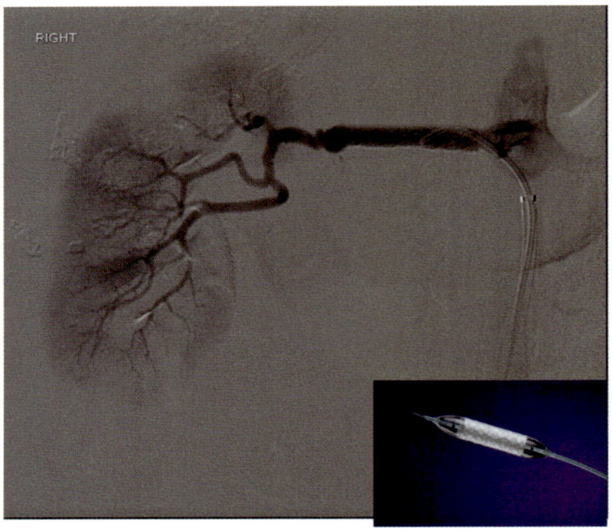

FIGURE 20.4
Completion renal angiography after placement of a 6- x 22-mm iCast stent (Atrium Med) shows complete sealing of the arterial rupture and preserved renal flow. The patient had a subsequent renal artery duplex study one month later showing normal velocities in the renal artery. The inset shows a balloon mounted and expanded iCAST stent.

Medical, Hudson, NH) was deployed across the main renal artery up to the level of its bifurcation. Completion angiography demonstrated resolution of extravasation with preserved flow through the bulk of the kidney, although there was segmental thrombosis of a small lower pole renal artery branch (Figure 20.4). Final pressure measurements reveal no residual trans-stenotic gradient.

CASE ANALYSIS

In this case, renal artery rupture occurred because of balloon oversizing combined with a buddy wire technique. Renal artery rupture is a rare complication of renal angioplasty and may occur due to wire perforation, dissection, or oversizing of the angioplasty balloon relative to the diameter of the renal artery. The diagnosis of rupture is made by the identification of contrast outside of the normal confines of the renal artery. Small wire induced cortical perforations may cause extravasation that is self-limited or more rarely require segmental coil embolization of the affected intrarenal branch. Similarly, subtle small and contained areas of rupture adjacent to the main renal artery may possibly be managed conservatively with observation, reversal of anticoagulation, and repeated angiography until extravasation is no longer demonstrated. Close follow-up and computed tomography imaging would be recommended to better identify the extent of injury and associated retroperitoneal blood loss. In contrast, overt disruption of the main renal artery necessitates immediate attention, temporary balloon occlusion, and definitive management. Historically, surgical repair has been the treatment of choice. Ice cooled saline can be intermittently infused through the balloon catheter lumen to help preserve renal viability pending surgical exploration.

Over the past decade, the commercial availability of polytetrafluoroethylene covered stent grafts has allowed renal artery rupture to be managed using endovascular techniques. Balloon expandable grafts are generally employed due to reliable positioning, short available lengths that are suitable for use in the renal artery, and predictable radial force to provide sealing of the arterial defect. In the United States in 2010, the iCAST (Atrium Medical) stent graft was the only commercially available device. The iCAST stent graft is a fully encapsulated stainless steel platform available in 5 to 7 mm diameters and lengths of 16 mm and 22 mm. Since renal artery rupture requiring urgent intervention is uncommon, there are limited descriptions of this technique, although high rates of success would be anticipated, as demonstrated in this case. However, in cases in which rupture occurs at the renal artery ostium, adequate sealing may not be possible, and rapid aortic occlusion and surgical repair are necessary.

LESSONS

- Oversizing of balloons can result in renal artery rupture.
- Small injuries may be conservatively managed; large tears require immediate endovascular intervention.
- Balloon occlusion should be secured while preparing a balloon expandable stent graft for definitive repair.
- Quick and coordinated team efforts are needed to upsize the delivery sheath and expediently deliver the stent graft to avoid hemodynamic compromise.

SUGGESTED READING

Ashenburg RJ, Blair RJ, Rivera FJ, Weigele JB. Renal arterial rupture complicating transluminal angioplasty: Successful conservative management. *Radiology.* 1990;174(3 Pt 2):983–985.

Rasmus M, Huegli R, Jacob AL, Aschwanden M, Bilecen D. Extensive iatrogenic aortic dissection during renal angioplasty: Successful treatment with a covered stent-graft. *Cardiovasc Intervent Radiol.* 2007;30(3):497–500.

Yeo KK, Rogers JH, Laird JR. Use of stent grafts and coils in vessel rupture and perforation. *J Interv Cardiol.* 2008;21(1):86–99.

CASE 20.2

Intrarenal Thrombus During Renal Artery Stenting

CLINICAL HISTORY AND DIAGNOSTIC TESTING RESULTS

A 62-year-old woman with history of type 2 diabetes, coronary artery disease with prior coronary artery bypass grafting and coronary stenting, prior stroke, and chronic lymphocytic leukemia in remission presents with two-block claudication and multidrug-resistant hypertension. Current blood pressure medications are amlodipine 5 mg daily, hydrochlorothiazide 25 mg daily, carvedilol 6.25 mg daily, and ramipril 10 mg twice daily. In addition, she took acetylsalicylic acid 81 mg daily. She had normal renal function (serum creatinine 0.57 mg/dL). On examination, blood pressure was 165/82 mmHg and heart rate 78 beats per minute. Heart sounds were normal. Computed tomography angiography demonstrated bilateral superficial femoral artery chronic total occlusions and a severe ostial right renal artery stenosis.

PLANNED PROCEDURE

Right renal artery direct stenting.

PROCEDURE

Through a right common femoral artery approach, a pigtail catheter was inserted and an abdominal aortogram and selective right renal arteriogram obtained, demonstrating severe ostial and proximal right renal artery stenosis (RAS) (Figure 20.5). Through a 7-Fr RDC (renal double curve) guide (Cordis Inc, Bridgewater, NJ), the lesion was crossed with a 0.014-inch Spartacore wire (Abbott Medical, Abbott Park, IL). Direct stenting was performed with a 5-mm diameter by 14-mm long Express SD stent (Boston Scientific, Natick, MA).

COMPLICATION AND MANAGEMENT

Selective angiography after stenting demonstrated complete resolution of the ostial and proximal RAS, with a "tram-track" appearing defect extending distal to the stent most consistent with intraluminal thrombus (Figure 20.6). An initial attempt at aspiration thrombectomy using an Export catheter (Medtronic Inc, Minneapolis, MN) did not result in any improvement. Therefore, a second 6-mm diameter by 14-mm long Express SD stent was deployed overlapping the first stent and covering the thrombus. This resulted in nearly complete exclusion of the thrombus with only a small residual filling defect and brisk renal perfusion (Figure 20.7). Follow-up angiography at the time of lower extremity revascularization 4 months later showed moderate in-stent stenosis without remaining thrombus (Figure 20.8).

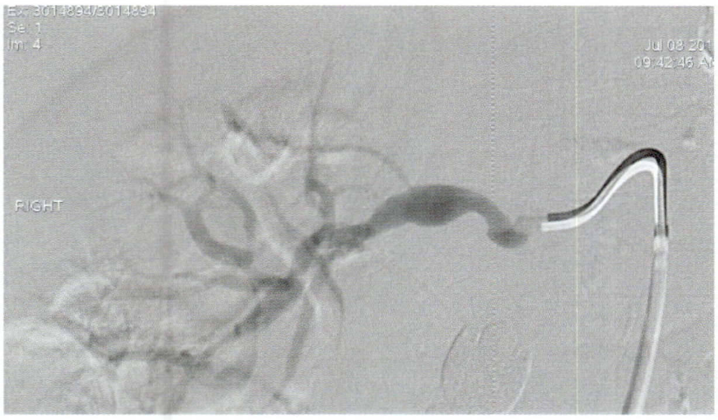

FIGURE 20.5
Selective arteriography demonstrates tight stenoses of the ostial and proximal right renal artery.

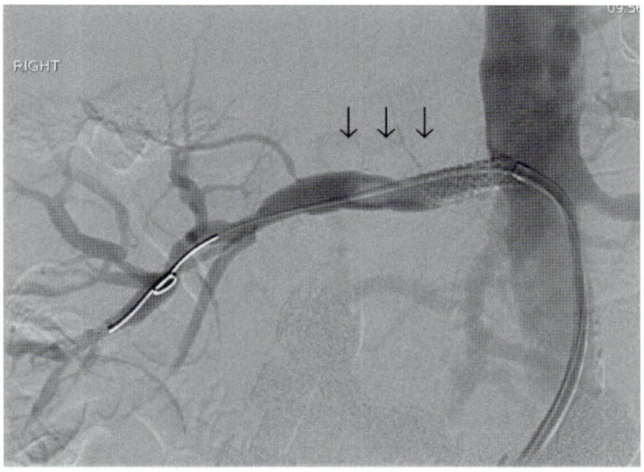

FIGURE 20.6
After stenting of the proximal stenosis, intraluminal thrombus is seen extending distal to the stent within the middle portion of the main renal artery (arrows).

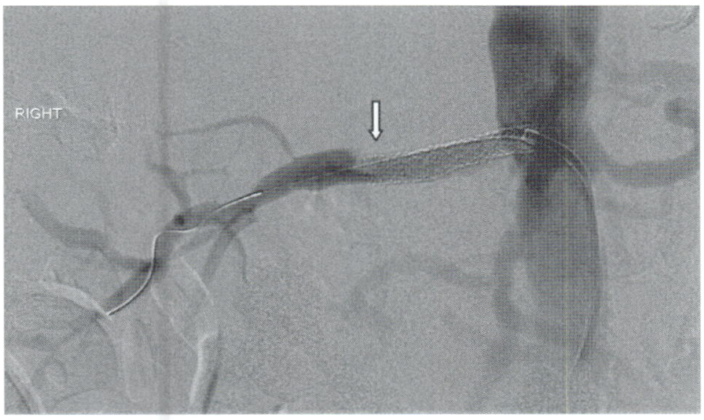

FIGURE 20.7
After placement of a second overlapping 6-mm stent, most of the thrombus is excluded, with only a small persistent defect noted at the terminal portion of the second stent. Renal perfusion is preserved. This was managed conservatively with 24 hours of intravenous unfractionated heparin and oral clopidogrel.

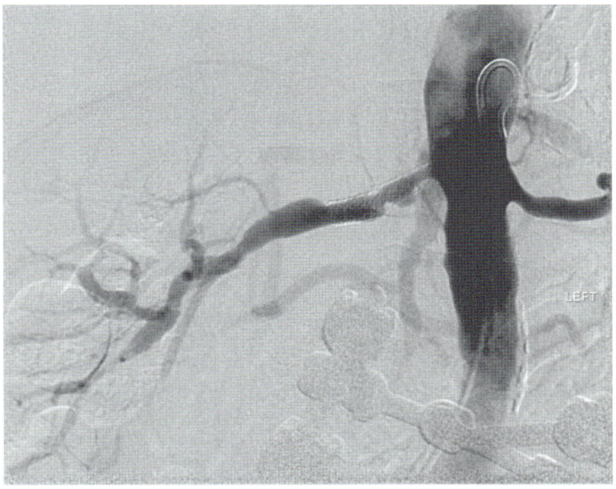

FIGURE 20.8
Follow-up aortography 4 months later at the time of lower extremity revascularization shows resolution of intraluminal thrombus or dissection with mild early in-stent restenosis. The patient's blood pressure remained clinically improved.

CASE ANALYSIS

Although the cause of intrarenal artery thrombus formation or atheroma in this case is uncertain, it is likely that it originated from the aorta. Review of the preprocedural computer tomography angiography (CTA) in this patient reveals a significant region of juxta-renal atheroma in the aorta. It is likely that during catheterization of the renal artery or advancement of the stent resulted in intrarenal thromboembolism. Although this was not a case of acute renal artery occlusion, aggressive management of acute thromboembolism is imperative to prevent further thrombosis and occlusion resulting in renal failure.

Acute renal artery occlusion during PRAI is rare, occurring in 2% to 3% of cases. The clinical significance and true incidence of nonocclusive atheroembolization during PRAI is unknown. Generally, atheroemboli result in progressive loss of renal function due to localized inflammation of arterioles rather than an acute embolus or thrombus in the main renal artery. While there is no specific treatment for atheroembolization, DPDs with or without the use of a glycoprotein 2b/3a inhibitor may play a role in preventing the devastating consequence of atheroembolization. It is not known at which point during PRAI atheroembolization occurs, however, embolization can be avoided by minimizing contact of the guide catheter to the renal artery ostium, by decreasing the number of passes and possibly by utilizing a "no touch" technique.

Percutaneous treatment options for intrarenal thromboembolism during PRAI would include aspiration thrombectomy, intraarterial pharmacologic thrombolysis, and/or direct stenting. Several studies and case reports have shown the benefit of thrombolysis with or without aspiration thrombectomy in restoring flow and preserving renal function for cases involving complete renal artery occlusion. In our case, immediate catheter directed aspiration thrombectomy was initially chosen, although no significant amount of thrombus was aspirated and there was no angiographic change. This led us to believe the thrombus was not acute but rather likely due to dislodged mural thrombus or atheroma. Furthermore, continued manipulation with the aspiration catheter and/or use of a mechanical thrombolytic device can possibly lead to further downstream embolization of material, resulting in worsening renal function due to occlusion of arterioles. Therefore, direct stenting of the lesion was the preferred treatment option, with the caveat that if renal blood flow was not improved then further techniques, such as pulse spray thrombolysis, mechanical thrombectomy, or overnight thrombolysis with an infusion catheter, might be considered.

LESSONS

- In contrast to microembolization or clinically silent cholesterol embolization, bulk atheroembolization of the kidney occurs rarely during PRAI.
- Intrarenal atheroembolization during PRAI may be clinically silent, indolent, or manifest itself acutely.
- Acute intrarenal embolus should be treated aggressively with various percutaneous techniques, such as aspiration thrombectomy, mechanical/pharmacologic thrombolysis, and/or stent placement.

SUGGESTED READING

Feldman R, Wargovich T, Bittl J. No-touch technique for reducing aortic wall trauma during renal artery stenting. *Catheter Cardiovasc Interv.* 1999;46:245–248.

Morris C, Bonnevie G, Najarian K. Nonsurgical treatment of acute iatrogenic renal artery injuries occurring after renal artery angioplasty and stenting. *AJR.* 2001;177:1353–1357.

Murphy T, Dubel G. Distal embolic protection for renal arterial interventions. *Cardiovas Intervent Radiol.* 2008;31:14–22.

Salam T, Lumsden A, Martin L. Local infusion of fibrinolytic agents for acute renal artery thromboembolism: Report of ten cases. *Ann Vasc Surgery.* 1993;7:21–26.

CASE 20.3

Dislodged Stent During Renal Artery Stenting

CLINICAL HISTORY AND DIAGNOSTIC TESTING RESULTS

A 75-year-old man had a history of hypertension and type 2 diabetes recently diagnosed with right renal artery stenosis.

PLANNED PROCEDURE

Direct renal artery stenting.

PROCEDURE

Through a femoral approach, the ostial right renal artery lesion was crossed, and a 0.035-inch Rosen wire secured in the distal artery utilizing a 7-Fr renal double curve (RDC) guide catheter, cobra catheter, and Bentson wire (Cook Medical, Bloomington, IN) (Figure 20.9). As direct stenting was planned, an earlier version 6-mm × 18-mm Genesis stent (Cordis, Bridgewater, NJ) was advanced over the wire but resistance was met during the attempt to cross the ostial lesion.

COMPLICATION AND MANAGEMENT

As the stent was being pushed through the lesion it inadvertently dislodged off the balloon, but it remained on the wire (Figure 20.10). The stenosis was dilated with the balloon to facilitate subsequent placement of a second stent. Keeping the wire tip in the renal artery, the balloon was then removed, and the loop portion of a 25-mm Amplatz Gooseneck snare (Microvena, White Bear Lake, MN) was placed around the wire and closed so that the loop and its attached constraining catheter could then be slid over the renal wire using the wire as a monorail system (Figure 20.11). The

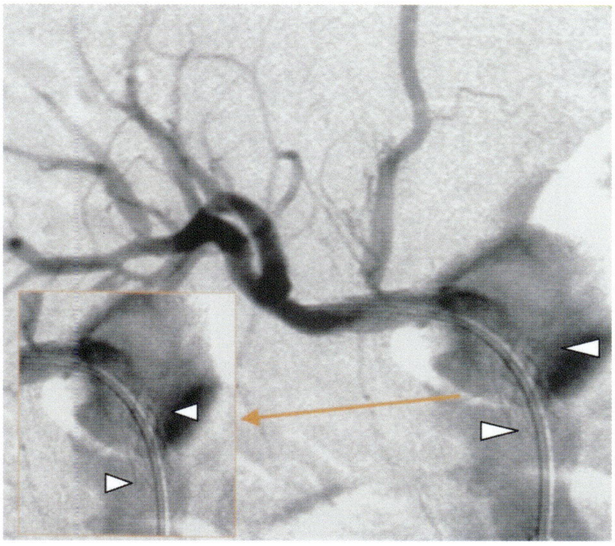

FIGURE 20.10
During attempted stent positioning, the partially dilated stent inadvertently dislodged from the balloon (arrowheads in figure and inset) due to unanticipated lesional severity and calcification.

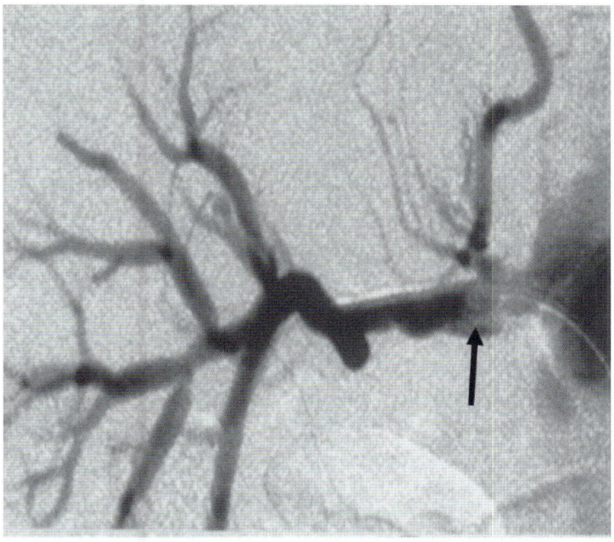

FIGURE 20.9
An ostial right renal artery stenosis is noted on selective angiography (arrow).

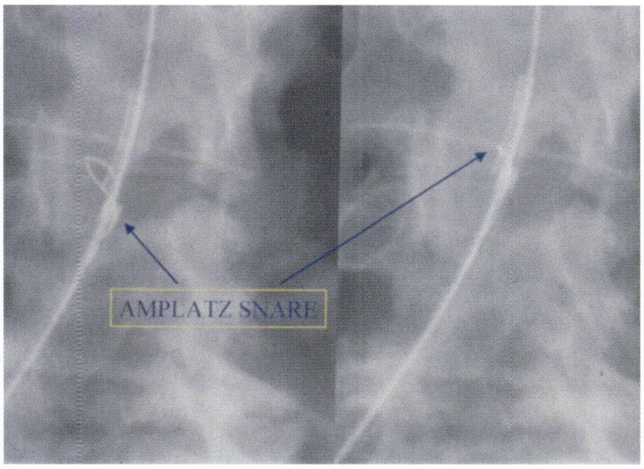

FIGURE 20.11
A nitinol loop snare advanced through the sheath with its loop over the wire and its restraining catheter parallel to the wire successfully captured and constrained the stent, which was then removed through the femoral sheath.

snare was then advanced through the sheath until it was positioned just below the stent, at which point the snare was opened and manipulated upward until it surrounded the lower stent edge (figure 3C). The stent was constrained and pulled downward into the sheath. Although most of the stent was captured within the sheath, a small portion protruded beyond the sheath and could not be entirely collapsed. Therefore, the entire sheath and stent were removed from the femoral access site, which resulted in loss of wire access across the renal artery. Once the stent was outside of the body, the sheath and its contained stent and snare were carefully taken off of the wire, allowing the wire to be pushed up into the aorta and the sheath to be replaced. The renal artery was again traversed and successfully stented.

CASE ANALYSIS

Stent dislodgment is infrequent with current generations of balloon premounted stents but may still occur in cases of heavily calcified renal artery origins, which may cause separation of the leading edge of the stent from the balloon and consequent engagement of the stent on the aortic lip of the renal plaque during attempted positioning. Dislodgment is also a risk when treating severe stenoses without predilation, particularly if the stent–balloon system prolapses above the renal artery during attempted advancement across the lesion. Careful observation during all manipulations, avoidance of excessive forward pressure, predilation when necessary, and optimized guide selection and positioning at the renal ostium are key to preventing stent dislodgement.

Once dislodgment occurs, it is critical to maintain wire access across the renal artery to avoid "losing" the stent off of the wire. Using the stent balloon to dilate the artery, as was done in this case, will allow easier placement of a later stent after the dislodged stent is retrieved, and at least assure that there has been therapeutic intervention for the target lesion in the event that a second stent cannot be placed. The technique of passing the nitinol loop snare over the wire affords co-axial positioning of the loop around the dislodged stent. Tightening of the loop then allows stent capture. In some cases, a repeated motion of opening and closing the snare along the length of the stent may be needed for complete constrainment. Alternatively, the stent can be pulled down to the iliac artery, released from the snare, recrossed with a fresh balloon, and deployed in the iliac artery. Clearly, the success of these maneuvers is case dependent and related to the diameter of the partially deployed stent, the degree to which it has been dilated (i.e., can another balloon be placed within the stent), and the tortuosity of the patients vasculature. Other potential strategies for engaging and retrieving dislodged stent have been described and include the use of stone baskets, forceps, and novel devices specifically designed to capture the trailing edge of nondeployed stents.

LESSONS

- For tight, calcified or markedly angulated renal artery stenosis, predilation may avoid the risk of stent dislodgment. Appropriately shaped and positioned guide catheters or sheaths should also reduce this.
- Initially, maintaining wire access across the renal artery is important to avoid distal stent embolization that may render retrieval to be more difficult or impossible. Do not "lose" the stent.
- Coaxial and parallel placement of a nitinol loop snare assures controlled stent capture in most cases.

SUGGESTED READING

Gabelmann A, Kramer S, Gorich J. Percutaneous retrieval of lost or misplaced intravascular objects. *Am J Roentgenol.* 2001;176(6):1509–1513.

Tsuchida M, Kawashiri MA, Uchiyama K, et al. An enhanced device for transluminal retrieval of vascular stents without surgical procedures: Experimental studies. *J Interv Cardiol.* 2010;23(3):264–270.

Wolf F, Schernthaner RE, Dirisamer A, et al. Endovascular management of lost or misplaced intravascular objects: Experiences of 12 years. *Cardiovasc Intervent Radiol.* 2008;31(3):563–568.

CASE 20.4

Renal Artery Dissection During Renal Artery Stenting

CLINICAL HISTORY AND DIAGNOSTIC TESTING RESULTS

A 75-year-old man with refractory hypertension recently diagnosed with bilateral renal artery stenosis seen on CTA.

PLANNED PROCEDURE

Bilateral renal artery stent placement.

PROCEDURE

An initial aortogram (not shown) demonstrated bilateral severe renal artery stenosis. After successful stent placement of the left renal artery with good result, the right renal artery was selectively catheterized with the aid of a 4-Fr Sos Omni (Angiodynamics, Queensbury, NY) catheter and Bentson guidewire. The Bentson wire was then exchanged for a stiff J-tipped wire. A 7-Fr RDC guide (Cordis Inc, Bridgewater, NJ) was advanced to the ostium and the Sos Omni was removed. A 6- × 18-mm Racer stent (Medtronic, Minneapolis, MN) was then deployed.

COMPLICATION AND MANAGEMENT

An initial poststent deployment angiogram (Figure 20.12) demonstrated widely restored patency of the renal artery ostium. However, a "double shadow" was noted at the distal touchdown point of the stent, adjacent to an early bifurcating lower pole renal artery branch. In addition, the patient complained of persistent pain after stent implantation and removal of the inflating deflation, and a focal dissection was therefore suspected. A 10-minute delayed poststent placement angiogram (Figure 20.13) was performed showing extensive antegrade dissection of the main renal artery distal to the stent. The segmental renal arteries and the early branching lower pole renal artery are no longer perfused. On the delayed image (Figure 20.14), contrast is seen filling the dissection plane. Based on the findings of the poststenting distal renal artery dissection, it was decided to place an additional stent to tack down the intimal flap and restore renal perfusion. A crucial point in the successful management of this case was the fact the guidewire was still in place across the dissection flap and in the true lumen. Therefore, a second 5- × 18-mm Racer stent (Medtronic, Minneapolis, MN) was deployed in an overlapping fashion and extending distal to the previously placed stent. A completion right renal angiogram demonstrated good perfusion of the main renal artery with exclusion of the dissection plane; however, the lower pole branch is no longer perfused, leading to loss of portion of the lower pole kidney (Figure 20.15). The blood pressure stabilized and the pain dissipated poststenting.

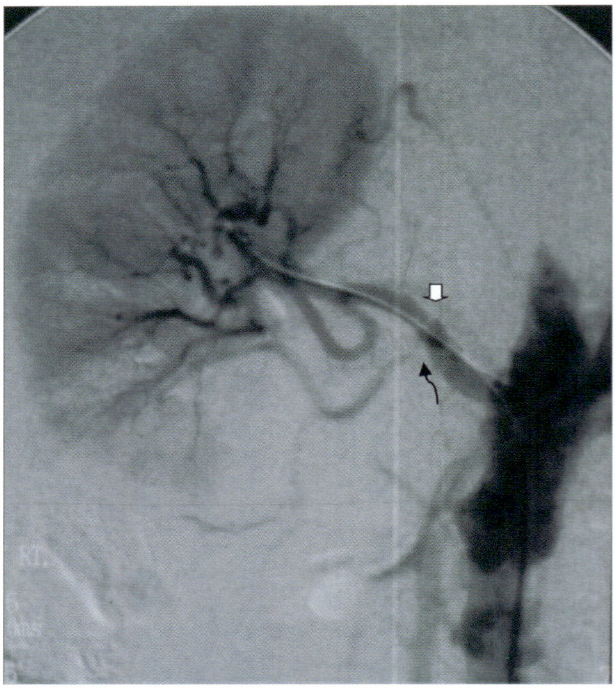

FIGURE 20.12
Initial poststenting angiography of the right renal artery. The presence of an unusual area of shadowing at the distal stent edge (arrowhead) and adjacent narrowing of a proximally branching lower pole renal artery branch (curved arrow) signaled potential dissection.

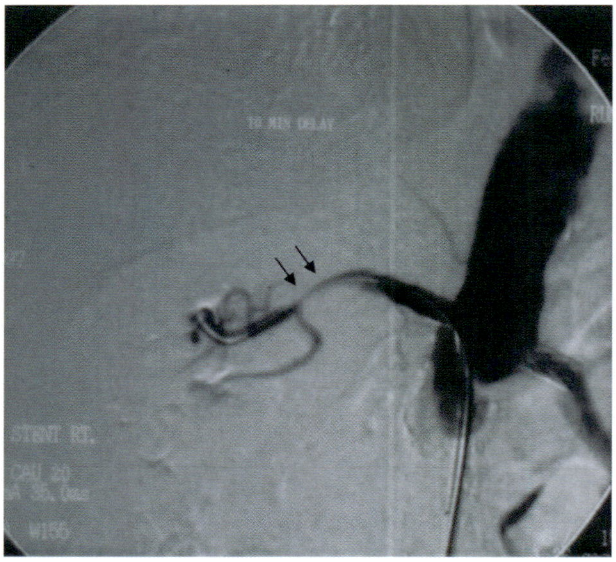

FIGURE 20.13
Dissection and narrowing of the distal renal artery is apparent on delayed angiography (arrows), which extends to the main renal bifurcation.

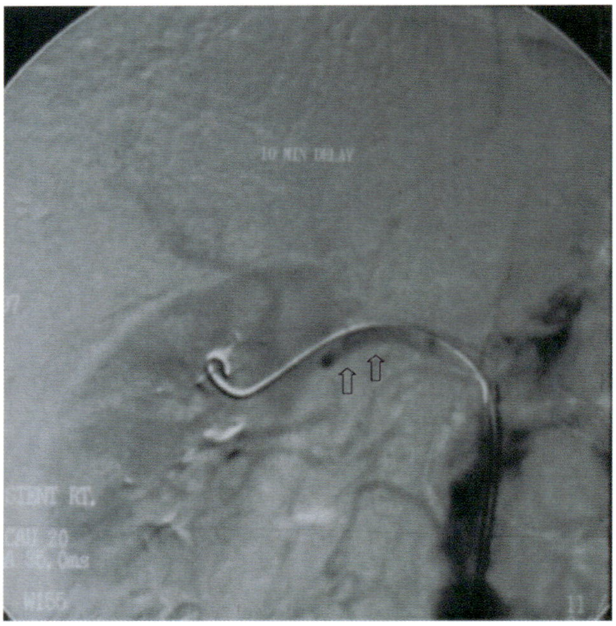

FIGURE 20.14
A late image from the angiogram shows contrast pooling in the dissection plane (open arrows).

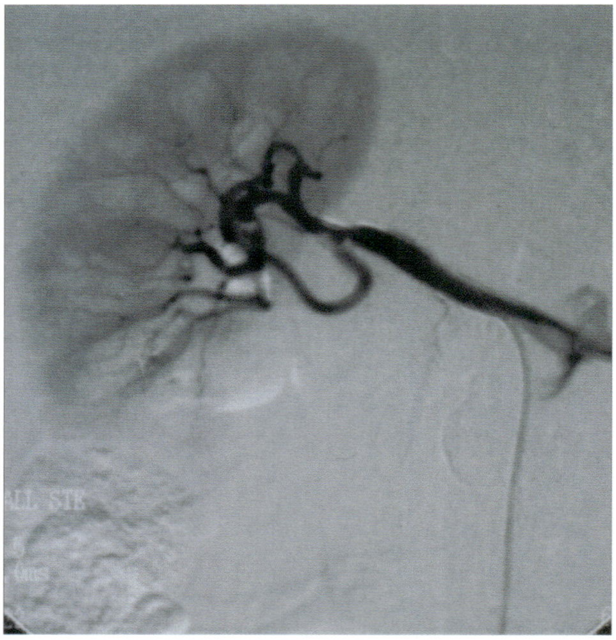

FIGURE 20.15
Completion angiography after placement of a second stent shows resolution of the dissection and restored renal perfusion. A small cortical perfusion defect at the inferior aspect of the kidney is related to dissection induced subsegmental branch artery occlusion.

CASE ANALYSIS

It is unclear when the antegrade dissection in this case occurred. Based on the persistence of pain after initial stent placement, it is likely that a subintimal plane was created during the injury of initial stent positioning and deployment. While the proximal portion of the dissection plane was successfully excluded by the stent, persistent pulsatile flow into the subintimal plane propagated the dissection distal to the stent edge. Less likely, dissection developed distal to the stent related to compliance mismatch and arterial injury during normal respiratory excursion of the artery. In this case, intervention was performed using an 0.035-inch based stent platform. Recent series suggest that utilizing low profile stents placed over 0.018-inch or 0.014-inch wires may reduce the risk of injury to the renal artery during PRAI.

Antegrade renal artery dissection is a known complication of PRAI and is believed to occur in as many as 7% of cases. Antegrade renal artery dissection may be benign without any associated symptoms or may present with symptoms such as flank pain, abdominal pain, nausea, vomiting, and elevated blood pressure. Typically, patients experience discomfort during balloon inflation, which resolves within 30 seconds; a persistence of pain is a warning sign for potential dissection of rupture requiring further evaluation. The exact mechanism of dissection is uncertain but may be related to catheter trauma, wire perforation of the intima, balloon and stent oversizing, or aggressive balloon dilation. Additionally, relatively rigid larger caliber and longer length stents may induce direct arterial trauma during introduction of the stent. Stable and non-flow-limiting dissections will generally heal spontaneously. Management options include conservative treatment with observation and delayed angiography, prolonged balloon angioplasty, or placement of an additional balloon expandable or self-expandable stent. Surgical bypass is reserved for failed endovascular treatment.

LESSONS

- Antegrade dissection of the renal artery is a well known complication of PRAI.
- Direct stenting is one of the several options available for percutaneous treatment of procedural related antegrade renal artery dissection.
- Careful examination of the angiographic images prior to removing vascular access coupled with attention to any changes in patient's symptoms can alert the interventionalist to possible complications, which can be managed effectively and safely without surgical intervention.

SUGGESTED READING

Morris C, Bonnevie G, Najarian K. Nonsurgical treatment of acute iatrogenic renal artery injuries occurring after renal artery angioplasty and stenting. *AJR*. 2001;177:1353–1357.

Smith B, Holcomb III G, et al. Renal artery dissection. *Ann Surg*. 1984;200:134–146.

Talner L, McLaughlin AP, Bookstein J. Renal artery dissection: A complication of catheter angiography. *Radiology*. 1975;117:291–295.

References

1. Martin LG, Rundback JH, Wallace MJ, et al. Quality improvement guidelines for angiography, angioplasty, and stent placement for the diagnosis and treatment of renal artery stenosis in adults. *J Vasc Interv Radiol.* 2010;21:421–430.
2. Beek FJ, Kaatee R, Beutler JJ, et al. Complications during renal artery stent placement for atherosclerotic ostial stenosis. *Cardiovasc Intervent Radiol.* 1997;20:184–190.
3. Dorros G, Jaff M, Mathiak L, et al. Four-year follow-up of Palmaz-Schatz stent revascularization as treatment for atherosclerotic renal artery stenosis. *Circulation.* 1998;98:642–647.
4. Leertouwer TC, Gussenhoven EJ, Bosch JL, et al. Stent placement for renal arterial stenosis: Where do we stand? A meta-analysis. *Radiology.* 2000;216:78–85.
5. Bakker J, Goffette PP, Henry M, et al. The Erasme study: A multicenter study on the safety and technical results of the Palmaz stent used for the treatment of atherosclerotic ostial renal artery stenosis. *Cardiovasc Intervent Radiol.* 1999;22:468–474.
6. Balk E, Raman G, Chung M. Comparative effectiveness of management strategies for renal artery stenosis. Rockville (MD): Agency for Healthcare Research and Quality (US); 2006 Oct.
7. Bax L, Woittiez AJ, Kouwenberg HJ, et al. Stent placement in patients with atherosclerotic renal artery stenosis and impaired renal function: A randomized trial. *Ann Intern Med.* 2009;150:840–841.
8. Laird JR, Rundback JH, Zierler E, et al. Safety and efficacy of renal artery stenting following suboptimal renal angioplasty for de novo and restenotic ostial lesions: Results from a nonrandomized, prospective multicenter registry. *J Vasc Interv Radiol.* 2010;21:627–637.
9. The ASTRAL investigators. Revascularization versus medical therapy for renal-artery stenosis. *N Engl J Med.* 2009;361(20):1953–1962.
10. ACR Manual on Contrast Media 2010, Version 7. http://www.acr.org/SecondaryMainMenuCategories/quality_safety/contrast_manual/FullManual.aspx. Accessed November, 2010.
11. Hawkins IF, Cho KJ, Caridi JG. Carbon dioxide in angiography to reduce the risk of contrast-induced nephropathy. *Radiol Clin North Am.* 2009;47(5):813–825.
12. Duong MH, MacKenzie TA, Malenka DJ. N-acetylcysteine prophylaxis significantly reduces the risk of radiocontrast-induced nephropathy: Comprehensive meta-analysis. *Catheter Cardiovasc Interv.* 2005;64(4):471–479.
13. Weisz G, Filby SJ, Cohen MG, et al. Safety and performance of targeted renal therapy: The Be-RITe! Registry. *J Endovasc Ther.* 2009;16(1):1–12.
14. Bates MC, Campbell JE, Stone PA, Jaff MR, Broce M, Lavigne PS. Factors affecting long-term survival following renal artery stenting. *Catheter Cardiovasc Interv.* 2007;69(7):1037–1043.
15. Sapoval M, Zähringer M, Pattynama P, et al. Low-profile stent system for treatment of atherosclerotic renal artery stenosis: The GREAT trial. *J Vasc Interv Radiol.* 2005;16(9):1195–1202.
16. Corriere MA, Pearce JD, Edwards MS, Stafford JM, Hansen KJ. Endovascular management of atherosclerotic renovascular disease: Early results following primary intervention. *J Vasc Surg.* 2008;48(3):580–587.
17. Edwards MS, Craven BL, Stafford J, et al. Distal embolic protection during renal artery angioplasty and stenting. *J Vasc Surg.* 2006;44(1):128–135.

21

Lawrence A. Garcia

Complications of Iliac and Superficial Femoral Artery Interventions

CASE 21.1

Thrombotic Embolization During Recanalization of a Chronically Occluded Viabahn Stent in the Superficial Femoral Artery

CLINICAL HISTORY AND DIAGNOSTIC TESTING RESULTS

A 68-year-old man had a history of extensive peripheral arterial disease and had undergone multiple prior percutaneous procedures, including revascularization of a right superficial femoral artery (SFA) occlusion 3 years prior with Viabahn covered stents (Gore Medical, Flagstaff, AZ). He presented to clinic with recurrent right calf claudication, Rutherford-Becker class III. Subsequent arterial duplex ultrasonography demonstrated complete occlusion of the SFA at the proximal edge of the prior stent.

PLANNED PROCEDURE

Recanalization of the chronic right SFA Viabahn stent occlusion.

PROCEDURE

Retrograde access was obtained in the left common femoral artery and a 5-Fr modified hook catheter was advanced to the contralateral common femoral artery. Initial angiography demonstrated a 80% stenosis at the bifurcation of the profunda femoris artery (PFA), and SFA and confirmed a total occlusion of the SFA at the level of the prior stents (Figure 21.1, Loop 21.1). We exchanged for an 8-Fr sheath and administered 4,500 units of unfractioned heparin. The occlusion was crossed with an angled Glidewire through a Quick-Cross catheter (Spectranetics, Colorado Springs, CO) and advanced to the below-knee popliteal artery, without restoration of flow. Initial balloon angioplasty was then performed with a 5-mm balloon with improved flow (Figure 21.2, Loop 21.2). We then performed additional angioplasty with a 7-mm balloon (Figure 21.3).

COMPLICATION AND MANAGEMENT

Repeat angiography after additional angioplasty showed no flow in the distal vessel (Figure 21.4, loop 21.4), which most likely resulted from distal embolization of laminated thrombus. The patient remained clinically stable and did not experience any significant leg discomfort. We treated this by excluding the thrombus with covered stenting using Viabahn stents deployed distally and proximally. Additionally, we performed balloon angioplasty in the below-knee popliteal artery at the site of the embolization. This resulted in restoration of normal flow and no residual stenosis in the SFA (Figure 21.5a–c).

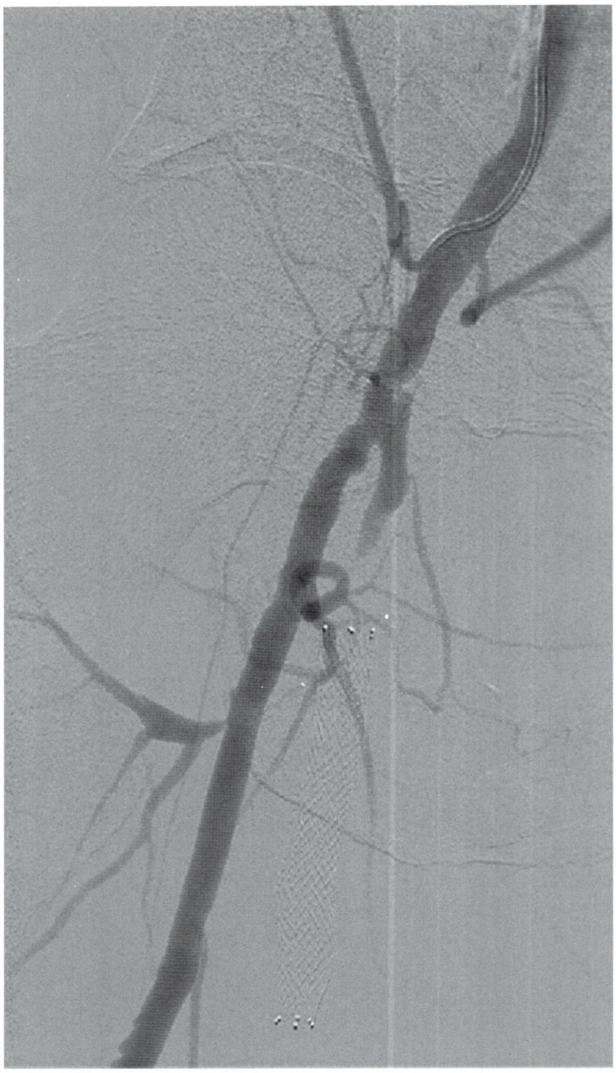

FIGURE 21.1

Baseline right lower extremity arterial angiography demonstrating an 80% stenosis at the bifurcation of the profunda femoris artery and SFA and total occlusion of the SFA at the level of the prior Viabahn stents. (LOOP 21.1)

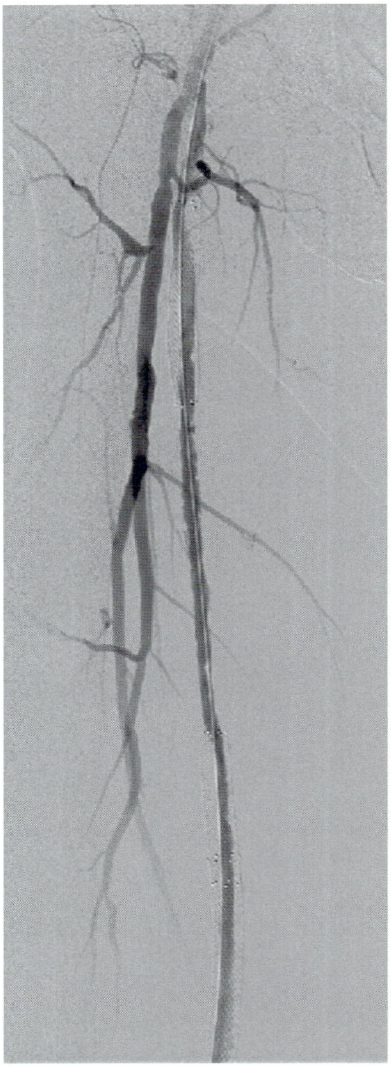

FIGURE 21.2

Angiography after initial balloon angioplasty with a 5-mm balloon with improved flow. (LOOP 21.2)

CASE ANALYSIS

In contrast to chronic total occlusions of native vessels which occur as a result of progressive, severe atherosclerosis, occlusion of peripheral stents often involves a significant amount of laminated thrombus. Performing aggressive balloon angioplasty can result in disruption of the thrombus and cause distal embolization, as it did in this case. If we had elected to exclude the thrombus with covered stents after our initial angioplasty with the 5-mm balloon, this complication would have most likely been avoided. Other potential measures that should be considered are thrombectomy or distal protection devices.

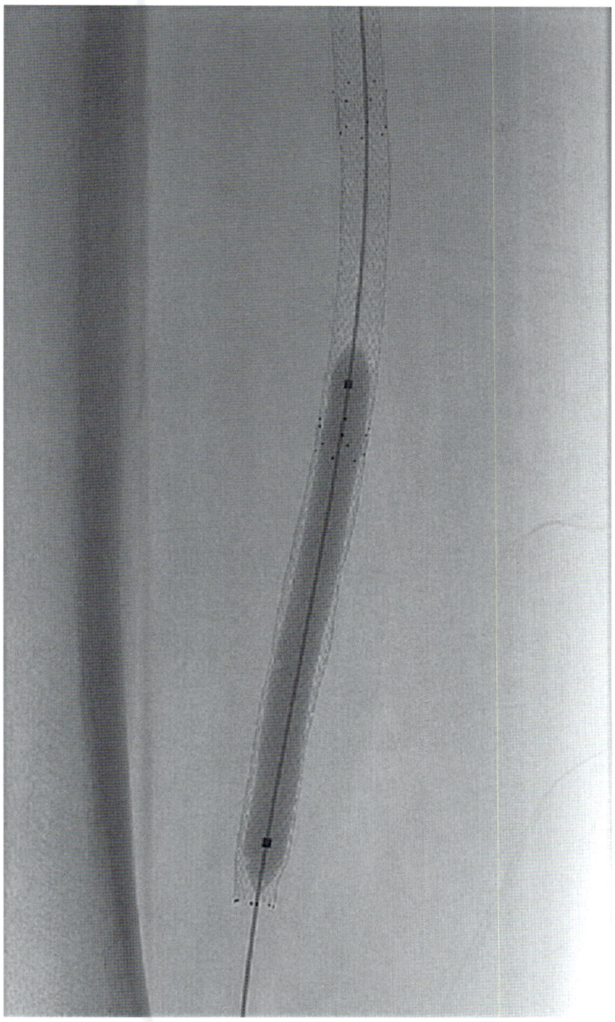

FIGURE 21.3
Additional balloon angioplasty with a 7-mm balloon.

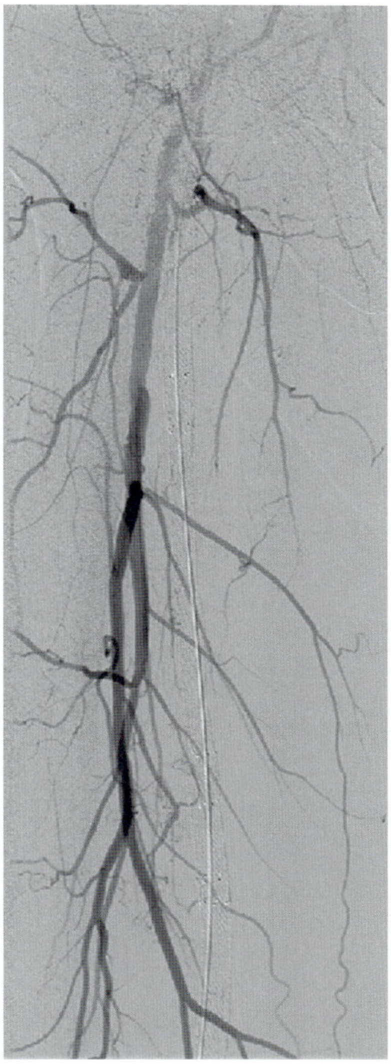

FIGURE 21.4
Repeat angiography after additional angioplasty with a 7-mm balloon showed no flow. (LOOP 21.4)

LESSONS

- Total occlusion of peripheral stents often involves a significant thrombus burden, which is typically laminated.
- Aggressive balloon angioplasty or other techniques that could result in dislodgement and distal embolization should be avoided.
- Thrombectomy, distal protection devices, or covered stents may reduce the probability of distal embolization.

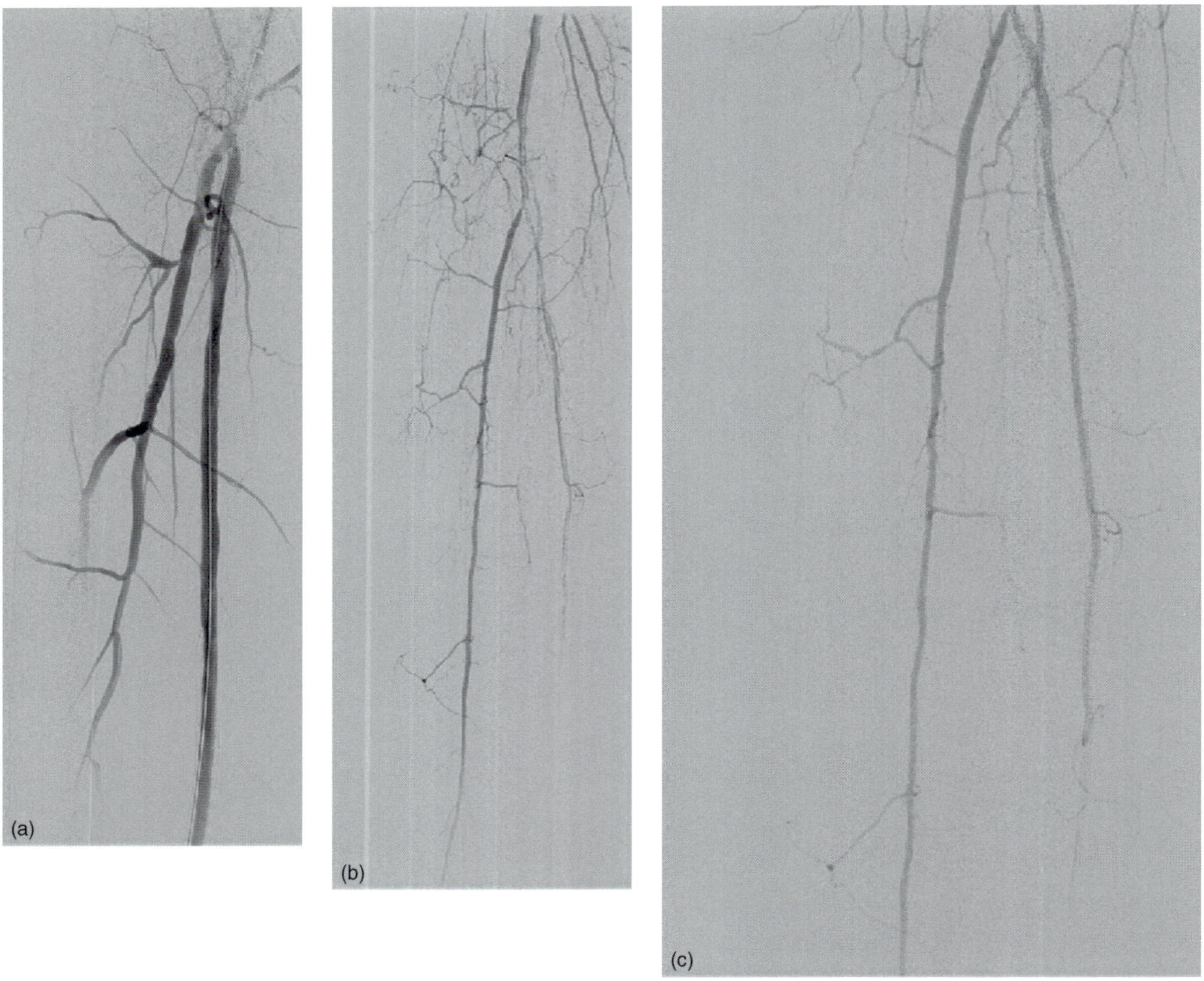

FIGURES 21.5 a–c

Repeat angiography showing normalized flow after implantation of more Viabahn stents and additionally balloon angioplasty in the below-knee popliteal artery. **(LOOPS 21.5a-c)**

SUGGESTED READING

Davie MG, Bismuth J, Saad WE, et al. Implications of in situ thrombosis and distal embolization during superficial femoral artery endoluminal intervention. *Ann Vasc Surg.* 2010;24:14–22.

Lam RC, Shah S, Faries PL, et al. Incidence and clinical significance of distal embolization during percutaneous interventions involving the superficial femoral artery. *J Vasc Surg.* 2007;46:1155–1159.

CASE 21.2

Iliac Perforation During Common Iliac Artery Stenting

CLINICAL HISTORY AND DIAGNOSTIC TESTING RESULTS

A 78-year-old woman had a history of hypertension, coronary artery disease, and peripheral arterial disease and had previously undergone revascularization of a left SFA occlusion. She was presented to clinic with recurrent bilateral claudication, Rutherford-Becker class III. Noninvasive evaluation demonstrated an ankle-brachial index of 0.24, and duplex ultrasonography suggested bilateral common iliac stenoses and infrainguinal disease.

PLANNED PROCEDURE

Bilateral common iliac stenting.

PROCEDURE

Access was obtained in the right common femoral artery, and initial angiography and hemodynamic assessment confirmed significant stenoses in both the right and left ostial common iliac arteries (Figure 21.6). We exchanged for an 8-Fr sheath and administered 3,000 units of unfractioned heparin. The left common iliac stenosis was successfully treated with an 8-mm balloon-expandable stent. The sheath was then withdrawn and the wire was redirected into the descending aorta (Figure 21.7). We then deployed another 8-mm balloon-expandable stent in the right common iliac artery.

COMPLICATION AND MANAGEMENT

Following deployment of the right ostial common iliac stent, the patient complained of back pain, and angiography revealed a perforation (Figure 21.8). The patient remained hemodynamically stable. At this point, we administered 10 mg of intravenous protamine and attempted to seal the perforation with a low-pressure inflation of an 8-mm balloon (Figure 21.9). Repeat angiography after balloon deflation demonstrated less dye extravasation but persistence of the perforation (Figure 21.10). Therefore, we elected to treat this by deploying an 8-mm covered wall-stent, which successfully sealed the perforation (Figure 21.11).

CASE ANALYSIS

Iliac perforation is a potentially fatal complication, as it results in retroperitoneal hemorrhage. It most commonly occurs as a result of over-aggressive balloon angioplasty or placement of oversized stents. In this case, the 8-mm stent was appropriate for the left common iliac artery but may have been slightly oversized for the right iliac artery. With prompt recognition, iliac perforation can typically be easily managed by reversal of anticoagulation, prolonged low-pressure balloon angioplasty, and if necessary, placement of a covered stent.

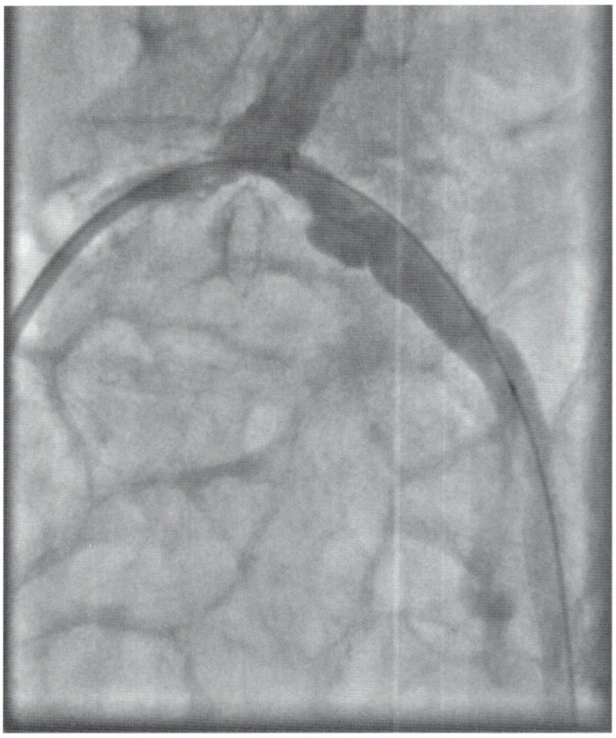

FIGURE 21.6

Baseline angiography shows bilateral stenoses in both the right and left ostial common iliac arteries. (LOOP 21.6)

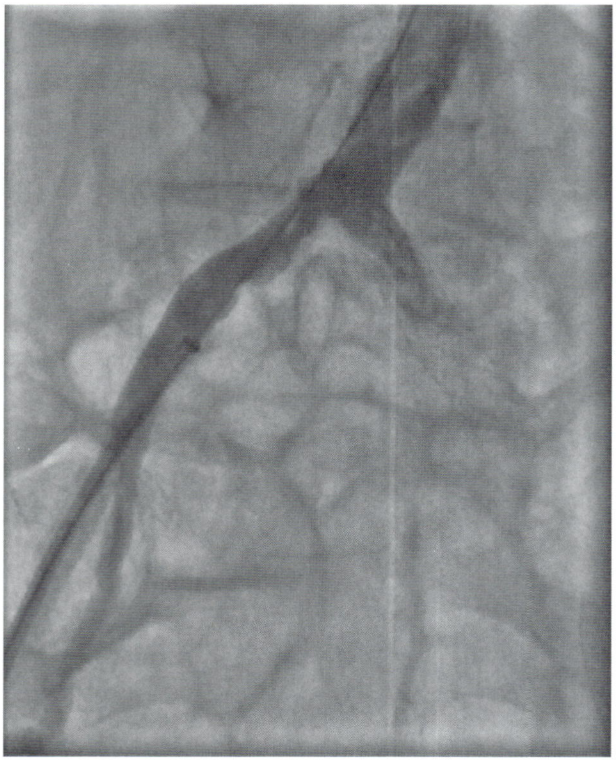

FIGURE 21.7

Right iliac angiography after successful implantation of an 8-mm balloon-expandable stent in the left common iliac artery. (LOOP 21.7)

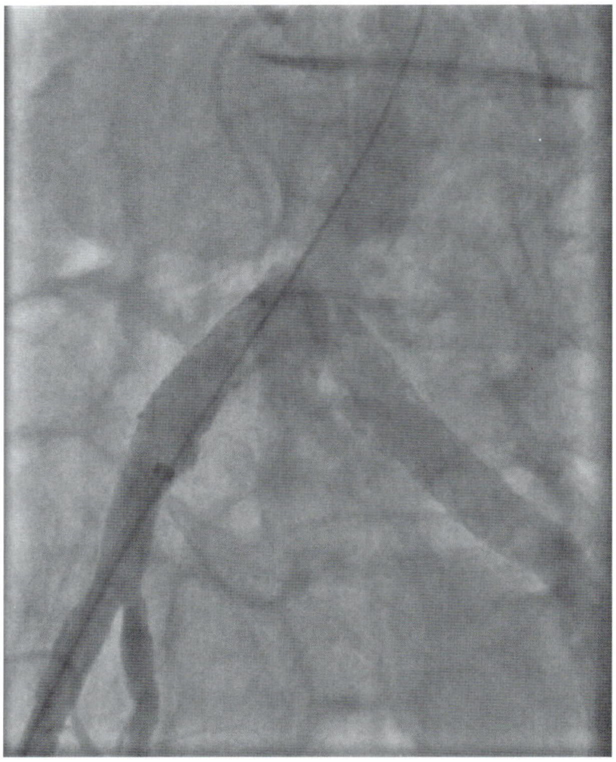

FIGURE 21.8

Right iliac angiography after implantation of an 8-mm balloon-expandable stent in the ostial right common iliac artery demonstrating a perforation. (LOOP 21.8)

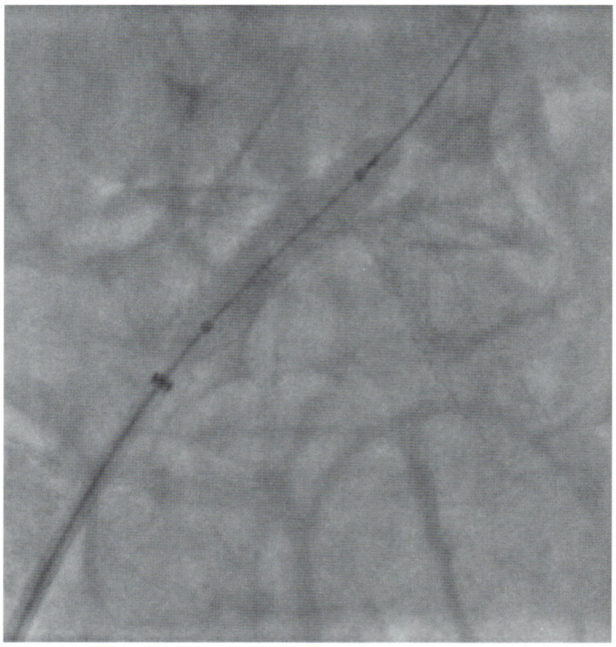

FIGURE 21.9

Low-pressure balloon inflation at the site of the perforation. (Loop 21.9)

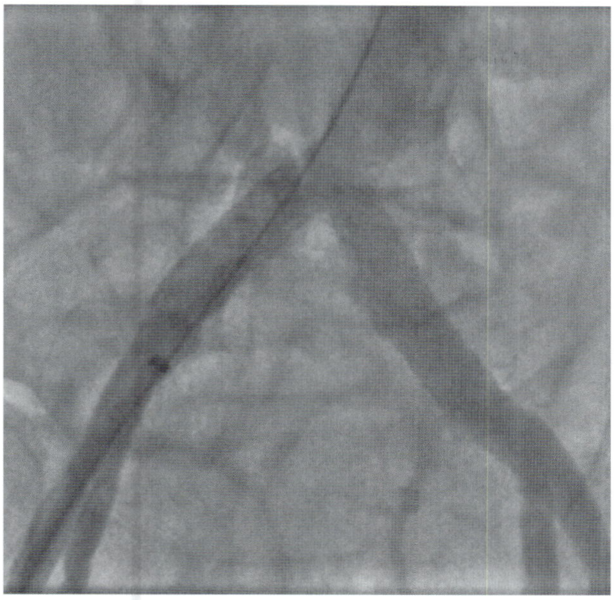

FIGURE 21.10

Repeat angiography after balloon deflation demonstrating persistence of the perforation. (LOOP 21.10)

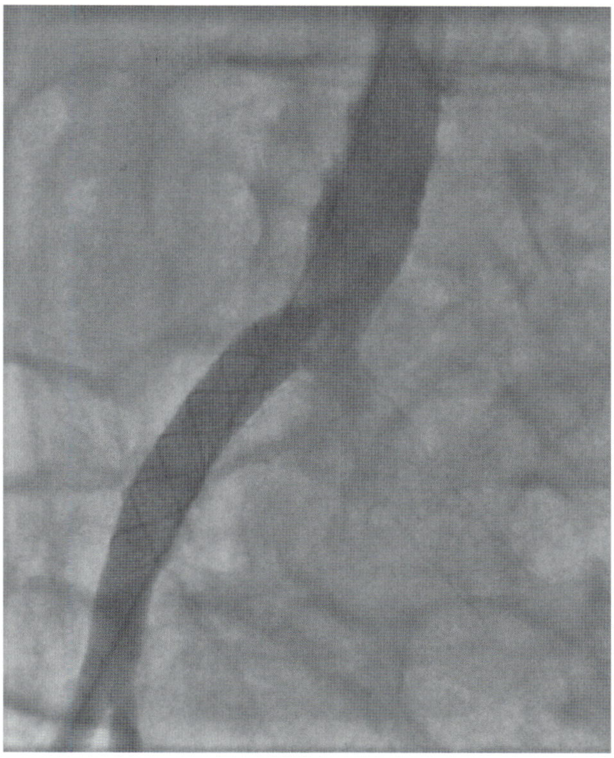

FIGURE 21.11

Right iliac angiography after implantation of an 8-mm covered wall-stent, which successfully sealed the perforation. (LOOP 21.11)

LESSONS

- Iliac perforation can result from deployment of oversized balloons or stents, and thus careful attention must be paid to proper assessment of the true vessel size.
- Prompt recognition of a perforation is critical to prevent a potentially fatal retroperitoneal bleed.
- Treatment consists of reversal of anticoagulation, prolonged low-pressure balloon angioplasty in attempt to seal the perforation or the placement of a covered stent.

SUGGESTED READING

Klein WM, van der Graaf Y, Seegers J, et al. Dutch iliac stent trial: Long-term results in patients randomized for primary or selective stent placement. *Radiology*. 2006;238:734–744.

Stockx L, Poncylijusz W, Krzanowski M, et al. Express LD vascular stent in the treatment of iliac artery lesions: 24-month results from the MELODIE trial. *J Endovasc Ther*. 2010;17:633–641.

Tetteroo E, van der Graff Y, Bosch JL, et al. Randomised comparison of primary stent placement versus primary angioplasty followed by selective stent placement in patients with iliac-artery occlusive disease. Dutch Iliac Stent Trial Study Group. *Lancet*. 1998;351:1153–1159.

CASE 21.3

Calcific Embolization During SilverHawk Atherectomy of a Severely Calcified SFA Stenosis

CLINICAL HISTORY AND DIAGNOSTIC TESTING RESULTS

A 71-year-old man with a history of tobacco abuse, diabetes mellitus, and hypertension presented to the clinic with progressive right calf claudication, Rutherford-Becker class II. An ankle-brachial index was not obtainable, and therefore, a magnetic resonance angiogram (MRA) was performed. The MRA demonstrated occluded and severely calcified right SFA.

PLANNED PROCEDURE

Right-SFA atherectomy with the SilverHawk device (FoxHollow Technologies, Redwood City, CA) followed by balloon angioplasty.

PROCEDURE

Contralateral access was obtained in the left common femoral artery. Baseline angiography showed severely stenosed (not occluded) and calcified right SFA (Figure 21.12). We exchanged for an 8-Fr sheath and administered 4,000 units of unfractionated heparin. A 5.0-mm Spider filter (ev3, Irvine, CA) was placed in the below-knee popliteal artery for embolic protection. Several runs were performed with the SilverHawk device, with a suboptimal result (Figure 21.13). We then elected to perform balloon angioplasty with a 6-mm balloon. Interval angiography revealed minimal residual stenosis in the SFA (Figure 21.14).

COMPLICATION AND MANAGEMENT

Runoff angiography showed a filling defect in the Spider filter (Figure 21.15). Despite the significant amount of embolic plaque burden in the filter, flow was preserved in this patient, and he did not experience any untoward events. The filter was removed, and angiography confirmed resolution of the filling defect and preserved outflow (Figure 21.16). Inspection of the filter device after retrieval revealed an extensive amount of atheroembolic and calcific debris (Figure 21.17).

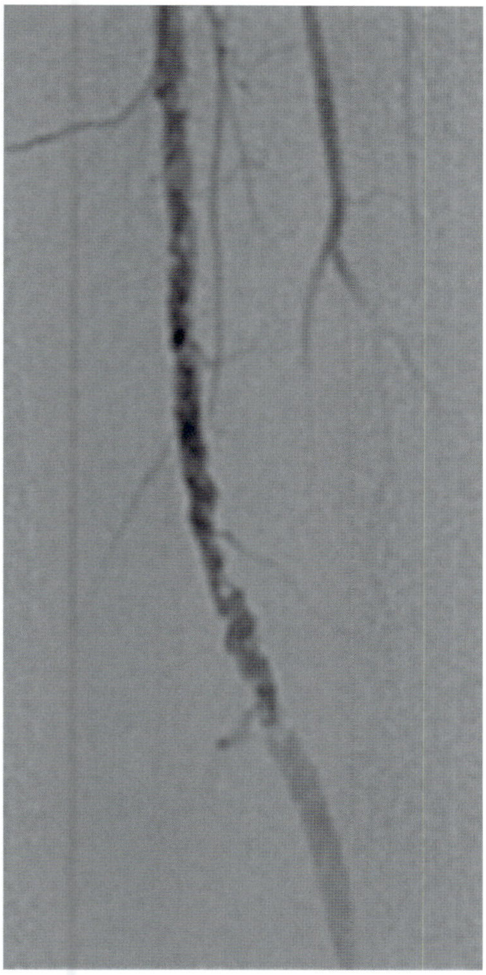

FIGURE 21.12

Baseline angiography shows severely stenosed and calcified right SFA. (LOOP 21.12)

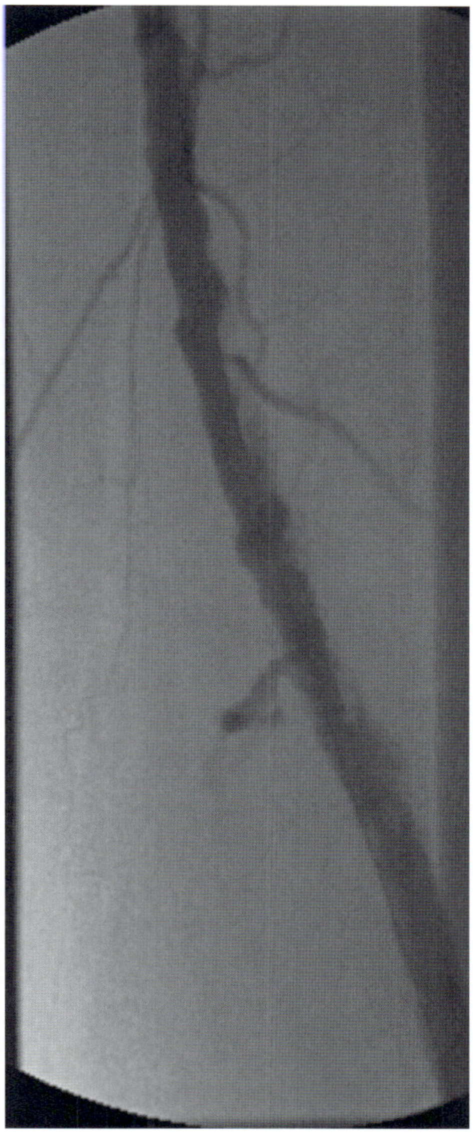

FIGURE 21.13

Angiography after SilverHawk atherectomy showing suboptimal result. (LOOP 21.13)

CASE ANALYSIS

Atherectomy devices often purport their ability to retain the removed plaque burden, thus obviating the need for embolic protection. However, despite these safeguards, a significant amount of embolization can often occur. In this case, the prophylactic placement of a distal embolic protection device avoided a potential serious complication.

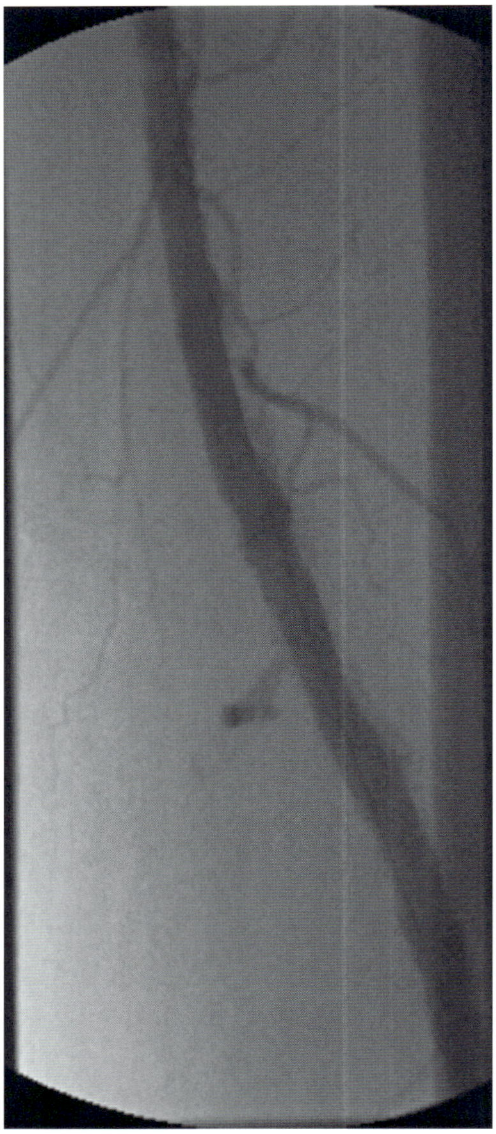

FIGURE 21.14

Angiography after balloon angioplasty with a 6-mm balloon showing improved residual stenosis. (LOOP 21.14)

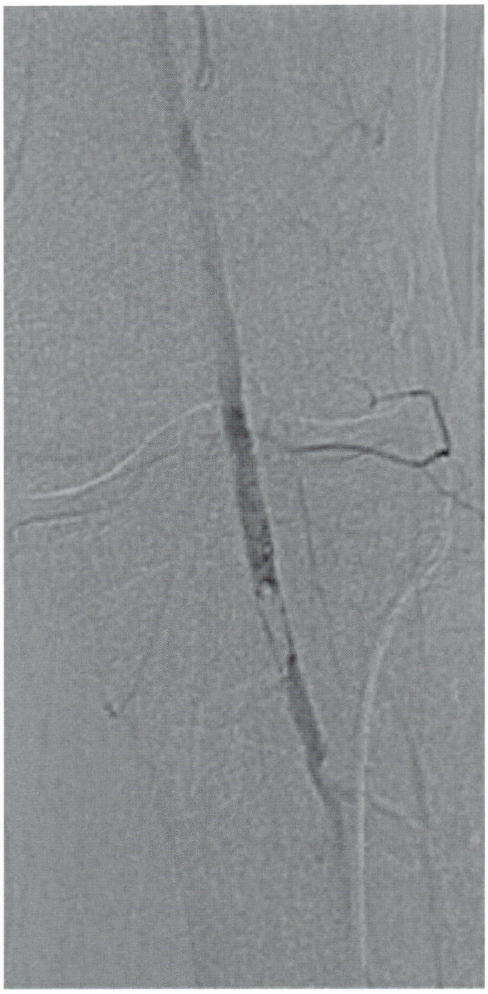

FIGURE 21.15

Runoff angiography after SilverHawk atherectomy and adjunct balloon dilation shows a filling defect in the Spider filter. (LOOP 21.15)

LESSONS

- Severe calcific disease in the SFA often requires the use of atherectomy devices for plaque reduction to allow for optimal angioplasty.
- Use of atherectomy devices often results in embolization of a significant amount of debris.
- Whenever possible, the use of distal embolic protection should be employed.

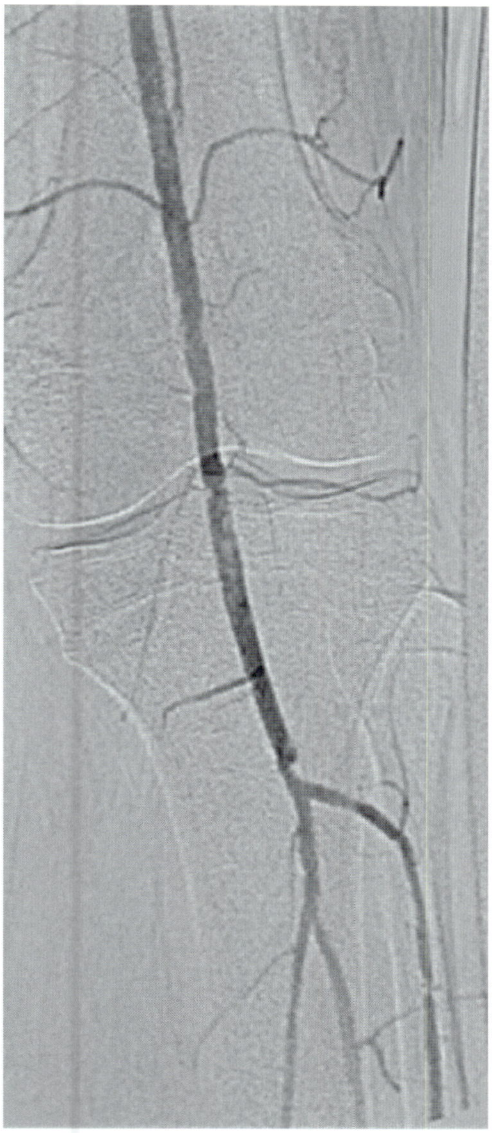

FIGURE 21.16

Final angiography after filter retrieval shows resolution of the filling defect and preserved outflow. **(LOOP 21.16)**

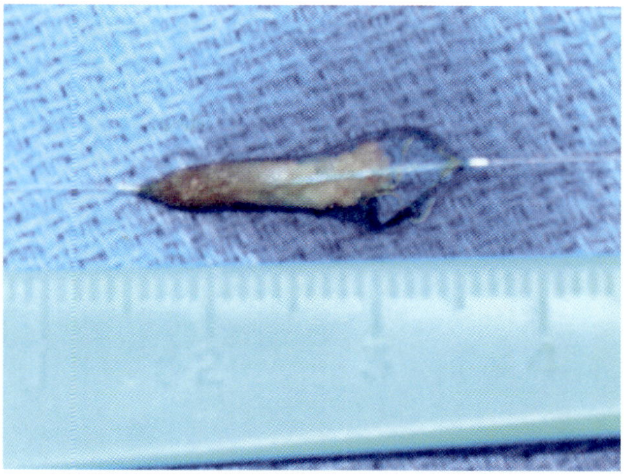

FIGURE 21.17

Inspection of the filter device after retrieval reveals an extensive amount of atheroembolic and calcific debris.

SUGGESTED READING

Shafique S, Nachreiner RD, Murphy MP, et al. Recanalization of infrainguinal vessels: Silverhawk, laser, and the remote superficial femoral artery endarterectomy. *Semin Vasc Surg.* 2007;20:29–36.

Shammas NW, Dippel EJ, Coiner D, et al. Preventing lower extremity distal embolization using embolic filter protection: Results of the PROTECT registry. *J Endovasc Ther.* 2008;15:270–276.

Suri R, Wholey MH, Postoak D, et al. Distal embolic protection during femoropopliteal atherectomy. *Catheter Cardiovasc Interv.* 2006;67:417–422.

22

Gary M. Ansel, Charles F. Botti, and Mitchell J. Silver

Complications of Infrapopliteal Complications

INTRODUCTION

Balloon angioplasty for the treatment of limb threatening ischemia has shown 1- to 3-year outcomes similar to bypass surgery when evaluated by amputation-free survival (1–3). The majority of these data were driven by the treatment of fairly short, simple tibial disease. The acute ability to treat much more diffuse disease has increased with advancements in balloon, atherectomy, and stent technology. Longer-term clinical success is dependent on careful surveillance with secondary interventions as needed, as well as multidisciplinary attention to wound care, nutritional status, and pharmacotherapy.

Complications of tibial intervention typically occur at the local intervention site. In our opinion, unless previously bypassed, tibial lesions are rarely thrombotic and distal embolization is uncommon. However, patients with critical limb ischemia have demonstrated an increased tendency for complications when compared to claudicants with major complications arising from tibial interventions reported in 2% to 6% of procedures (4,5). Infrapopliteal disease is more closely aligned with diabetes and is therefore more associated with calcific medial disease than the subintimal atheroma and thrombus seen in the femoropopliteal vascular bed. Dissection leading to flow disturbance and possibly acute vessel occlusion is the most common complication of balloon angioplasty in the infrapopliteal arterial system. Additionally, as more aggressive technology, such as high-pressure balloons, cutting/scoring balloons, and atherectomy, becomes available, perforation and embolization can be expected to follow. If a significant perforation occurs, one should deal with the leakage promptly, generally with anticoagulation reversal and prolonged balloon inflation of 2 to 5 minutes, and close clinical follow-up for compartment syndrome will need to be done so that fasciotomy can be completed if needed. When endovascular complications do occur, over 86% are typically diagnosed in the endovascular suite (6). Amputation should be seen in <1% of procedures, with major amputation usually limited to patients with preexisting critical limb ischemia (7).

Popliteal Artery Perforation During Atherectomy

CLINICAL HISTORY AND DIAGNOSTIC TESTING RESULTS

A 38-year-old diabetic man presented with a 9-month history of a nonhealing ulcer of the left foot first digit and rest pain. There was pain at the ulcer site but no erythema or cellulitis. The past medical history included premature coronary artery disease and aortic valvular stenosis treated with coronary artery bypass and mechanical aortic valve replacement. Preinterventional noninvasive studies demonstrated a noncompressible left ankle-brachial index and toe waveforms of 2 mm in amplitude. Angiography from an outside institution demonstrated severe calcified stenoses of the left distal popliteal artery with only one vessel runoff to the foot (the peroneal artery) (Figure 22.1).

PLANNED PROCEDURE

Due to the anatomic location behind the knee and the significant calcification, atherectomy and balloon angioplasty were to be utilized in an effort to debulk the lesion and allow for restoration of flow without the use of a stent.

PROCEDURE

The patient was already off warfarin and on full-dose intravenous heparin, as well as dual antiplatelet therapy, including aspirin 325 mg and clopidogrel 75 mg. A braided, kink resistant sheath was introduced from the right (contralateral) common femoral artery access. A rotational type atherectomy device was used to debulk the popliteal lesion prior to balloon angioplasty. (Figure 22.2) During the first pass of atherectomy, the device appeared to bind on the lesion twice, so the device was removed and angiography repeated.

COMPLICATION AND MANAGEMENT

Postatherectomy angiography demonstrated a moderate arterial perforation with free-flowing contrast into the extravascular space (Figure 22.3). Low-pressure balloon inflation was applied, and heparin anticoagulation was reversed with protamine. To reduce the likelihood of distal thrombus formation, the guidewire was removed during balloon inflation with flushing of the balloon lumen. After two 10-minute inflations were completed, persistent contrast extravasation was still evident (Figure 22.4). A self-expanding polytetrafluoroethylene covered stent was then placed with resultant sealing of the perforation (Figure 22.5). The patient was discharged the following day on coumadin and low-molecular-weight heparin without subsequent events.

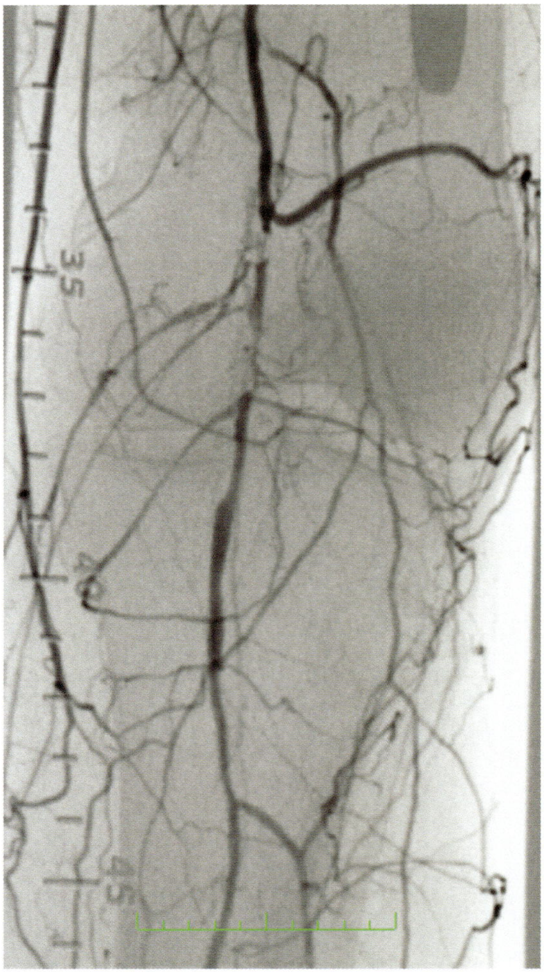

FIGURE 22.1

Baseline angiogram demonstrating severe stenosis of the popliteal artery.

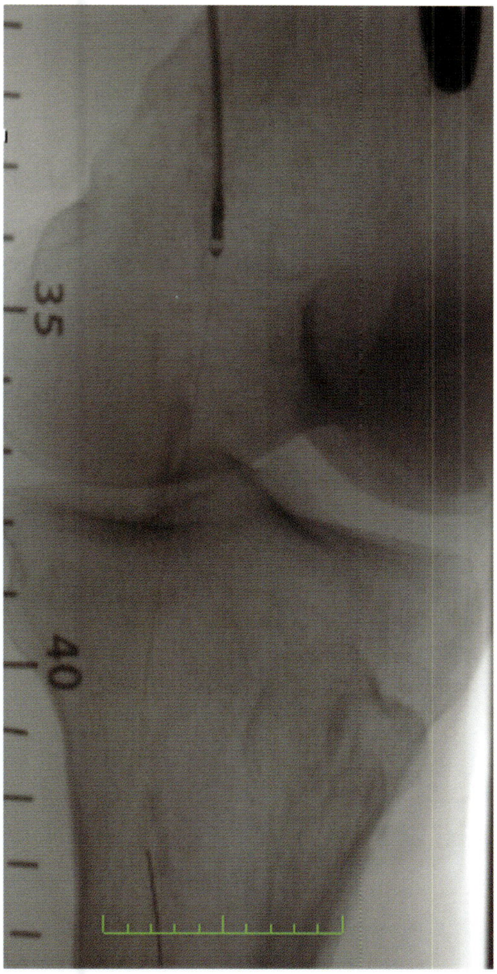

FIGURE 22.2
Digital picture of the atherectomy device utilized for debulking of the popliteal artery.

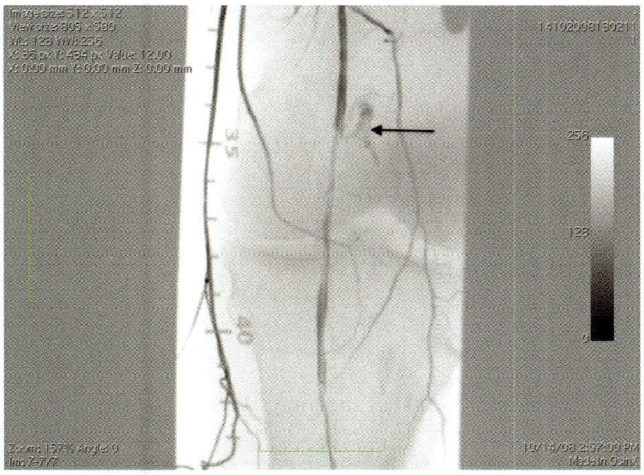

FIGURE 22.3
Angiogram postatherectomy demonstrating an arterial perforation (arrow).

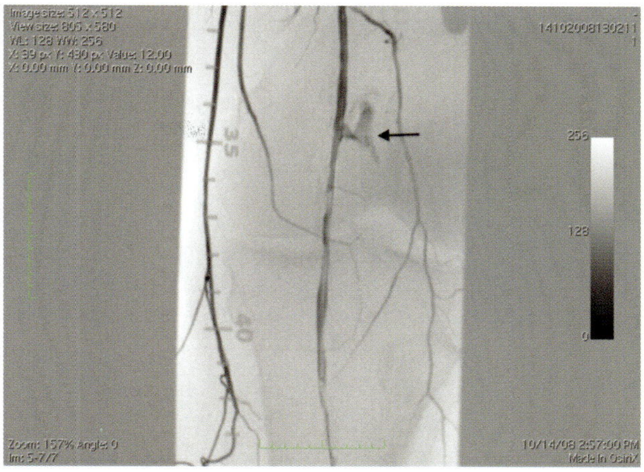

FIGURE 22.4
Repeat angiogram demonstrating continued contrast extravasation after two prolonged balloon angioplasty inflations.

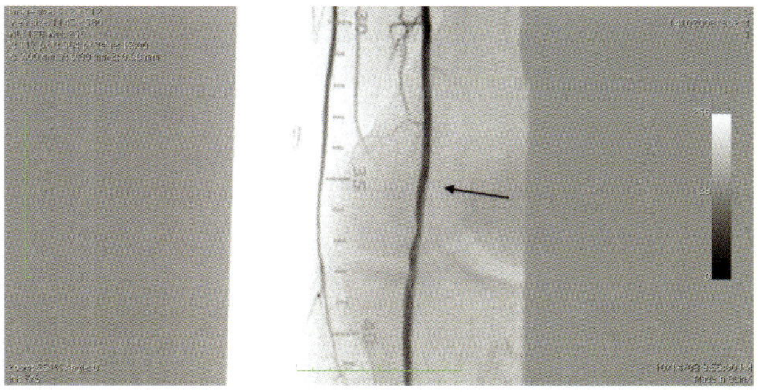

FIGURE 22.5
Final angiogram after placement of a self-expanding stent graft and successful treatment of the perforation.

CASE ANALYSIS

In retrospect, this complication was potentially avoidable. The atherectomy catheter utilized was somewhat oversized in comparison to the true vessel size.

LESSONS

- In heavily calcified lesions, downsizing the atherectomy device at the first pass may reduce the possibility of perforation.
- When treating severely calcified infrapopliteal stenoses, always prepare an angioplasty balloon of appropriate diameter to tamponade a potential perforation while anticoagulation is reversed.
- Stent grafts are invaluable tools for sealing of perforations.

CASE 22.2

External Compression of a Balloon-Expandable Stent in the Popliteal Artery

CLINICAL HISTORY AND DIAGNOSTIC TESTING RESULTS

An 82-year-old woman presented with rest pain of the right lower extremity. The patient's past medical history was significant for a femoral to below knee popliteal venous bypass 6 years earlier, utilizing reversed saphenous vein conduit. The patient had also undergone previous coronary bypass utilizing the contralateral saphenous vein. The patient had the resting pain symptoms for 1.5 months. Noninvasive vascular testing revealed an ischemic right lower limb with an ankle-brachial index of 0.38. Angiography demonstrated total occlusion of the bypass as well as the proximal to distal superficial femoral artery (Figure 22.6a). The popliteal artery reconstituted just above the knee and there was two-vessel tibial runoff.

PLANNED PROCEDURE

Due to the patient's age and lack of venous bypass conduit, endovascular treatment was offered as the first therapeutic alternative. Since the bypass was more than 6 years old, we did not feel reopening it would be a good long-term alternative. The native vessel was a long chronic total occlusion, and it was anticipated that we would open the vessel subintimally followed by stenting.

PROCEDURE

The patient underwent subintimal wiring with intraluminal reentry gained via a reentry device just above the knee. Angioplasty and stenting of the superficial femoral artery were completed with wide patency. However, a new intraluminal filling defect was noted in the area of the previous distal graft anastomosis (Figure 22.6b). A balloon-expandable stent was then placed with an excellent angiographic result (Figure 22.7). Post procedure the patient's rest pain resolved, and she was able to ambulate without claudication. At the time of discharge, the ankle-brachial index was 0.94. At 6 months follow-up, the patient's foot ulcer had resolved, and she denied any claudication of the treated extremity. The pedal pulse was normal. The ankle-brachial index was 0.92, and the stents were patent on duplex scanning.

COMPLICATION AND MANAGEMENT

Three days later, the patient contacted the office complaining of painful "purple toes." On examination,

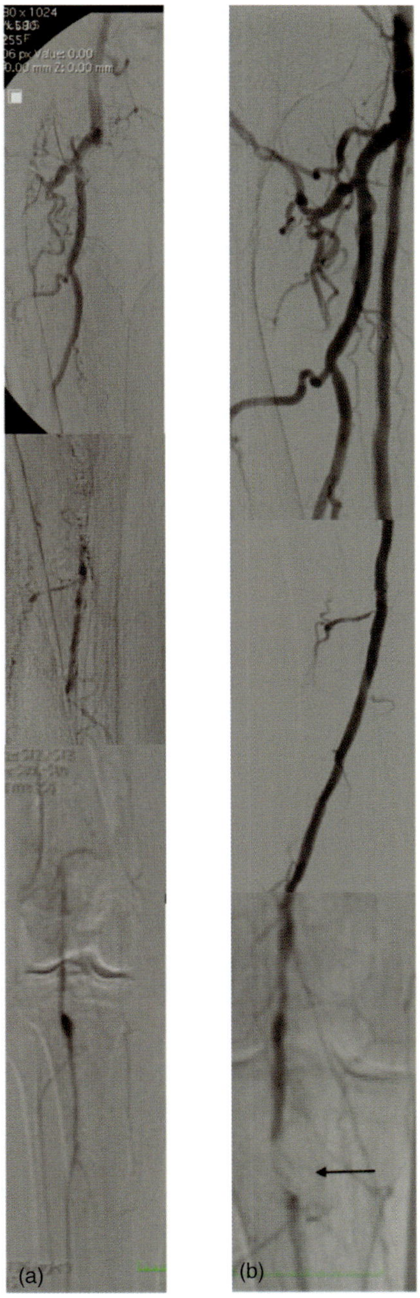

FIGURE 22.6 a,b

(a) Composite baseline angiogram of the right lower extremity. Note the normal appearing popliteal artery below the knee. (b) Composite angiogram after traversal of the superficial femoral artery and placement of stents. Note the new narrowing in the popliteal artery. (arrow)

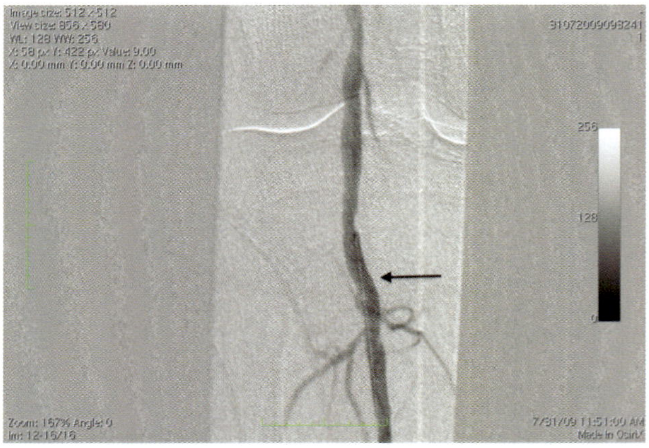

FIGURE 22.7
Repeat angiogram after placement of a balloon-expandable stent in the popliteal artery.

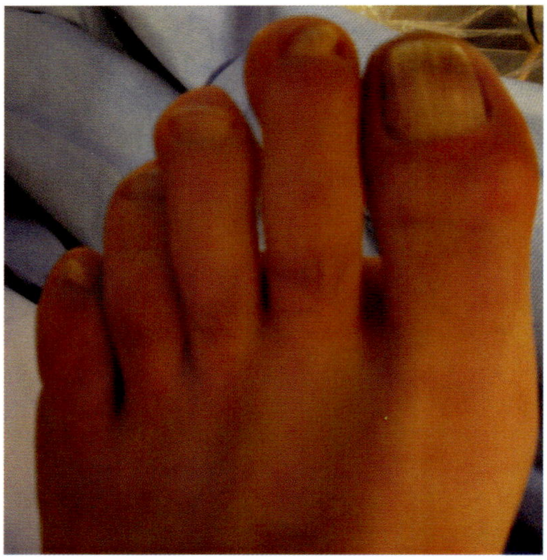

FIGURE 22.8
Digital photograph of the forefoot upon presentation for pain in the toes 3 days after normal noninvasive testing. Note the patchy ischemia pattern intermixed with normal tissue that is characteristic of embolization.

there were no palpable pulses and the patient had a classic pattern of distal embolization ("blue toe syndrome") (Figure 22.8). Duplex ultrasound demonstrated a monophasic Doppler waveform. Angiography demonstrated severe narrowing at the stent site and what appeared to be stent compression (Figure 22.9). Intravascular ultrasound demonstrated that the previously implanted balloon-expandable stent was compressed (Figure 22.10). We speculate that cuff pressure placed during the noninvasive study led to stent compression. Subsequently, we implanted a self-expandable heparin coated stent graft at the side of the previous stent. Hand compression was utilized during balloon dilation to help crush the previous stent, with an excellent final angiographic result (Figure 22.11). Follow-up surveillance 6 months later demonstrated a clinically asymptomatic foot with an ankle-brachial index of 0.92.

CASE ANALYSIS

In this case, the cause of leg ischemia at follow-up was stent compression and thrombus formation and embolization. With a normal duplex scan and distal ankle pressure 3 days before the onset of symptoms, it was felt that the blood pressure cuff at the time of noninvasive study may have compressed the previously implanted balloon-expandable stent, leading to thrombosis. In retrospect, placement of a balloon expandable stent in the juxta-popliteal position during the index procedure was inappropriate. Cases of compression of balloon-expandable stents in the infrainguinal region have been known to occur.

LESSONS

- Implantation of balloon-expandable stents in the popliteal artery region should be avoided.
- Intravascular ultrasound of new intraluminal filling defects may lead to unexpected beneficial information.
- More information is needed on the effects of external pressure on infrapopliteal stents.

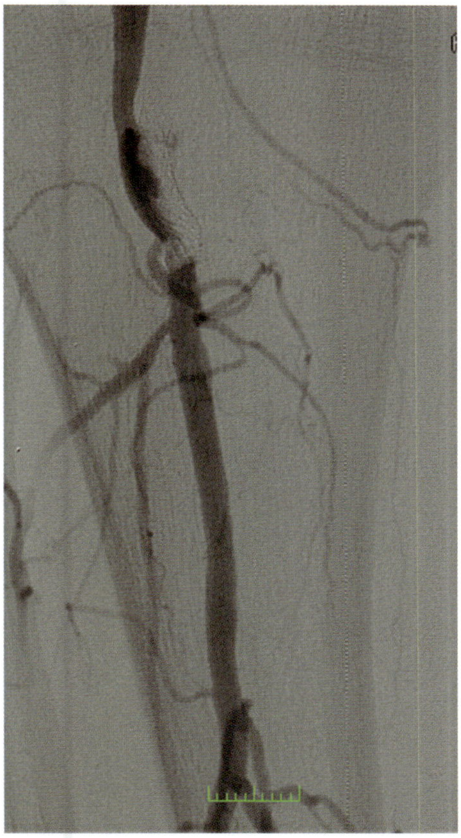

FIGURE 22.9
Angiogram of the popliteal artery. Note that the stent appears to be compressed.

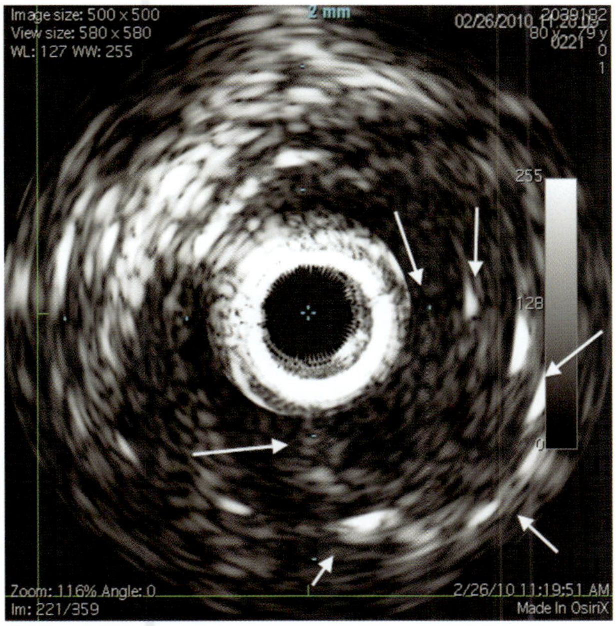

FIGURE 22.10
Intravascular ultrasound of the popliteal artery at the previous stent site. Note that the stent (arrows) is compressed.

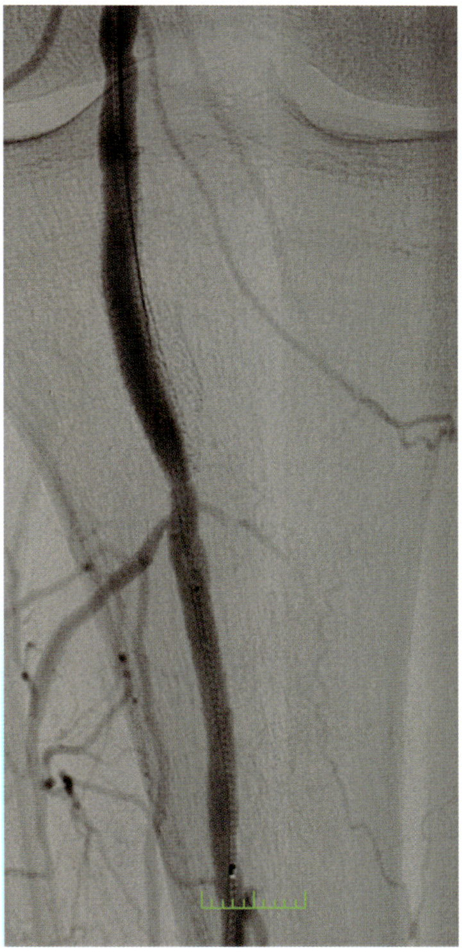

FIGURE 22.11
Final angiogram of the popliteal artery after crushing of the balloon-expandable stent and placement of a self-expanding stent.

CASE 22.3

Reperfusion Injury After Successful Revascularization

CLINICAL HISTORY AND DIAGNOSTIC TESTING RESULTS

A 56-year-old man presented with 11 hours of increasing left leg pain and 4 hours of paralysis and numbness of the leg. Past medical history is significant for left femoropopliteal bypass with synthetic conduit 6 months earlier. On examination, there was a palpable femoral pulse bilaterally. The left leg was cool to touch, there was absence of light touch sensation, the fine motor movement of the toes was absent, and the foot motor strength was <1. The left leg below the level of the femoral artery demonstrated only venous Doppler signal.

PLANNED PROCEDURE

It was felt that the most likely cause of patient's presentation (acute limb ischemia) is thrombosis of the left femoropopliteal synthetic graft. Our plan was to do immediate angiography and endovascular revascularization of the graft.

PROCEDURE

The patient was anticoagulated with intravenous heparin and emergently taken to the angiographic suite. Percutaneous contralateral femoral access was obtained. Preintervention angiography revealed thrombotic occlusion of the femoropopliteal bypass graft with continued thrombus formation in the popliteal and infrapopliteal vessels (Figure 22.12). A braided sheath was placed across the iliac bifurcation, and a 0.035-inch hydrophilic wire was placed through the graft and into the tibial vessels. A 4-Fr catheter was advanced over the 0.035-inch guidewire to the distal popliteal artery to exchange it for a 0.014-inch guidewire. Mechanical thrombectomy with a rheolytic device was completed in "powerpulse" fashion utilizing 6 units of reteplase. The device was advanced through the graft, popliteal artery, and tibial vessels with clearance of the thrombus to the foot via the posterior tibial vessel. Then, we performed balloon angioplasty of the distal graft anastomosis (Figure 22.13). After procedure completion, the patient was closely monitored with frequent blood analysis (for potential hyperkalemia and rhabdomyolysis) and compartment pressures for early detection of compartment syndrome. He was also hydrated with intravenous bicarbonate solution.

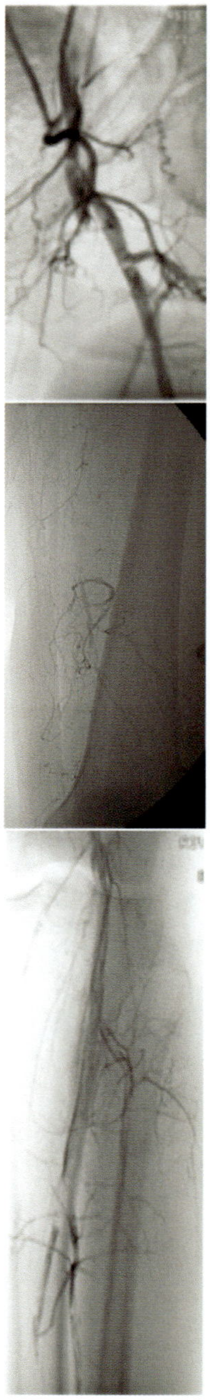

FIGURE 22.12
Composite baseline angiogram demonstrating diffuse occlusion with thrombus of the femoral, popliteal, and infrapopliteal arteries.

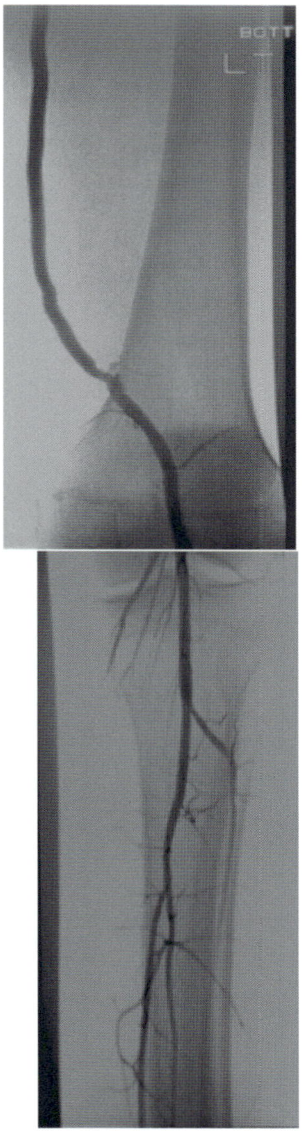

FIGURE 22.13
Angiogram after treatment of the femoropopliteal bypass, popliteal, and infrapopliteal vessels. Note the wide patency of the posterior tibial and peroneal arteries.

COMPLICATION AND MANAGEMENT

The patient developed rising anterior compartment pressures and subsequently was taken to the operating room for fasciotomy (Figure 22.14). Subsequently, the patient underwent closure of the fasciotomy site with a skin graft from the thigh. At 6 month follow-up, the femoropopliteal graft remained patent with complete healing of the fasciotomy site (Figure 22.15). The patient was ambulating with residual mild foot drop.

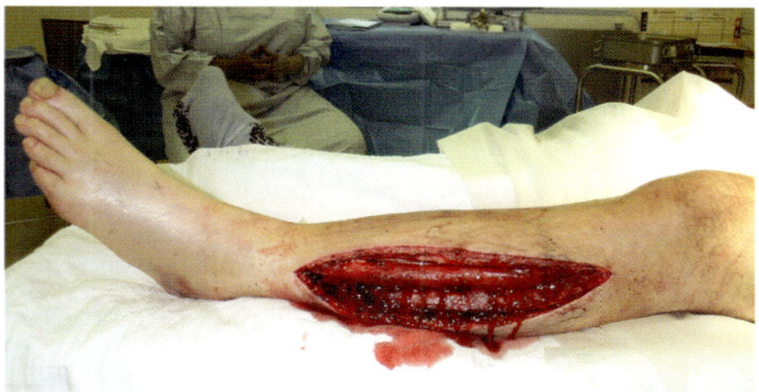

FIGURE 22.14
Digital photograph during fasciotomy for treatment of compartment syndrome.

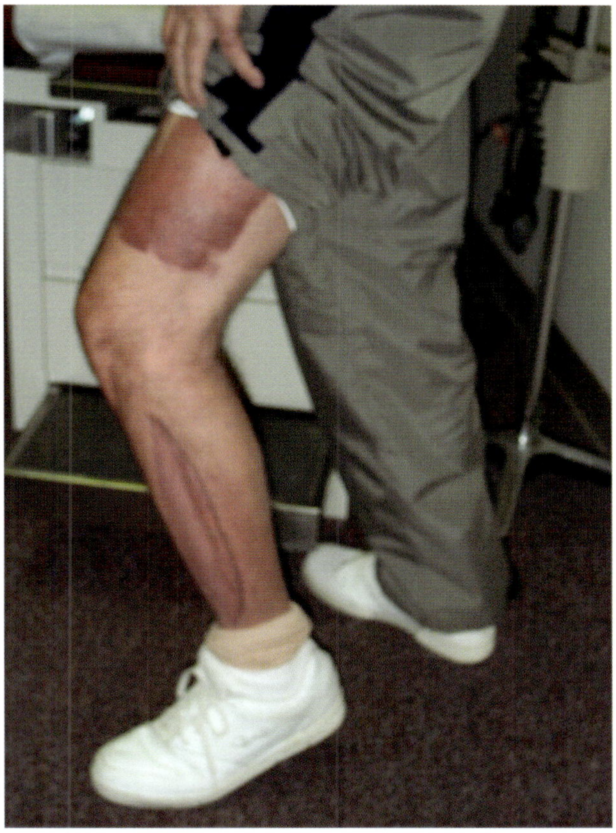

FIGURE 22.15
Digital photograph at 6 month clinical follow-up demonstrating the healed lower leg fasciotomy site as well as the upper thigh tissue donor site.

CASE ANALYSIS

Although the patient's ischemic limb was quickly reperfused, compartment syndrome (an uncommon event with percutaneous revascularization) occurred. Patients with more than 4 hours of acute limb ischemia should be monitored for the development of several potentially life-threatening events, including hyperkalemia, rhabdomyolysis, and compartment syndrome. In case of compartment syndrome, fasciotomy is the procedure of choice and must be performed early to limit muscle necrosis, arterial closure, and nerve damage.

LESSONS

- Prolonged acute limb ischemia may lead to muscle infarction and compartment syndrome.
- After successful revascularization of an acutely ischemic limb, patients should undergo close monitoring of cardiac rhythm, potassium level, myoglobin, compartment pressures, and serial limb examination.
- If a compartment syndrome diagnosis is made, fasciotomy should be performed expeditiously.

References

1. Schwarten DE, Cutliff WB. Arterial occlusive disease below the knee: Treatment with percutaneous transluminal angioplasty performed with low-profile catheters and steerable guidewires. *Radiology.* 1988;169:71–74.
2. Bull PG, Mendel H, Hold M, Schlegl A, Denck H. Distal popliteal and tibioperoneal transluminal angioplasty: Long-term follow-up. *JVIR.* 1992;3:45–53.
3. Wagner HJ, Klose KJ. Infrapopliteal angioplasty for limb-salvage: A 4-year experience. *J Vasc Interv Radiol.* 1997;8(suppl):247.
4. Wagner HH, Rager G. Infrapopliteal angioplasty: A forgotten region? *Rofo Fortschr Geb Rontgenstr Neuen Bildgeb Verfahr.* 1998;168(5):415–420.
5. Matsi PJ, Manninen HI. Complications of lower-limb percutaneous transluminal angioplasty: A prospective analysis of 410 procedures on 295 consecutive patients. *Cardiovasc Intervent Radiol.* 1998;21:361–366.
6. Burns BJ, Phillips AJ, Fox A, Boardman P, Phillips-Hughes J. The timing and frequency of complications after peripheral percutaneous transluminal angioplasty and iliac stenting: Is a change from inpatient to outpatient therapy feasible? *Cardiovasc Intervent Radiol.* 2000;23:452–456.
7. Axisa B, Fishwick G, Bolia A. Complications following peripheral angioplasty. *Ann R Coll Surg Engl.* 2002;84:39–42.

Index

Note: Page references followed by "*f*" and "*t*" denote figures and tables, respectively.